Evolutionary Biology of Primitive Fishes

NATO ASI Series

Advanced Science Institutes Series

A series presenting the results of activities sponsored by the NATO Science Committee, which aims at the dissemination of advanced scientific and technological knowledge, with a view to strengthening links between scientific communities.

The series is published by an international board of publishers in conjunction with the NATO Scientific Affairs Division

A	**Life Sciences**	Plenum Publishing Corporation
B	**Physics**	New York and London
C	**Mathematical and Physical Sciences**	D. Reidel Publishing Company Dordrecht, Boston, and Lancaster
D	**Behavioral and Social Sciences**	Martinus Nijhoff Publishers
E	**Engineering and Materials Sciences**	The Hague, Boston, and Lancaster
F	**Computer and Systems Sciences**	Springer-Verlag
G	**Ecological Sciences**	Berlin, Heidelberg, New York, and Tokyo

Recent Volumes in this Series

Volume 96—Epidemiology and Quantitation of Environmental Risk in Humans from Radiation and Other Agents
edited by A. Castellani

Volume 97—Interactions between Electromagnetic Fields and Cells
edited by A. Chiabrera, C. Nicolini, and H. P. Schwan

Volume 98—Structure and Function of the Genetic Apparatus
edited by Claudio Nicolini and Paul O. P. Ts'o

Volume 99—Cellular and Molecular Control of Direct Cell Interactions
edited by H.-J. Marthy

Volume 100—Recent Advances in Nervous System Toxicology
edited by Corrado L. Galli, Liugi Manzo, and Peter S. Spencer

Volume 101—Chromosomal Proteins and Gene Expression
edited by Gerald R. Reeck, Graham H. Goodwin, and Pedro Puigdomènech

Volume 102—Advances in Penicillium and Aspergillus Systematics
edited by Robert A. Samson and John I. Pitt

Volume 103—Evolutionary Biology of Primitive Fishes
edited by R. E. Foreman, A. Gorbman, J. M. Dodd, and R. Olsson

Series A: Life Sciences

Evolutionary Biology of Primitive Fishes

Edited by

R. E. Foreman

Bamfield Marine Station
Bamfield, British Columbia, Canada

A. Gorbman

University of Washington
Seattle, Washington

J. M. Dodd

University College of North Wales
Bangor, United Kingdom

and

R. Olsson

University of Stockholm
Stockholm, Sweden

Plenum Press
New York and London
Published in cooperation with NATO Scientific Affairs Division

Proceedings of a NATO Advanced Research Workshop on
Evolutionary Biology of Primitive Fishes,
held April 14–17, 1985,
at Bamfield Marine Station, Bamfield, British Columbia, Canada,
co-sponsored by the Natural Sciences
and Engineering Research Council of Canada
and the Western Canadian Universities
Marine Biological Society

Library of Congress Cataloging in Publication Data

NATO Advanced Research Workshop on Evolutionary Biology of Primitive Fishes (1985: Bamfield, B.C.)
Evolutionary biology of primitive fishes.

(NATO ASI series. Series A, Life sciences; v. 103)
"Proceedings of a NATO Advanced Research Workshop on Evolutionary Biology of Primitive Fishes, held April 14–17, 1985, at Bamfield Marine Station, Bamfield, British Columbia, Canada"—T.p. verso.
"Published in cooperation with NATO Scientific Affairs Division."
Includes bibliographies and index.
1. Fishes—Evolution—Congresses. 2. Fishes, Fossil—Congresses. I. Foreman, R. E. (Ronald Eugene), date. II. North Atlantic Treaty Organization. Scientific Affairs Division. III. Title. IV. Series.
QL618.2.N37 1985 597'.038 85-31168
ISBN 0-306-42224-7

A Division of Plenum Publishing Corporation
233 Spring Street, New York, N.Y. 10013

Printed in the United States of America

PREFACE

What, precisely, is a primitive fish? Most biologists would agree that the living cyclostomes, selachians, crossopterygians, etc. cannot be considered truly primitive. However, they and the fossil record have served to provide the information which forms the basis for speculation concerning the nature of the original vertebrates. This symposium of biologists from a variety of disciplines was called together to create collectively, from the best available current evidence, a picture of the probable line of evolution of the prototype primitive fishes. The symposium was designed to follow one that took place in Stockholm in 1967, convened for a similar purpose, with about the same number of participants. It is a matter of interest that almost the entire 1967 symposium (Nobel Symposium 4) dealt only with the hard tissues, whether fossil or modern.

In charting the course of the present symposium it was felt that the intervening years have produced numerous lines of new evidence that could be employed in the same way that a navigator determines his position. Each field, be it adult morphology, geology, ecology, biochemistry, development or physiology, generates evidence that can be extrapolated backward from existing vertebrate forms and forward from invertebrate forms. If the intersect of only two lines of evidence produces a navigational "fix" of rather low reliability, then an intersect, however unfocussed, of multiple guidelines from more numerous disciplines might provide a better position from which to judge early vertebrate history. Accordingly, we have recorded here information from behaviorist-ecologists who have tried to see the early vertebrates in their own prevailing environments and subject to the exacting restraints of these environments. The biochemists and immunocytochemists can trace particular peptide combinations from the established vertebrate taxa clear across the *terra* (or *mare*) *incognita* into the invertebrate domain. Developmental information hopefully supplies even more insight than adult structure, and we have tried to obtain as much of this as is available and appropriate. The large body of accumulated physiological lore now can be drawn upon to give us some understanding of how the early vertebrates may have solved their adaptive functional problems.

At any rate, we have here as good a picture as is currently available of the prevailing circumstances and probable structural and functional features of the truly primitive fishes, if that is what these aquatic creatures may be called. For whatever it is worth, we present this crystallization, or condensation, of current information as it applies to early vertebrate phylogeny.

We gratefully acknowledge the editorial assistance of Dr. William S. Wheeler and Dr. Christine E. Milliken, and typing assistance of Miss Sandra Kschischang and Mrs. Linda Mather. The technical software support group of Lexisoft, Inc. of Davis, California, was always there when we needed their assistance, for which we are very appreciative.

We are most grateful to Dr. M. di Lullo, Director of NATO ARW Programme, and the North Atlantic Treaty Organization for their support of the workshop. Financial support was also provided by the Natural Sciences and Engineering Research Council of Canada and the Western Canadian Universities Marine Biological Society. The sponsoring organizations greatly contributed to the success of the workshop, as did Mrs. Linda Mather, Miss Sabina Leader and Miss Anne Bergey.

R. E. Foreman
A. Gorbman
J. M. Dodd
R. Olsson

September, 1985

CONTENTS

SCENARIOS: WHY?

Carl Gans

Division of Biological Sciences
The University of Michigan
Ann Arbor, Michigan 48109-1048

Introduction

In beginning this symposium on the patterns disclosed by primitive fishes, we should perhaps ask what it is that we are trying to achieve. Some of us hope to generate schemes for the taxonomic placement of certain Recent animals and for mapping the shifting pattern of their phenotypes through time. However, another part of our agenda might involve the generation of scenarios, *i.e.* efforts to reconstruct the functional changes producing the process of vertebrate evolution. Obviously, there are two sets of evidence that can be used to achieve these aims. The first derives from fossils and was emphasized in the previous symposium. The second derives from the Recent and is the topic here.

At the start, we may wish to remind ourselves about the guidelines for making decisions about the past events that we wish to reconstruct. Specifically, what is it that we can observe and what is it that we may conclude from it? Obviously, comparison is the key of this symposium, and we hope to enhance the potential for it by assembling specialists on different groups of organisms and of distinct organ systems. We operate less by absolute determinations of conditions in one kind of system or animal, than by analyzing the similarities and differences disclosed by observation of diverse species. Hence, the rules of comparison apply to our system as well as to most others in biology, and we must keep them in mind.

Aspects in comparison

Animals provide us with three sets of data, their adult phenotype, the pattern by which the phenotype develops after fertilization and the way the phenotype is utilized by the organism. Thus, structure, development and function form three sets of descriptors of currently observable phenomena (Fig. 1). These descriptors

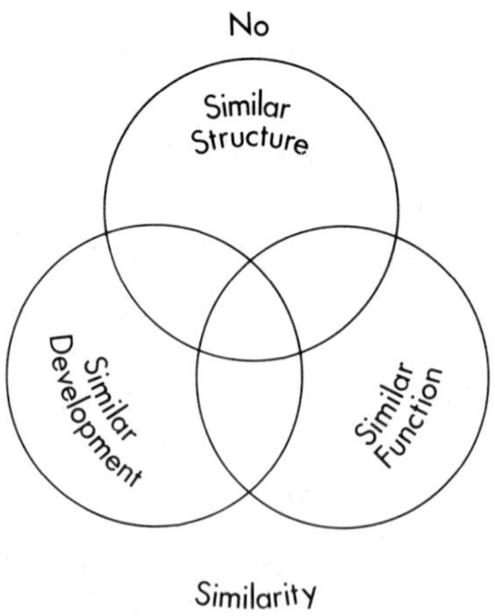

Fig. 1. Venn diagram to show the three kinds of current similarities likely to be exhibited by organisms and the combined states that these may display. Note that similarity of function is not an aspect generated by the phenotype, but one that is permitted by the phenotype. (After Gans, 1985, Amer. Zool., in press).

may be compared, and the similarities and differences thus disclosed may be refined by incorporating more specimens and species and improving the reliability of the observations.

However, the similarities and differences obtained by the study of individuals of any single or pair of species may have multiple causes and permit only limited conclusions about affinity. More is needed, because similarities of morphology and physiology may reflect closeness of derivation from a common ancestor, matching of different phenotypes to a common environment or both. Hence analysis of affinity must take into account the potential pitfalls posed by the convergence of characters. This difficulty requires matching our findings against phylogenetic schemes, or cladograms. These let us test whether a particular condition seen in several species represents a single invention (*i.e.* appears in a single evolutionary line) or whether it has been invented independently a number of times (*i.e.* it appears in several separate evolutionary lines; Fig. 2).

The origin of vertebrates involves another set of complicating problems. There are few obvious "outgroups" against which the vertebrates, and for that matter the chordates, may be compared; too many of the presumably intermediate forms appear to have become extinct. Also, there are no immediately obvious "ancestors" from which "descendents" are derivable in a single, or relatively few steps. Indeed, we see an array of vertebrate characteristics, all of which are shared and derived, and all of which appear in the fossil record almost simultaneously, not shared with any other group. Such a situation suggests either that much time has passed (with the intermediate forms having all become extinct) or that there may be a common denominator for some of the set.

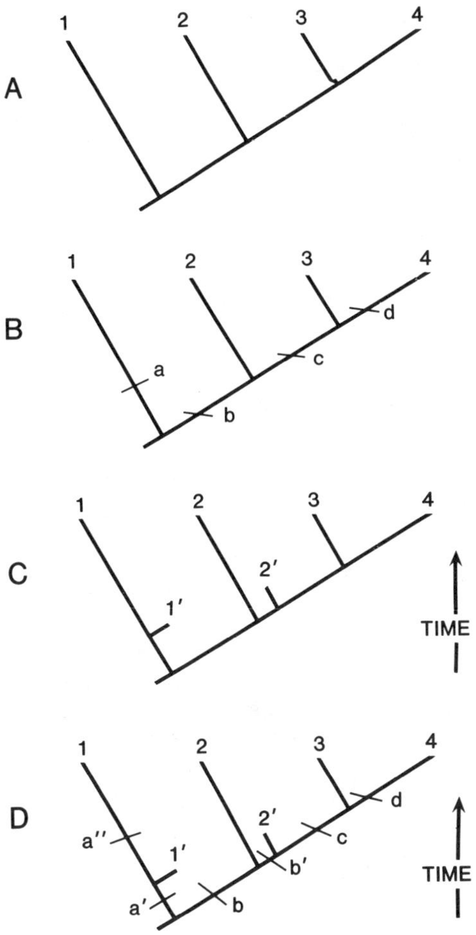

Fig. 2. A set of cladograms labelled and modified to show the pattern of character states of recent organisms (A), and the way this pattern would be modified if the vertical axis is explicitly made to represent time and fossils mapped into the appropriate places (C). The ecological, behavioral, physiological states seen in the Recent have been mapped onto one cladogram (B); whereas, the time-associated diagram indicates the potential for functional (as well as phenotypic) shifts in each line leading to members of a pair of sister groups (D). Obviously, selection for the transition must have been effected by the function-associated demands existing at the time of bifurcation.

Common denominators are of interest because it is obviously easier to posit evolution by means of a limited number of changes than by positing multiple, coincident, but supposedly independent, events. Incidentally, this is one reason for our interest in the association between placodes and neural crest on the one hand, and the many shared-derived states of vertebrates on the other. Discovery of this developmental association greatly simplified our analysis of the possible evolutionary changes. Instead of a multiplicity of states that seem to be independent, there is a single associated set. This makes it possible to consider the mode of life history and the origins of ancestral forms.

Adaptive causes

The kinds of analyses indicated above suggest that we should begin by generating statements of phylogeny based upon descriptions of the extant phenotypes (1,2,3,4 in Fig. 2A). One may amplify such diagrams by plotting on them the current functional, *i.e.* ecological/behavioral/physiological/biochemical characteristics (a,b,c,d in Fig. 2B). However, such diagrams do not indicate *causes*, as cladistic arrangements are generated seemingly independent of information concerning such causes that produced the changed phenotypes. Moreover, vertical and horizontal distances on our diagrams correlate absolutely neither with time nor with degree of change. Thus, the physiological conditions disclosed by each of two sister groups need not be equivalent, or of similar value to those that pertained at the time that their lines bifurcated.

At this point we should also note that the analysis is often simplified by considering the evolution of individual characteristics (limb structure, CNS pathways, blood pigments). In such comparison it seems appropriate to refer to some characteristic of an early fish as "primitive" and to the more developed state attained by some Recent form as "derived". However, we must apply such terms to characteristics only; if a modern fish retains the condition seen in the early species, the state is primitive. In contrast, the concept that a currently living fish is "primitive" does not make sense, as the fish is unlikely to have retained in stasis all early characteristics without further evolution.

It is possible to modify the initial cladogram by adding a time dimension (Fig. 2C). One can then add fossils to the scheme and this will often indicate whether the present functional aspects (establishing selective influences) could or could not have applied at the time of bifurcation of the ancestral line. Not only this, but the diagram permits extrapolation to the functional conditions pertaining at the time of bifurcation. Questions, such as what was the mode of life of the earliest hagfish, may thus be opened to discussion. Mode of life is obviously significant as it presumably defines the selective effects at the time of bifurcation that led to the phenotypes we see. Implicit in this analysis is the occurrence of adaptation, *i.e.* the assumption that the environment of the fossils was among the range of environments in which the observed phenotype could have operated. Of course, some critics argue that such causal explanations incorporate so many uncertainties that they constitute story telling rather than a useful approach to science. Obviously I do not share this view nor do I accept the position that the process of adaptation is rare.

There are three possible causes for changes in aspects of the phenotype through time (Fig. 3). The first is, obviously, direct adaptation of the character, selected because it matched a particular aspect of the environment. The second is that the

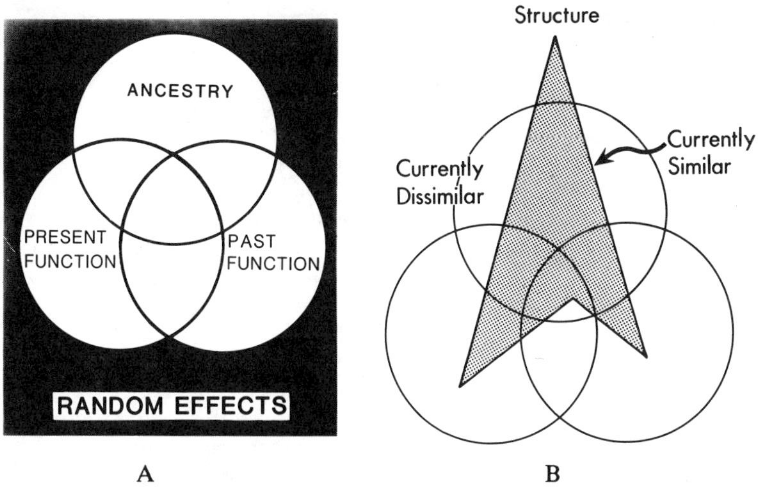

Fig. 3. Venn diagrams to illustrate the causes that may account for the observed phenotypic similarities. A. The association of ancestry, and past and present function with various phenotypes. B. The same diagram with an overlay indicating the current level of similarity. (After Gans, 1985, Amer. Zool., in press).

expression of the phenotype is linked to adaptations of some other feature, possibly a pleiotropic or developmental one. Both of these items leave open the time at which this adaptation took place, and whether or not it is now maintained. A third possible cause of change is apparently independent of adaptation, representing a neutral or non-adaptive influence.

Non-adaptive changes in particular aspects of the phenotype are difficult to document on the macro-level at which we are examining characteristics in fossils. The difficulty reflects the fact that many properties of an organism's structure obviously at least "permit" it to occupy their current environment. Even if an individual animal seems to bear demonstrably non-adaptive features, we should remember that comparison should be among populations, not individuals. It may be possible to show that an aspect of a specimen's phenotype is non-adaptive at a particular moment, but it is much more difficult to show this is the case for the population or species from which the individual was sampled.

Presence of adaptation is often more obvious, particularly for phenotypic characteristics associated with major influences of the environment. Also, there is the second explanatory argument, that of association. This implies constraint, *i.e.* that the phenotype is shaped by partly conflicting influences. Selection likely optimizes totality and does not perfect unitary features. Hence, animal constructions may be excessive in individuals at some time of their life span. However, it is interesting that recent tests of the functional performance of structures generally indicate that performance tends to vary less than do individual morphometric features. Perhaps we have been trapped by a tendency to analyze separate aspects of morphology instead of considering the functioning totality of the organism.

In short, I propose that it may be appropriate to assume that adaptation should represent the null hypothesis for any particular property of an organism. However, it is clear that we must expect noise in the system and we must recognize that, at any instant, the congruence of phenotype and role should be expected to be imperfect. What needs testing is the closeness of the match, and if possible, determination of the basis for differences in degree of matching among multiple phenotypic features.

Technique for scenarios

The preceding statements concern the mechanism for establishing hypotheses or scenarios for the several ways in which particular structures might have arisen at a specific point in time. Naturally, such hypotheses of organismic transition need to be tested against the structure, ecology, behavior and physiology of existing groups. Occasionally, one may be lucky enough to know of relevant fossils that occupied ancestral positions at critical stages in time. More often, it will be possible to ask how often parallel phenotypic changes have occurred in phylogeny and to use the relative frequency of the associated functional or ecological changes as a basis for testing our answer.

Recently, we have seen much emphasis on the formulation and testing of "hypotheses". However, it is important to remember that refutation of one or more hypotheses does not represent proof of validity of the remaining one; it implies only that the first was unlikely, and not that the remaining one is true. The correct hypothesis may not have been included in the set of hypotheses subjected to test.

Also, the search for the most plausible of several options does incur the risk that nature may not have been parsimonious. However, this risk is unavoidable; unless the evidence is equivocal, we must use "Occam's razor". Here, knowledge of morphological and developmental principles may well be decisive. Uncritical numerical counts of multiple byproducts of a single developmental event may lead to an inappropriate phylogeny; some evolutionary transitions may be viewed as having been more complex than was actually the case.

Hence, there is merit to comparing multiple character sets and to testing whether the phylogenies they permit are congruent. One hopes that the noncongruent sets will stand out and allow one to examine more closely the particular characteristics on which they are based. Hopefully too, the greater the congruence, the more robust the conclusions that are generated.

As we are using phenotypes for analysis, and as structural elements are likely to be all that is left of fossils, there are several classes of adaptation that are likely to be invisible. Populational interactions, secondary sexual characters and purely behavioral responses to predators and prey are among these. Their existence may limit test of the the structure-"function" congruence, as they often represent an unrecognized portion of function.

At another level one should ask whether the posited scenario explains aspects of different systems, perhaps aspects not previously recognized as being pertinent to the analysis, or aspects previously assumed to bear on quite different situations. Do the conclusions deriving from the analysis of one period in history have explanatory power at a later time?

In short, the approach described entails the development of statements about changes in ecology-behavior-physiology. These are derived from the sequentially changing phenotypic patterns in time (upon which our classifications are based). It is assumed that functional changes produced the phenotypic shifts, and that we may use the latter to aid reconstruction of the conditions that led to them. Also, we assume that currently observed biochemistry, physiology and geology, indeed current cosmology, applied in prehistoric times as well.

Examples

I would like to clarify my position regarding the uses of scenarios by giving two examples deriving from an ongoing series of discussions with R. Glenn Northcutt. They pertain to the origin of the notochord and second, to the origin of the branchiomeric muscle.

Considering the notochord, one may question whether it started in the trunk or in the tail. Indeed, what was its earliest role?

There are four possible hypotheses regarding sites of origin. The notochord might have arisen in the trunk and extended into the tail. The notochord might have developed in the tail and grew into the trunk. It might have formed at the caudal region of the trunk and developed in both directions. Finally, it may have arisen simultaneously along the full length of the trunk and tail. Looking at available organisms, we see the first condition in hemichordates and nemerteans, the second in urochordates, the third in no known group and the fourth in cephalochordates and vertebrates.

Functional analysis would argue that burrowing-associated stiffening of the anterior end of the organism represented the functional role for the first hypothesis, in which the notochord originated anteriorly. Rapid lateral displacements of the caudal appendage are associated with the second hypothesis, whether or not these related to sculling propulsion or another role. No mechanism known to us is associated with the third developmental pattern. Locomotion by undulation of the entire trunk and tail represents the functional role for the fourth. There are good reasons for not accepting the first (burrowing) hypothesis, as the coelomic and muscular patterns observed in tunicates and cephalochordates do not match functional expectations. A difficulty with the fourth hypothesis is that simultaneous development would require a sudden major change forcing the entire trunk and post-trunk region to be reorganized. However, the second hypothesis proposing that the notochord arose in association with the caudal appendage has attractive aspects.

Stiffening of the caudal process appears in urochordates, thus phylogenetically earlier than does a chord in the trunk (*i.e.* a caudal chord appears in the phylogenetically "correct" place). More important is the assumption that the caudal flapper initially served not so much for continuous, directed propulsion (which might require advanced motor coordination), but for sudden, even asymmetrical, flapping movements that would shift the position of the animal or distract the strike of a predator. Such a mechanism has the appeal that any degree of stiffening of the appendage would have an immediate advantage; further selection might lead to supplementary modifications that could improve the system.

Stiffening by budding off a rod-like pseudocoelomic space from the ectoderm-endoderm would provide a mechanical function with a relatively simple developmental process. What is most attractive is that the hypothesis is predictive of observations in development. Thus, the notochordal anlage of *Branchiostoma* forms from the blastoporal lip and one sees epiboly and involution of the presumptive notochordal tissue. Its development is hence back to front. The notochordal tissue, of course, serves as the primary organizer for the other elements of the dorsal array that comprises the vertebrate propulsive system. In contrast, the somites start to form near the front of the anlage and develop posteriorly, *i.e.* in a direction opposite to that of the notochord itself.

A second example concerns the branchiomeric muscle of vertebrates, namely the constrictors and adductors of the pharynx, which are homologous to much of the masticatory and other cephalic musculature of gnathostomes. This musculature has been historically interpreted as an anterior extension of the muscular wall of the gut. However, the observation that it is striated, that it is directly innervated from the CNS, that it lacks second order motor neurons and that it is innervated by dorsal rather than ventral root nerves, has always made this interpretation confusing and perplexing. Remarks that the advent of striation reflects the need for active rather than passive motor control do not explain these observations. The argument that the branchiomeric muscle is an anterior extension of the visceral mass derives from the idea that the plan of the cranial nerves reflects the organization of the spinal nerves in lampreys. Also, there is the assumption that the axial mass of *Branchiostoma* represents muscle homologous and equivalently organized to that of vertebrates, whereas these animals lack a precursor for vertebrate branchiomeric and hypaxial muscles.

However, the axial muscle of *Branchiostoma* is connected to the CNS by non-contractile processes of the muscle cells; these synapse directly onto the nerve cord and there are no nerve roots *per se*. In contrast, the striated subpterygial "coughing" (reverse flow or "cleaning") muscles of *Branchiostoma* are innervated directly by neurons of the CNS, that send their axons out of the central nervous tube *via* a dorsal path.

This leads to the hypothesis that the subpterygial muscles of *Branchiostoma* are homologous to the branchiomeric muscles of vertebrates. The functional basis for the change from one to the other may then relate to a shift in the role from coughing to muscle-powered ventilation that may have been advantageous with a change to a free-living predacious life-style. Here again, the hypothesis is supported by recently generated developmental evidence. Witness the demonstration that the branchiomeric muscle derives not from hypomeric tissues but from the presomitic dorsal mesoderm referred to as somitomeres.

Conclusions

I hope that these brief remarks have persuaded you to consider my view that the merit of scenarios is not that they may happen to provide a "correct" reconstruction of prehistory. The ultimate correctness of the two scenarios described above, as well as other possible scenarios is much less important than the fact that they force us to re-examine our basic conclusions. Scenarios also force us to re-examine the evidence regarding functional systems upon which they are based.

The questions generated by scenarios make us realize that we know much less about many animals than is commonly assumed. For instance, developmental studies of many early fishes are lacking. Indeed, many generalizations about the fate of neural crest tissues derive entirely from the recent elegant studies on birds and remain to be confirmed in anamniotes. Much of our information on the biology and embryology of invertebrates, in particular of protochordates, derives from studies carried out during the last century. Many of these studies were beautifully done but had to be carried out with tools that today we would judge totally inadequate. They deserve repetition and amplification.

In short, the major merit of scenarios is that they oblige us to determine what we need to know, and they lead us to ask new and different questions which are likely to improve our understanding of the biology of organisms.

Acknowledgements

I thank R.G. Northcutt for permission to refer to our joint studies and D. Carrier and P. Pridmore for many comments on versions of this manuscript. Its preparation was supported by NSF DEB 8121229

GENERAL ECOLOGY OF PRIMITIVE FISHES

Gunnar Bertmar

Department of Ecological Zoology
University of Umeå
Sweden

Evolution of the ecology discipline

One of the satisfactions that ecology can offer to the nonecologist is an appreciation of nature's complex patterns and the biological forces that produce them. The progress of ecology over the last few years has emphasized that a deep, intimate knowledge of natural history is essential to understand these complex patterns. Early ecological studies were largely descriptive and the experimental approach to the study of function was rare. Animals were described as to the form of their organs "designed" to perform a purposeful function. A growing recognition of the dynamic and diverse nature of the phenomena in nature has been accompanied by a diminished reliance on broad generalizations and a greater emphasis on qualifying special cases. This has created a greater appreciation of the strengths and limitations of ecological principles. Over the last few years these changes have provided the stimulus for the development of more precise hypotheses and an increasing reliance on experimentation, both in the laboratory and in the natural environment, as a means of testing hypotheses. The growth of experimentation is a reflection of ecology's increasing maturity as a science.

Ecology has been variously defined, but most biologists continue to regard it in the same light as those who defined it more than a century ago as the study of the total relations between the organisms and their natural environments. Ecologists may utilize methods of other biological disciplines, like morphology and physiology, or even other scientific disciplines like chemistry and physics, but all attempt to understand how organisms are integrated into nature.

Sensory ecology

Plant and animal ecology, autecology, pure and applied ecology, population and community ecology, evolutionary ecology, are all subdisciplines of ecology which have contributed to the vitality of a single, unified science. However, sensory organs are essential for the interplay between the organism and its environment. Research on chemoreception in fishes has been growing at a remarkable rate over the last few decades. This has greatly expanded our understanding of the structure and function of the olfactory organs, and of their role for the control of behavior (Hasler, 1966; Kleerekoper, 1969, 1982; Hara, 1975). Some of this research has been directed towards the primary sensory processes in olfaction and taste. Other research has been devoted to the role of taste and its application to artificial baits, alarm substances and fright reactions. Yet another approach has been to study the interactions between aquatic pollutants, chemoreceptors and behavior (Bertmar, 1982). Part of the chemosensory research in fishes recently has become in this way more ecological. To some extent this ecological trend is seen in chemosensory research in all vertebrates (Stoddart, 1980). However, even research on senses other than olfaction has become more ecological (Bertmar, 1979) (Table I). For example, there has recently been presented an olfaction-vision theory, indicating that there may be an integrated hierarchical orientation model in homing anadromous fishes (Bertmar, 1979, 1982) (Fig. 1). A new branch of autecology therefore can be designed, called Sensory Ecology (Bertmar, 1983). The goal of this subdiscipline is to develop a sensory perspective of the whole organism in its environment. This goal may be achieved by studies on feeding relations, reproductive ecology, ecological distribution, social organization, ability of an organism to give warning and defend itself, and mechanisms for migration and orientation. Sensory ecology may have applications to animal husbandry, pest control and crop protection.

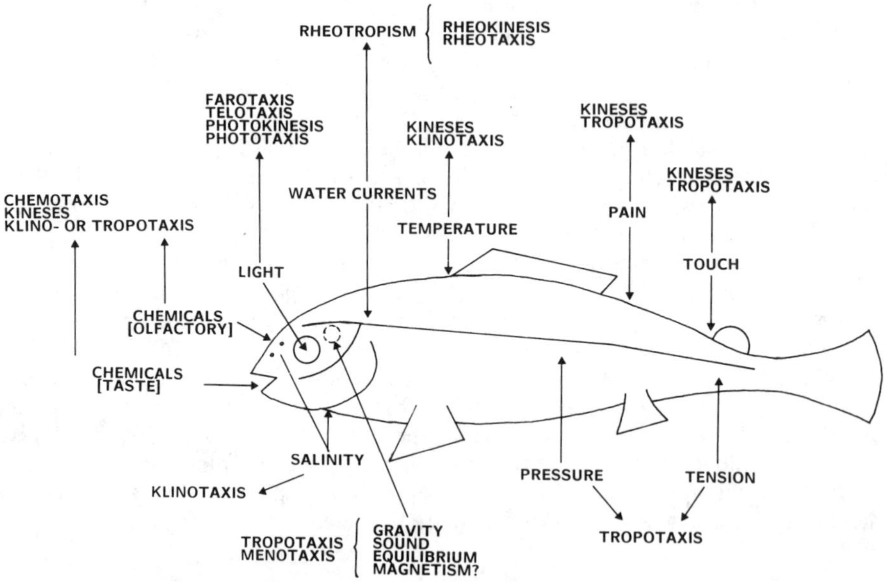

Fig. 1. Sensory ecology gives a sensory perspective of the organism in relation to the environment. Different external stimuli are the basis for various direct or indirect orientation movements. From Bertmar (1979, 1982).

Table I. Sense organs and their functions in orientation and orientation behaviour (modified from Bertmar, 1979,1982).

Main group of orienting mechanisms	Orienting receptor organs	Orientation behaviour
Orientation in fixed-space reference system: stimulus sources provide the coordinates and/or serve to maintain the normal position, and they are not the goal of the orientation.	Gravity and proprioceptive organs	Maintenance of physical balance. Control of position and direction of action in space.
	Eyes	Orientation related to light. Horizontal near-orientation to landmarks.
	Latero-sensory organs	Tactile, kinesthetic registration and repetition of own movements. Orientation in currents.
Stabilization of posture and movement (locomotion) independent of locality.	Semicircular canals utriculus-sacculus (inner ear)	Orientation related to equilibrium.
	Eyes	Optomotoric (kinetic) control
Object orientation: stimulus sources are the objects of orientation; frequently locating processes (goal and direction is considered).	Eyes	Optical target orientation
	Lagena (inner ear)	Acoustical orientation
	Skin receptors	Tactile orientation to other fish *etc.*
	Gustatory receptors	Chemo-sensory near-orientation to food *etc.*
	Olfactory organs	Chemo-sensory near-orientation to different water qualtities in feeding areas. Homing orientation.

This new branch of ecology has recently evolved in different parts of the world, but the data have been presented and discussed under other headings, for example, Behavioral Ecology and Sensory Physiology. In the following, this new branch will be exemplified by data on distribution, feeding, migration and orientation in lampreys.

There are tensions and conflicts between competing hypotheses and theories, and the dynamic interaction between them. One way to resolve them is to have a problem-solving approach that relies on the interplay between theory and data to reveal the reality of nature. One has to be suspicious of theory that purports to prove something in the absence of empirical support and of data collected without a clear, hypothesis-testing objective.

An integrated approach to the relationship between evolution and ecology is also essential. Answers to questions about why an ecological pattern takes a certain form ultimately rest on an understanding of the evolutionary forces that shape interactions between organisms and the environment. Evolutionary ecology is a very dynamic field at present.

Lampreys

The originator of the name and classification of Cyclostomata was Dumeril (1807), the foremost ichthyologist in France at the beginning of the 19th century. That paper also was the first one dedicated exclusively to the olfactory sense of fishes, but it took more than 100 years for science to prove that olfaction was functional in water as well as air (Matthes, 1924). Well before the term "pheromone" was coined, Roule (1931) described the release and perception of specific odor involved in nest site selection, sexual attraction and courtship positioning in *Lampetra*. Modern work on these problems has its origin and stimulation in the work of these and other pioneers.

Distribution

The distribution of lamprey populations is able to satisfy the divergent ecological requirements of adult and ammocoete. The upstream migration into the higher reaches provide suitable conditions for spawning. The subsequent slow but continuous downstream drift and/or migration of the larvae brings them into the slower currents and more silted bottoms of the middle and lower courses. There, conditions are conducive to the feeding and burrowing activities of the ammocoete.

After the absorption of the yolk, the young ammocoetes leave the nest at night to swim. They then usually drift downstream (Malmquist, 1983b) but may also actively seek out more favourable areas for colonization (Hardisty and Potter, 1971a). Different factors determining the larval distribution have been suggested for several species of lampreys, for example, current velocity (Hardisty, 1944; Applegate, 1950; Potter, 1970), shade (Schroll, 1959) and organic material in the sediment (Enequist, 1937; Sterba, 1962). By discriminant analysis Malmquist (1980a) showed that most larvae of the brook lamprey *Lampetra planeri* selected habitats with low current velocity, low water depth, a low number of particles in the

0.5-1 mm range, and with low chlorophyll *a* content, whereas organic content, shade and presence of algae did not improve the discriminant model. Stream bed stability was considered to be of great importance although it was not possible to estimate quantitatively.

Feeding

Evidence suggests that larvae mainly feed on microscopic organisms, especially diatoms, and fine particulate detritus (Schroll, 1959; Manion, 1967). Moore and Potter (1976a) demonstrated that larval *Lampetra planeri* grow better on diatoms than on bacteria, and better on bacteria than on detritus with its microorganisms. They also found (1976b) that all species of non-filamentous algae found in the water and on the sediment of Highland Water (New Forest, England) contributed to the diet of larval lampreys (*Lampetra planeri*).

The filtration rate of different sized larval *Lampetra planeri* was recently estimated by Malmquist and Brönmark (1982). They found that large larvae had a higher absolute filtration rate than small ones and were less dependent on temperature. The most "economic" filtration was achieved below 10^{0}C. This is in accordance with the low mean annual temperature of typical *Lampetra planeri* streams. A high ratio of filtration to respiration was seen to coincide with maximum food availability in the stream. Low particle concentrations were compensated for by an increased filtration rate. In the interval between 30 and 100 mg dry weight of suspended yeast per litre, larvae increased their rates of filtration.

They also found that intraspecific food competition must be minimal. Abiotic factors, in combination with predation and parasitism, are probably the main regulators of larval abundance. Generally, burrowing animals cannot exhibit as high seston capture efficiencies as those that are able to utilize a three-dimensional substratum of aquatic macrophytes or a rough bottom surface. The increased cross sectional area permits large numbers of blackflies and netspinning caddisflies to occur. Their greater efficiency in seston removal can be attributed to high densities rather than to high removal rates per individual.

The efficiency of the stream community in utilizing the organic material within a given reach of a stream is, however, far less than 100%. Insect species downstream seem to be adapted to capitalize on the inefficiency of the upstream species in processing the organic material (Vannote *et al.*, 1980). The efficiency of the filter feeders therefore must not be exaggerated, either in large rivers (Cudney and Wallace, 1980) or in small woodland streams (Malmquist and Brönmark, 1982). The latter authors found that the importance of *Lampetra planeri* larvae in depleting the water of particles is minimal. Less than 1×10^{-4}% of the water passing each metre of stream length is filtered by the lampreys.

As the ammocoetes generally feed on the microflora and microfauna in the regions surrounding their burrows, there must be mechanisms controlling the size of the organisms ingested. It is widely agreed that this size discrimination is imposed by the meshwork of branched cirri at the posterior end of the oral hood, acting as a sieve through which water must pass before entering the pharynx. The larger particles accumulate in the oral hood where they become enmeshed in mucus and are periodically expelled by a kind of "coughing action" (Applegate, 1950).

In addition to this purely mechanical limitation based on particle size, Manion (1967) observed differences in the types of diatoms taken by smaller (33-55 mm) and larger (70-72 mm) ammocoetes, and differences were also found between the frequencies with which the various diatom genera occurred in the water and in the ammocoete gut. For example, *Fragillaria* was found to be less frequent in the gut than in the water. On the other hand, *Navicula* made up only 7.7-11.5% of the diatoms in the water, but constituted 32.9% of the diatoms taken by the larger ammocoetes and 19.1% of those ingested by the group of smaller larvae.

The sensory basis for this selective feeding is largely unknown. The ammocoete olfactory organs are certainly not highly developed (Kleerekoper, 1971) but they may possibly be well provided with gustatory receptors (Schroll, 1959); the presence of temperature receptors was indicated by observations on recolonizing behavior (Thomas, 1962).

During metamorphosis, which lasts for several months, the animal is generally not feeding (Potter and Beamish, 1977) and therefore there is some loss of weight (but not length). There seems to be a degree of synchrony, when considered in relation to the seasonal nature of metamorphosis, which suggests that the internal mechanisms involved may be very sensitive to the triggering effect of environmental factors. Temperature may be one operating factor as shown by the observation that the timing of metamorphosis in the laboratory can be altered by temperature differences (Potter, 1970). There may also be a correlation with changes in water level (Sjöberg, 1980).

There may be species differences in the feeding habits of adult parasitic lampreys. These may vary with the stage in the life cycle and the food available. Analyses of gut contents have shown material other than blood, for example muscle tissue, scales and fish eggs. These indications of a carnivorous habit of feeding have been found in, for example, *Lampetra japonica*, which attacks fish, gnawing out tissues and even internal organs (Nikolskii, 1956). It has therefore been suggested that the term "predatory" is much more appropriate than "parasitic" (Grossu *et al.*, 1962).

While lamprey attacks may cause some mortality among smaller teleosts, any effect on salmon is probably indirect through causing increased susceptibility to infection and stress (Potter and Beamish, 1977).

Lampreys may rely on vision to locate potential hosts (Lennon, 1954). However, the evidence that they often feed in deep water indicates that other senses may be more important. Studies on diurnal rhythms have shown that the endogenous cycles of activity in *Petromyzon marinus*, which are gradually lost in constant conditions of dim light, may be rapidly reestablished by a short period of sensory stimulation by the scent of fish (Kleerekoper, 1971). Sensory ecology tests on *Eudontomyzon danfordi* showed that they approached the bait (whitefish) from downstream and were equally attracted whether the bait was on a light or a dark background (Chappuis, 1939). The importance of the olfactory sense has been further emphasized by the behavioral response of lampreys to fish odour and to one or two of its various amine components (Kleerekoper *et al.*, 1961; Kleerekoper and Mogensen, 1963).

Nutrition and contamination

Studies on lamprey nutrition have recently acquired a new ecological aspect. In the Great Lakes, the sea lamprey is an external parasite of larger fishes, particularly the salmonid and coregonid species (Farmer and Beamish, 1973). Laboratory studies on the adult lamprey showed that its gross food conversion efficiency averages 40-50% (Farmer *et al.*, 1975). It was also demonstrated that the lamprey lives almost entirely on the blood of the host fishes, with intake of muscle tissues being less than 2% of the blood consumed. Assuming an average weight of 250 g for the adult lamprey, and a given blood content of 3.13 % of the host fish (Conte *et al.*, 1963), the total weight of fish destroyed by one lamprey could be 20 kg. This is probably a conservative estimate as it assumes the ingestion of all the host's blood by the lamprey. Given an average weight of the teleost as 2 kg, it is apparent that a lamprey will feed on a minimum of 10 host fish before it reaches maturity.

During the feeding period, from spring to fall, the organochlorine contamination (OC) body burdens of host fishes are accumulated primarily from their diet. This has been shown for lake trout with reference to DDT (Reinert *et al.*, 1974), and is supported by field observations on the correlation of contaminant and fat levels in other species (Kelso and Frank, 1974). From feeding experiments on channel catfish, *Ictalurus punctatus*, it is also known that the concentration of PCB isomers in fish blood are about 10% of those in the total body (Hansen *et al.*, 1976). Therefore, in the growth period, lamprey accumulate contaminants from the hosts blood which reflects the recent dietary exposure of the host specimens rather than the hosts total body burdens, as might be the case in periods of lipid mobilization (Kaiser 1982). Because of the small weight of the ammocoete, any contaminants accumulated by ammocoetes contribute negligibly to that of the fully grown individual.

The interspecies quotients of the contaminant concentrations in the lamprey and host tissue are even more sensitive to changes in the lake water than the actual concentrations in lamprey tissue. This can be demonstrated in more detail by determining intraspecies contaminant ratios and their interspecies quotients. The unique biological relationship of the lamprey and its host can therefore be used for early trend determination of levels of PCB, DDT, DDE, dieldrin and other contaminants.

Migration

Metamorphosed animals of the European river lamprey *Lampetra fluviatilis* migrate and drift downstream during the nights between March and May (Hardisty and Potter, 1971b; Fogelin, 1972; Sjöberg, 1980). Like downstream migrants of other lamprey species, they do not feed during this phase. Major downstream movements of *Petromyzon marinus* larvae of the 1960-year class in the Big-Garlic River, Michigan, occurred during high water in April and May, and of transformed lampreys in mid-October through November (Manion and Smith, 1978). Each year about 40% of the annual production of transformed lampreys migrated from the Big-Garlic River system in one 12-h period, and 82% by the end of October. Metamorphosis of a single year class occurs over a number of years. Spring migratory synchrony of salmonid, catostomid and cyprinid fishes with juvenile

Petromyzon marinus has been found in Canada during May-June 1980 and June-July 1982 (Montgomery *et al.*, 1983).

Large numbers of the Southern Hemisphere lamprey, *Geotria australis*, were found in the regurgitated food of albatrosses breeding on South Georgia (South Atlantic Ocean) (Potter *et al.*, 1979). This lamprey apparently is found in large groups at sea, presumably associated with its host, and can travel very large distances from its natal streams.

In all lamprey species there is an upstream migration for spawning. By upstream migration the adult lampreys compensate for downstream drift and/or migration in younger stages (Thomas, 1962). The brook lampreys migrate over comparatively short distances, whereas the anadromous species which spend one or several years in the sea may migrate over long distances. A number of different environmental factors are believed to affect this migration. While the information on the landlocked sea lamprey shows a clear correlation between migratory activity and temperature (Applegate, 1950), most observations on other species have tended to emphasize the importance of high water levels (Hardisty and Potter, 1971b). However, catches made at river barriers may tend to produce misleading results because of a build-up of migratory populations during low water levels (Lanzing, 1959). There may also be seasonal differences in the characteristic timing of migration.

Energy expended in migration and reproduction has been determined from measurements of caloric concentration and body and gonadal weight for nontrophic sea lampreys (*Petromyzon marinus*) collected from different sites along the St. John River, New Brunswick, Canada (Beamish, 1979). The estimated cost of locomotion in swimming the 140 km which separates the estuary from the spawning redds was 300 and 260 kcal for males and females, respectively. The actual distance which lampreys swam and mean swimming speed were estimated. Energy expenditure for breeding was considerably greater than that catabolized throughout the upstream migration. Data on upstream migrants indicate that males and females undergo length reductions of at least 11 and 15%, respectively, between the time of their entry into fresh water and the completion of spawning (Potter and Beamish, 1977).

The spawning migration of the brook lamprey *Lampetra planeri* was investigated in a South Swedish lake and stream system (Malmquist, 1980b). In the first season, characterized by frequent rain storms, water level was the most important factor, whereas in the following year when the migration period was unusually dry, temperature and on-shore winds at the stream mouth could explain 50% of the behavior changes. However, when data were combined for two years, only temperature showed a significant influence. The critical temperature for the onset of migration was 7.5°C. This species mainly migrates at night, but late in the season diurnal migration may occur.

Several authors have studies the spawning migration of the river lamprey *Lampetra fluviatilis*. In this species Tesch (1967) did not find any influence of hydrographical factors in the River Elbe, but he suggested that the phase of the moon may initiate the migration. Lunar influence was also documented by Ryapolova (1964), who noted that fewer river lampreys were caught on moon lit nights than on nights with no moon. This was confirmed by Asplund and Södergren (1975), but they also noted that the length of the night and the water level influenced the upstream migration in a North Swedish river (Rickleån). In a later study on the same stream Sjöberg (1980) found that in the early spring only a few river lampreys were caught in a trap, and therefore he assumed that the lampreys are quite inactive under the ice cover, but as soon as the ice had gone at the end of April or early May, the water temperature rose and there was a peak in the number of lampreys caught.

The ecology of the very early stages in the upstream migration of the river lamprey was studied using samples taken from the cooling water intake screens of the Olsbury Power Station in the Severn Estuary (England). Examination of the numbers of lampreys caught at different times indicates that an increase in freshwater discharge is the predominant environmental factor responsible for initiating the movement from the sea into the estuary, although temperature may also be a contributory factor (Abou-Seedo and Potter 1979).

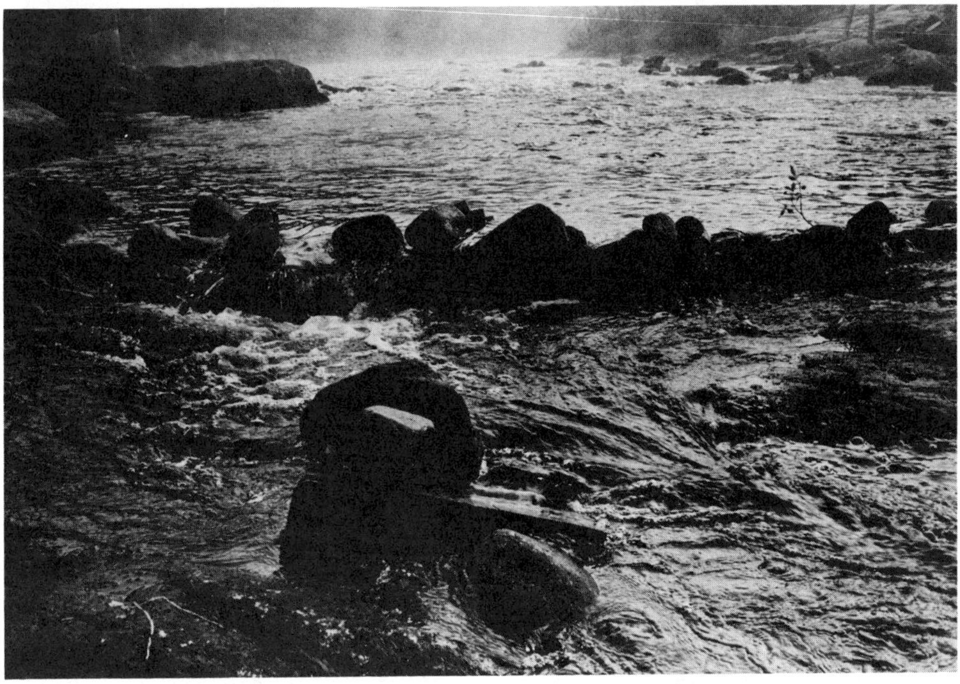

Fig. 2. Typical habitat for the river lamprey *Lampetra fluviatilis* in the River Rickleå, September 1983. A single unit of fishing gear (in the foreground) and a "raft" of units are anchored between stones. The traps are made of wooden laths and catch the lampreys migrating along the sides of the river. Documentation photo: Sune Jonsson, County Museum of Västerbotten, Umeå.

The factors that influence the later stages in upstream migration are not known. In general, however, the migrating animals are nocturnal (Wikgren, 1954; Sjöberg, 1977) and move along the edges of the main stream in comparatively shallow water (Fig. 2). Particularly difficult stretches or obstacles are surmounted by short bursts of intense activity followed by periods of rest when they attach themselves to convenient structures by means of their oral suckers (Applegate, 1950). They are able to pass quite high barriers by a series of wriggling movements, although they seldom jump more than about 0.5 m vertically.

There is no conclusive evidence that upstream migrant lampreys tend to home into the same streams as those in which they were borne. Only 14 of 159 marked spawning-run *Petromyzon marinus* from the Pancake River returned home, whereas the others were found mainly in other streams nearest to the point of release (Skidmore, 1959). Only two out of 50 marked spawning-run *Lampetra planeri* were found in the home tributary (Malmquist, 1980b). Applegate (1950) suggested that lampreys might find their way into the spawning tributaries by a rheotactic response to the outflow current, since streams with a stronger or more sustained outflow tend to have larger spawning populations.

Spawning

At the approach of spawning, the negative response to light that was characteristic of the sexually immature lamprey changes quite sharply to an apparent tolerance or even preference for lighted areas during the spawning act (Sterba, 1962). The general pattern of nesting and spawning activity appears to be similar in all species of the Northern Hemisphere (Applegate, 1950; Hagelin, 1959; Sterba, 1962; Lohnisky, 1966). In non-parasitic and many parasitic lamprey species spawning tends to be performed in groups. The assembly on the spawning grounds may be facilitated by olfactory signals (Hardisty and Potter, 1971b). Joining a group will improve the chances of females of finding fit partners as competition among males will be high in a group (Gosling and Petrie, 1981). Since the females spawn vigorously and usually are spent within a day there is a pronounced surplus of males in the nests (Malmquist, 1978; Bird and Potter, 1979). Such conditions may favour aggressive behavior when the density of adult lampreys is low which may occur very early or late in the spawning season (Malmquist, 1983a). Since spawning takes place in daylight the risk of falling victim to a predator is obvious.

At high altitudes (62-64°N) in Sweden, the river lamprey *Lampetra fluviatilis* is shown to have a 24 h locomotor activity during its spawning period just before midsummer (Sjöberg, 1977). This activity is caused by addition of diurnal spawning activity to the basic nocturnal activity and is not caused by weak Zeitgeber conditions which might be suspected just before midsummer at these high altitudes, as it is described for many other species (Müller, 1973; Eriksson, 1975). By keeping lampreys in cold water, spawning was delayed about a month, but by keeping them at normal (10°C) temperature and in total darkness the spawning time was normal (Sjöberg, 1977). Water temperature may therefore indirectly determine time of spawning of the river lamprey.

Experiments on activity and orientation

As the factors that influence the upstream migration in winter are unknown, and as the reasons for the non-homing behavior are obscure, we have studied the circadian rhythm of River Rickleå lampreys, *Lampetra fluviatilis*, during the winter, and their response to two kinds of natural water.

The working hypothesis for the activity experiments was that temperature is the decisive factor, as it seems to be for initiating both the movement from the sea into the estuary and spawning (see above). By using running tap water in the aquarium it was possible to keep a constant 10°C (=spawning temperature). As Sjöberg (1977) showed that individuals of this river have a 24 h locomotor activity during the spawning period, and that the individuals are nocturnal in May, prior to the spawning period, one could predict that our experimental animals from the same river, besides their normal nocturnal activity, would show signs of diurnal activity.

The experimental animals were 20-30 cm long and were acclimatized for about two months prior to testing. They were caught at night during their spawning run in September, about 1 km from the estuary of River Rickleå (64°05' N). Lampreys are still caught in the old way, by wooden traps placed between stones at the bottom of the rapids (Fig. 2). Dark rainy nights without moonlight and with wind resulting in high sea level are said to give the best catches (Sjöberg, 1982).

A new type of aquarium was used and this has been described in detail (Bertmar, 1985). It consists of three arms, each arm at 120° to the other arms (Fig. 3). The terminal part of each arm has an inlet for tap water; the stream velocity and temperature (10°C) were the same in all three arms. Two of these inlets could be shut off and another kind of water with the same stream velocity and temperature could be introduced at random into one of the arms. In this way water from the sea and from another river (R. Umeälven) were tested. The locomotor activity was continuously registered by two photocells in the distal third of each arm. No bottom material was present. The aquarium was placed in a cold green house at the university, about 40 km south of the place where they were caught. The animals received natural light from roof windows. Between experiments the lampreys were kept in the same room in a 300 l aquarium with running tap water of the same temperature as in the experimental aquarium. During the activity experiments in November, five individuals were registered individually for two days each (Fig. 4 A-E). The tests showed that the activity certainly was nocturnal but also that each animal had some diurnal activity. No arm was preferred and therefore no special orientation direction was chosen.

The next experiments were designed to see if an animal could adapt to the water at 10° C and return to a solely nocturnal activity. The results showed that this was not possible (Fig. 5). They also showed that the nocturnal activity had a certain rhythm which sometimes could be interrupted at full moon and which could sometimes continue after sunrise. However, there were also separate bursts of diurnal activity. There were still no signs of a particular orientation direction, or release of gonadal products.

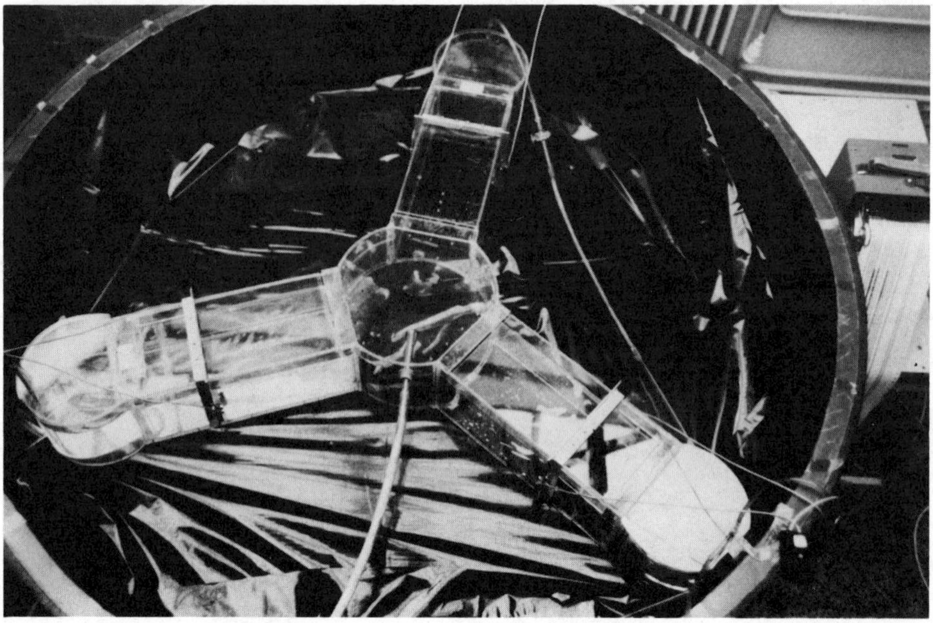

Fig. 3. Three-armed locomotor activity and orientation experiment aquarium in a green house, University of Umeå. Natural light through roof windows, and temperature (10°C), current velocity and pH were stable during mid winter 1984-1985. Documentation photo: Nils Häggström, University of Umeå.

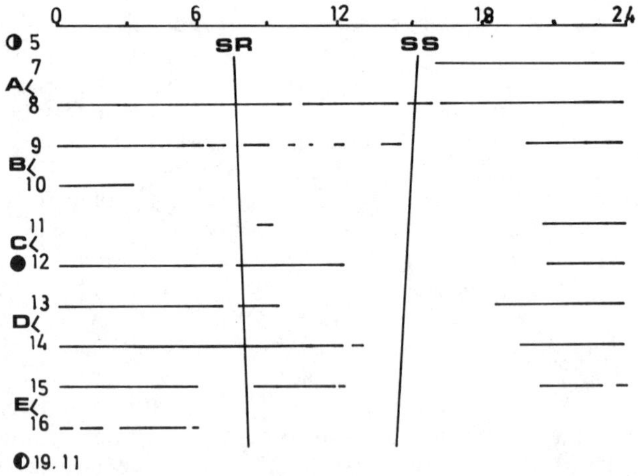

Fig. 4. Locomotor activity of *Lampetra fluviatilis* from the River Rickleå during the spawning migration phase in November 1984, natural light and 10°C water temperature. Sunrise (SR), sunset (SS) and moon cycle are shown. Five individuals (A-E) were tested.

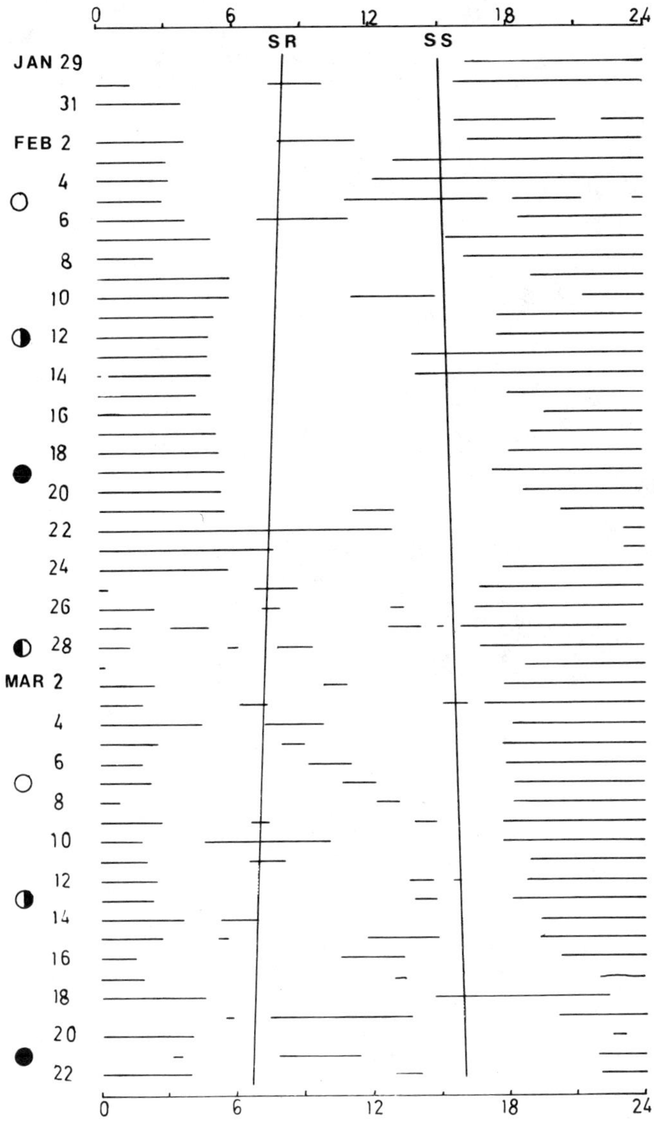

Fig. 5. Locomotor activity of *Lampetra fluviatilis* from the River Rickleå during the spawning migration phase in January-March 1985, natural light and 10°C water temperature. Sunrise (SR), sunset (SS) and moon cycle are shown.

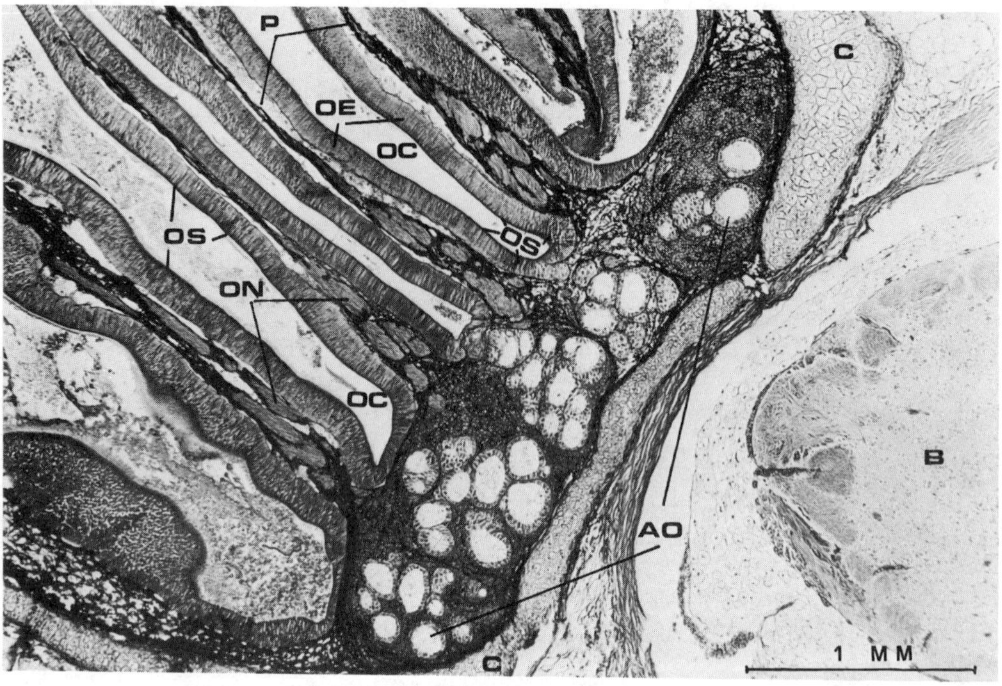

Fig. 6. Longitudinal section of parts of the olfactory organ and accessory olfactory organ (*AO*) in *Lampetra fluviatilis* from the River Rickleå during the spawning migration in November 1984; Bouin fixation, Azan-Mallory staining of paraffin sections 6 microns thick. *B*, brain; *C*, cartilage: *OC*, olfactory cavity; *OE*, olfactory epithelium; *ON*, olfactory nerve; *OS*, olfactory sensory cells; *P*, primary nasal fold. Microphoto: Frank Johansson, DE zoology project work.

The activity experiments thus showed that spawning temperature can certainly produce some diurnal activity in immature lampreys (as was predicted), but not a continuous 24 h activity. At this period of the cycle the temperature is not the decisive factor, and the lampreys cannot be lured into spawning by temperature manipulation.

The chemosensory orienting experiments were conducted in November. In order to ascertain that the migrating lampreys of this population at this time of the year can smell, the histology of the nose was studied. It was found that both the olfactory organ and the accessory olfactory organ that has evolved from it (Bertmar, 1969, 1981) are well developed and functioning (Fig. 6).

The orientation technique and kinds of test water were described above. Three animals were observed and registered individually over a period of 15-20 minutes. The experiments were preceded by a blank (control) test for 15-20 minutes using

Table II. Orientation experiments with three *Lampetra fluviatilis* during the spawning migration phase in November 1984. Blank and seawater tests. Observation time: 1 h. (3 animals, 20 min. each).

Type of water	# of visits in arm		
	A	B	C
Blank tests	72	64	63
Seawater into arm A	55[a]	80	72

[a]Not significant at $p<0.05$, x^2-test.

Table III. Orientation experiments with three *Lampetra fluviatilis* during the spawning migration phase in November 1984. Blank tests with strange river water (R. Umeälven). Observation time: 45 min. (3 animals, 15 min. each).

Type of water	# of visits to each arm		
	A	B	C
Blank tests	63	47	55
River Umeälven water into arm A	39[a]	73	56

[a]Significant at $p<0.05$ x^2-test.

only tap water in all arms. All tests were performed between 2000h and 2200 h. One observator was used throughout.

The results show that during the control tests the animals (as usual) swam at random, but when seawater or water from the River Umeälven was introduced they seemed to increase the swimming speed a little to avoid the unknown water (Tables II,III).

Thus, these pilot tests indicate that, during the period of the spawning migration, lampreys do not show the kind of direction orientation that might indicate the involvement of the stars or of magnetic fields. However, they are able to sense water of another quality and to avoid this unknown water. Therefore, it is possible that the chemical quality of the water is an ecological factor of equal or even greater importance than temperature for their orientation ability. It may be the case that migrating lampreys have integrated hierarchical orientation of the same type suggested for salmonid fishes (Bertmar, 1979, 1982) (Fig. 1). However, it is not known whether they have homing abilities.

Literature cited

ABOU-SEEDO, F.S., and I.C. POTTER. 1979. The esturarine phase in the spawning run of the river lamprey *Lampetra fluviatilis*. J. Zool. (Lond.) **188**: 5-26.

APPLEGATE, V.C. 1950. Natural history of the sea lamprey, *Petromyzon mariunus* in Michigan. Spec. Scient. Rep. U.S. Fish. Wildl. Serv. **55**: 1-237.

ASPLUND, C., and S. SÖDERGREN. 1975. Flodnejonögats (*Lampetra fluviatilis* L.) lekvandring i Rickleån. Zool. Revy **36**: 111-119. (Swedish with Engl. summary).

BEAMISH, F.W.H. 1979. Migration and spawning energetics of the anadromous sea lamprey *Petroymyzon marinus*. Environ. Biol. Fishes. **4**: 3-8.

BERTMAR, G. 1969. The vertebrate nose, remarks on its structural and functional adaptation and evolution. Evolution **23**: 131-152.

BERTMAR, G. 1979. Home range, migrations and orientation mechanisms of the River Indalsälven trout *Salmo trutta* L. Report Inst. Freshwater Research (Drottningholm). **58**: 5-26.

BERTMAR, G. 1981. Evolution of vomeronasal organs in vertebrates. Evolution **35**: 351-366.

BERTMAR, G. 1982. Structure and function of the olfactory mucosa of migrating Baltic trout under environmental stresses, with special reference to water pollution. pp. 395-422 *In* Hara, T.J. [ed.] Chemoreception in fishes, vol. 8. Developments in aquaculture and fisheries science. Elsevier, Amsterdam.

BERTMAR, G. 1983. Sinnesekologi hos renar och laxfiskar. Fauna och Flora **78**: 223-229. (In Swedish with Engl. summary and Figure texts).

BERTMAR, G. 1985. A new type of chemical choice aquarium for testing Salmonid fishes. *In* Johannson, N. [ed.] Int. Symp. Baltic Salmon Problems (Lulea) (In press).

BIRD, D.J., and I.C. POTTER. 1979. Metamorphosis in the paired species of lampreys, *Lampetra fluviatilis* L. and *Lampetra planeri* (Bloch). 2. Quantitative data for body proportions, weights, lengths and sex ratios. J. Linn. Soc. (Lond.) Zool. **65**: 145-160.

CHAPPUIS, P.A. 1939. Über die Lebensweise von *Eudontomyzon danfordi* (Regan). Arch. Hydrobiol. **34**: 645-658.

CONTE, F.P., WAGNER, H.H., and T.O. HARRIS. 1963. Measurement of blood volume in the fish *Salmo gairdneri*. Amer. J. Physiol. **205**: 503-540.

CUDNEY, M.D., and J.B. WALLACE. 1980. Life cycles, microdistribution and production dynamics of six species of netspinning caddisflies in a large southeastern (USA) river. Holarctic Ecol. **3**: 169-182.

DUMERIL, C. 1807. Mémoire sur l'odorat des poissons. Magasin Enclopédique (Paris) **5**: 99-113.

ENEQUIST, P. 1937. Das Bachneunauge als ökologische Modification des Flussneunauges. Über die Flussneunaugen und Bachneunaugen Schwedens. Ark. Zool. **29**: 1-22.

ERIKSSON, L.O. 1975. Diel and annual locomotor activity rhythms in some freshwater fish species, with special reference to the inversion in Salmonids. Ph.D. thesis, Univ. of Umeå.

FARMER, G.J., and F.W.H. BEAMISH. 1973. Sea lamprey (*Petromyzon marinus*) predation on freshwater teleosts. J. Fish Res. Bd. Can. **30**: 60-605.

FARMER, G.J., F.W.H. BEAMISH, and G.A. ROBINSON. 1975. Food

consumption of the adult landlocked sea lamprey *Petromyzon marinus* L.. Comp. Biochem. Physiol. **50A**: 753-757.

FOGELIN, P. 1972. Studier över drift av larver och nymetamorfoserade ungar av flodnejonoga *Lampetra fluviatilis* L. in Indalsälven och Rickleån. Report from Rickleå Field Station **20**: 28. (In Swedish).

GOSLING, L.M., and M. PETRIE. 1981. The economics of social organisation. *In* Townsend, C.R., and P. Calow [eds.]. Physiological ecology: an evolutionary approach to resource use. Blackwell, Oxford.

GROSSU, A., V. HOMEI, P. BARBU, and A. POPESCU. 1962. Contribution à l'étude des Pétromyzontides de la République Populaire Roumaine. Trav. Mus. Hist. Nat. Gr. Antipa **3**: 253-279.

HAGELIN, L.-O. 1959. Further aquarium observations on the spawning habits of the river lamprey, *Petromyzon fluviatilis*. Oikos **10**: 50-64.

HANSEN, L.G.,W.B. WIEKHORST, and J. SIMON. 1976. Effects of dietary Aroclor 1242 on channel catfish (*Ictalurus punctatus*) and the selective accumulation of PCB components. J. Fish. Res. Bd. Can. **33**: 1243-1352.

HARA, T.J. 1975. Olfaction in fish. Prog. Neurobiol. (Oxford) **5**: 271-335.

HARDISTY, M.W. 1944. The life history and growth of the brook lamprey *Lampetra planeri*. J. Anim. Ecol. **13**: 110-122.

HARDISTY, M.W., and I.C. POTTER. 1971a. The behavior, ecology and growth of larval lampreys. pp. 85-135 *In* Hardisty, M.W., and I.C. Potter [eds.]. The biology of lampreys, vol. 1. Academic Press, London.

HARDISTY, M.W., and I.C. POTTER. 1971b. The general biology of adult lampreys. pp. 127-206 *In* Hardisty, M.S., and I.C. Potter [eds.] The biology of lampreys, vol. 1. Academic Press, London.

HASLER, A.D. 1966. Underwater guideposts. Univ. of Wisconsin Press, Madison, 155 pp.

HUBBS, C.L., and I.C. Potter. 1971. Distribution, phylogeny and taxonomy. pp. 1-65 *In* Hardisty, M.W., and I.C. Potter [eds.] The biology of lampreys, vol. 1. Academic Press, London.

KAISER, K.L.E. 1982. Early trends of organochlorine contamination from residue ratios in the sea lamprey *Petromyzon marinus* and its lake whitefish *Coregonus clupeaformis* host. Can. J. Fish. Aquat. Sci. **39**: 571-579.

KELSO, J.R.M., and R. FRANK. 1974. Organochlorine residues, mercury, copper and cadmium in yellow perch, white bass and smallmouth bass, Long Point Bay, Lake Erie. Trans Amer. Fish. Soc. **103**: 577-581.

KLEEREKOPER, H. 1969. Olfaction in fishes. Indiana Univ. Press, Bloomington, Indiana.

KLEEREKOPER, H. 1971. The sense organs. pp. 373-404 *In* Hardisty, M.W., and I.C. Potter [eds.] The biology of lampreys, vol. 2. Academic Press, London.

KLEEREKOPER, H. 1982. The role of olfaction in the orientation of fishes. pp. 201-225 *In* Hara, T.J. [ed.] Chemoreception in fishes, vol. 8. Developments in aquaculture and fisheries science. Elsevier, Amsterdam.

KLEEREKOPER, H., and J.A. MOGENSEN. 1963. Role of olfaction in the orientation of *Petromyzon marinus*. I. Response to a single amine in prey's body odor. Physiol. Zool. **36**: 347-360.

KLEEREKOPER, H., G. TAYLOR, and R. WILTON. 1961. Diurnal periodicity in the activity of *Petromyzon marinus* and the effects of chemical stimulation. Trans. Amer. Fish. Soc. **90**: 73-78.

LANZING, W.J.R. 1959. Studies on the river lamprey *Lampetra fluviatilis* during its anadromous migration. Uitsgeversmaatschappij Neerlandia, Utrecht.

LENNON, R.E. 1954. Feeding mechanisms of the sea lamprey and its effect on host fishes. Fish. Bull. U.S. **56**: 247-293.

LINNÉ (Linnaeus), C. 1735. Systema Natura. Lugduni Batavorum.

LOHNISKY, K. 1966. The spawning behaviour of the brook lamprey, *Lampetra planeri*. Vestn. csl. spol. zool. **30**: 289-307.

MALMQUIST, B. 1978. Population structure and biometry of *Lampetra planeri* (Bloch) from three different watersheds in South Sweden. Arch. Hydrobiol. **84**: 65-86.

MAMLQUIST, B. 1980a. Habitat selection of larval brook lampreys (*Lampetra planeri*, Bloch) in a South Swedish stream. Oecologia (Berl.) **45**: 35-38.

MALMQUIST, B. 1980b. The spawning migration of the brook lamprey, *Lampetra planeri* (Bloch) in a South Swedish stream. J. Fish. Biol. **16**: 105-114.

MALMQUIST, B. 1983a. Breeding behavior of brook lampreys (*Lampetra planeri*): experiments on mate choice. Oikos. **41**: 43-48.

MALMQUIST, B. 1983b. Growth, dynamics, and distribution of a population of the brook lamprey *Lampetra planeri* in a South Swedish stream. Holarctic Ecol. **6**: 404-412.

MALMQUIST, B., and C. BRÖNMARK. 1982. Filter feeding in larval *Lampetra planeri*: effects of size, temperature and particle concentration. Oikos **38**: 40-46.

MANION, P.J. 1967. Diatoms as food of larval sea lampreys in a small tributary of Northern Lake Michigan. Trans. Amer. Fish. Soc. **96**: 224-226.

MANION, P.J., and B.R. SMITH. 1978. Biology of larval and metamorphosing sea lampreys (*Petromyzon marinus*) of the 1960 year class in the Big Garlic River, Michigan, Part II, 1966-72. Tech. Rep. 30. Great Lakes Fish Comm. 35 pp.

MATTHES, E. 1924. Das Geruchvermögen von Triton beim Aufenhalt under Wasser. Z. vgl. Physiol. **1**: 57-83.

MONTGOMERY, W.L., S.D. McCORMIC, R.J. NAIMAN, F.G. WHORISKEY, and G.A. BLACK. 1983. Spring migratory synchrony of salmonid, catostomid and cyprinid fishes in Riviere á la Truite, Quebec, Canada. Can. J. Zool. **61**: 2495-2502.

MOORE, J.W., and I.C. POTTER. 1976a. A laboratory study on the feeding of larvae of brook lampreys, *Lampetra planeri* (Bloch). J. Anim. Ecol. **45**: 81-90.

MOORE, J.W., and I.C. POTTER. 1976b. Aspects of feeding and lipid deposition and utilization in the lampreys *Lampetra fluviatilis* and *Lampetra planeri*. J. Anim. Ecol. **45**: 669-712.

MÜLLER, K. 1973. Circadian rhythms of locomotor activity in aquatic organisms in the subarctic summer. Aquilo, Ser. Zool. **14**: 1-18.

NIKOLSKII, G.V. 1956. Some data on *Lampetra japonica* (Martens) during the period of sea life. Zool. Zh. **35**: 589-591.

POTTER, I.C. 1970. The life cycles and ecology of Australian lampreys of the genus *Mordacia*. J. Zool. (Lond.) **161**: 487-511.

POTTER, I.C., and F.W.H. BEAMISH. 1977. The freshwater biology of adult anadromous sea lampreys *Petromyzon marinus*. J. Zool. (Lond.) **181**: 113-130.

POTTER, I.C., P.A. PRINCE, and J.P. CROXALL. 1979. Data on the adult marine and migratory phases in the life cycle of the Southern Hemisphere lamprey *Geotria australis*. Environ. Biol. Fishes **4**: 65-70.

REINERT, R.E., L.J. STONE, and H.L. BERGMAN. 1974. Dieldrin and DDT: accumulation from water and food by lake trout *Salvelinus namaycush* in the laboratory. Proc. 17th Conf. Great Lakes Res. pp. 52-58.

ROULE, L. 1931. Les poissons et la monde vivant des eaux. Vol. 4. Librairie Delagrave (Paris) pp. 63-67.

RYAPOLOVA, N.I. 1964. *Lampetra fluviatilis* L. in Latvian rivers. Trudy vses. natuchnoissled. Inst. morsk. ryb. khoz. Okeanogr. **1964**: 66-69, (in Russian).

SCHROLL, F. 1959. Zur Ernährungsbiologie der steirischen Ammocöten *Lampetra planeri* (Bloch) und *Eudontomyzon danfordi* (Regan). Int. Revue Ges. Hydrobiol. Hydrogr. **44**: 395-429.

SJÖBERG, K. 1977. Locomotor activity of river lamprey *Lampetra fluviatilis* L. during the spawning season. Hydrobiologia **55**: 265-270.

SJÖBERG, K. 1980. Ecology of the European river lamprey *Lampetra fluviatilis* in Northern Sweden. Can. J. Fish. Aquat. Sci. **37**: 1974-1980.

SJÖBERG, K. 1982. Exploitation of lampreys in Europe. Ethnol. Scand. 1982.

SKIDMORE, J.F. 1959. Biology of spawning-run sea lampreys (*Petromyzon marinus*) in the Pancake River, Ontario. M.Sc. thesis, Univ. Western Ontario.

STERBA, G. 1962. Die Neunaugen Petromyzonidae. pp. 263-352 *In* Demoll, R., H. N. Maier *et al.* [eds.]. Handbuch der Binnenfischerei Mitteleuropas, vol. 3. E. Schweizerbart, Stuttgart.

STODDART, D.M. 1980. The ecology of vertebrate olfaction. Chapman and Hall, London, 234 p.

TESCH, F.W. 1967. Aktivität und Verhalten wandernder *Lampetra fluviatilis, Lota lota* und *Anguilla anguilla* im Tidegebiet der Elbe. Helgoländer wiss. Meeresunters. **16**: 92-111.

THOMAS, M.L.H. 1962. Observations on ecology of ammocoetes *Petromyzon marinus* L. and *Entosphenus lamottei* (La Sueur). Thesis, Univ. Toronto, Canada.

VANNOTE, R.L., G.W. MINSHALL, K.W. CUMMINS, J.R. SEDELL, and C.E. CUSHING. 1980. The river continuum concept. Can. J. Fish. Aquat. Sci. **37**: 130-137.

FACTS AND THOUGHTS ON PISCINE PHYLOGENY

Hans C. Bjerring

Department of Palaeozoology
Swedish Museum of Natural History
S-104 05 Stockholm, Sweden

Introduction

Craniate animals, it is estimated, are represented today by some 50,000 species, about half of which constitute the piscine world. Their fossil record extends back to the Upper Cambrian. Although craniate animals have many forms and shapes, they are readily subdivided into ten large groups: osteolepipods, urodelomorphs, struniiforms, actinopterygians, brachiopterygians, coelacanthiforms, dipnoans, elasmobranchiomorphs, pteraspidomorphs, and cephalaspidomorphs (Fig. 1).

The cephalaspidomorphs have a dorsal nasohypophyseal opening; the pteraspidomorphs have a nasopharyngeal duct. Their living representatives, the lampreys and the hagfishes, are collectively known as cyclostomes. Cephalaspidomorphs and pteraspidomorphs have entodermal gills directed towards the pharynx; together, therefore, they are termed entobranchiates. The eight other groups of craniate animals have outwardly directed gills of ectodermal derivation; accordingly they are referred to as ectobranchiates. They also have jaws formed from branchial-arch elements. Consequently ectobranchiates are commonly called gnathostomes.

At the very beginning of their known history the ectobranchiates had already subdivided into two major phylogenetic lines, termed plagiostomes and teleostomes. The former are characterized by an utricular diverticulum; the latter, by a dental arcade, *i.e.* by dentigerous dermal bones around the jaw apparatus.

Plagiostomes comprise the elasmobranchiomorphs, which have open endolymphatic ducts, and the dipnoans, which have pseudotrabecles (*cf.* Bjerring, 1977). The six other ectobranchiate groups constitute the teleostomes. Each of these may be characterized thus: the osteolepipods have an occipital artery; the urodelomorphs have an intracerebral olfactory bulb; the actinopterygians have a swimbladder; the brachiopterygians have a multipinnulate dorsal fin; the

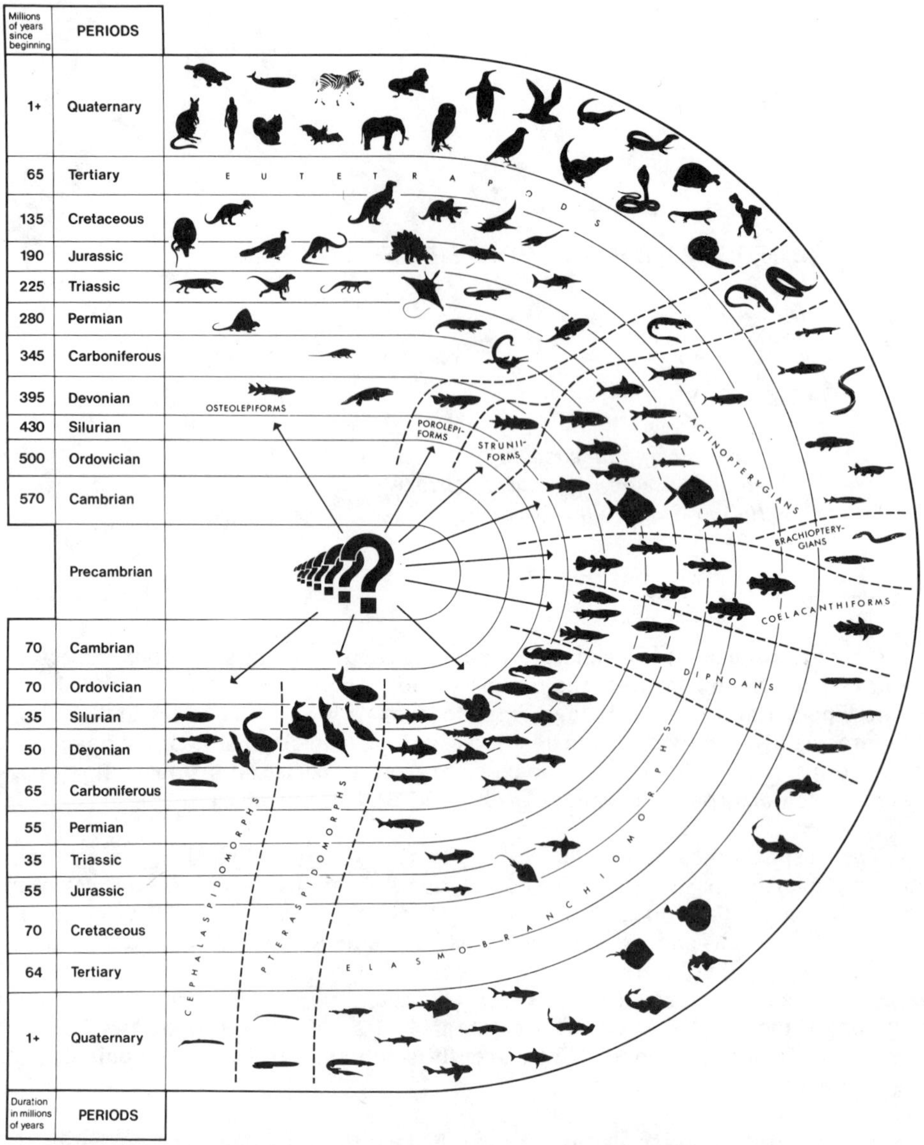

Fig. 1. Panorama of the documented history of craniote evolution. (From Bjerring, 1984a).

coelacanthiforms have an electroreceptive rostral organ; and the struniiforms have a single, long submandibular between the lower jaw and the ipsilateral gular.

From their beginnings to the present day, all ten groups of craniate animals show a relatively advanced anatomical organization which changes only moderately.

Thus, during their documented history, craniate animals have undergone merely small-scale evolution. To put it differently, all the major steps towards craniotedness were taken during the Precambrian (*cf.* Bjerring, 1984a).

The following account, emphasizing coelacanthiforms and osteolepipods, shows that many of the morphological specializations found in living craniate animals already occurred at the time of their earliest occurrence as fossils. Attention is also directed to the commonly-made statement that the brachiopterygian fishes are actinopterygians.

Comparison between a living and a fossil coelacanthiform

Anatomically the sole Recent coelacanthiform, *Latimeria chalumnae*, or the Comoro tufttail, is well-known (Fig. 2). This is due in a great measure to the three volumes of "Anatomie de *Latimeria chalumnae*" by J. Millot, J. Anthony and D. Robineau (1958, 1965, 1978). The cranial anatomy of *Nesides schmidti* of the European late Upper Devonian is also well-known. Its cephalic skeleton has been serially ground by Stensiö (1932, 1937) and wax models from these sections are on deposit in the Swedish Museum of Natural History, Stockholm.

Comparison of these two tufttails indicates that many specializations have existed without any appreciable change for some 350 million years (*cf.* Jarvik, 1964, 1980).

The intracranial juncture apparatus and its basicranial muscles

The Comoro tufttail is unique amongst its contemporaries in possessing an intracranial juncture apparatus. This articulatory complex consists of two

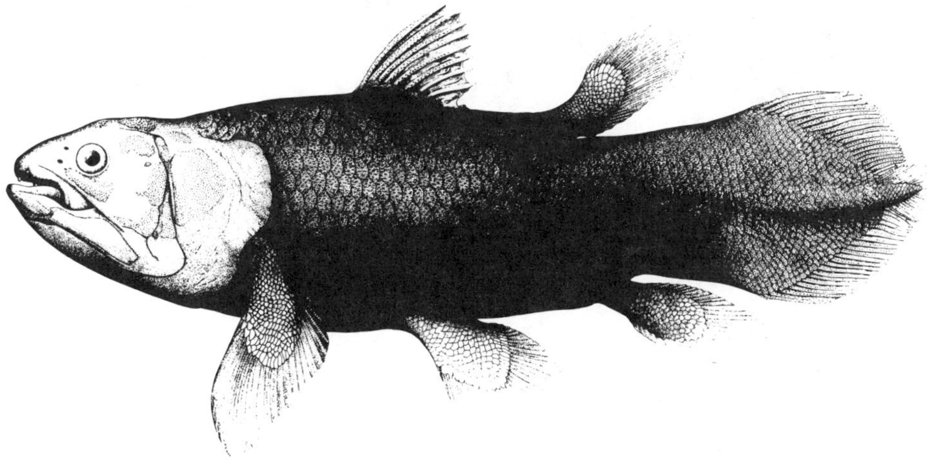

Fig. 2. *Latimeria chalumnae*. Lateral view of male specimen on deposit in the Swedish Museum of Natural History, Stockholm.

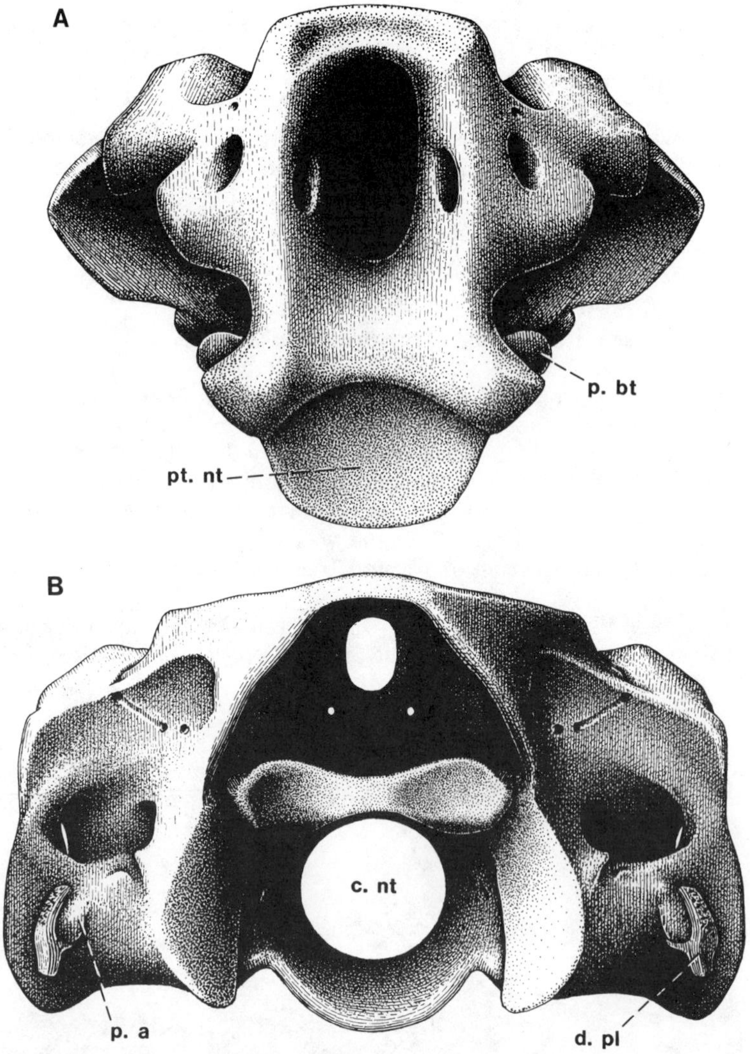

Fig. 3. *Nesides schmidti*. A, posterior view of ethmosphenoid; B, anterior view of otoccipital. *c.nt*, canal for notochord; *d.pl*, dental plate; *p.a.*, affacial process; *p.bt*, basipterygoid process; *pt.nt*, pit for anterior end of notochord.

divisions, infracerebral and supracerebral. The former is a paired triple joint, formed between an anazygal, the ethmosphenoid and the otoccipital. The latter, more forwardly located, is a paired joint, formed between the parietal shield and the ethmosphenoid. Except for a median, supracerebral syndesmosis between the ethmosphenoid and the otoccipital, *Nesides schmidti* exhibits an intracranial juncture apparatus (Fig. 3) which tallies with that of *Latimeria chalumnae* (Bjerring, 1967, 1973, 1977). A ligamentous connection of the Comoro tufttail is homologous to the supracerebral syndesmosis of the Devonian tufttail.

The intracranial juncture apparatus of *Latimeria chalumnae* is spanned ventrally by a paired basicranial muscle. This muscle arises from an oblong area on the otoccipital and is inserted, by a strong tendon, into the lateral side of the parasphenoid. As pointed out elsewhere (Bjerring, 1967), *Nesides schmidti* displays impressions for muscular attachments on the ventral parts of the otic and hypophyseal divisions of its cranium. These impressions suggest that a paired basicranial muscle acting upon the intracranial juncture apparatus already existed during the earliest known phase of coelacanthiform phylogeny. In contrast with the basicranial muscle of the Comoro tufttail that of the Devonian tufttail lacked an anterior tendinous part; it did not extend backwards to the posterior limit of the cranium but ended underneath the otic capsule.

It may be mentioned that the basicranial muscle which spanned the intracranial juncture apparatus in osteolepiforms and porolepiforms extended for a shorter posterior distance, being mainly confined to the third (mandibular) metamere of the body. In these fishes the muscle arose from a depressed area on the anteroventral part of the otic capsule and was inserted into a pit-like impression on the posterior part of the parasphenoid (Bjerring, 1967). This short basicranial muscle has the same positional relations as does the polar cartilage, which is an embryonic structure occurring in craniate animals lacking an intracranial junctural apparatus. In as much as the polar cartilage in elasmobranchs develops from the myotome of the mandibular somite, it has been concluded that the basicranial muscle and the polar cartilage are homologous (Bjerring 1967, 1968). Thus, as the otic and orbitotemporal regions of the endocranium in a number of craniate animal phylogenies became ankylosed, the myotomic source of the basicranial muscle gained a skeletogenous ability which led to the rise of the polar cartilage. This change of the prospective fate of the third-metamere myotome from the basicranial muscle to the polar cartilage is seen in the embryology of *Squalus acanthias*; here the posterodorsal part of the mesial wall of the mandibular somite, besides the polar cartilage, gives origin to the transient muscle *e* of Platt (1891). This embryonic muscle has been observed in *Squalus acanthias* (Lamb, 1902; Neal, 1918) in *Squalus canicula* (Dohrn, 1906), and in *Chelydra serpentina* (Johnson, 1913); it later degenerates and disappears. Finally, the Lower Devonian osteolepiform *Youngolepis praecursor* of China lacks the intracranial juncture apparatus (Chang, 1982). In this fossil fish, interestingly enough, the anteroventral part of the otic region of the endocranium is connected with the hypophyseal part of the orbitotemporal region of the endocranium by a skeletal bridge, here called the ansilla basicranialis (Fig. 4). Most likely, therefore, *Youngolepis praecursor* had a polar cartilage; this cartilage subsequently formed the basicranial ansilla strengthening the endocranial base.

The rostral organ

Latimeria chalumnae agrees with most other living fishes in having a pair of nasal sacs, each of which opens to the exterior by an incurrent and an excurrent nostril and has lost the choana. However, *Latimeria chalumnae* is unique among

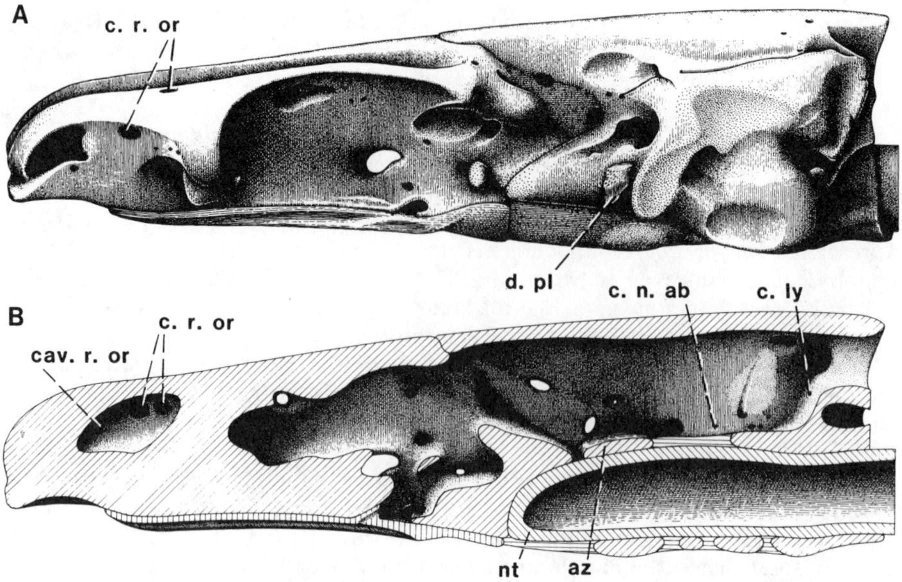

Fig. 5. *Nesides schmidti.* A, endocranium with parasphenoid in lateral view; B, endocranium and parasphenoid in midsagittal section. *az*, anazygal plate; *cav.r.or*, cavity for rostral organ; *c.ly*, canal for lymphatic vessel; *c.n.ab*, canal for abducens nerve; *c.r.or*, canals for tubes of rostral organ; *d.pl*, dental plate; *nt*, notochord.

therefore, that this Devonian fish had a rostral organ which probably functioned as an electroreceptor.

The nervus abducens

The abducens nerve pursues a most unusual course in *Latimeria chalumnae* (Millot and Anthony 1965, fig. 23). It emerges ventrally from the posterior part of the medulla oblongata, below the roots of the glossopharyngeal and vagus nerves. Almost immediately the nerve enters the saccular portion of the otic capsule through a narrow canal. It then continues downward to the floor of the cavity of the otic capsule and bends abruptly anteriorly to reach a canal which tunnels through the anteroventral part of the otic capsule. As it emerges from this canal, the nerve passes anteriorly above the basicranial muscle and supplies the external rectus muscle of the eye.

In *Nesides schmidti* the cranial cavity communicates with the cavity of the otic capsule *via* a narrow canal which is equidistant from the foramen for the acoustic nerve and the canal for the glossopharyngeal nerve (Bjerring, 1972). Moreover, in this Devonian tufttail, the floor of the otic capsule is perforated anteriorly by a minute canal which opens externally mesial to the oblong depression that has been interpreted as the area of origin of the basicranial muscle (Bjerring, 1967).

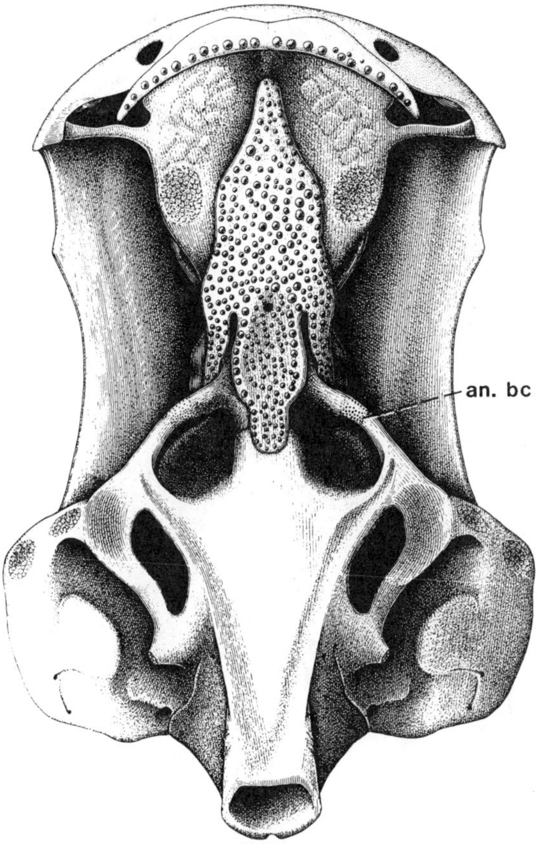

Fig. 4. *Youngolepis praecursor*. Endocranium with some exoskeletal elements in ventral view (from wax model made by Mee-man Chang). *an.bc*, ansilla basicranialis (formed from the polar cartilage).

living fish in having a rostral organ (Millot and Anthony, 1956, 1965). This structure, accommodated by a cavity in the ethmoidal region of the endocranium, consists of three pairs of unconnected tubes that open to the exterior and lead to a system of crypts invaginated into a median sac composed of connective tissue. The tubes contain a gelatinous substance and, like the median sac, they are separated from the endocranium by a conspicuous layer of adipose tissue. On the basis of its morphology and the fact that it is innervated by ophthalmic lateralis fibers terminating in the dorsal octavolateralis nucleus, the rostral organ has recently been ascribed an electroreceptive function (Hetherington and Bemis, 1979; Northcutt, 1980).

As reported elsewhere (Bjerring, 1972, 1973, 1977), *Nesides schmidti* exhibits an unpaired cavity in the ethmoidal region of the endocranium that communicates with the exterior by three pairs of canals (Fig. 5). It seems reasonably certain,

Consequently, the abducens nerve in the Devonian tufttail is similar to that of the Comoro tufttail in emerging from the brain as far back as the vagal portion of the medulla oblongata, running through the otic capsule and innervating an extrinsic eye muscle which arises from the hypophyseal part of the endocranium.

The ductus communicans saccularis

In *Latimeria chalumnae*, the right and left sacculus are interconnected by a tubular endolymphatic passage, the saccular communicating duct (Millot and Anthony, 1965, fig. 47). This duct lies in a transverse groove on the occipital region of the endocranium, above the notochord and below the rear of the medulla oblongata (Fig. 6A). On either side it enters the cavity for the membranous labyrinth through a foramen in the posteromesial part of the otic capsule and joins the sacculus between the ampulla of the posterior semicircular duct and the lagena.

As seen in Fig. 6B, the occipital region of the endocranium of *Nesides schmidti* displays a transverse groove which is situated between the foramen magnum and the canal for the notochord and which laterally opens into the cavities of the otic capsules. Therefore, this Devonian coelacanthiform was equipped with a ductus communicans saccularis.

Mention should also be made of a paired, narrow canal which in the Comoro tufttail leads from the cranial cavity to the groove for the saccular communicating duct and provides passage for a lymphatic vessel. This canal was already present in the Devonian tufttail (Fig. 5B).

The hyomandibula

In *Latimeria chalumnae*, the hyomandibula is pentagonal and platelike. Anterodorsally it is expanded into two eminences, the upper and lower condyles, which articulate with the endocranium. Posterodorsally it bears a distinct process which articulates with the opercular. Ventrally it presents a concave facet for articulation with the stylohyal. It is perforated by a canal for the hyomandibular trunk of the facial nerve and by one for the hyoid branch of the same nerve. The element is acted upon by an adductor muscle which is inserted into its mesial surface. The hyomandibula also gives attachment to three ligaments which extend, respectively, to the pterygoquadrate division of the palatoquadrate, the lower jaw, and the symplectic (Millot, Anthony and Robineau, 1978), fig. 4).

As pointed out elsewhere (Bjerring, 1977), the hyomandibula of *Nesides schmidti* resembles that of *Latimeria chalumnae* and, no doubt, was suspended in exactly the same way.

The palatoquadrate

Typically, in most gnathostome fishes, the palatoquadrate consists of three major parts forming one unit: the pterygoquadrate, the vinculum, and the autopalatine. Of these, the pterygoquadrate belongs to the mandibular arch and the autopalatine to the premandibular arch; the vinculum has been interpreted as modified epal gill rays of the premandibular arch (Bjerring, 1977). In *Latimeria*

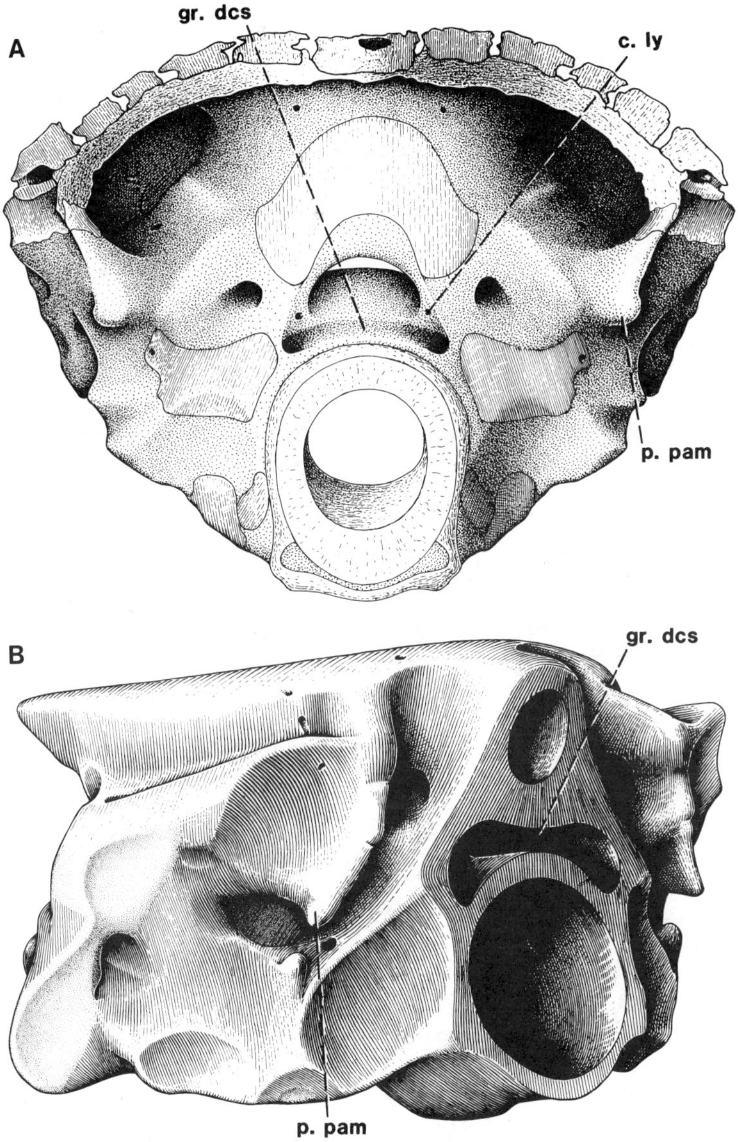

Fig. 6. A, the Comoro tufttail, *Latimeria chalumnae*; otoccipital with the extrascapular bones in posterior view. B, *Nesides schmidti*; otoccipital in oblique posterior view (From Bjerring 1984b). *c.ly*, canal for lymphatic vessel; *gr.dcs*, groove for ductus communicans saccularis; *p.pam*, parampullary process.

chalumnae, the vinculum is lacking and the palatoquadrate consists of two separate parts: the pterygoquadrate and the prepterygoquadrate. The pterygoquadrate is divisible into a body, an ascending process, and an otic process. The body represents the epimandibular, the ascending process represents the suprapharyngomandibular, and the otic process is to be regarded as a modified mandibular gill-ray component. The prepterygoquadrate is an osseocartilaginous rodlike structure which anteriorly is raised into a triangular lamelliform process received in a depression on the external surface of the postnasal wall. This anterior parethmoidal process of the prepterygoquadrate probably represents the infrapharyngopremandibular, whereas the rest of the prepterygoquadrate is an epipremandibular.

In the Devonian coelacanthiform *Nesides schmidti*, the palatoquadrate, (as seen in Bjerring, 1977, fig. 24) agrees in most essentials with that of *Latimeria chalumnae*, except that it articulates with the basipterygoid process of the endocranium (*cf*. Fig. 3). This process is totally reduced in *Latimeria chalumnae.*

The affacial process with its dental plate, the prefacial eminence, the prefacial ligament, and the orbital artery.

Both *Latimeria chalumnae* and *Nesides schmidti* have an affacial process with a dental plate, a prefacial eminence, a prefacial ligament, and an orbital artery (Figs. 3, 5). The affacial process - as first designated by Bjerring (1972) - juts out of the otical shelf, anteroventral to the canal for the jugular vein. Its apex carries a small, curved dental plate that is visible in the spiracular pouch. The prefacial eminence (Bjerring, 1972) is a small, endoskeletal elevation situated just dorsal to the affacial process and immediately ventral to the groove for the palatine ramus of the facial nerve. This eminence serves for the attachment of the ventral extremity of the prefacial ligament which extends upwards outside the jugular vein and may be pierced at its base by the palatine ramus of the facial nerve. Moreover, in *Nesides schmidti* the affacial process presents a distinct groove anteroventrally. This suggests that, as in *Latimeria chalumnae*, the orbital artery passed upwards close in front of the affacial process and then continued lateral to the palatine ramus of the facial nerve and the jugular vein (Bjerring, 1972, fig. 5; Jarvik, 1980, p. 276).

The parampullary process

Lateral to the ampulla of the posterior semicircular duct and immediately above the posterior part of the groove for the jugular vein, the otic capsule of *Latimeria chalumnae* presents a distinct projection, to which branchial levator musculature is attached. This endocranial projection, the parampullary process (Bjerring, 1972), probably represents the suprapharyngobranchial element of the fifth metamere which has fused secondarily with the endocranium (Bjerring, 1973). A parampullary process was well developed already in *Nesides schmidti* (Fig. 6B).

The above examples, as well as others (*cf*. Jarvik, 1964, 1980), demonstrate that the earliest coelacanthiforms were highly organized anatomically, and that many structures have remained practically unchanged during the known history of coelacanthiforms (approx. 350 million years). In fact, since the Devonian, coelacanthiforms have undergone merely small-scale evolution.

Comparison between the appendicular skeleton of osteolepiforms and tetrapods

Under this heading follows another illustration of small-scale evolution that directly relates to our own phylogeny.

It has been suggested recently that tetrapods and lungfishes are collateral relatives (Rosen *et al.*, 1981). However, the evidence remains clearly in favor of a porolepiform origin of the urodeles and an osteolepiform origin of the remaining tetrapods. Lungfishes are plagiostomes and lack choanae. Osteolepiforms and porolepiforms are teleostomes and are the only fishes with choanae.

It is generally agreed that the pectoral and pelvic appendages stem from a pair of long folds running the length of either flank. These integumentary folds subsequently underwent muscularization through myomeric muscle-buds. Each myomere produced two muscle-buds; these subdivided into dorsal and ventral radial muscles. Later, an endoskeletal radial arose between each dorsal and ventral radial muscle (*cf.* Jarvik, 1965a). Accordingly, there are two endoskeletal radials in each metamere and twice as many endoskeletal radials as the spinal nerves that innervate the fin or limb.

The endoskeleton of the paired fins of porolepiforms is practically unknown. However, it is well known in the osteolepiform *Eusthenopteron foordi* of the Upper Devonian (Jarvik, 1964, 1965a, 1965b, 1980).

In *Eusthenopteron foordi*, the endoskeleton of the pectoral fin includes four mesomeres; that of the pelvic fin, three (Figs. 7,8). All the pectoral mesomeres, except the second, carry a winglike projection. The first pelvic mesomere lacks this, whereas each of the others has one. In both appendages, the first mesomere articulates distally with a ray that supports the ventrolateral margin of the fin. The rest of the endoskeletal elements of the paired fins are arranged so that they radiate towards the second mesomere. The first mesomere of the pectoral fin presents a canal tunnelling through the base of its winglike projection. It also presents a distinct lateral ridge which bends downward anteriorly and merges into a forwardly and upwardly directed crest. The middle part of the lateral ridge is pierced by a few canals which admit nerves and vessels to the extensor side of the fin. The first mesomere of the pelvic fin is moderately expanded proximally and distally. The distal end is partly divided into two condyles; between these there lies a short, groove-like intercondylar fossa on the ventromesial surface of the element. Its dorsolateral surface presents an oblique ridge which is broader and more prominent anterodorsally than ventrolaterally.

In man, the pectoral limb is innervated by six spinal nerves, the pelvic limb by seven (Gray, 1973). Thus, the endoskeleton of these limbs is composed of twelve and fourteen radial rays, respectively. Five of these rays are represented by the digital phalanges. The hand and the foot of the human embryo contain, respectively, two and four more radial rays. In the pectoral limb, the remaining radial rays might be represented by the humeral epicondylar, supracondylar, and deltoid processes; in the pelvic limb they might be represented by the femoral epicondylar processes and the trochanters.

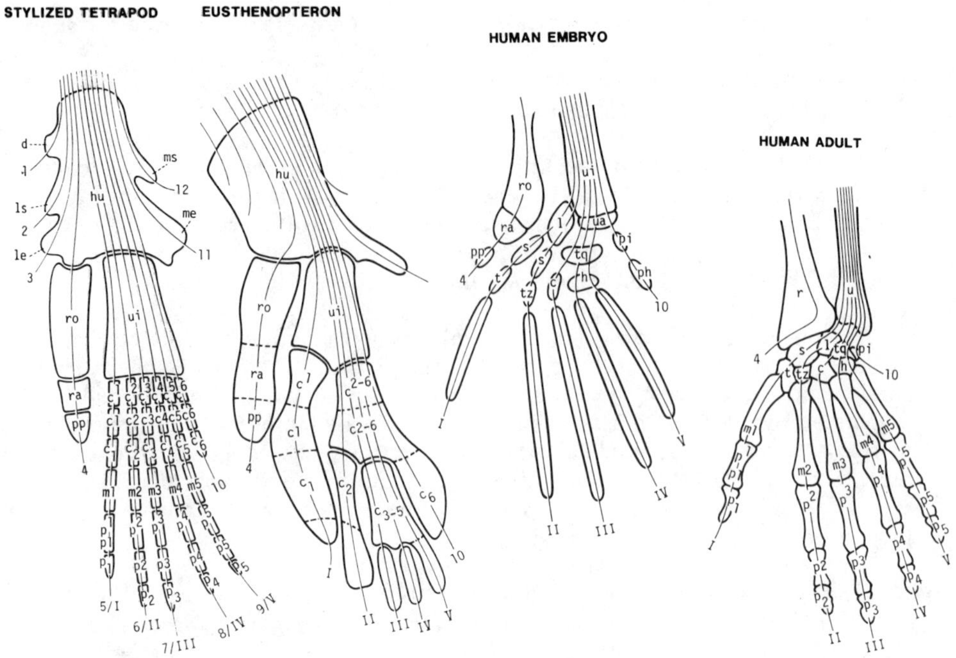

Fig. 7. **Membrum Anterius.** Pectoral appendicular endoskeleton (from various sources, mainly Jarvik, 1980, and Schmidt-Ehrenberg, 1942). *c*, capitatum (c_3); c^1-c^6, proximal carpals; *c1-c6*, middle carpals; c_1-c_6, distal carpels; *d*, deltoid process; *h*, hamatum (c_4-c_5); *hu*, humerus; *l*, lunatum (c^1-c^2); *le*, lateral epicondylar process; *ls*, lateral supracondylar process; *m1-m5*, metacarpels; *me*, medial epicondylar process; *ms*, medial supracondylar process; p^1-p^5, proximal phalanges; *p1-p5*, middle phalanges; p_1-p_5, distal phalanges; *ph*, posthamatum (c_6); *pi*, pisiforme (*c6*); *pp*, prepollex; *r*, radius; *ra*, radials; *ro*, radiolus; *s*, scaphoideum (*c1-c2*); *t*, trapezium (c_1); *tq*, triquetrum (*c3-c5*); *tz*, trapezoideum (c_2); *u*, ulna; *ua*, ulnare (c^3-c^6); *ui*, ulnilla; *1-12*, rays or radials; *I-V*, digiti I-V.

The distal portion of the appendicular endoskeleton of *Eusthenopteron foordi* has seven pectoral radial rays and nine pelvic radial rays (*cf. Ichthyostega*, Fig. 10). In the first pectoral mesomere, the winglike projection, perforated by a canal, represents the humeral medial epicondylar and supracondylar processes. Distally, the perforated lateral ridge represents the humeral lateral epicondylar process; proximately, it represents the humeral lateral supracondylar (supinator) process. The crest lying anterior to the lateral ridge represents the humeral deltoid process. In the first pelvic mesomere, the somewhat expanded distal extremity represents the femoral epicondylar processes; the anterodorsal part of the oblique ridge represents the fourth trochanter; the slightly expanded proximal extremity represents the greater and lesser trochanters.

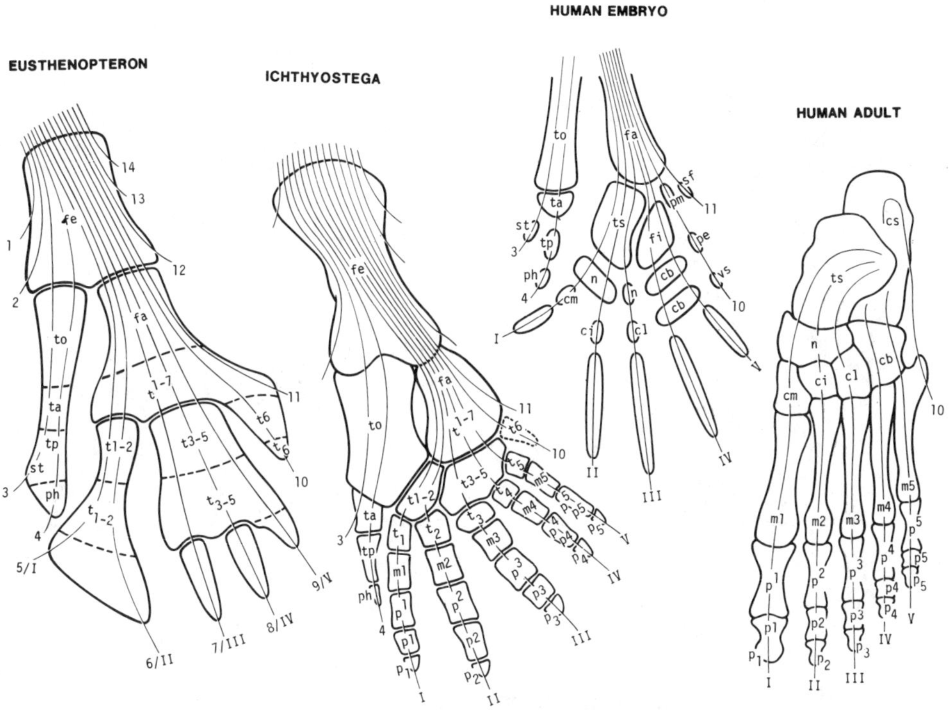

Fig. 8. **Membrum Posterius**. Pelvic appendicular endoskeleton (from various sources, manily Jarvik, 1980, and Schmidt-Ehrenberg, 1942). *cb*, cuboid; *ci*, intermediate cuneiform; *cl*, lateral cuneiform; *cm*, medial cuneiform; *cs*, calcaneus; *fa*, fibula; *fe*, femoris; *fi*, fibulare; *m1-m5*, metatarsals; *n*, navicular; p^1-p^5, proximal phalanges; *p1-p5*, middle phalanges; p_1-p_5, distal phalanges; *pe*, peroneum; *ph*, prehallux; *pm*, postminimus; *sf*, subfibulare; *st*, subtibiale; t^1-t^7, proximal tarsals; *t1-t6*, middle tarsals; t_1-t_6, distal tarsals; *ta*, tibiale; *to*, tibiola; *tp*, prehallucal tarsal; *ts*, talus; *vs*, vesalianum.

Thus, as in humans, the endoskeleton of each pectoral and pelvic appendage of *Eusthenopteron foordi* was composed of twelve and fourteen radial rays, respectively (Fig. 9). Moreover, the radial rays, which correspond to the phalangeal skeleton, radiate towards the second mesomere as does the digital skeleton in the human embryo. In this respect the arrangement of the appendicular endoskeletal elements differs radically from that seen in lungfishes.

All the above shows that very little has happened to the pectoral and pelvic endoskeleton of the Paleozoic osteolepiforms during its evolution into the bones of the human limbs.

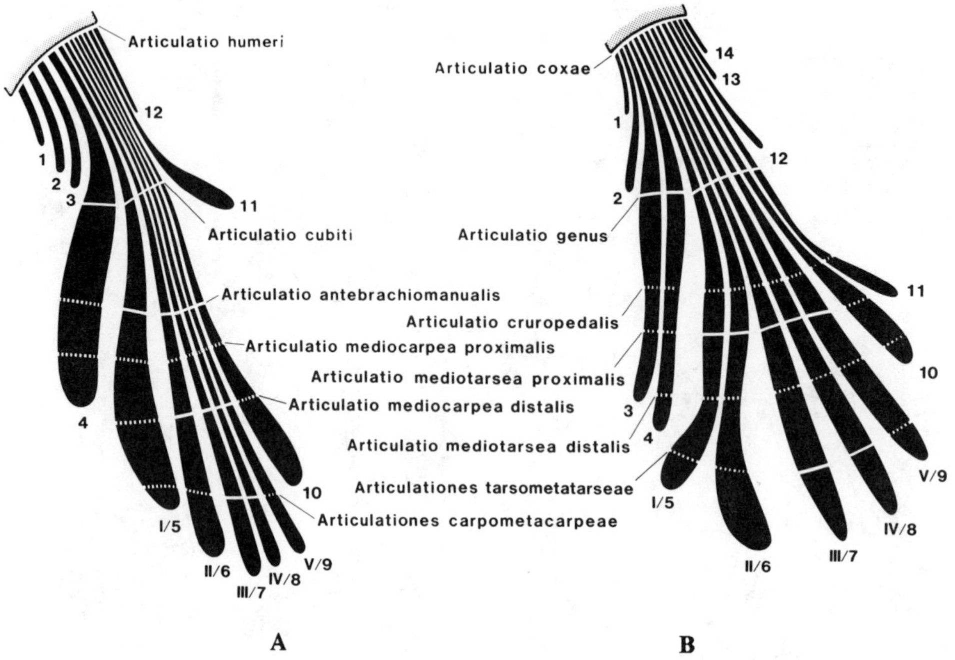

Fig. 9. Schema of appendicular endoskeleton of *Eusthenopteron foordi*. A. Membrum Anterius; B. Membrum Posterius.

Whereas the articulatio antebrachiomanualis has its counterpart in the pectoral fin of *Eusthenopteron foordi*, the articulatio cruropedalis lacks this (Fig. 9). The latter articulation is also lacking in the Devonian tetrapod *Ichthyostega* (Fig. 8); this and other facts (neuromasts situated in canals within the cephalic exoskeleton; presence of gill cover; caudal fin with lepidotrichia) indicate that *Ichthyostega* was an aquatic animal that hardly could walk (Fig. 10).

The question of the relationships of the genus *Polypterus*

We have virtually no fossil record for the polypterids (Greenwood, 1974); hence comparisons like those above are impossible. However, it is possible to compare them with other fishes, provided that the anatomy is adequately known. Toward that end, embryos of *Polypterus senegalus* have been sectioned and wax models have been made of one of them (32 mm). Also, adult specimens have been dissected.

Since the late 1920s it has been customary to regard *Polypterus* as an actinopterygian (Goodrich, 1928). A few dissenting voices included Holmgren and Stensiö (1936) and Jarvik (1942), who considered *Polypterus* and its close relative, *Calamoichthys*, as representing a separate group of teleostome fishes of high systematic rank, the Brachiopterygii. Recently Patterson (1982) and Gardiner (1984) have each presented their own list of characters said to be valid for both

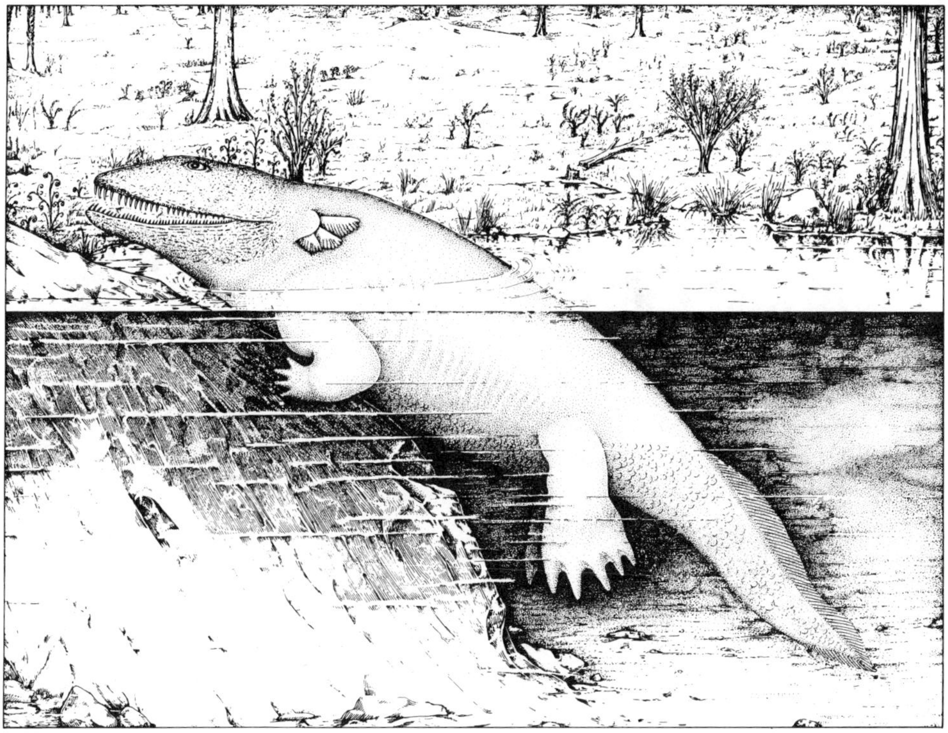

Fig. 10. Reconstruction of *Ichthyostega*.

actinopterygians and *Polypterus*. Ten characters are common to both lists. In this section these lists will be discussed.

Pectoral propterygium

In actinopterygians, the pectoral propterygium is short and broad and strongly articulated to the shoulder girdle. It is perforated by a canal for nerves and blood vessels. *Polypterus* lacks such a propterygium, in this respect resembling *Squalus* (Fig. 11).

Pelvic plate and two series of radials

If this statement is correct, the pelvic plate of *Acipenser* should resemble that of *Polypterus* more than that of *Squalus*. It is indeed just the reverse (Fig. 12). Moreover, in *Amia*, the pelvic plates overlap each other anteriorly whereas those of *Polypterus* are connected by separate cartilages. Furthermore, each pelvic fin of *Amia* contains three radials: a hook-like mesial one and a bipartite lateral one. During embryology one more radial element arises which becomes incorporated into the pelvic plate (Sewertzoff, 1934), and the hooklike radial arises from four elements. Thus, the pelvic endoskeleton of *Polypterus* clearly differs from that of *Amia*.

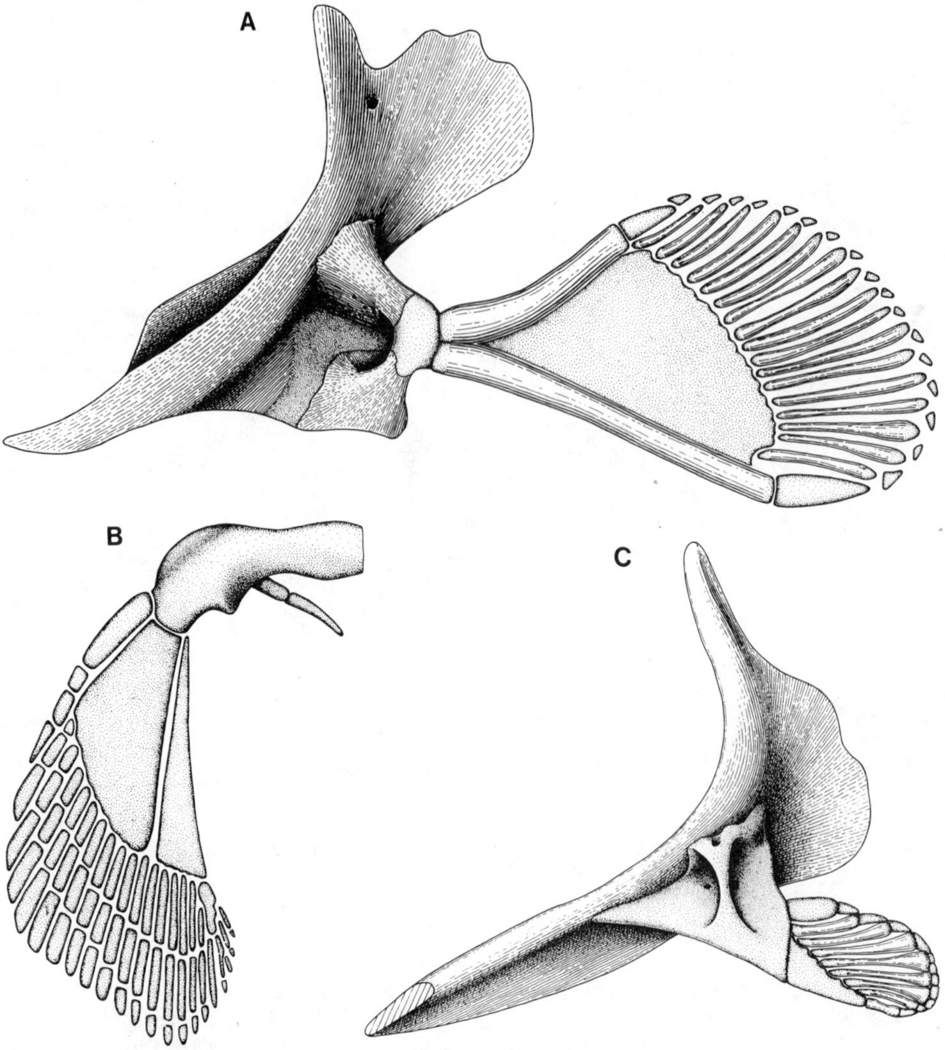

Fig. 11. Shoulder girdle and endoskeleton of pectoral fin in (A) *Polypterus bichir*, (B) *Squalus acanthias*, and (C) *Amia calva*. (A, mainly after Jessen, 1972; B, from Jarvik, 1965a; C, from Jessen, 1972).

Ganoin

As pointed out by Ørvig (1978a) the so-called ganoin of the scales of *Polypterus* is histologically of a type of its own. In fact, the "ganoin" in the dermal bones, in the scales and in the fin spines of *Polypterus*, differs from the ganoin of paleonisciforms.

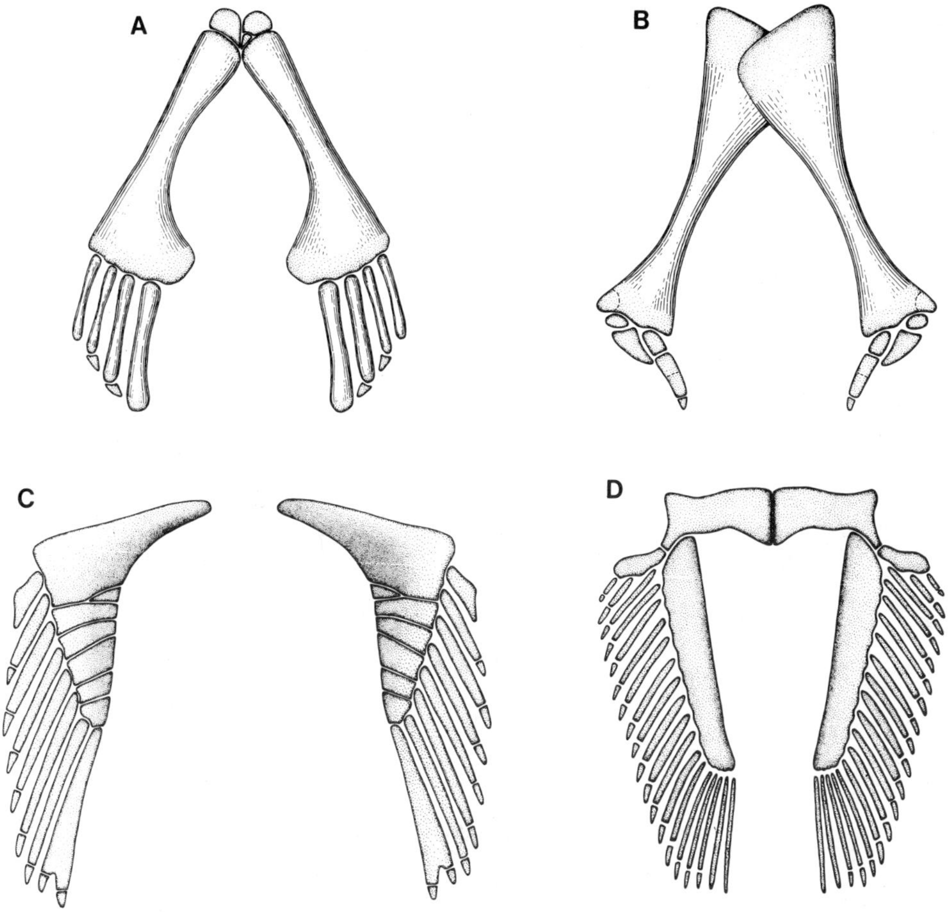

Fig. 12. Pelvic girdle and endoskeleton of pelvic fin in (A) *Polypterus bichir*, (B) *Amia calva*, (C) *Acipenser ruthenus*, and (D) *Squalus acanthias*. (A, from Goodrich, 1930; B, after Sewertzoff, 1934, and Jarvik, 1980; C, after Wiedersheim, 1892, and Marinelli and Strenger, 1973; D, after Marinelli and Strenger, 1959, and Jarvik, 1965a).

Peg-and-socket articulations between scales

In addition to actinopterygians and *Polypterus*, this type of articulation between scales of the same row also occurs in porolepiforms, osteolepiforms, and dipnoans (Fig. 13).

Anterodorsal angle or process of scales

This scarf-jointing of the suture between scales of the same row, occurring in actinopterygians and polypterids as well as in osteolepiforms, appears to have the role of equalizing the distribution of the transmitted load.

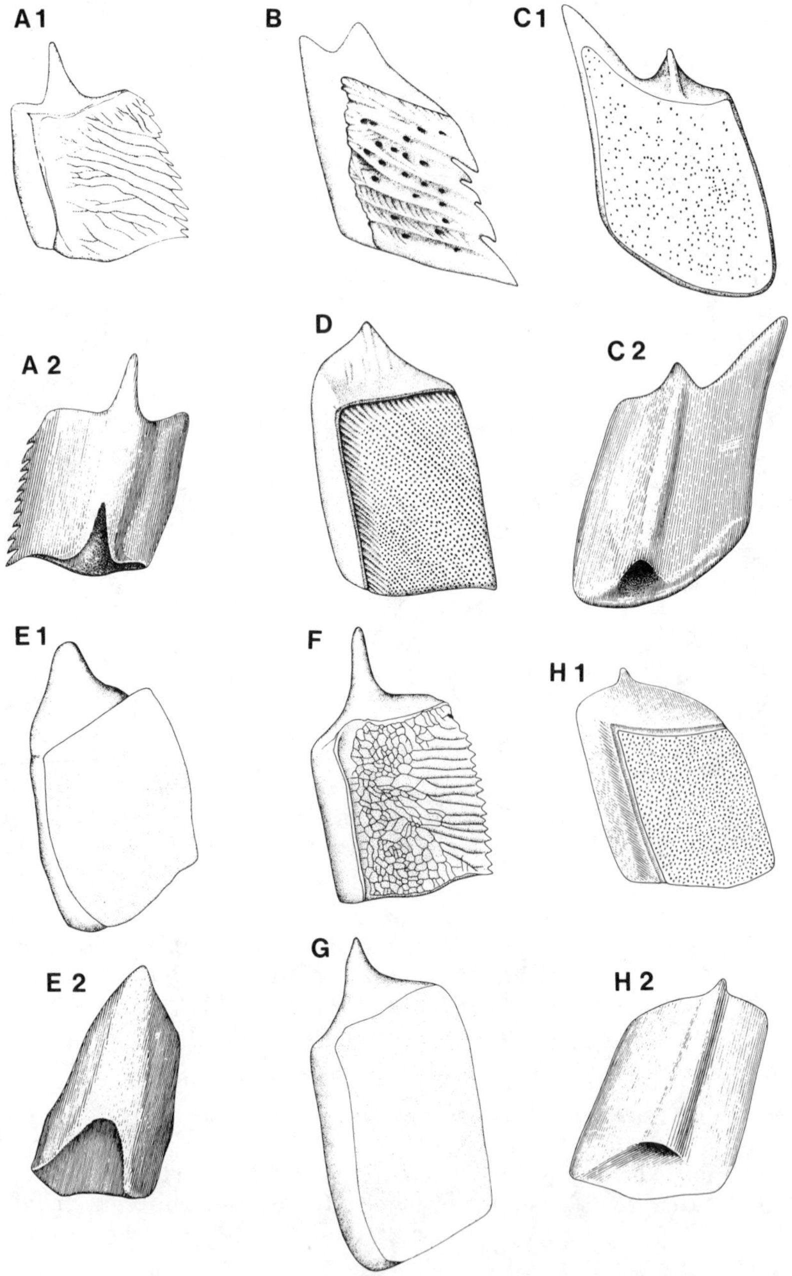

Fig. 13. Scales. A, B, F, G, actinopterygians; C, polypterids; D, porolepiforms; E, lungfish; H, osteolepiforms. (Based on data from Schultze, 1966; Gross, 1966; Denison, 1968; and Jarvik, 1948).

Squamosal absent and jugal canal reduced to a pit-line

Polypterids, osteolepiforms, porolepiforms, and paleonisciforms agree in having a complete external cheek plate. Hence nothing is absent. In osteolepiforms, this plate consists of seven bones, namely the lacrimal, jugal, postorbital, maxilla, squamosal, preopercular, and quadratojugal. In porolepiforms the makeup of the external cheek plate agrees in most essentials with that of the osteolepiforms, except that the postorbital consists of anterior and posterior parts, and the squamosal, of upper and lower parts (Jarvik, 1972). The external cheek plate of paleonisciforms is easily accounted for as fusions of lower squamosals with maxilla, and upper squamosals with the preopercular (Fig. 15B). This explains the anterodorsal direction of the jugal neuromast canal and anteroventral direction of the squamosal pit-line. In the external cheek plate of *Polypterus* (Fig. 15A1), the maxilla and the jugal are united with one another, the preopercular is fused with the squamosal, and the upper part of the cheek plate has become fragmented into a row of spiracular bones (prespiraculars and juxtaspiraculars). By this, the jugal neuromast canal has been directed upwards and somewhat forwards; however,the squamosal pit-line has retained its horizontal position. This interpretation is in full agreement with what is known about the embryology of the external cheek plate in *Polypterus* (Pehrson, 1947; own observations).

Dentary with enclosed mandibular neuromast canal

The lateral aspect of the Meckelian bone (ceratomandibular), in adult polypterids, is covered by two dermal bones (Fig. 15A1). Embryologically, the anterior of these bones develops from an upper tooth-bearing element, the dentary, and three lower elements, the infradentaries, which enclose the mandibular neuromast canal (Pehrson, 1947; own observations). Hence this bone is a dentalo-infradentary.

Dermohyal

Discovered and defined by Nielsen (1936) in *Pteronisculus* of the Greenland Triassic, the dermohyal is known to occur generally in paleonisciforms. It rests upon the upper part of the outer surface of the hyomandibula (Fig. 14). As pointed out by Nielsen (1936), the dermohyal represents fused dental plates comparable to those occurring on the lateral surface of the hyomandibula in *Eusthenopteron foordi*. In *Polypterus* (Fig. 14), the anterior postspiracular is firmly attached to the upper aspect of the hyomandibula by descending inner and outer laminae. Accordingly it is called the accessory hyomandibular by some writers (Traquair, 1870; Jarvik, 1980). Embryologically, this spiracular bone arises in the line of the other spiraculars and only secondarily establishes contact with the hyomandibula. Therefore, it is not homologous with the dermohyal, and the latter bone is absent in *Polypterus*.

Hyomandibular articulation single, above jugular canal

The hyomandibula in osteolepiforms (*cf*. Jarvik 1954) is proximally provided with dorsal and ventral articular heads which fit into articular areas on the otoccipital. One of these areas is above the jugular vein, the other is below that vein. The osteolepiform hyomandibula is also provided with an opercular process. In actinopterygians and *Polypterus*, the hyomandibula has only one articular head and an opercular process (Fig. 14). The articulation between the hyomandibular head and the endocranium is above the jugular vein and thus corresponds to the dorsal articulation between the hyomandibula and the endocranium in osteolepiforms. This type of articulation between the hyomandibula and the endocranium above the jugular vein, however, is not restricted to actinopterygians and *Polypterus*. It also occurs in lungfishes (Jarvik, 1980), the hyomandibula of which has one articular head as well as an opercular process.

Acrodin caps on all teeth

The teeth of many actinopterygians have an apical cap of a special, hypermineralized hard tissue called acrodin (Ørvig, 1973, 1978b, 1978c). Similar caps occur in *Polypterus*; however, it remains to be determined whether these caps really are made up of acrodin.

Presupracleithrum

The presupracleithrum is an exoskeletal pectoral element (Fig. 15) that occurs in Paleozoic and Mesozoic actinopterygians. It has been equated with the posterior post-spiracular in *Polypterus*. Since the posterior postspiracular is an opercular element, it cannot be homologous with the presupracleithrum. *Polypterus* lacks a presupracleithrum (Bjerring, 1985).

Clearly, then, none of the foregoing characters are tenable. Also, this study has failed to disclose any other derived character common to *Polypterus* and actinopterygians. However, many known dissimilarities exist between *Polypterus* and actinopterygians (*cf*. Jarvik, 1980). These include: (1) distinct differences in the morphology of the ethmoidal region of the endocranium; (2) the lack in *Polypterus* of a posterior myodome, an interorbital septum, a pila lateralis, a supra-auditive fossa (for this term see Bjerring, 1984b) accommodating somatic musculature, a spiracular canal, and a spiracular sensory organ; (3) only four branchial arches in *Polypterus* (five in actinopterygians) and only one large element of the basibranchial series (several in actinopterygians); (4) the absence of supra-angular dermal bones and independent branchiostegic rays and submandibulars in *Polypterus*, but the presence of a large retroarticular process; (5) the existence of a frontal pit-line in *Polypterus* (absent in actinopterygians); (6) the endoskeleton of the shoulder girdle as well as of the pectoral and pelvic fins of *Polypterus* is fundamentally different from that of actinopterygians; (7) the subdivision of the nasal sac of *Polypterus* is unknown in actinopterygians; (8) larval stages of *Polypterus* exhibit external gills (external gills do not occur in actinopterygians); (9) the lung arises from the midventral part of the foregut in *Polypterus*, whereas the swimbladder in actinopterygians connects with the middorsal part of the foregut. Moreover, *Polypterus* displays a number of unique features, *e.g.* numerous spiracular plates, a special construction of the anterior part of the palate, and a complex posterior ascending process of the parasphenoid. Furthermore, in *Polypterus*, the dorsal fin is highly specialized (finlets) and the caudal fin is heterocercal. Because of these many differences, the present writer adopts the position that *Polypterus* cannot be classified as an actinopterygian.

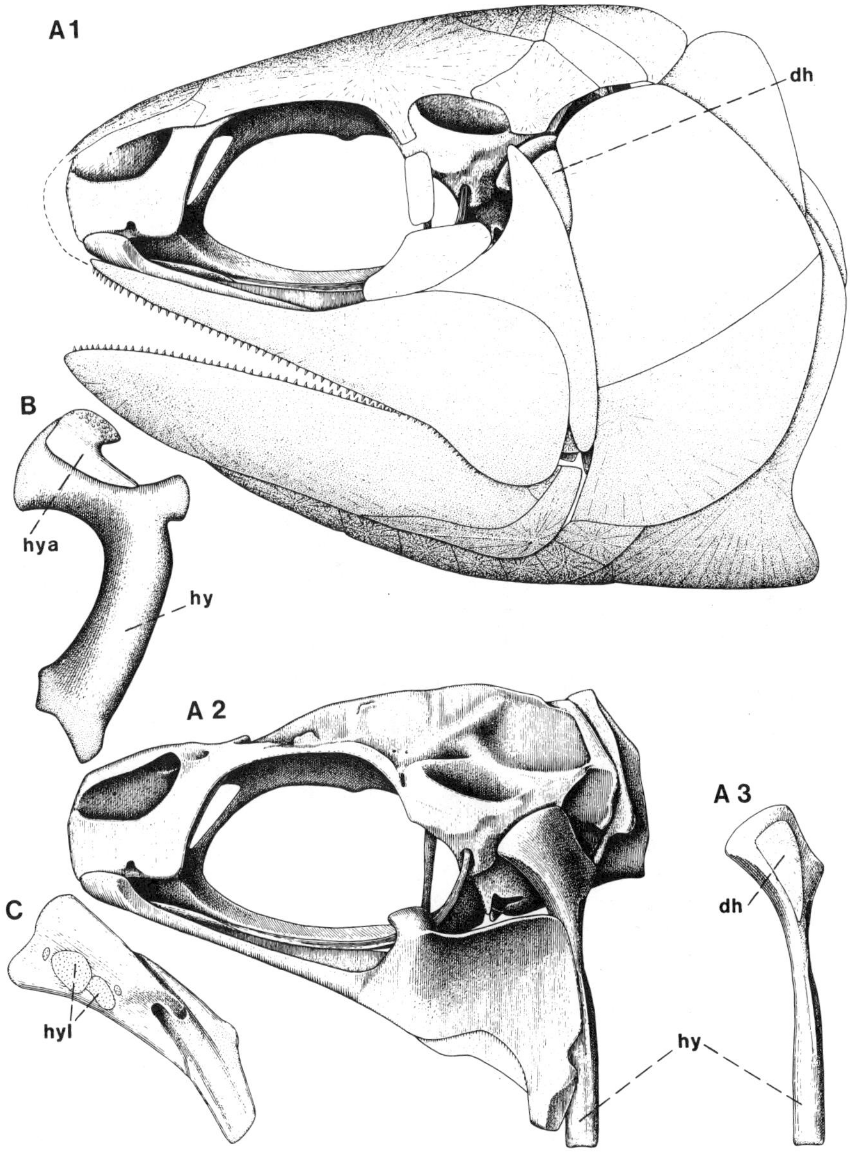

Fig. 14. A1, A2, A3, cranial elements of *Australosomus kochi* in lateral view (from Nielsen, 1949); B, hyomandibula and associated postspiracular of *Polypterus bichir* in lateral view (from Allis, 1922); C, hyomandibula with tooth-plates of *Eusthenopteron foordi* in lateral view (from Jarvik, 1954). *dh*, dermohyal; *hy*, hyomandibula; *hya*, accessory hyomandibular (anterior post-spiracular); *hyl*, lateral hyomandibular dental plates.

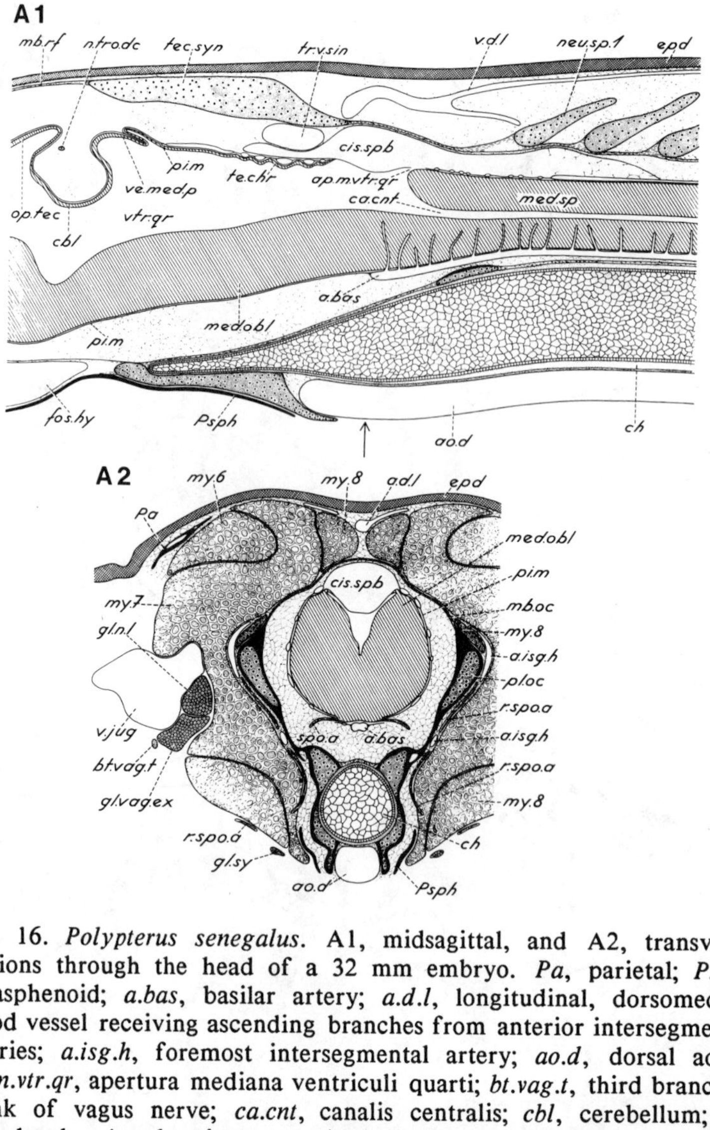

Fig. 16. *Polypterus senegalus*. A1, midsagittal, and A2, transverse sections through the head of a 32 mm embryo. *Pa*, parietal; *Psph*, parasphenoid; *a.bas*, basilar artery; *a.d.l*, longitudinal, dorsomedian blood vessel receiving ascending branches from anterior intersegmental arteries; *a.isg.h*, foremost intersegmental artery; *ao.d*, dorsal aorta; *ap.m.vtr.qr*, apertura mediana ventriculi quarti; *bt.vag.t*, third branchial trunk of vagus nerve; *ca.cnt*, canalis centralis; *cbl*, cerebellum; *ch*, notochord; *cis.spb*, cisterna spinobulbaris; *edp*, epidermis; *fos.hy*, hypophyseal fossa; *gl.n.l*, ganglion of lineal nerve of lateralis system; *gl.sy*, sympathetic ganglion; *gl.vag.ex*, main extracranial ganglion of vagus nerve; *mb.oc*, membranous part of occipital endocranial region; *mb.rf*, membranous roof of endocranial region; *med.obl*, medulla oblongata; *med.sp*, medulla spinalis; *my6–my8*, myomeres of metameres 6 to 8; *neu.sp.1*, first neural spine; *n.troc.dc*, trochlear nerve decussation; *op.tec*, optic tectum; *pi.m*, pia mater; *pl.oc*, occipital pila; *spo.a*, first occipital nerve; *te.chr*, tela chorioidea; *tec.syn*, synotic tectum; *tr.v.sin*, transversal vein sinus; *v.d.l*, dorsolateral vein; *ve.med.p*, posterior medullary vellum; *v.jug*, jugular vein; *vtr.qr*, ventriculus quartus.

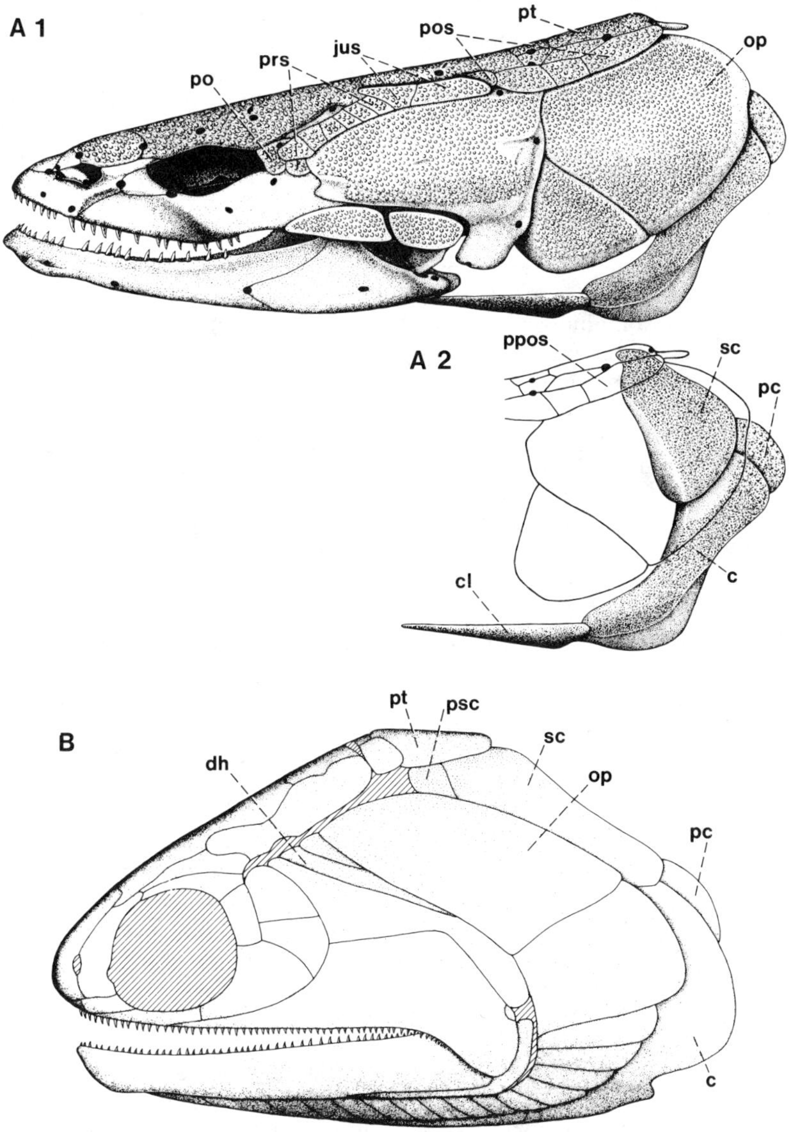

Fig. 15. A1, A2, *Polypterus bichir*; based on data from Allis (1922), Jarvik (1944b), and specimens in the Swedish Museum of Natural History. B, *Pteronisculus stensioei*; after Nielsen (1942). A1, cranium and exoskeletal shoulder girdle in left lateral view. A2, exoskeletal shoulder girdle in relation to part of the cranium (the latter drawn as if transparent). B, sinistral view of cranium. *c*, cleithrum; *cl*, clavicle; *dh*, dermohyal; *jus*, juxtaspiraculars; *op*, opercular; *pc*, postcleithrum; *po*, postorbital; *pos*, postspiraculars; *ppos*, posterior postspiracular; *prs*, prespiraculars; *psc*, presupracleithrum; *pt*, posttemporal; *sc*, supracleithrum.

This view is further supported by the following observation. In *Polypterus*, dorsal to the choroid tela of the medulla oblongata and the anterior part of the spinal cord, there exists a space formed by the meningeal membranes and filled with cerebrospinal fluid (Fig. 16). This intermeningeal space, previously unknown in fishes, is referred to here as the cisterna spinobulbaris. It resembles the cisterna cerebellomedullaris in man and other mammals and, like this, it communicates with the fourth ventricle by a small opening, the apertura mediana ventriculi quarti (Magendie's foramen).

In actinopterygians, the release of a cerebrospinal fluid probably takes place by diffusion *via* the dorsal sac of the diencephalon. Thus, these fishes are not equipped with a spinobulbar cistern. Instead, above the medulla oblongata, a number of extant actinopterygians (*Acipenser*, *Polyodon*, *Lepisosteus*, and *Amia*) have a lymphomyeloid organ which may be provided with a paired lateral diverticulum extending into the dorsoposterior part of the ipsilateral otic capsule (*cf.* Bjerring, 1984b). Inasmuch as the cranial cavity in certain paleoniscids (Nielsen, 1942; Poplin, 1974) widens dorsally between the posterior parts of the otic capsules and continues laterally on both sides into a tubular space which occasionally communicates with the ipsilateral sphenopterotic fossa, it can be concluded that these extinct fishes, like the living actinopterygians mentioned above, probably had an epimyelencephalic lymphomyeloid organ with a median main body and paired lateral diverticula. These lateral diverticula most likely occupied the sphenopterotic fossae in such paleoniscids where the said fossae were in communication mesially with the cranial cavity.

In *Polypterus*, the upper parts of the anterior trunk myomeres occupy a paired endocranial depression situated between the upper back parts of the otic capsules. This depression, termed fossa tectosynotica, also appears in the Devonian tufttail *Nesides schmidti* as well as in embryos of *Amia calva* (Bjerring, 1984b). However, in the embryology of *Amia*, somatic musculature shifts from the tectosynotic fossa to the supra-auditive fossa. Therefore, it seems likely that the presence of somatic musculature in the supra- auditive fossa is a secondary specialization. Thus, from what has been said earlier, it appears that originally the supra-auditive fossa came about for accomodation of lymphomyeloid tissue. In *Polypterus*, as well as in the Devonian tufttail *Nesides schmidti*, the supra-auditive fossa is secondarily occupied by exoskeleton enclosing the temporotic neuromast canal (Bjerring, 1984b).

In summary, all of the above evidence suggest that *Polypterus* is not to be classified as an actinopterygian or a descendent of the paleoniscids. Hence, for the present, *Polypterus* must be placed in a group of teleostomes of its own.

Literature cited

ALLIS, E.P. 1922. The cranial anatomy of *Polypterus*, with special reference to *Polypterus bichir*. J. Anat. **56**: 189-294.

BJERRING, H.C. 1967. Does a homology exist between the basicranial muscle and the polar cartilage? Colloques int. Cent. natn. Rech. scient. **163**: 223-267.

BJERRING, H.C. 1968. The second somite with special reference to the evolution of its myotomic derivatives. Nobel Symp. **4**: 341-357.

BJERRING, H.C. 1971. The nerve supply to the second metamere basicranial muscle in osteolepiform vertebrates, with some remarks on the basic composition of the endocranium. Acta Zool. (Stockh.) **52**: 189-225.

BJERRING, H.C. 1972. The nervus rarus in coelacanthiform phylogeny. Zool. Scripta **1**: 57-68.

BJERRING, H.C. 1973. Relationships of coelacanthiforms. Zool. J. Linn. Soc. (suppl. 1) **53**: 179-205.

BJERRING, H.C. 1977. A contribution to structural analysis of the head of craniate animals. Zool. Scripta **6**: 127-183.

BJERRING, H.C. 1984a. Major anatomical steps toward craniotedness: a heterodox view based largely on embryological data. J. Vert. Paleontol. **4**: 17-29.

BJERRING, H.C. 1984b. The term "fossa bridgei" and five endocranial fossae in teleostome fishes. Zool. Scripta **13**: 231-238.

BJERRING, H.C. 1985. The question of a presupracleithrum in brachiopterygian fishes. Acta Zool. (Stockh.) (in press).

CHANG, M. 1982. "The brain case of *Youngolepis*, a Lower Devonian crossopterygian from Yunnan, southwestern China." Department of Geology, University of Stockholm, and Section of Palaeozoology, Swedish Museum of Natural History, Stockholm.

DENISON, R.H. 1968. The evolutionary significance of the earliest known lungfish, *Uranolophus*. Nobel Symp. **4**: 247-257.

DOHRN, A. 1906. Studien zur Urgeschichte des Wirbeltierekörpers, 23, die Mandibularhöhle der Selachier. Pubbl. Staz. zool. Napoli **17**: 1-116.

GARDINER, B.G. 1984. The relationships of the palaeoniscid fishes, a review based on new specimens of *Mimia* and *Moythomasia* from the Upper Devonian of Western Australia. Bull. Br. Mus. nat. Hist. (Geol.) **37**: 173-428.

GOODRICH, E.S. 1928. *Polypterus* a palaeoniscid? Palaeobiologica **1**: 87-92.

GOODRICH, E.S. 1930. Studies on the structure and development of vertebrates. Macmillan, London.

GRAY, H. 1973. Anatomy of the human body. C.M. Goss [ed.], Lea and Febiger, Philadelphia, Pennsylvania.

GREENWOOD, P.H. 1974. Review of Cenozoic freshwater fish faunas in Africa. Ann. Geol. Surv. Egypt **4**: 211-232.

GROSS, W. 1966. Kleine Schuppenkunde. N. Jb. Geol. Paläontol. Abh. **125**: 29-48.

HETHERINGTON, T.E., and W.E. BEMIS. 1979. Morphological evidence of an electroreceptive function of the rostral organ of *Latimeria chalumnae*. Amer. Zool. **19**: 976.

HOLMGREN, N., and E. STENSIÖ. 1936. Kranium und Visceralskelett der Akranier, Cyclostomen und Fische. *In* Bolk, L. *et al.* [eds.] Handbuch der vergleichenden Anatomie der Wirbeltiere. Urban and Schwarzenberg, Berlin.

JARVIK, E. 1942. On the structure of the snout of crossopterygians and lower gnathostomes in general. Zool. Bidr. Upps. **21**: 235-675.

JARVIK, E. 1944a. On the dermal bones, sensory canal and pit-lines of the skull in *Eusthenopteron foordi* Whiteaves, with some remarks on *E. saeve-soederberghi* Jarvik. K. svenska VetenskAkad. Handl. **21**: 1-48.

JARVIK, E. 1944b. On the exoskeletal shoulder-girdle of teleostomian fishes, with special reference to *Eusthenopteron foordi* Whiteaves. K. svenska Vetensk-Akad. Handl. **21**: 1-32.

JARVIK, E. 1948. On the morphology and taxonomy of the Middle Devonian osteolepid fishes of Scotland. K. svenska VetenskAkad. Handl. **25**: 1-301.

JARVIK, E. 1954. On the visceral skeleton in *Eusthenopteron* with a discussion of the parasphenoid and palatoquadrate in fishes. K. svenska VetenskAkad. Handl. **5**: 1-104.

JARVIK, E. 1964. Specializations in early vertebrates. Annls. Soc. r. zool. Belg. **94**: 1-95.

JARVIK, E. 1965a. Die Raspelzunge der Cyclostomen und die pentadactyle Extremität der Tetrapoden als Beweise für monophyletische Herkunft. Zool. Anz. **175**: 101-143.

JARVIK, E. 1965b. On the origin of girdles and paired fins. Isreal J. Zool. **14**: 141-172.

JARVIK, E. 1972. Middle and Upper Devonian Porolepiformes from East Greenland with special reference to *Glyptolepis groenlandica* n. sp. Meddr Grønland **187**: 1-295.

JARVIK, E. 1980. Basic structure and evolution of vertebrates. Academic Press, London.

JESSEN, H. 1972. Schultergürtel und Pectoralflosse bei Actinopterygiern. Fossils Strata **1**: 1-101.

JOHNSON, C.E. 1913. The development of the prootic head somites and eye muscles in *Chelydra serpentina*. Amer. J. Anat. **14**: 119-185.

LAMB, A.B. 1902. The development of the eye muscles in *Acanthias*. Amer. J. Anat. **1**: 185-202.

MARINELLI, W., and A. STRENGER. 1959. Vergleichende Anatomie und Morphologie der Wirbeltiere, vol. 3. F. Deuticke, Wien.

MARINELLI, W., and A. STRENGER. 1973. Vergleichende Anatomie und Morphologie der Wirbeltiere, vol. 4. F. Deuticke, Wien.

MILLOT, J., and J. ANTHONY. 1956. L'Organe rostral de *Latimeria* (Crossoptérygien, Coelacanthidé). Annls. Sci. nat. (Zool.) **11**: 381-389.

MILLOT, J., and J. ANTHONY. 1958. Anatomie de *Latimeria chalumnae*, vol. 1. Cent. natn. Rech. Scient., Paris.

MILLOT, J., and J. ANTHONY. 1965. Anatomie de *Latimeria chalumnae*, vol. 2. Cent. natn. Rech. scient., Paris.

MILLOT, J., J. ANTHONY, and D. ROBINEAU. 1978. Anatomie de *Latimeria chalumnae*, vol. 3. Cent. natn. Rech. scient., Paris.

NEAL, H.V. 1918. Neuromeres and metameres. J. Morphol. **31**: 293-315.

NIELSEN, E. 1936. Some few preliminary remarks on Triassic fishes from East Greenland. Meddr Grønland **112**: 1-55.

NIELSEN, E. 1942. Studies on Triassic fishes from East Greenland, 1, *Glaucolepis* and *Boreosomus*. Meddr Grønland **138**: 1-403.

NIELSEN, E. 1949. Studies on Triassic fishes from East Greenland, 2, *Australosomus* and *Birgeria*. Meddr Grønland **146**: 1-309.

NORTHCUTT, R.G. 1980. Anatomical evidence of electroreception in the coelacanth (*Latimeria chalumnae*). Zbl. Vet. Med. C. Anat. Histol. Embryol. **9**: 289-295.

ØRVIG, T. 1973. Fossila fisktänder i svepelektronmikroskopet. Gamla frågeställningar i ny belysning, (Fossil fish teeth in the scanning electron microscope; old question in new light). Fauna Flora (Stockh.) **68**: 166-173.

ØRVIG, T. 1978a. Microstructure and growth of the dermal skeleton in fossil actinopterygian fishes: *Nephrotus* and *Colobodus*, with remarks on the dentition in other forms. Zool. Scripta 7: 297-326.

ØRVIG, T. 1978b. Microstructure and growth of the dermal skeleton in fossil

actinopterygian fishes: *Birgeria* and *Scanilepis*. Zool. Scripta : 33-56.
ØRVIG, T. 1978c. Microstructure and growth of the dermal skeleton in fossil actinopterygian fishes: *Boreosomus, Plegmolepis* and *Gyrolepis*. Zool. Scripta 7: 125-144.
PATTERSON, C. 1982. Morphology and interrelationships of primitive actinopterygian fishes. Amer. Zool. **22**: 241-259.
PEHRSON, T. 1947. Some new interpretations of the skull in *Polypterus*. Acta Zool. (Stockh.) **28**: 399-455.
PLATT, J.B. 1891. Further contribution to the morphology of the vertebrate head. Anat. Anz. **6**: 251-265.
POPLIN, C. 1974. Étude de quelques Paléoniscidés pennslyvaniens du Kansas. Cah. Paléont. Cent. natn. Rech. scient., Paris, pp. 1-151.
ROSEN, D.E., P.L. FOREY, B.G. GARDINER, and C. PATTERSON. 1981. Lungfishes, tetrapods, paleontology, and plesiomorphy. Bull. Amer. Mus. Nat. Hist. **167**: 159-276.
SCHMIDT-EHRENBERG, E.C. 1942. Die Embryogenese des Extremitätenskelettes der Säugetiere. Ein Beitrag zur Frage der Entwicklung der Tetrapodengliedmassen. Rev. Suisse Zool. **49**: 33-131.
SCHULTZE, H.-P. 1966. Morphologische und histologische Untersuchungen an Schuppen mesozoischer Actinopterygier (Übergang von Ganoid- zu Rundschuppen). N. Jb. Geol. Paläont. Abh. **126**: 232-314.
SEWERTZOFF, A.N. 1934. Evolution der Bauchflossen der Fische. Zool. Jb. (Anat.) **58**: 415-500.
STENSIÖ, E. 1932. Triassic fishes from East Greenland collected by the Danish expeditions in 1929-1931. Meddr Gronland **83**: 1-305.
STENSIÖ, E. 1937. On the Devonian coelacanthids of Germany with special reference to the dermal skeleton. K. svenska VetenskAkad. Handl. **16**: 4-56.
TRAQUAIR, R.H. 1870. On the cranial osteology of *Polypterus*. J. Anat. Physiol. (Lond.) **5**: 166-183.
WIEDERSHEIM, R. 1892. Das Gliedmassenskelet der Wirbeltiere. Gustav Fischer, Jena.

RECONSTRUCTING THE LIFE CYCLE AND THE FEEDING OF ANCESTRAL VERTEBRATES

Jon Mallatt

Department of Zoology
Washington State University
Pullman, Washington

One goal of this symposium is to examine the earliest evolution of the vertebrates. This problem can be approached from an ecological perspective, by considering possible habitats and feeding modes of ancestral Paleozoic fish. This chapter will expand and re-evaluate some ideas put forth recently (Mallatt, 1984b). It deals with the initial vertebrate adaptive radiation, which occurred between the Cambrian and the Devonian periods, from about 550 to 375 million years ago. Fossil documentation of this radiation is fragmentary, so extant animals and habitats must be used to help interpret their Paleozoic ancestors and analogues. Except for its latest phase, this earliest radiation of fishes was probably confined to shallow marine environments (Denison, 1956; Spjeldnaes, 1967; Ritchie and Gilbert-Tomlinson, 1977; Repetski, 1978; Darby, 1982). The fossil record, while incomplete, is unambiguous on this point: there are no demonstrably freshwater fossil vertebrates known until the late Silurian (Denison, 1956).

The fish groups of interest to this discussion (Fig. 1) include the ancestors of hagfish, lampreys, and various ostracoderm groups (extinct), and gnathostome fish. The earliest known vertebrates lived in the late Cambrian period, and ancestral vertebrates will be viewed in this chapter as a middle to late Cambrian group. The classification scheme of Figure 1 is adopted from Janvier and Blieck (1979) and Mallatt (1984a). It has gained support from detailed cladistic analyses (Janvier, 1981; Hardisty, 1982).

Some terms and concepts

A number of terms should be presented defining the feeding modes that could have been employed by early fish groups. Aquatic *suspension feeders* use specialized food-trapping surfaces to remove large quantities of suspended food particles from the ambient water. They tend to be non-selective feeders, with only limited abilities to reject non-nutritious particles or to select preferentially for the

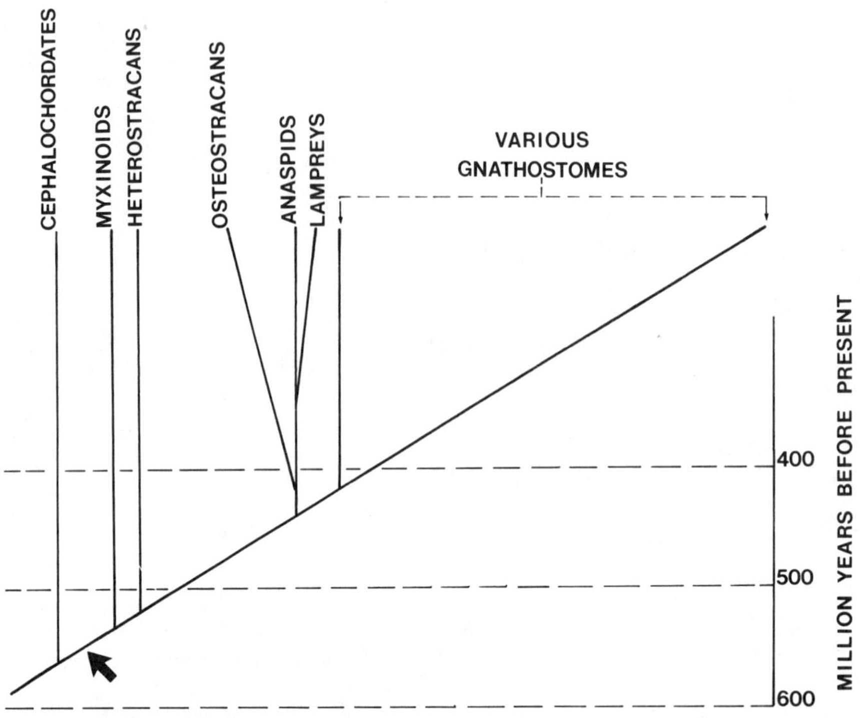

Fig. 1. Classification scheme followed in this chapter, with a time scale showing dates at which various groups may have arisen. The large arrow at lower left indicates the age and the phylogenetic position of the ancestral vertebrates considered in this paper. Two fossil jawless groups are omitted from this figure, Galeaspids and Thelodonts, although I follow Janvier's (1981) interpretation of the relationships of these forms (see his Fig. 16).

most nutritious particles in a suspension (Jørgensen, 1966). *Raptorial feeders* (Parsons, 1980), by contrast, take individual food particles and tend to be highly selective in the food items sought. The distinction between suspension and raptorial feeding blurs in animals whose mouths do not much exceed in diameter the largest available suspended food particles. For example, small zooplankton like copepods can ingest either single or multiple particles, and thus operate as either raptorial or suspension feeders (Jørgensen, 1966; but for new interpretation of copepod feeding, see Koehl and Strickler, 1981).

Alternatively, feeding types in aquatic animals can be classified according to the size of food items taken. *Micro*phagy involves the ingestion of the smallest food particles, such as bacteria, unicellular algae (phytoplankton), and fine detritus. *Macro*phagous feeders on the other hand, utilize macroscopic food items, the size of crustacean zooplankton and larger. The dividing line between microscopic and macroscopic food particles can be set at about 100 micrometers in diameter. It is a mistake to correlate suspension feeding rigidly with microphagy and raptorial feeding with macrophagy. Some suspension feeders are macrophagous: anchovies, paddlefish, and baleen whales feed on zooplankton, which can reach several centimeters in length in the case of krill ingested by whales (Harden Jones, 1980; Rosen and Hales, 1981). Likewise, some raptorial feeders are microphagous: the very youngest larvae of many bony fish seize individual phytoplankton particles, before they graduate to larger zooplankton prey as they grow (Harden Jones, 1980, p. 126).

Another feeding type to consider is *deposit feeding*. This involves the ingestion of sediment for the extraction of contained organic matter. ("Deposit feeders . . . consume a specific fraction or the whole of the surrounding sediment": Barnes, 1980.) The term 'detritus feeding' is often used as a synonym of 'deposit feeding', but this is not strictly correct. Detritus (fragments of plants or animal bodies) can occur suspended in the water column, as well as in the substrate.

Other aquatic animals can be classified as scavengers, herbivores, and omnivores (See Fauchald and Jumars, 1979, for examples among marine worms). Although such feeders need not actively pursue prey, they all resemble macrophagous raptorial feeders in taking macroscopic individual food items with some degree of selectivity.

Ancestral vertebrate feeding mode

Microphagous suspension feeding is employed by many nonvertebrate chordate groups (Barrington, 1965) and by larval lampreys, so ancestral vertebrates are often suggested to have utilized this feeding mode (Berrill, 1955; Young, 1962; Romer, 1966). I have studied the intricate pattern of ciliary tracts in the pharynx of lamprey larvae (Mallatt, 1981) and found this to correspond in detail to ciliary tracts in ascidian tunicates and amphioxus. These tracts are intimately related to suspension feeding, functioning in all three chordate groups to propel thick strands of food-trapping mucus. This evident homology between feeding structures in nonvertebrate and vertebrate chordates implies that ancestral fish were suspension feeders at some point in their life cycle. Unfortunately, as pointed out by Jollie (1982) and Northcutt and Gans (1983), the life cycle of protovertebrates probably was complex, because larval and adult stages characterize most tunicates, cephalochordates, hemichordates and extant fish. The question thus arises as to which stage of the protovertebrate life cycle employed suspension feeding. Jollie (1982) and Northcutt and Gans (1983) placed suspension feeding in the larval stage, and modelled the adult protovertebrates as predators, while I (Mallatt, 1984b) envisage the adults as suspension feeders. I view the larvae as raptorial feeders upon small zooplankton and phytoplankton particles. The differences between these two life cycle models are summarized in Figure 2.

The relative merits of these alternate models will be considered below. First, it should be noted that, independent of feeding modes proposed, the two schemes agree in picturing a pelago-benthic life cycle for ancestral fish (Fig. 2), with pelagic, dispersive larvae, and benthic adults. It seems reasonable to propose this,

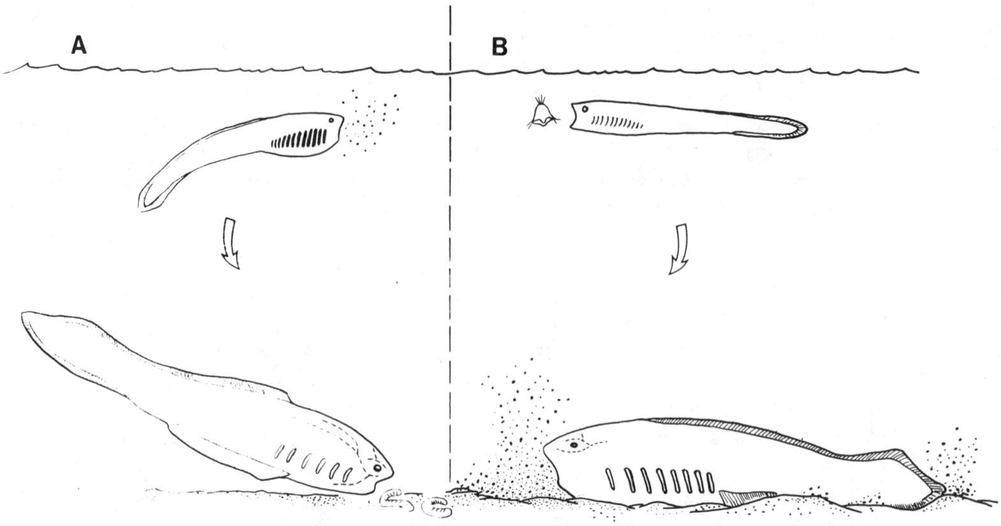

Fig. 2. Alternative pictures of the ancestral vertebrate life cycle. Model 'A' at left, proposed by Northcutt and Gans (1983), pictures the larvae as pelagic suspension feeders and the adults as benthic predators (also see Jollie, 1982). Model 'B' at right (Mallatt, 1984b) places suspension feeding in the ancestral adult, and proposes the larvae were planktonic raptorial feeders. Reconstructions of the external appearance of the protovertebrates are strictly my own, and they may differ in detail from the anatomical interpretations of Northcutt, Gans and Jollie. It is possible to propose that suspension feeding characterized both the larval and the adult stages of the ancestral vertebrate, but such a model is not illustrated here.

for such a life cycle occurs very frequently among extant marine metazoans, and it is probably primitive for the whole metazoan group (Jägersten, 1972).Cephalochordates (Gosselck and Kuehner, 1973), many urochordates (ascidians), and hemichordates (*e.g.*, *Balanoglossus*) have pelagic larvae and benthic adults. Neither lampreys nor hagfish show these stages, but their life cycles need not be considered primitive for vertebrates. Assuming a littoral marine ancestry for vertebrates, lamprey and hagfish ancestors subsequently appear to have invaded special habitats where pelagic larvae tend to be selected against. Pelagic larvae seldom occur among animals inhabiting streams, the home of sand-dwelling lamprey larvae, because unidirectional currents threaten to sweep plankton out to sea; likewise, larval stages tend to be abbreviated or eliminated among animals in the deep sea, the hagfish habitat, because the supply of food particles in the overlying water column is severely limited (Mann, 1980). Amphioxus has a pelago-benthic life cycle, which can be considered basically like that proposed for the protovertebrates. (However, neither I, nor Northcutt and Gans, considered the benthic protovertebrate adult to have been a burrowing form.)

Larval feeding

The larvae of ancestral vertebrates were modelled as suspension feeders by Northcutt and Gans (1983) and by Jollie (1982), while I have proposed they were raptorial feeders on phyto- and zooplankton (Mallatt, 1984b). It is difficult to choose between these two proposed feeding modes, because both are broadly represented among surviving chordates. Larvae of most extant fishes are raptorial planktivores (Harden Jones, 1980), but very many larval marine invertebrates are microphagous suspension feeders, including the larvae of deuterostomes related most closely to vertebrates (tornaria larvae of hemichordates, dipleurula larvae of echinoderms: Strathmann and Bonar, 1976). With present evidence, it is not possible to pinpoint when in the invertebrate-to-vertebrate transition the larvae may have switched from suspension to raptorial feeding. No known extant fish, with the single exception of lampreys, has a microphagous suspension feeding larva (Bone and Marshall, 1982, ch. 7). The reason for this is not known, however, so it is unwise to conclude that early Paleozoic fish likewise produced no suspension feeding larvae.

Perhaps the protovertebrate larva utilized both suspension and raptorial feeding. This seems to be the condition in larval amphioxus (*Branchiostoma*). Suspension feeding on microscopic particles has been directly documented in these larvae (Jørgensen, 1966; Gosselck and Kuehner, 1973; Olsson, 1983), but Webb (1969) found particles among the gut contents that reached the size of the mouth and included copepods. Gosselck and Kuehner (1973, p. 72) found no copepods, but did find copepod-sized detritus fragments in the gut, confirming that some macroscopic items can be ingested. These studies indicate that larval cephalochordates can take macroscopic food particles one at a time, and in this they resemble raptorial feeders. It is not known, however, how active or selective the larvae are in obtaining these food items. In larval amphioxus, due to the small size of the animal (under 1 cm long) and its mouth, the lines blur between raptorial and suspension feeding. Raptorial feeding in extant fish larvae could readily have descended from such a condition.

Adult feeding

I proposed (Mallatt, 1984a,b) that adult ancestral vertebrates were microphagous suspension feeders, with the switch to predation in the vertebrate lineage only coming later, in the Silurian, with the evolution of gnathostomes (see also Romer, 1966; Denison, 1956; Young 1962). This idea has been criticized on the grounds that a suspension feeding lineage could not have evolved the characteristic fish features of active existence, such as segmented trunk musculature and spinal cord, the brain, and the special sensory organs for distance reception (Jollie, 1982). This criticism seems to stem in part from equating suspension feeding with a highly sedentary to sessile existence. Suspension feeders need not be inactive, however, as shown by the many swimming zooplankton groups (Jørgensen, 1966). In theory, suspension feeders can experience selection for increased motility in those environments where the quality and concentration of suspended food varies markedly in time and space (Mallatt, 1984b). I proposed that early fish moved about the ocean bottom to find appropriately rich patches of suspended food. In theory, such an existence might lead to the evolution of sensory organs for detecting both food patches and predators. In actuality, however, it is not clear that receptors such as image-forming eyes have ever evolved *de novo* in any suspension feeding metazoans. The theory that ancestral adult vertebrates were suspension feeders cannot at present refute the assertion (Northcutt and Gans, 1983, p. 14) that "only aggressive and carnivorous members of the arthropods, cephalopods, and gastropods show an analogous evolution" to vertebrate special sense organs. Scallops (*Pecten*) are the most active suspension feeders among the bivalves (Barnes, 1980) and possess image-forming eyes that superficially resemble the lateral eyes of vertebrates (Gardiner, 1972, p. 639-640.). However, on the retina of the scallop eye where the image is focused, light does not excite the receptor cells, but inhibits them (Land, 1968; McReynolds and Gorman, 1970). Scallop eyes are primarily elaborate shadow detectors for sensing the approach of predators --- and thus, are very unlike fish eyes.

Northcutt and Gans (1983) and Jollie (1982) proposed that ancestral adult vertebrates were incipient predators (*i.e.* macrophagous raptorial feeders, by my terminology). While this view can explain the evolution of special sense organs in protovertebrates, it does not seem to fit what is known about fossil jawless fish. Under the classification scheme presented in Figure 1, which does not recognize the Agnatha as a monophyletic taxon, each of the jawless fish groups is as important an indicator of primitive vertebrate characters as is the entire gnathostome assemblage. The potential difficulty with viewing ancestral vertebrates as predacious is that no clearly predatory forms are known until the late Silurian strata, with the first known bony and cartilaginous jawed fish occuring over 100 million years after the earliest recorded appearance of vertebrates in the Cambrian. Among jawless fish groups, the earliest and presumably most primitive genera of osteostracans (*Tremataspis*) and heterostracans (*Arandaspis*, plus various cyathaspid genera) were heavily armored, lacked paired fins, and were not streamlined for swimming, as they were round in transverse section (Moy-Thomas and Miles, 1971; Ritchie and Gilbert-Tomlinson, 1977). It is difficult to view these fish as anything except benthic forms that remained mostly on the substrate and swam only in short spurts. These animals have been interpreted as relatively inactive predators that took only slow moving prey (Northcutt and Gans, 1983), but the implied long sedentary periods are more consistent with suspension feeding. It should be mentioned that *anaspid* ostracoderms were not heavily armored and were just as likely to have been predators as suspension feeders; Ritchie (1968) proposed that anaspids fed by scraping algae from rock surfaces.

To be sure, the fossil record for early vertebrates is incomplete, and it must be considered biased toward the preservation of the most heavily armored jawless groups. Even so, there can be no support for a theory of a carnivorous vertebrate ancestry in a record where the earliest known vertebrates show the least evidence of active existence. Based on the sizes of the orbits, the eyes of ostracoderms appear to have been quite small, at least in the less derived fossil groups. The orbits of heterostracans, thelodonts, and tremataspid ostreostracans average only about 2 mm in diameter in animals of 5 to 10 cm body length (see figures in Moy-Thomas and Miles, 1971).

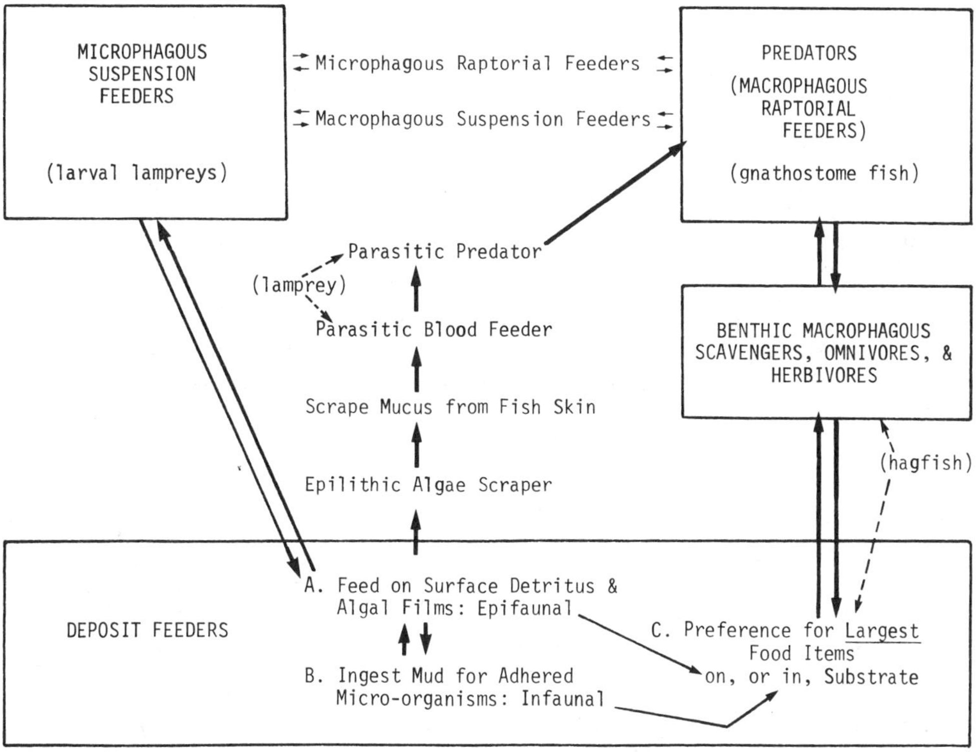

Fig. 3. Feeding types employed by aquatic metazoan animals, with the proposed interrelationships between them. It is proposed that ancestral vertebrates used one (or more) of the feeding modes given in the rectangles, and that all of these feeding niches were subsequently entered by various jawless and jawed fish during the early Paleozoic. Extant groups (larval lampreys, adult lampreys, hagfish, gnathostome fish) are assigned to their appropriate feeding types. All the feeding types are discussed in the text, except the sequence in the center of the diagram (epilithic algal scraper to parasitic predator), which models the derivation of the adult lamprey feeding type. This diagram is an expanded and corrected version of the scheme presented as Fig. 2 in Mallatt (1984b).

It might be suggested that a predacious ancestry for vertebrates is reflected in the predacious habits of hagfish, adult lampreys, and early gnathostomes. (Arguments that hagfish are predators as well as scavengers are presented by Shelton, 1978, and the markedly carnivorous nature of most Devonian gnathostomes is noted by Mallatt, 1984b.) Prey uptake, however, is achieved by dissimilar mechanisms in each of these three fish groups. Gnathostome fish rely on horizontally-oriented jaws to bite prey, and on strong suction to draw prey items into the pharynx. This suction results from a rapid pharyngeal expansion produced by hypobranchial muscles pulling on a jointed branchial skeleton (Moss, 1977; Lauder, 1982). Adult lampreys produce suction for attaching to prey fish and for then sucking in blood and flesh, but the pharynx is not involved: the negative pressure results from the actions of an oral hood and a specialized tongue (Randall, 1972). Hagfish apparently produce no suction for feeding and rely on the biting and tugging performance of horny, vertically oriented 'jaws' (Dawson, 1963). Observations of feeding Pacific hagfish (*Eptatretus stouti*) in our laboratory suggest that the hagfish feeding apparatus is extremely efficient at reeling in long worms, as the jaws alternately flick in and out of the oral cavity. There seems to be no shared structural basis for prey capture among hagfish, parasitic lampreys, and jawed fishes, and this suggests an independent derivation of carnivory in each. It might be hypothesized that an inability of the pharynges of jawless vertebrates to produce strong suction limited their evolutionary potential as carnivores, because the hypobranchial apparatus is considered an important factor in the success of gnathostome fish as predators (Lauder, 1982).

In conclusion, it is difficult at present to decide whether adult protovertebrates were microphagous suspension feeding animals or incipient predators. Both views seem to have weaknesses, the suspension feeding model explaining the evolution of special vertebrate sense organs, and the predator model explaining the fossil record for early fish. This is a paradoxical situation that current knowledge cannot resolve. New methods should be devised for testing these two models against each other, and the possibility of still other feeding modes might be considered for ancestral fish (omnivorous benthic scavengers?). No matter what course future investigation takes, it will require a clear outline of the range of feeding types found among aquatic metazoan animals. Therefore, Figure 3 summarizes the range of feeding niches that could have been available to early Paleozoic fish.

Literature cited

BARNES, R.D. 1980. Invertebrate zoology, 4th ed. Saunders, Philadelphia.

BARRINGTON, E.J.W. 1965. The biology of the Hemichordata and Protochordata. W.H. Freeman and Co., San Francisco.

BERRILL, N.J. 1955. The origin of vertebrates. Clarendon Press, Oxford.

BONE, Q., and N.B. MARSHALL. 1982. Biology of fishes (Tertiary level biology). Blackie, London.

DARBY, D.G. 1982. The early vertebrate *Astraspis*, habitat based on a lithographic association. J. Paleontol. **56**: 87-1196.

DAWSON, J.A. 1963. The oral cavity, the 'jaws', and the horny teeth of *Myxine glutinosa*. pp. 231-255 *In* Brodal, A., and R. Fänge [eds.] The biology of *Myxine*. Universitetsforlaget, Oslo.

DENISON, R.H. 1956. A review of the habitat of the earliest vertebrates. Fieldiana:Geology **11**: 359-457.

FAUCHALD, K., and P.A. JUMARS. 1979. The diet of worms: a study of polychaete feeding guilds. Oceanogr. mar. Biol. Ann. Rev. **17**: 193-284.

GARDINER, M.S. 1972. The biology of invertebrates. McGraw-Hill, New York.

GOSSELCK, K., and E. KUEHNER. 1973. Investigations on the biology of

Branchiostoma senegalense larvae off the northwest African coast. Mar. Biol. **22**: 67-73.

HARDEN JONES, F.R. 1980. The nekton: production and migration patterns. pp. 119-142 *In* Barnes, R.S.K., and K. Mann [eds.] Fundamentals of aquatic ecosystems. Blackwell, Boston.

HARDISTY, M.W. 1982. Lampreys and hagfishes: analysis of cyclostome relationships. pp. 166-260 *In* Hardisty, M.W., and I.C. Potter [eds.] The biology of lampreys. Academic Press, London.

JÄGERSTEN, G. 1972. Evolution of the metazoan life cycle. Academic Press, New York.

JANVIER, P. 1981. The phylogeny of craniata, with particular reference to the significance of fossil "agnathans". J. Vert. Paleontol. **1**: 121-159.

JANVIER, P. and A. BLIECK. 1979. New data on the internal anatomy of the Heterostraci (Agnatha), with general remarks on the phylogeny of the craniata. Zoologica Scripta **8**: 287-296.

JOLLIE, M. 1982. What are the "Calcichordata"? and the larger question of the origin of the chordates. Zool. J. Linn. Soc. **75**: 167-188.

JØRGENSEN, C.B. 1966. Biology of suspension feeding. (International Series of monographs in pure and applied biology/zoology division, 27) Pergamon Press, Oxford.

KOEHL, M.A.R., and J.R. STRICKLER. 1981. Copepod feeding currents: food capture at low Reynolds number. Limnol. Oceanogr. **26**: 1062-1073.

LAND, M.F. 1968. Functional aspects of the optical and retinal organization of the mollusc eye. Symp. Zool. Soc. (Lond.) **23**: 75-96.

LAUDER, G.V. 1982. Patterns of evolution in the feeding mechanism of actinopterygian fishes. Amer. Zool. **22**: 275-285.

MALLATT, J. 1981. The feeding mechanism of the larval lamprey *Petromyzon marinus*. J. Zool. (Lond.) **194**: 103-142.

MALLATT, J. 1984a. Early vertebrate evolution: pharyngeal structure and the origin of gnathostomes. J. Zool. (Lond.) **204**: 169-183.

MALLATT, J. 1984b. Feeding ecology of the earliest vertebrates. Zool. J. Linn. Soc. **82**: 261-272.

MANN, K. 1980. Benthic secondary production. pp. 103-118 *In* Barnes, R.S.K., and K. Mann [eds.] Fundamentals of aquatic ecosystems. Blackwell, Boston.

McREYNOLDS, J.S., and A.L.F. GORMAN. 1970. Photoreceptor potentials of opposite polarity in the eye of the scallop, *Pecten irradians*. J. gen. Physiol. **56**: 376-391.

MOSS, S.A. 1977. Feeding mechanisms in sharks. Amer. Zool. **17**: 355-364.

MOY-THOMAS, J.A., and R.S. MILES. 1971. Palaeozoic fishes, 2nd ed. Saunders, Philadelphia.

NORTHCUTT, R.G., and C. GANS. 1983. The genesis of neural crest and epidermal placodes: a reinterpretation of vertebrate origins. Quart. Rev. Biol. **58**: 1-28.

OLSSON, R. 1983. Club-shaped gland and endostyle in larval *Branchiostoma lanceolatum* (Cephalochordata). Zoomorphology **103**: 1-13.

PARSONS, T.R. 1980. Zooplankton production. pp. 46-66 *In* Barnes, R.S.K., and K. Mann [eds.] Fundamentals of aquatic ecosystems. Blackwell, Boston.

RANDALL, D.J. 1972. Respiration. pp. 287-306 *In* Hardisty, M.W., and I.C. Potter [eds.] The biology of lampreys, vol. 2. Academic Press, London.

REPETSKI, J.E. 1978. A fish from the upper Cambrian of North America.

Science **200**: 529-531.

RITCHIE, A. 1968. New evidence on *Jamoytius kerwoodi* White, an important ostracoderm from the Silurian of Lanarkshire, Scotland. Paleontolology **11**: 21-39.

RITCHIE, A., and J. GILBERT-TOMLINSON. 1977. First Ordovician vertebrates from the Southern hemisphere. Alcheringa **1**: 351-368.

ROMER, A.S. 1966. Vertebrate paleontology, 3rd ed. University of Chicago Press, Chicago.

ROSEN, R.A., and D.C. HALES. 1981. Feeding of paddlefish, *Polyodon spathula.* Copeia **1981**: 441-455.

SHELTON, R.G.J. 1978. On the feeding of the hagfish *Myxine glutinosa* in the North Sea. J. mar. biol. Assoc. U.K. **58**: 81-86.

SPJELDNAES, N. 1967. The paleoecology of the Ordovician vertebrates of the Harding Formation (Colorado, U.S.A.). Colloques int. natn. Centre Rech. Scient. **163**: 11-20.

STRATHMANN, R., and D. BONAR. 1976. Ciliary feeding of tornaria larvae of *Ptychodera flava* (Hemichordata: Enteropneusta). Mar. Biol. **34**: 317-324.

WEBB, J.E. 1969. On the feeding and behavior of the larva of *Branchiostoma lanceolatum.* Mar. Biol. **3**: 58-72.

YOUNG, J.E.Z. 1962. The life of vertebrates. Oxford University Press, Oxford.

HABITAT, PHYLOGENY AND THE EVOLUTION OF OSMOREGULATORY STRATEGIES IN PRIMITIVE FISHES

Robert W. Griffith

Department of Biology
Southeastern Massachusetts University
North Dartmouth, MA 02747

Introduction

The application of physiological features to phylogenetics has been regarded with enthusiasm by some authors (e.g. Løvtrup, 1977; Lagios, 1979a) while being seriously questioned by others (Simpson, 1960; Scheer, 1964; Hoar, 1983). Without a doubt, many physiological features show such a degree of convergence that they are useless for phylogenetic studies at higher taxonomic levels, whereas other physiological features are sufficiently stable to provide information at least as useful as morphological data. It is difficult to predict *a priori* whether a particular character will show a high degree of convergence, and this problem is likely to be especially serious for physiological features where the perspective provided by prior use in systematics is generally absent. It is worth noting Nelson's (1970) contention that the application of characters of a physiological nature to systematics is best accomplished by physiologists who most fully understand the nature of their data and the source of its variability, rather than by the "professional" systematist whose bias towards a particular "system" might prevent the physiological data from acting as a truly independent test of the conventional phylogenetic scheme.

One category of physiological characters that has seen widespread application to fish phylogenetics is osmotic and ionic regulatory mechanisms. The stability of osmoregulatory features is suggested by the restriction of a number of major taxa of fishes to freshwater or to seawater, as evidenced by the zoogeographical classifications of Myers (1938, 1949), Mayr (1944) and Darlington (1957). Further evidence for the stability of osmoregulatory features might include the contention of the eminent comparative renal physiologist, Homer Smith, based upon the apparently universal possession of osmotic regulation by urea retention in elasmobranch and holocephalan fishes. Smith considered that, because of the apparent restriction of the mechanism to this group, urea retention is more diagnostic systematically than morphological features and that the taxon possessing this feature should be renamed appropriately (Smith, 1959). Subsequent demonstrations that the urea retention habitus is neither ubiquitous in chondrichthians (Thorson *et al.*, 1967) nor unique to them (Pickford and Grant, 1967; Gordon *et al.*, 1961) have not prevented the application of this character to taxonomic studies (*cf.* Løvtrup, 1977; Thorson and Watson, 1975).

Of course, osmoregulatory mechanisms cannot be thought to be solely a product of a fish's phylogenetic history. These mechanisms are specific solutions to the problems that are imposed by environmental salinity. Whenever a fish moves from freshwater to a marine environment or *vice versa*, it faces a reversal of osmotic and ionic gradients and, in response, it undergoes fundamental changes in its osmoregulatory physiology. These physiological changes might be transient; they might occur in conjunction with development as they do in many diadromous fishes, or, if the exposure to a particular range of salinities persists over many generations, the species might evolve towards or away from euryhalinity. Although the close relationship of osmoregulatory mechanisms to environmental salinity might appear to limit the usefulness of such characters in phylogenetic studies, we might suggest that a thoughtful and detailed analysis of such characters is likely to provide a unique insight into the environmental conditions under which the various groups of fish evolved. We propose to survey here the array of osmoregulatory strategies that occur in primitive fishes and to attempt to trace the interplay of phylogeny and environmental history that was responsible for the evolution of these patterns.

An overview of osmoregulatory strategies and their occurrence in primitive fishes

The osmotic, ionic and organic composition of the blood has been investigated for a large number of fish species representing all major extant taxa and most major environmental situations (see reviews by Smith, 1959; Holmes and Donaldson, 1969; Prosser, 1973; Pang *et al.*, 1977; Griffith and Pang, 1979; and Griffith, 1981). In general, four patterns can be discerned, one in freshwater and three in seawater. The physiological mechanisms responsible for the maintenance of these osmoregulatory patterns are described in numerous reviews including those of Smith (1959), Potts and Parry (1963), Conte (1969), Hickman and Trump (1969), Maetz (1974), Pang *et al.* (1977), Griffith and Pang (1979) and the most recent volume of *Fish Physiology* (Hoar and Randall, 1984).

With but a handful of exceptions, fishes living in freshwater possess hyperosmotic body fluids (in the range of 200-400 mOsm) with inorganic ions accounting for most of the osmolarity. Typically, hyperosmotic regulation in fishes involves branchial uptake of electrolytes and renal elimination of excess fluid. The hyperosmotic strategy is characteristic of freshwater lampreys, polypterids, lungfishes, chondrosteans, holosteans, teleosts and one family of freshwater elasmobranchs, the Potamotrygonidae. Euryhaline elasmobranchs in freshwater differ a bit by possessing moderately high urea (around 100 mM) and high urea may also occur in some species of lungfishes during prolonged estivation.

In the sea, where high ion content results in an environmental osmolarity of around 1000 mOsm, three different osmoregulatory strategies occur in fishes. Marine teleosts and, from available evidence, lampreys and chondrosteans in high salinities have blood that is hypo-osmotic to their environment (usually blood values are from 350-500 mOsm) with most of the osmolarity being due to Na^+ and Cl^-. This hypo-osmotic regulation is accomplished by drinking seawater to maintain fluid balance and secreting salts branchially to offset passive epithelial and active gut ion uptake. Marine elasmobranchs, holocephalans and the coelacanth, *Latimeria chalumnae*, maintain blood osmolarity close to that of seawater. Electrolyte levels account for only about half of the total osmolarity, with the remainder being due to urea (around 400 mM) and trimethylamine oxide (around 100 mM usually). *Latimeria* differs somewhat from chondrichthians in being slightly hypo-osmotic to seawater and having lower ion levels, whereas the holocephalans differ from elasmobranchs proper in possessing higher electrolyte levels. In the ureo-osmotic fishes high blood urea is maintained by a combination of low epithelial permeability, renal conservation and hepatic synthesis *via* the ornithine-urea cycle. Excess salts appear to be excreted *via* a "rectal" gland or, in some species, through branchial mechanisms. The third marine strategy is found in the myxinoid agnathans and is characterized by blood osmolarity, Na^+ and Cl^- concentrations that differ little from those of the seawater environment. This ionosmotic strategy is also typical of most strictly marine invertebrates. Although its use in the regulation of water and NaCl balance is moot, the hagfishes possess a fairly well developed glomerular kidney which appears to function in the regulation of divalent ions and the removal of wastes.

Euryhaline fishes that can live in freshwater, estuarine and marine environments should not be thought to fall into a special fifth category of osmoregulatory strategies. All such fishes display hyperosmotic regulation while in freshwater and either hypo-osmotic or ureo-osmotic regulation while in the sea. The variety of control mechanisms that are involved in the switchover from one strategy to another represents a potentially rich source of information of phylogenetic and evolutionary importance that has been insufficiently pursued from these viewpoints.

Hyperosmotic regulation: the obligatory strategy of freshwater animals

The most notable aspect of osmoregulation in freshwater fishes is that the basic strategy of hyperosmotic regulation, with the branchial uptake of ions and renal excretion of water, is essentially the same regardless of phylogenetic affinity. This strategy is also found in freshwater amphibia and in freshwater invertebrates, although the sites for ion uptake and fluid elimination obviously differ from those of fishes. It should not be surprising that freshwater animals are uniform in maintaining higher blood osmolarity and ion levels than their very dilute environment. Many enzymes are dependent upon ions for their activity, and excitable cells such as neurons and muscles rely upon ionic gradients between the intra- and extracellular fluids for their operation.

The biochemical and physiological necessity to maintain high blood ion levels results in an osmotic gradient that causes the passive influx of water. This influx makes opposing mechanisms for water excretion necessary. All freshwater fishes, except a handful of aglomerular species, accomplish water excretion by using a high volume ultrafiltration device, the glomerular kidney. High blood ion levels also entail passive losses of electrolytes across the epithelia and *via* renal filtration which must be offset by active, energy-requiring ion uptake involving a variety of ion exchange pumps, and by the active reabsorption of ions in the kidney tubules. It is worth noting that the energy required for water and electrolyte balance will be lessened if the ionic gradient between the animal and freshwater is reduced and, therefore, there is a strong selective pressure for freshwater animals to have the lowest blood ion levels consonant with suitable enzyme and excitable cell activity.

Freshwater animals differ considerably in the osmotic and ionic concentrations of their extracellular fluids, with low values (<100 mM) occurring in rotifers, coelenterates, sponges and lamellibranchs, and high values being found in arthropods and fishes (Potts and Parry, 1963; Prosser, 1973). Two considerations likely account for much of this variability. Animals that are inactive and have low neuromuscular function can probably tolerate lower ion levels than active animals. Secondly, animals that have existed in freshwater for long periods of time are likely to have evolved lower ion levels than more recent migrants or euryhaline species.

Hypo-osmotic and ureo-osmotic regulation: two alternative marine strategies for fishes with a freshwater ancestry

The only reasonable explanation for the possession of blood ion levels much lower than those of seawater in both hypo-osmotic and ureo-osmotic regulators is that the ancestors of animals with these strategies lived in freshwater, had hyperosmotic regulation, and evolved an intolerance to internal electrolyte levels as high as those of seawater. This intolerance was then retained when the fishes adapted to a marine environment. The notion that low blood electrolytes might be necessary for an active existence is invalidated by the ionosmotic condition of highly active cephalopods and arthropods. The idea that hypo-osmotic regulation might evolve as a mechanism to achieve neutral buoyancy (see for example Blaxter *et al.*, 1971) is unlikely to apply to the development of this feature in fishes, although it could be a factor selecting for the retention of hypo-osmotic regulation in midwater teleosts (Griffith, 1981).

Given the likelihood that ureo-osmotic and hypo-osmotic regulation represent two alternative strategies for animals derived from hyperosmotic regulators for living in the marine environment, it is natural to ask why one or the other was adopted by a particular taxon. Although such considerations are by nature highly speculative, in earlier publications I have pointed out a variety of predisposing features that would influence whether one or the other strategy would be likely to evolve (Griffith and Pang, 1979; Griffith, 1981). Characteristics favoring the development of the hypo-osmotic strategy in fishes include: continued euryhalinity and association with a dilute environment, small size, active metabolism, and reproduction *via* oviparity with a 'non-cleidoic' egg. A constant marine environment, relatively large adult size, sluggish metabolism, and reproduction *via* viviparity, ovoviviparity or presence of a 'cleidoic' egg (with, of course, internal fertilization) would be characteristics conducive to the evolution of ureo-osmotic regulation.

It is logical to consider that hypo-osmotic regulation is energetically beneficial to euryhaline species since the osmotic gradient is much lower when the animals are in freshwater than is the case with ureo-osmotic regulators, and less energy needs to be spent for water balance and solute retention. Of course, the endocrine and neural mechanisms necessary to control water balance might need to be more elaborate for hypo-osmotic regulators than for ureo-osmotic regulators that remain in positive water balance regardless of environmental salinity. The correlations of large size, relatively low metabolism, and internal fertilization with ureo-osmotic regulation in fishes have a common physiological basis. In ureo-osmotic fishes such as elasmobranchs most urea is lost across the respiratory epithelia (Smith, 1959), but it is manufactured in the liver. Consequently, animals with a large surface area relative to their volume (which would include small animals, embryos, and those with a high metabolic rate) will find it energetically impractical to synthesize urea rapidly enough to replace that which is lost.

Several other factors that could play major roles in the choice between ureo-osmotic and hypo-osmotic regulation are tolerance to elevated urea levels and the presence or absence of a complete ornithine-urea cycle. Urea tolerance does not appear to be a very serious impediment to the evolution of ureo-osmotic regulation (Griffith *et al.*, 1979). One aspect of urea tolerance may relate to the physiological regulation of other solutes such as TMAO (Yancey and Somero, 1980). Activity levels of enzymes of the ornithine-urea cycle may be below detectable limits in many teleosts and agnathans (Brown and Cohen, 1960; Read, 1968, 1975) yet they can be substantial, or even quite high, in others (Read, 1971; Huggins, *et al.*, 1969). Urea levels and activities of ornithine-urea cycle enzymes are much higher in the embryos of teleosts than in adults, particularly in the live-bearing *Poecilia reticulata* (Depeche *et al.*, 1979). This finding may explain the anomalously high urea cycle activity in some teleosts, and may suggest the rather intriguing possibility that ureo-osmotic regulation evolved *via* paedogenesis.

As well as considering why some groups evolved hypo-osmotic, and others evolved ureo-osmotic regulation, we may wonder whether the possession of ureo-osmotic regulation in chondrichthians and *Latimeria* represents convergence, persistence of a primitive feature, or unique specialization. Likewise, we may question whether hypo-osmotic regulation arose independently in the lampreys and in the diverse groups of ray-finned fishes possessing this feature. We have earlier (Griffith and Pang, 1979; Griffith, 1980) expressed our opinion that ureo-osmotic regulation arose independently in *Latimeria* and the chondrichthians, although an opposite conclusion has been reached by others (Lagios, 1979a, 1979b). The bases for our assessment were: (1) the apparent use of different mechanisms for urea retention in the kidneys of the two groups, renal urea reabsorption [involving a complex loop-of-Henle-like countercurrent exchange (Lacy *et al.*, 1985)] in chondrichthians, and low urine output because of a slightly hypo-osmotic state in *Latimeria*; (2) the accomplishment of internal fertilization, a necessary concomitant of ureo-osmotic regulation, by strikingly different mechanisms in the chondrichthians (*via* pelvic claspers) and *Latimeria* (*via* erectile cloacal caruncles); and (3) the obviously independent occurrence of ureo-osmotic regulation in the euryhaline amphibian, *Rana cancrivora*. We cannot totally exclude the possibility that ureo-osmotic regulation is homologous in *Latimeria* and chondrichthians. Nevertheless, the arguments listed above, together with the considerations that the capability of urea synthesis is virtually ubiquitous in jawed vertebrates and that very high urea levels occur with dehydration in lungfishes, amphibia and reptiles makes the idea that ureo- osmotic regulation is an apotypic character of much systematic usefulness a highly dubious one.

Relatively little consideration has been given to the question of whether hypo-osmotic regulation has arisen once or many times in fishes. Little convincing data exist for either hypothesis, and one suspects that most people implicitly accept the idea that hypo-osmotic regulation has arisen independently in the lampreys, and that it has arisen a number of times within rayfins, simply because the lampreys are so "distinctive" and because the teleosts are so "diverse". It is at least worth noting the possibility that euryhalinity, with a switchover from hyperosmotic to hypo-osmotic regulation, is a very ancient phenomenon in vertebrates, that may have been lost in certain lines that became stenohaline freshwater or stenohaline marine, but which is essentially homologous in many distantly related euryhaline fishes.

The ionosmotic strategy of hagfishes: plesiotypic or degenerate? (and its relevance to the environmental habitat of the earliest vertebrates)

The ionosmotic strategy of the hagfishes, with major blood electrolytes differing little from those of seawater and with little capability of regulation (Munz and McFarland, 1964) represents a striking contrast to the osmoregulatory patterns of all other vertebrates where ion levels are much lower and well regulated. On the other hand, ionosmotic "regulation" is nearly universal in marine invertebrates. Since it is generally accepted that the hagfishes are the most primitive of living vertebrates, it is a natural and parsimonious conclusion that they have simply retained the plesiotypic condition of the chordate ancestor of the vertebrates. A less parsimonious alternative is that the ionosmotic condition of the hagfishes is secondarily derived from the freshwater hyperosmotic strategy or from one of the marine regulatory strategies, ureo-osmotic or hypo-osmotic regulation.

It is obvious that the question of the origin of the hagfish strategy is, in essence, tied to the question of the habitat of the earliest vertebrates. If the hagfish ionosmotic habitus evolved unchanged from the ancestral vertebrate, then the habitat of the earliest vertebrate was doubtless marine. If it is secondarily derived, then it evolved from a situation characterized by low ion levels that developed in freshwater. It must be pointed out that in terms of osmoregulatory strategies, "freshwater" need not necessarily mean that the fishes had a permanent freshwater habitat. An estuarine environment with exposure to freshwater, or a diadromous life history would probably be sufficient to select for low blood electrolytes, and regulation of these ions at relatively constant levels would also be favored by selection. Since the habitat of the earliest vertebrates is a question that has engendered considerable discussion over the past few decades, we might consider the major lines of evidence and arguments that have been presented thus far, and see whether a convincing case can be made one way or the other.

Although it is hardly a novel hypothesis, the strongest recent advocation of a freshwater origin for the vertebrates was based upon the physiological work of Homer Smith and the paleontological reviews of A.S. Romer. In a series of papers, Smith (Smith, 1930, 1932, 1959) set forth the argument that the glomerular kidney of vertebrates is perfectly designed to produce a large volume of urine, necessary in a freshwater environment, but it is of marginal usefulness in the sea where water balance is negative (hypo-osmotic regulators) or neutral (ureo-osmotic or ionosmotic regulators). The aglomerular status of various marine teleosts buttressed

Smith's argument. A.S. Romer's review of the pertinent paleontological information led him to conclude that the earliest vertebrate finds were from freshwater deposits (Romer, 1966; Romer and Grove, 1935).

Rebuttals of the freshwater hypothesis also used both paleontological and physiological arguments. Dennison (1956) and Halstead (1973) presented seemingly unequivocal evidence that the earliest known marine vertebrate fossils, Ordovician heterostracans, were of strictly marine habitat, and that freshwater vertebrates did not occur in the fossil record until much later. The recent finding of Cambrian heterostracans, also in marine deposits (Repetski, 1978), presents no contradiction. In a very compelling paper, J.D. Robertson (1957) demonstrated that the most primitive living vertebrate, *Myxine*, has an osmoregulatory pattern consistent with a strictly marine ancestry and, further, he noted that ultrafiltration devices similar in function to the glomerular kidney of vertebrates occur in a variety of strictly marine invertebrates. Robertson suggested that ultrafiltration kidneys play a role in divalent ion regulation and in the the removal of wastes, and he suggested that the glomerular kidney was preadapted for, rather than a consequence of, life in freshwater. Munz and McFarland (1964) concluded from their studies on renal function in hagfishes that Robertson's arguments were valid, although McInerney (1974) disagreed, based on his findings, and held that the data were inconclusive regarding the freshwater or marine origin of vertebrates.

Recent years have seen the balance of opinion swing towards the side advocating a marine origin of the vertebrates and for the myxinoid osmoregulatory pattern. Nevertheless, several serious objections can be raised to the arguments that have thus far been proposed in favor of a marine origin. First, the principle of parsimony as an argument for the hagfish pattern being plesiotypic cannot be regarded as carrying much weight when applied to a group as ancient as the hagfishes and when applied to a pattern of osmoregulation. We have seen that the other three osmoregulatory patterns likely have been independently acquired a number of times. Certainly the ionosmotic strategy is energetically the most favorable strategy in the marine habitat and, given sufficient time, a tolerance to high ion levels would likely evolve. Marine fishes of ancient lineages (holocephalans and deep sea eels, for instance) seem to have much higher ion levels than more recently evolved teleosts (Robertson, 1976; Griffith, 1981). Second, Smith's argument that the glomerular kidney is best designed to excrete large volumes of excess water is not invalidated by the fact that some marine invertebrates possess ultrafiltration devices. Such devices are not found in invertebrate chordates, and I believe that the development of such an elegantly designed water excretion device is more explicable as an adaptation evolved in response to life in a dilute environment, than as a preadaptation for it. Finally, the paleontological data must be regarded as fragmentary bits of information that are unlikely to provide a meaningful answer to the freshwater *vs.* marine origin question since the fossil record only preserves certain types of habitats and certain stages of a fish's life history. The earliest heterostracans are known only from adult specimens and we have absolutely no knowledge of the biology of early developmental stages (Halstead, 1973). The fact that the earliest known vertebrates were Silurian in Romer's day, and Cambrian now, underlines how truly fragmentary is our knowledge of the earliest fossil vertebrates.

Perhaps one approach that might prove helpful in addressing what seems to be an impenetrable problem is to follow Nelson's (1970) suggestion to construct an ancestral 'physiotype' that is consistent with the physiological status of living vertebrates and logical in terms of life in early paleozoic environments. The construction of such a physiotype should involve not only the osmoregulatory pattern but also the general way of life of the 'protovertebrate' and the reasons for the evolution of bone. I believe that these considerations are intimately intertwined with osmoregulation in the early vertebrates.

A suggested physiotype for the protovertebrate

A physiotype of the protovertebrate may very easily be constructed by a simple set of premises; that the animal lived in freshwater, that it lacked bone, and that it had a natural history very similar to that of the ammocoete larva of living lampreys. Some explanation of its derivation and subsequent evolution is necessary.

The origin of this protovertebrate would clearly have been from a marine cephalochordate-like form that invaded estuaries during the Cambrian, evolved a glomerular kidney in response to the water influx inherent in dilute media, and eventually adapted to a fully freshwater habitat, where it lived by filter feeding on microalgae. The blood electrolyte levels would be low, as in all freshwater animals, and active ion pumps for the accumulation of ions would have developed. The breeding location of the animal would also shift to freshwater, favored by the absence of predators and competitors for the developing larvae.

After successful adaptation to freshwater, the adult of derivatives of the protovertebrate reinvaded the estuaries and the seas to exploit the food resources available to larger animals. In effect, they became anadromous fish. We suggest that it might not have been necessary for all stages of the protovertebrate to have been exclusively freshwater, and that tolerance of seawater could have been retained. Anadromy would likely permit the production of more or larger gametes, but increased gamete production would require the provision of more inorganic minerals, particularly calcium and phosphate which are vital to gonadal maturation (Love, 1970). Although the tissues and body fluids of animals contain quantities of these materials, the elaboration of bone as a storage site would provide a much larger reservoir of calcium and phosphate that would be of selective advantage.

Once bony anadromous vertebrates had evolved, a variety of avenues for specialization led to the diversity of early vertebrates. With the omission of the freshwater phase and prolonged selection under marine conditions for high electrolyte levels, the hagfish with its ionosmotic condition is readily derived. If the freshwater phase were retained, and the marine phase became specialized for parasitism on other fishes, the *Petromyzon* habitus would have evolved. It is possible to derive the various gnathostome life histories from our protovertebrate. No imagination is necessary to derive gnathostome osmoregulatory strategies since hyperosmotic, hypo-osmotic and ureo-osmotic regulation are not only derivable from a freshwater ancestor, but require one.

Our hypothesis of a freshwater origin of vertebrates, with the development of bone occurring in the marine adult phase of an anadromous species, provides satisfactory explanations for two thorny problems that have confronted students of the earliest vertebrates. Halstead (1973) pointed out the patchy and infrequent nature of early vertebrate fossil deposits that is problematical in light of the high fossilization potential of bone. The problem only exists if one assumes the vertebrates were successful and widely distributed marine animals at this time; if they were anadromous with a transient and scarce marine phase the distribution pattern is exactly what one would expect. The function that required the origin of the bone has been an issue of contention for many decades (Halstead, 1969). I believe that our physiotype, involving a specific and obviously important physiological role for bone (*i.e.* the provision of calcium and phosphate for gonadal development in freshwater) accounts for the origin of bone far better than prior explanations which tended either to be far-fetched or vague concerning the real need for bone.

Further evidence for a freshwater origin of vertebrates

Two recent physiological studies provide highly persuasive evidence for the idea that the vertebrates had their origin in freshwater. In the Nobel symposium, Moss (1968) pointed out that current theoretical models held that the deposition of calcium phosphate in bone cannot occur in a medium of high ionic strength. Moss carried this idea to its natural conclusion, suggesting that the early vertebrates possessing bone had dilute body fluids. As we have seen, a pattern of low blood ion levels is explicable only in a freshwater animal or one derived from freshwater ancestors. Experimental studies by Nancollas and Tomazik (1974) clearly demonstrate that high (yet within the 'physiological' range) levels of 'neutral' salts such as NaCl inhibit calcium phosphate deposition, making bone formation much more difficult. The paleontologists have shown that bone first was found in animals that lived in the marine environment, but they were animals that came from freshwater.

Recently Evans (1984) demonstrated the presence of ion uptake mechanisms involving Cl^-/HCO_3^- and Na^+/H^+ exchange pumps in the hagfish, *Myxine*. Such pumps do not occur in strictly marine invertebrates (Kirschner, 1983) but are found in freshwater animals, where they are necessary for ion balance, and in marine elasmobranchs and teleosts. Because of the presence of these branchial ion uptake mechanisms in the (supposedly) primitively marine hagfish, Evans recanted his own logical assumption that such pumps are evidence of a freshwater ancestry, and concluded that they must be preadaptations for freshwater, perhaps useful somehow in acid-base balance. Evans should not have believed the conventional marine hypothesis more than his own data, which provide direct evidence for the hypothesis that the hagfish ionosmotic pattern is secondarily derived, not primitive.

It is time for the marine hypothesis for the origin of vertebrates to be discarded. It has provided no insight into the evolution of the vertebrates, and it is no longer the most parsimonious explanation for the derivation of osmoregulatory patterns in fishes.

Literature Cited

BLAXTER, J.H.S., C.S. WARDLE, and B.L. ROBERTS. 1971. Aspects of the circulatory physiology and muscle systems of deep-sea fish. J. mar. biol. Assoc. U.K. **51**: 991-1006.

BROWN, G.W., and P.P. COHEN. 1960. Comparative biochemistry of urea synthesis 3. Activities of urea-cycle enzymes in various higher and lower vertebrates. Biochem. J. **75**: 82-91.

CONTE, F.P. 1969. Salt secretion. pp. 241-292 *In* Hoar, W.S., and D.J. Randall [eds.] Fish physiology. Academic Press, New York.

DARLINGTON, P.J. 1957. Zoogeography: the geographical distribution of animals. John Wiley and Sons, New York.

DENNISON, R.H. 1959. A review of the habitat of the earliest vertebrates. Fieldiana: Geol. **11**: 357-457.

DEPECHE, J., R. GILLES, S. DAUFRESNE, and H. CHIAPELLO. 1979. Urea content and urea production *via* the ornithine-urea cycle during the ontogenic development of two teleost fishes. Comp. Biochem. Physiol. **63A**: 51-56.

EVANS, D.H. 1984. Gill Na^+/H^+ and Cl^-/HCO_3^- exchange systems evolved before the vertebrates entered fresh water. J. exp. Biol. **113**: 465-469.

GORDON, M.S., K. SCHMIDT-NIELSEN, and H.M. KELLY. 1961. Osmotic regulation in the crab-eating frog *Rana cancrivora*. J. exp. Biol. **38**: 659-678.

GRIFFITH, R.W. 1980. Chemistry of the body fluids of the coelacanth, *Latimeria chalumnae*. Proc. R. Soc. (Lond.) B. **208**: 329-347.

GRIFFITH, R.W. 1981. Composition of the blood serum of deep-sea fishes. Biol. Bull. **160**: 250-264.

GRIFFITH, R.W., and P.K.T. PANG. 1979. Mechanisms of osmoregulation in the coelacanth: evolutionary implications. Occ. Pap. Calif. Acad. Sci. **134**: 79-93.

GRIFFITH, R.W., P.K.T. PANG, and L.A. BENEDETTO. 1979. Urea tolerance in the killifish, *Fundulus heteroclitus*. Comp. Biochem. Physiol. **62A**: 327-330.

HALSTEAD, L.B. 1969. The origin and early evolution of calcified tissue in the vertebrates. Proc. Malacol. Soc. (Lond.) **38**: 552-553.

HALSTEAD, L.B. 1973. The heterostracan fishes. Biol. Rev. **48**: 279-332.

HICKMAN, C.P., and B.F. TRUMP. 1969. The kidney. pp. 91-329 *In* Hoar, W.S., and D.J. Randall. [eds.] Fish physiology, Vol. 1. Academic Press, New York.

HOAR, W.S. 1983. General and comparative physiology, 3rd ed. Prentice Hall, Inc., Englewood Cliffs, N.J.

HOAR, W.S., and D.J. RANDALL [eds.]. 1984. Fish physiology. vol. 10. Gills, Part B: ion and water transfer. Academic Press, Orlando, Fl.

HOLMES, W.N., and E.M. DONALDSON. 1969. The body compartments and the distribution of electrolytes. pp. 1-89 *In* Hoar, W.S., and D.J. Randall, [eds.] Fish physiology, vol. 1. Academic Press, New York.

HUGGINS, A.K., G. SKUTCH, and E. BALDWIN. 1969. Ornithine-urea cycle enzymes in teleost fishes. Comp. Biochem. Physiol. **28**: 587-602.

KIRSCHNER, L.B. 1983. Sodium chloride absorption across the body surface: frog skins and other epithelia. Amer. J. Physiol. **244**: R249-R443.

LACY, E.R.; E. REALE, D. SCHLUSSELBERG, W.K. SMITH, and D.J. WOODWARD. 1985. A renal countercurrent system in marine elasmobranch fish: a computer assisted reconstruction. Science **227**: 1351-1354.

LAGIOS, M.D. 1979a. The coelacanth and the Chondrichthyes as sister groups: a review of shared apomorph characters and a cladistic analysis and reinterpretation. Occ. Pap. Calif. Acad. Sci. **134**: 25-44.

LAGIOS, M.D. 1979b. Reply to the rebuttal of Leonard Compagno, "Coelacanths: shark relative or bony fishes". Occ. Pap. Calif. Acad. Sci. **134**: 53-55.

LOVE, R.M. 1970. The chemical biology of fishes. Academic Press, New York.

LØVTRUP, S. 1977. The phylogeny of vertebrata. John Wiley and Sons, London.

MAETZ, J. 1974. Aspects of adaptation to hypo-osmotic and hyperosmotic environments. pp. 1-167 *In* Malins, D.C., and J.R. Sargent [eds.] Biochemical and biophysical perspectives in marine biology, vol. 1. Academic Press, New york.

MAYR, E. 1944. Wallace's line in the light of recent zoogeographic studies. Quart. Rev. Biol. **19**: 1-14.

McINERNEY, J.E. 1974. Renal sodium reabsorption in the hagfish, *Eptatretus stouti*. Comp. Biochem. Physiol. **49A**: 273-280.

MOSS, M.L. 1968. The origin of vertebrate calcified tissues. Nobel Symp. **4**: 359-371.

MUNZ, F.W., and W.N. McFARLAND. 1964. Regulatory function of a primitive vertebrate kidney. Comp. Biochem. Physiol. **13**: 381-400.

MYERS, G.S. 1938. Freshwater fishes and West Indian zoogeography. Smithsonian Rep. **1937**: 339-364.

MYERS, G.S. 1949. Salt tolerance of freshwater groups in relation to zoogeographic problems. Bijdr. Dierk. **28**: 315-322.

NANCOLLAS, G.H., and B. TOMAZIK. 1974. Growth of calcium phosphate on hydroxyapatite crystals: effect of supersaturation and ionic medium. J. phys. Chem. **78**: 2218-2225.

NELSON, G.J. 1970. Outline of a theory of comparative biology. Syst. Zool. **19**: 373-384.

PANG, P.K.T., R.W. GRIFFITH, and J.W. ATZ. 1977. Osmoregulation in elasmobranchs. Amer. Zool. **17**: 365-377.

PICKFORD, G.E., and F.B. GRANT. 1967. Serum osmolality in the coelacanth, *Latimeria chalumnae*: urea retention and ion regulation. Science **155**: 568-570.

POTTS, W.T.W., and G. PARRY. 1963. Osmotic and ionic regulation in animals. Pergamon Press, Oxford.

PROSSER, C.L. [ed.]. 1973. Comparative animal physiology. W.B. Saunders Co. Philadelphia, Penn.

READ, L.J. 1968. A study of ammonia and urea excretion in the fresh-water-adapted form of the Pacific lamprey, *Entosphenus tridentatus*. Comp. Biochem. Physiol. **26**: 455-466.

READ, L.J. 1971. The presence of high ornithine-urea cycle enzyme activity in the teleost, *Opsanus tau*. Comp. Biochem. Physiol. **39A**: 409-413.

READ, L.J. 1975. Absence of ureogenic pathways in liver of the hagfish, *Bdellostoma cirrhatum*. Comp. Biochem. Physiol. **51B**: 139-141.

REPETSKI, J.E. 1978. A fish from the upper Cambrian of North America. Science **200**: 529-531.

ROBERTSON, J.D. 1957. The habitat of the earliest vertebrates. Biol. Rev. **32**: 156-187.

ROBERTSON, J.D. 1976. Chemical composition of the body fluids and muscle of the hagfish *Myxine glutinosa* and the rabbitfish *Chimaera monstrosa*. J. Zool. (Lond.) **178**: 261-277.

ROMER, A.S. 1966. Vertebrate paleontology, 3rd ed. Universty of Chicago Press, Chicago, Ill.

ROMER, A.S., and B.H. GROVE. 1935. Environment of the early vertebrates. Amer. Midl. Nat. **16**: 805-856.

SCHEER, B. 1964. The uses of comparative physiology. pp. 101-117 *In* Leone, C.A. [ed.]. Taxonomic biochemistry and serology. The Ronald Press, New York.

SIMPSON, G.G. 1960. Principles of animal taxonomy. Columbia University Press, New York.

SMITH, H.W. 1930. The absorption and excretion of water and salts by marine teleosts. Amer. J. Physiol. **93**: 480-505.

SMITH, H.W. 1932. Water regulation and its evolution in the fishes. Quart. Rev. Biol. **7**: 1-26.

SMITH, H.W. 1959. From fish to philosopher. CIBA edition, CIBA Pharmaceutical Products Inc., Summit, New Jersey.

THORSON, T.B., C.M. COWAN, and D.E. WATSON. 1967. *Potamotrygon* spp.: elasmobranchs with low urea content. Science **158**: 375-377.

THORSON, T.B., and D.E. WATSON. 1975. Reassignment of the African freshwater stingray, *Potamotrygon garonaensis*, to the genus *Dasyatis*, on physiologic and morphologic grounds. Copeia **1975**: 701-712.

YANCEY, P.H., and G.N. SOMERO. 1980. Methylamine osmoregulatory solutes of elasmobranch fishes counteract urea inhibition of enzymes. J. exp. Zool. **212**: 205-213.

THE BRAIN AND SENSE ORGANS OF THE EARLIEST VERTEBRATES: RECONSTRUCTION OF A MORPHOTYPE

R. Glenn Northcutt

Division of Biological Sciences
University of Michigan
Ann Arbor, Michigan

Introduction

Speculations on the nature of the brain and sense organs in the earliest vertebrates have traditionally been based on two different strategies. One approach has been to examine the brain and sense organs in living hagfishes and lampreys, with the assumption that these taxa are primitive and thus represent the starting point of vertebrate phylogeny (Worthington, 1906; Ariens Kappers, 1929; Heier, 1948; Stahl, 1977). This approach is confounded by considerable differences in the organization of the brain and sense organs in hagfishes and lampreys themselves, so that a single pattern of organization can not be recognized, and it also ignores the fact that these living taxa have a long evolutionary history during which many changes have obviously occurred.

A second strategy has been to reconstruct the brain and sense organs of the earliest vertebrates (ostracoderms) based on their fossil remains (Stensiö, 1927, 1932, 1963; Denison, 1964; Whiting and Tarlo, 1965). This approach is severely limited as, at best, one is restricted to estimating the external shape and size of the brain and sense organs based on the cast of an endocranial cavity, and it is further confounded by the fact that endocranial cavities can be interpreted only in light of soft anatomy as seen in living taxa. Thus there is an element of circular reasoning: fossils are examined to determine the primitive condition and are then interpreted in terms of the anatomy of living taxa, which are then concluded to be primitive also.

A third approach involves the reconstruction of a morphotype, *i.e.* the characters believed to be present in the common ancestor, based on a determination of shared primitive characters of the stem taxa. This approach, a cladistic analysis, requires that one determine the polarity (*i.e.* primitive versus derived condition) of the characters being examined. Out-group and ontogenetic criteria are considered the most reliable for determining this polarity (Eldredge and Cracraft, 1980; Wiley, 1981; Patterson, 1982).

In this paper various characters of the brain and sense organs of hagfishes, lampreys and gnathostomes will be examined, and an attempt will be made to establish the polarity of these characters. Those that can be argued to be shared primitive characters (symplesiomorphies) of hagfishes, lampreys and gnathostomes constitute characters that, by definition, must have been present in the common ancestor of these three groups. Wherever possible, characters of extinct groups will also be considered, but the conditions in living taxa are considered more heavily, as there is less ambiguity in interpreting their anatomy.

A cladistic analysis is strongly influenced by the hypothesis of the phyletic relationship of the taxa involved, and frequently it also involves distinguishing among various hypotheses of phyletic relationship. The present analysis, however, assumes valid the hypothesis (Fig. 1A) that lampreys are the sister group of gnathostomes and that lampreys and gnathostomes (myopterygians) are the sister group of hagfishes (Løvtrup, 1977; Janvier, 1978; Hardisty, 1979). Furthermore, cephalochordates are accepted as the sister group of craniates (Northcutt and Gans, 1983). Finally, Janvier's (1981) hypothesis of the relationship of fossil "agnathans" to living vertebrates (Fig. 1B) is assumed to be valid. Janvier (1981) argued that heterostracans are the sister group of myopterygians on the basis of four shared derived characters (synapomorphies): two vertical semicircular canals, a well developed lateral line system, the presence of arcual elements, and a mineralized

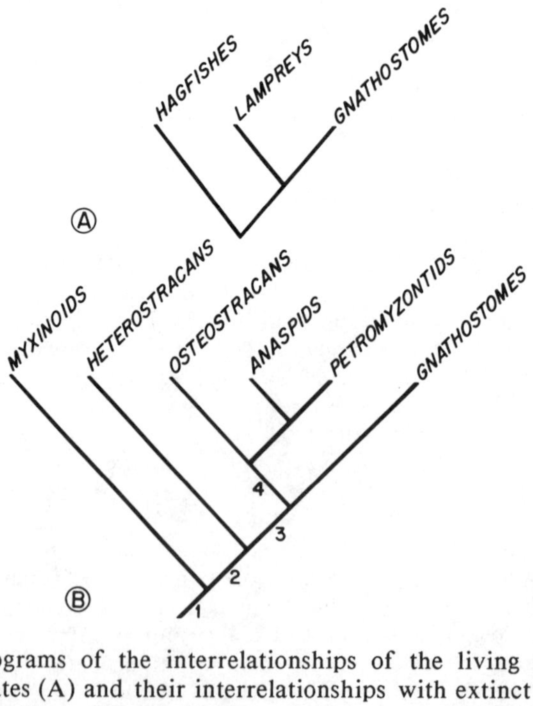

Fig. 1. Cladograms of the interrelationships of the living groups of craniates (A) and their interrelationships with extinct groups of jawless fishes (B). 1, Craniata; 2, Vertebrata; 3, Myopterygii; 4, Cephalaspidomorphi.

exoskeleton. These characters are absent in myxinoids, and their absence is assumed to represent the primitive condition. However, if their absence represents an apomorphic condition, the relationship of myxinoids and heterostracans is unresolved.

Reconstruction of a morphotype has additional benefits beyond speculating on the anatomy of a common ancestor or resolving different hypotheses of phyletic relationships. Recognition of primitive and derived characters represents a first step in constructing a scenario of the sequence and biological significance of the changes that have occurred in phylogeny. Such scenarios frequently reveal gaps in our knowledge and, in the process of envisioning how changes may have occurred, reveal correlations and contradictions that would not otherwise be apparent. A number of such gaps and contradictions are revealed in the follow analysis of myxinoid characters.

Special sense organs

All living craniates possess olfactory, optic, otic, lateralis, and gustatory sense organs that arise in development primarily or in part from neurogenic ectodermal placodes, whereas many of these special sense organs are absent in cephalochordates and urochordates, the obvious out-groups of craniates, or they are distinctly different in their anatomy and embryology (Northcutt and Gans, 1983). Thus it is probable that the earliest craniates were characterized by all of the special sense organs found in living craniates and that these organs arose with the origin of craniates.

Olfactory organs

In many gnathostomes the organs mediating olfaction arise from paired olfactory placodes that give rise to main olfactory organs, accessory olfactory organs (vomeronasal organs) and terminal nerves (Seydel, 1895; Locy, 1905a). Vomeronasal organs appear to have arisen phylogenetically as a secondary evagination of the main olfactory epithelium and are restricted to tetrapods (Northcutt, 1981), and terminal nerves do not appear to exist in hagfishes or lampreys (Demski, 1984). In gnathostomes, the terminal nerve consists of at least two classes of ganglion cells usually located beneath or among the axons of the olfactory nerve. The peripheral processes of these neurons arborize among the axons of the olfactory nerve (Springer, 1983) and may even reach the olfactory epithelium (Locy, 1905b; Demski and Northcutt, 1983), whereas their central processes enter the forebrain and retina (Munz *et al.*, 1981; Demski and Northcutt, 1983; Springer, 1983). Many of the centrally-projecting fibers of the terminalis nerve contain LHRH, which has facilitated their determination in many vertebrate groups. Studies of the distribution of LHRH in lampreys and hagfishes (Crim *et al.*, 1979) have not revealed a terminal nerve, nor have earlier descriptive anatomic studies (Johnston, 1902; Bone, 1963). These studies suggest that the terminal nerve arose with the origin of gnathostomes or, if this nerve occurred in the earliest craniates, it must have been lost in hagfishes and lampreys. Whichever hypothesis is correct, there is no basis for using the presence of a terminal nerve to support a hypothesis of multiple premandibular head segments in the earliest vertebrates (Jarvik, 1980; Bjerring, 1984).

The main olfactory organ in all living craniates consists of a hemispherical epithelial sheet comprising receptor cells, support or sustentacular cells, and basal cells. The receptor cells are characterized by ciliated apical surfaces and basally arising axons (0.1 to 0.4 μm in diameter) that form the olfactory nerve (Kleerekoper, 1969). The support cells are columnar epithelial cells that lie adjacent to receptor cells, and both receptor and support cells lie above a cuboidal layer of basal cells which appear to give rise to new receptor and support cells throughout life.

Although there are only minor differences in the histology of the olfactory epithelium, the overall morphology of the olfactory organs is distinctly different in the three groups of living craniates. Most gnathostomes possess paired olfactory organs that are located laterally on the head and open directly, or via short ducts, to the outside. In lampreys (Kleerekoper, 1969) and, apparently, fossil osteostracans (Stensiö, 1927, 1932; Janvier, 1974a) a single opening, the nasohypophyseal opening (Fig. 2C), located high on the dorsal surface of the head, gives rise to a caudoventrally-directed blind tube, the hypophyseal tube, that opens dorsally into the olfactory organ. The olfactory organ or sac in lampreys is housed within a single cartilaginous capsule but comprises left and right convoluted epithelial surfaces divided by a medial lamella or septum. Each epithelium gives rise to an olfactory nerve that terminates in the ipsilateral olfactory bulb of the telencephalon.

The olfactory apparatus of adult lampreys appears to be characterized by an autapomorphic glandular system. A series of gland-like vesicles develops caudally as diverticulae from the olfactory organ (Kleerekoper, 1969). These diverticulae consist of low cuboidal epithelium and are embedded in a blood sinus. They are believed to be innervated by fibers of the olfactory nerve, but their function is presently unknown.

In hagfishes, a single tubular prenasal sinus opens to the outside rostrally, above the mouth, and leads posteriorly to a short nasohypophyseal atrium which opens dorsally to the olfactory sac and caudally into the pharynx as a nasopharyngeal duct. The side-walls and roof of the olfactory sac are thrown into folds and divided by a median pair of lamellae that only partially separate the olfactory sac into left and right halves. However, as in lampreys, left and right olfactory nerves issue from the olfactory epithelium and terminate ipsilaterally in paired olfactory bulbs of the telencephalon.

The morphology of the olfactory apparatus in fossil heterostracans is uncertain, as the fossils consist only of a calcified dermal skeleton and no neurocranium (Stensiö, 1927; White, 1935; Denison, 1964; Janvier and Blieck, 1979). Stensiö (1927) and Janvier (1974a) postulated that paired depressions in the caudal rostrum (intrarostral space) housed paired olfactory organs that opened ventrally into a short nasohypophyseal duct separated from the pharynx by a presumed cartilaginous palato-subnasal lamina. Subsequently, Stensiö (1968) argued that only a single olfactory organ existed more caudally in a position that other workers have interpreted as a cavity that housed the telencephalon. Finally, Kiaer (1930) and Halstead (1973) have argued that the intrarostral space housed paired olfactory organs that opened directly into the roof of the mouth, or laterally and externally as in gnathostomes.

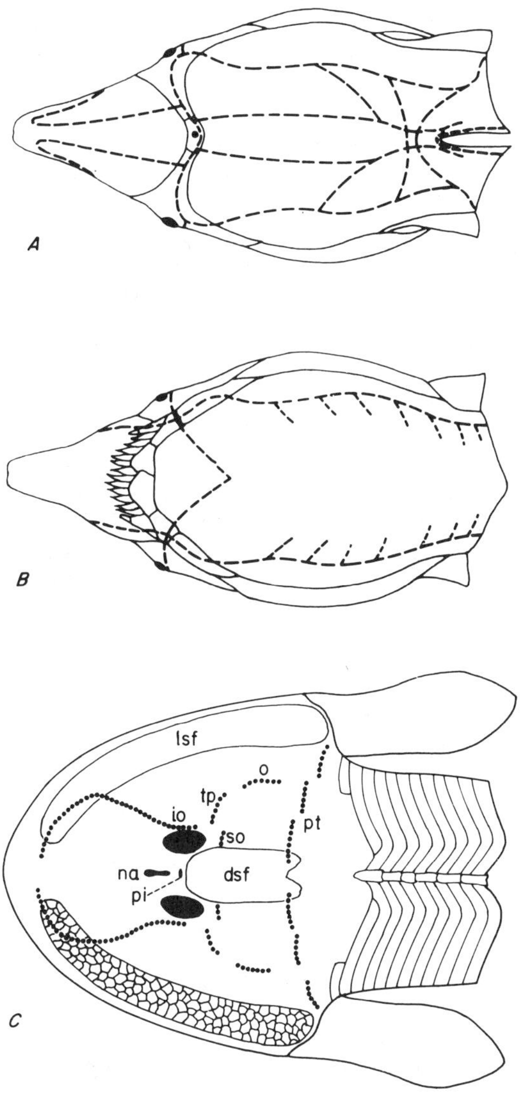

Fig. 2. Dorsal (A) and ventral (B) views of the dermal armor of the heterostracan *Pteraspis* showing the distribution of lateral lines (modified from White, 1935). Dorsal view (C) of the cephalic shield of the osteostracan *Hemicyclaspis* showing the distribution of lateral lines (modified from Stensiö, 1932). *Dsf*, dorsal sensory field; *io*, infraorbital line; *lsf*, lateral sensory field; *na*, nasohypophyseal opening; *o*, otic line; *pi*, pineal foramen; *pt*, posterior transverse zonal lines; *so*, supraorbital or postpineal line; *tp*, transverse postorbital line.

The lack of a complete median septum dividing the olfactory epithelium into two separate organs in hagfishes, and the development of the olfactory organ and adenohypophysis from a single placode in hagfishes and lampreys (Dohrn, 1883; von Kupffer, 1894; Damas, 1944) led to speculation that a monorhinic condition characterized the earliest craniates (von Kupffer, 1894; Fürbringer, 1897; Plate, 1924). The presence of paired olfactory nerves and bulbs in all living craniates strongly suggests that the presence of paired olfactory organs represents the original craniate condition and that the partial fusion of the olfactory epithelia in hagfishes is a derived condition.

The disposition and openings of the olfactory organs in the earliest craniates is more problematic. The dorsocaudal position of a naso-hypophyseal foramen and duct in osteostracans and lampreys is most likely a derived condition and diagnostic of cephalaspidomorphs, as the nasohypophyseal duct arises immediately dorsal to the mouth in the larvae of lampreys. It is unlikely that the olfactory organs opened into the roof of the pharynx in heterostracans, as this pattern does not occur in the embryonic or adult form of any living craniate. It is more likely that the olfactory organs initially opened separately and dorsorostral to the mouth, as in living gnathostomes, or into a short prenasal sinus associated with a nasohypophyseal duct, as has been postulated for heterostracans (Janvier, 1974a). The embryology of hagfishes and lampreys suggests that the olfactory organs and adenohypophysis may have been closely associated initially and that a short prenasal sinus may have existed in the earliest craniates. A corollary of this hypothesis is that the extremely long prenasal sinus in hagfishes may have arisen by fusion of cartilaginous plates supporting nasal tentacles as an adaptation to burrowing (Janvier, 1974a). In this context, gnathostomes would exhibit a derived condition in which development of a prenasal sinus is suppressed, and the olfactory organ and adenohypophysis develop from separate placodal centers.

Optic organs

In gnathostomes, evaginations of the embryonic diencephalon occur dorsally and ventrolaterally and give rise to the optic organs (Eakin, 1973). A right pineal eye and a left parapineal (parietal) eye frequently form as dorsal evaginations, whereas paired lateral eyes develop from more ventrally located evaginations. In lampreys, both pineal and parapineal evaginations form photoreceptor organs, with the better developed pineal eye located dorsal to the parapineal eye (Eddy, 1972). Each eye forms a hollow vesicle with a thin roof and a thick floor. The floor, or retina, of both the pineal and parapineal organs comprises sensory, supportive (pigment), and ganglion cells (Collin, 1969; Eakin, 1973). An apical expansion of the sensory cells protrudes into the central lumen and consists of lamellae similar to the cone receptors in the retina of the lateral eyes in other vertebrates. The basal surfaces of the receptor cells make contact with dendrites of the ganglion cells and form synaptic ribbons similar to those of lateral eyes. The pigment cells lie adjacent to individual sensory cells and contain granules and, on their apical surfaces, microvilli which extend into the central lumen. Ganglion cells occur scattered throughout the deeper two-thirds of the retina and give rise to axons that innervate either right (pineal) or left (parapineal) diencephalic centers. Experimental studies of the pineal-parapineal complex in lampreys suggest that this complex affects diurnal color rhythms (Eddy and Strahan, 1968), metamorphosis (Eddy, 1969) and reproduction (Eddy, 1970).

Adult hagfishes do not possess any trace of pineal or parapineal organs (Bone, 1963). Osteostracans (Stensiö, 1932) and some heterostracans (White, 1935) are believed to have possessed median photoreceptor organs, as the dermal shields of these taxa possess a median "pineal" foramen (Fig. 2A, C). It is assumed that this foramen housed at least a pineal eye, as this organ is usually the more dorsal of the two medial eyes in lampreys.

There are two possible hypotheses regarding the origin of median eyes in craniates: 1) median eyes arose with the origin of craniates and were subsequently lost in living hagfishes, perhaps in association with adaptations for burrowing; 2) median eyes arose in the common ancestor of heterostracans and myopterygians. The diencephalon in embryonic hagfishes should be examined for evidence of transient evaginations which, if present, would support the first hypothesis. In this context, Conel (1931) claimed that embryos of *Eptatretus* are characterized by a transient epiphysis. However, Holmgren (1946) was not able to confirm such an evagination in *Myxine*.

The lateral eyes of lampreys are similar to those of gnathostomes in most respects, however they differ in a number of features that are more similar to the eyes of embryonic or larval gnathostomes and are likely plesiomorphic features common to myopterygians (Kleerekoper, 1972). In lampreys, the cornea consists of an outer dermal segment, devoid of pigmentation, glands and blood vessels, and an inner mesodermal segment which is a continuation of the sclera. The two corneal layers are closely associated but separated by a capillary space. The nuclei of the cells composing the lens are diffuse, unlike the nuclei of lens cells in gnathostomes, and there are no ciliary muscles or a muscular iris. The iris consists of a single layer of epithelium, and accomodation occurs by changes of the scleral cornea affected by extrinsic eye muscles. The retina in lampreys consists of pigmented and neural layers, as in other myopterygians, and the neural retina appears to possess classes of receptor cells comparable to the rods and cones of other retinas. The usual cellular layers of the neural retina can be recognized, except that a distinct ganglion cell, along with bodies of the bipolar and amacrine cells, form the internal nuclear layer.

In hagfishes, the lateral eyes are poorly developed and are most similar to the eyes of gnathostomes that are highly degenerate (Fernholm and Holmberg, 1975). Eptatretids exhibit prominent eyespots of skin with reduced pigmentation over the eyes, whereas myxinoids do not possess recognizable eyespots. Similarly, the eyes of eptatretids and myxinids lack a cornea, lens, and iris, whereas the eyes of eptatretids do possess a central vitreous body which appears to have been lost in myxinids. The neural retina of eptatretids is differentiated into an outer receptor layer and inner and outer fibrous layers separated by an inner cell layer. The receptor cells contain outer segments with well organized discs and basal synaptic bodies similar to those of the hair cells of the lateral line organs in gnathostomes. The neural retina of myxinids consists of the same layers, but the outer segments of the receptor cells consist of disordered membranous whirls, and these cells do not appear to possess synaptic ribbons. Similarly, extrinsic eye muscles and their accompanying cranial nerves are absent in all hagfishes.

The lateral eyes of osteostracans were likely similar to those of lampreys and gnathostomes, based on the relative size of the orbits (Fig. 2C). Extrinsic eye muscles were likely present, as osteostracans possessed a myodome on the posterodorsal walls of the orbit, comparable to the trochlear innervated eye muscle of lampreys (Janvier, 1981), as well as foramina in the calcified neurocranium whose positions are comparable to foramina for the oculomotor, trochlear, and abducens nerves in lampreys (Stensiö, 1927).

The lateral eyes of heterostracans must have been relatively small, as their orbits are poorly developed (Fig. 2A) or absent (White, 1935; Denison, 1964; Halstead, 1973; Janvier, 1981). It is uncertain whether heterostracans possessed extrinsic eye muscles. Their neurocrania were apparently uncalcified, and there is essentially no information on the course of their cranial nerves. In some fossil heterostracans, the internal surface of the dorsal shield bears impressions of soft anatomy which have been variously interpreted. In some cyathaspids (Denison, 1964; Halstead, 1973; Janvier and Blieck, 1979) a series of oval impressions occur lateral to the impressions believed to be due to the pineal organ, midbrain, semicircular canals and medulla. These lateral impressions have been purported to mark the position of head myomeres (Halstead, 1973) or the dorsalmost portions of the branchial arches (Denison, 1964; Janvier and Blieck, 1979). If these impressions are due to myomeres, the lateral eyes occur rostral to all but the most anterior myomere (premandibular), which suggests that the pro-otic myomeres did not form extrinsic eye muscles. If the impressions are due to the dorsal portions of the branchial arches, there is no space for myomeres between these arches and the dermal skeleton, which suggests that head myomeres were either lost or had not yet evolved.

The existence of paired lateral eyes in all living craniates, and the presence of orbits in some members of all the extinct groups, suggests that lateral eyes arose with the origin of craniates. However, the overall organization of these eyes, and whether or not extrinsic eye muscles arose at the same time, is uncertain. One of two hypotheses is likely: 1) the eyes of hagfishes represent a plesiomorphic condition for craniates, and accessory optic structures such as the cornea, lens, iris, and extrinsic eye muscles developed subsequently; 2) the eyes of hagfishes are degenerate (apomorphic) and related to a burrowing habitat, and the eyes of the earliest craniates were more similar to those of lampreys. The second hypothesis could account for extrinsic eye muscle in at least two ways: 1) extrinsic eye muscles developed later than the other accessory organs (i.e. they arose with the common ancestor of cephalaspidomorphs and gnathostomes); 2) extrinsic eye muscles arose with the origin of craniates and were lost independently in myxinoids and heterostracans. The similarity of the eyes of hagfishes to those of blind cave or burrowing gnathostomes suggests that the simple condition in hagfishes is likely apomorphic. Additional information on the origin of extrinsic eye muscles might accrue from developmental studies of head somites in hagfishes or may never be forthcoming. In this context, Holmgren (1946) described a number of the muscle rudiments in the head of embryos of two different stages of development in *Myxine* but did not comment on head myotomes.

Otic organs

In gnathostomes the inner ear, labyrinth or otic organ, and its innervation arise from a tear-shaped ectodermal placode which invaginates to form three semicircular canals (anterior and posterior vertical canals and a lateral horizontal canal). These canals are arrayed around a central epithelial sac that is divided into a rostral chamber (utricle) and a posterior chamber subdivided into a rostral saccule and a caudal lagena (Ayers, 1892; Wilson and Mattocks, 1897; Rubel, 1978). One or more sensory organs composed of support cells and receptor or hair cells bearing kinocilia and microvilli on their apical surfaces form within each of the major otic chambers. A sensory organ is termed a crista when it occurs in an expanded ampullary portion of a semicircular canal, and a macula when it occurs in the utricle, saccule, or lagena. Thus in most anamniotic gnathostomes, there are three semicircular cristae and utricular, saccular, and lagenar maculae. An additional sensory macula, termed the macula neglecta, frequently occurs in a duct running from the saccule to the crista of the posterior semicircular canal.

The ganglion cells of the eighth (otic or octaval) cranial nerve arise from a restricted portion of the otic placode (Yntema, 1937); their peripheral processes innervate the various otic sensory organs, whereas their central processes enter the medulla of the brain. In most anamniotic gnathostomes the octaval nerve is divided into anterior and posterior rami and ganglia. The anterior ramus innervates the anterior horizontal semicircular cristae, the utricular macula, and a small part of the saccular macula, whereas the posterior ramus innervates the bulk of the saccular macula, the lagenar macula, and the macula neglecta, as well as the posterior semicircular crista (Meredith and Butler, 1983; Popper and Northcutt, 1983).

The otic organ of lampreys (Lowenstein *et al.*, 1968; Thornhill, 1972) differs from that of gnathostomes in that only anterior and posterior vertical semicircular canals and cristae are present, and the maculae are restricted to a median chamber. The ampullae of the vertical semicircular canals contain complex cristae with three sensory arms running in different planes, roughly perpendicular to each other. The spatial arrangement of these arms suggests that the two semicircular cristae of lampreys may cover a spatial range for response to angular acceleration that is dealt with in gnathostomes by the addition of a horizontal semicircular canal (Lowenstein *et al.*, 1968).

The labyrinth of lampreys consists of a median crescent-shaped chamber that houses a macula communis basally, and two large dorsal and lateral chambers whose walls are ciliated. The macula communis is divided into anterior, vertical, and posterior subdivisions which are believed to be homologous to the utricular, saccular, and lagenar maculae in gnathostomes (Lowenstein *et al.*, 1968). An additional macula (macula neglecta) occurs in a small recess on the dorsomedial face of the labyrinth, close to the region where the endolymphatic duct emerges from the ciliated chambers. Thus, although the otic organ of lampreys is simpler than that of gnathostomes in not possessing a horizontal semicircular canal and separate otolithic maculae, it is also unique among living craniates in possessing dorsal and lateral ciliated chambers that are almost as large as the remainder of the labyrinth. These chambers may be remnants of the extensive dorsal and lateral sensory fields of osteostracans (Jarvik, 1965).

In osteostracans the neurocranium was calcified, and several details are known regarding the otic capsule (Stensiö, 1927). Reconstructions of the labyrinth suggest that osteostracans possessed an otic organ similar to that of modern lampreys in that the labyrinth possessed two vertical semicircular canals but no horizontal canal.

Unlike in other craniates, a series of canals passed from the dorsal and lateral walls of the otic capsule toward the exterior of the shield, where they ended as shallow fossae that were covered by a mosaic of small dermal elements (Fig. 2C). Interpretation of the soft structures that occupied these cavities is problematical. Stensiö (1927) proposed that the dorsal and lateral fossae housed electric organs and suggested that they were innervated by cranial motor nerves running from the labyrinth. This interpretation appears unlikely, as such organs would probably have been innervated by postotic branchiomeric nerves rather than by nerves exiting the neurocranium ventral to the membranous labyrinth. Similarly, the extensive nature of these organs would suggest a sizable nerve supply, and living craniates that possess electric organs of this magnitude clearly reflect this specialization in greatly expanded brain stem centers related to the branchiomeric motor column. Endocasts of the neurocranium of osteostracans do not evince any trace of such central neural specializations. It is far more likely that these peripheral fossae housed extensive evaginations of the membranous labyrinth, and these structures may or may not have been mechanoreceptive in nature. Clearly, the ciliated chambers of the labyrinth in lampreys are the only structures among living craniates that bear any resemblance to the dermal "sensory" fields of osteostracans, and determination of the function of these ciliated chambers should improve our understanding of these unique osteostracan structures.

The membranous labyrinth in *Myxine* is enclosed in a kidney-shaped cartilaginous capsule and is toroidal in shape, with the cartilage penetrating the center of the torus (Lowenstein and Thornhill, 1970). The membranous labyrinth houses a single macula communis, covering the medioventral wall of the base of the torus, and two ampullae formed as dilations in the wall of the torus on either end of the macula communis. The ampullae, in turn, are connected by a single semicircular canal which forms the dorsolateral half of the torus.

Although the labyrinth in *Myxine* contains a single macula, the kinocilia of its hair cells have different orientations across its length. This hair-cell map resembles that of lampreys at either end of the macula, and Lowenstein and Thornhill (1970) suggested that the macula of *Myxine* contains subdivisions homologous to the utricular and lagenar maculae of gnathostomes but that a subdivision comparable to the saccular macula is not present.

The labyrinth of myxinoids, unlike that of other craniates, is innervated by separate utricular and saccular nerves. In the absence of ontogenetic information or a relevant out-group, it is impossible to evaluate the polarity of these characters. Recordings from octaval fibers that innervate the cristae of the two vertical ampullae demonstrate that the cristae are sensitive to angular accelerations in all planes of space, as are the semicircular cristae in lampreys and gnathostomes (Lowenstein and Thornhill, 1970). No response to vibrational stimuli could be elicited from any branch of the octaval nerve, as predicted by the absence of a saccular macula and a macula neglecta. Given the absence of a macular subdivision sensitive to vibrational stimuli in hagfishes, it is possible that the dorsal and lateral sensory fields of osteostracans represent primitive vibration detectors.

There is little information on the morphology of the labyrinth in heterostracans, as the neurocranium was not calcified. Impressions on the inner surface of the dorsal shield of some cyathaspids indicate that they possessed anterior and posterior vertical semicircular canals (Stensiö, 1963; Denison, 1964). However, it is impossible to decide whether these taxa possessed a horizontal semicircular canal, for even if present, it would have left no impression on the dorsal shield (Halstead, 1973).

Given the variation in the organization of the labyrinth in living craniates, two hypotheses concerning the origin and subsequent phylogeny of the labyrinth should be considered. The first assumes that the membranous labyrinth of the earliest craniates possessed a macula communis, homologous to the utricular and lagenar maculae of gnathostomes, and two vertical cristae. A macula neglecta and a saccular macula arose with the origin of myopterygians, and a horizontal semicircular canal arose with gnathostomes. This hypothesis assumes that the labyrinth of myxinoids represents a plesiomorphic condition for craniates. A second hypothesis assumes that the labyrinth of the earliest craniates was like that of living lampreys in possessing a macula communis, with subdivisions comparable to the utricular, saccular, and lagenar maculae of gnathostomes, as well as a macula neglecta and two vertical semicircular canals. In this case, the absence of a saccular division of the macula communis and a macula neglecta in myxinoids is viewed as a loss (apomorphic condition) and, again, the presence of a horizontal canal is linked to the origin of gnathostomes. Clearly, the absence of a reasonable out-group for these characters complicates the analysis, and rejection of either hypothesis will probably be based on whether myxinoids are believed to represent an early grade of craniate organization, prior to mineralization of the dermis, or whether they represent a highly modified burrowing form derived from armored craniates.

Lateral line systems

The sensory lateral line system in gnathostomes arises from a series of ectodermal placodes that may number thirteen pairs primitively (Pehrson, 1949). These placodes appear to give rise to at least three classes of morphological receptors as well as the cranial nerves (anterior and posterior lateral line nerves) that innervate these receptors. These classes of morphological receptors are mechanoreceptive neuromasts, mechanoreceptive spiracular organs, and electroreceptive ampullary organs. Mechanoreceptive neuromasts occur within lines or canals (canal neuromasts) as well as on the surface of the head and trunk (free neuromasts).

The canal neuromasts usually occur within tubes surrounded by dermal bone. The canals periodically open to the surface as pores, with a single neuromast located between adjacent pores. The primitive pattern of canal distribution in gnathostomes consists of paired supraorbital and infraorbital canals passing above and below the eyes and fusing caudally to form a temporal (otic) canal, which passes around the otic capsule to course caudally onto the trunk as a main lateral line canal (Northcutt, 1985). A mandibulo-preopercular canal runs from the tip of the lower jaw over the cheek to connect with the temporal canal, and a supratemporal canal or commissure interconnects the temporal canals near the caudal end of the head. More variable oral canals course dorsally to the mandibular canals, and jugal and additional cheek canals are seen in many fossil groups (Holmgren, 1942; Stensiö, 1947). Similarly, the trunk of the earliest gnathostomes was characterized by dorsal and ventral lateral lines in addition to the main lateral line of the trunk (Stensiö, 1947).

Free neuromasts occur primitively as a limited series of short lines (pit lines) in close association with the main canals. The exact number and position of these pit lines on the head is still not clear, however many gnathostomes possess at least three pairs of lines (anterior, middle and posterior) dorsally, two or three series on the cheek, and one or two series on the ventral surface of the head (Northcutt, 1985).

Paired spiracular organs occur as diverticula of the hyoid pouches and house a neuromast-like sensory organ (Barry and Boord, 1984). A spiracular organ has not been described in hagfishes or lampreys and likely arose with the origin of gnathostomes.

The ampullary organs or electroreceptors occur singly or in clusters as tube-like invaginations of the epidermis. Primitively, they are restricted to the head and exhibit the highest density on the snout and around the eyes. Ampullary organs are generally closely associated with the main canals of the ordinary lateral line, and their distribution and innervation by lateral line nerves strongly suggest that they arise embryonically from the same placodes that give rise to the neuromasts and ganglion cells of the lateral line nerves (Northcutt, 1985), but this has not been demonstrated.

Traditionally, the lateral line organs were said to be innervated by branches of the facial, glossopharyngeal, and vagal nerves. More recent studies (McCready and Boord, 1976; McCormick, 1982; Bullock *et al.*, 1983) have demonstrated that the lateral line organs are innervated by separate cranial nerves whose embryonic origin and central termination are distinct from the branchiomeric nerves. All lateral line organs of the head are innervated by a pair of anterior lateral line nerves, whereas all lateral line organs of the trunk and tail are innervated by a pair of posterior lateral line nerves.

The primitive pattern of innervation of lateral line organs in gnathostomes appears to consist of an anterior lateral line nerve with the following rami: a superficial ophthalmic ramus that innervates the neuromasts of the supraorbital canal, the anterior pit line, and ampullary organs on the rostral snout; a buccal ramus that innervates the neuromasts of the infraorbital canal and ampullary organs below the eye and on the upper jaw; a spiracular ramus that innervates the spiracular organ; an otic ramus that innervates the neuromasts in the rostral half of the temporal canal and ampullary organs on the dorsal head caudal to the eye. In addition, a hyomandibular trunk divides into mandibular and jugal or opercular rami. The mandibular ramus innervates the neuromasts of the mandibular and oral canals and the ampullary organs on the rostral half of the ventral surface of the head. The jugal or opercular ramus innervates the neuromasts of the opercular canals and ampullary organs on the lateral and caudoventral half of the head. Rami of the hyomandibular trunk also innervate the pit lines located on the cheek and gular regions as well as the middle pit line of the head.

The posterior lateral line nerve also consists of several rami: a squamosal ramus innervates the neuromasts in the caudal portion of the temporal canal and the posterior pit line; a lateral or main trunk ramus innervates the neuromasts in the main lateral line canal; a supratemporal-dorsal accessory ramus innervates the neuromasts of the supratemporal and dorsal trunk lines or canals; and a ventral accessory ramus innervates the neuromasts of the ventral trunk lines or canals.

The distribution of neuromasts and their innervation has been examined in the lampreys *Lampetra* and *Petromyzon* (Johnston, 1905; Holmgren, 1942; Marinelli and Strenger, 1954). In these taxa the neuromasts are not located within canals but occur as free neuromasts arranged as various lines on the skin surface. One such line runs from the caudal border of the eye forward, immediately beneath the eye, to the rostral tip of the oral hood; it is probably homologous to the infraorbital line in gnathostomes, based on its topography and innervation by a buccal ramus of the anterior lateral line nerve. Above the eye there is a short series of neuromasts, termed the postpineal row, which is innervated by a distinct ramus closely associated with the deep ophthalmic ramus. The postpineal row may be homologous to part of the supraorbital line and/or the anterior pit line in gnathostomes. Both series in gnathostomes arise from a single placode (Pehrson, 1949) and are innervated by branches of the supraorbital ramus, so a precise determination is impossible.

A third line of neuromasts occurs on the skin surface over the otic capsule and is innervated by a ramus lateralis communicans interconnecting the ganglia of the anterior and posterior lateral line nerves (Johnston, 1905). This ramus probably forms from a fusion of the otic ramus of the anterior lateral line nerve and the squamosal ramus of the posterior lateral line nerve in gnathostomes. However, most of the fibers in the ramus lateralis communicans arise from ganglion cells of the anterior lateral line nerve and innervate electroreceptors on the trunk (Ronan and Northcutt, 1982). There is no homologue of these electroreceptive related fibers in gnathostomes.

The remaining neuromasts in lampreys form four longitudinal lines, most of which are distributed caudal to the eye. A dorsal line begins caudal to the postpineal groups and courses caudally onto the trunk. This line, called the longitudinal dorsal line, is innervated by a dorsal ramus of the posterior lateral line nerve (Johnston, 1905). It is presently unclear whether this line is homologous to the dorsal accessory or main trunk line of gnathostomes.

Two additional longitudinal lines occur dorsal to the gill slits in adult lampreys; the more dorsal of the two runs caudal to the otic line, and a more ventral line runs immediately adjacent to the gill slits themselves. Both lines terminate at the level of the last gill slit. Only the ventral line appears to be present in ammocoetes. Johnston (1905) illustrated this line, but not the more dorsal one, and indicated that it was innervated by a branchial branch of the posterior lateral line nerve (branchial branch of vagus). It is probable that both the ventral and dorsal lines are innervated by the branchial ramus (more preferably termed the epibranchial or suprabranchial ramus), but additional studies are needed. The homologue(s) of these lines in gnathostomes, if any, is unclear. It is possible that they correspond to the main trunk line, although lungfishes exhibit a transient row of placodes, immediately dorsal to the gill slits, that have been suggested to represent a remnant of this series (Pehrson, 1949). If so, it is probable that gnathostomes have lost the suprabranchial neuromasts.

A fourth longitudinal line of neuromasts occurs ventral to the gill slits in lampreys. This row begins immediately ventral to the last gill slit and runs rostrally onto the ventrocaudal surface of the oral hood. Johnston (1905) indicated that the rostral neuromasts of this line are innervated by the hyomandibular trunk of the anterior lateral line nerve, whereas the intermediate and caudal neuromasts are innervated by the squamosal and branchial rami, respectively, of the posterior lateral line nerve. The rostral and intermediate segments of this ventral line of neuromasts are likely homologous to comparable lines innervated by the hyomandibular and squamosal rami in gnathostomes. It is possible that the caudal segment has been lost in gnathostomes, but additional studies are clearly needed to resolve the problems of comparison between lampreys and gnathostomes.

Adult lampreys have recently been demonstrated to be electroreceptive (Bodznick and Northcutt, 1981; Bodznick and Preston, 1983; Fritzsch *et al.*, 1984). The exact number and distribution of the electroreceptors is still uncertain, but it is known that they are located on both the head and trunk and are innervated only by the anterior lateral line nerve (Ronan and Northcutt, 1982). The receptors have also been identified as the ectodermal end buds (Ronan and Bodznick, 1984) of the older literature (Johnston, 1902). Although their morphology is considerably different from that of the ampullary organs of gnathostomes--the end buds are not located at the base of ectodermal invaginations, nor do they possess kinocilia as do the electroreceptors in gnathostomes--their physiology (Bodznick and Preston, 1983) and central projections (Ronan and Northcutt, 1982) strongly suggest that these electroreceptors are homologous to those of gnathostomes.

Ammocoetes exhibit a photokinetic response to light falling on the head or tail (Young, 1935a, b). This dermal light sense is dependent on an intact lateral line nerve, which suggests that the lateral line nerves of ammocoetes innervate photoreceptors in the skin. Recently Whitear and Lane (1983a) identified bipolar cells, which they termed multivillous cells, in the skin of ammocoetes. These cells contain dense masses of cylindrical organelles associated with a suspected photopigment, and the basal surface of the cells shows a presynaptic pattern comparable to that of the receptor cells in the ampullary organs of gnathostomes. Whitear and Lane also noted the similarity of multivillous cells in ammocoetes to the receptor cells of the end buds in adult lampreys. These observations suggest that multivillous cells may be the skin photoreceptors of ammocoetes and that they are reorganized at metamorphosis to form the electroreceptors (end buds) of adult lampreys. Similar skin photoreceptors associated with the lateral line system have not been described in other craniates, but *Myxine* also exhibits locomotory and burrowing responses evoked by light (Newth and Ross, 1955). Light sensitivity was found to be highest on the anterior end of the head and in the clocal region, and removal of the skin from these regions destroyed the light response, suggesting that photoreceptors are located in the skin.

Osteostracans apparently possessed a well developed lateral line system, comparable to that of lampreys in many features (Stensiö, 1932; Janvier, 1974b). The cephalic shield of *Hemicyclaspis* (Fig. 2C) and many other osteostracans shows shallow open grooves whose topography is comparable to that of the lines or canals of neuromasts found in living craniates. The most extensive sensory line on the dorsal surface of the shield is an infraorbital line (io, Fig. 2C) which appears to have been innervated by a buccal ramus of the anterior lateral line nerve (Janvier, 1974b), as in other craniates. Osteostracans, like lampreys, do not exhibit a well developed supraorbital line. A short postpineal line (so, Fig. 2C) may correspond to the postpineal row in lampreys or to the supraorbital-anterior pit line in gnathostomes. A transverse postorbital line (tp, Fig. 2C) occurs in many osteostracans and may have been innervated by the otic ramus or by a branch of the hyomandibular trunk of the anterior lateral line nerve (Janvier, 1974b). Its homology, if any, with lines in other craniates is uncertain. An otic or temporal line (o, Fig. 2C) occupies a position comparable to that of the same-named line in lampreys and gnathostomes and was probably similarly innervated.

The caudal zone of the dorsal shield of many osteostracans exhibits an extensive series of transverse lines, posterior transverse zonal lines, that must have been innervated by rami of the posterior lateral line nerves, as these lines occur caudal to the otic capsule (Janvier, 1974b). Their relationship to the lateral lines in other craniates is problematic. They may be homologous to part of the suprabranchial rows of lampreys and/or to the supratemporal and posterior pit lines of gnathostomes.

In some osteostracans, there are traces of more caudal longitudinal lines that may have continued onto the trunk. *Cephalaspis* exhibits a dorsal longitudinal line that arises rostrally at the level of the posterior transverse zonal line and continues caudally on the shield. Similarly, *Boreaspis* exhibits a more lateral longitudinal line that arises at the level of the posterior transverse zonal line and passes caudally in a position comparable to that of the main trunk line in gnathostomes. Janvier (1974b) argued that the dorsal longitudinal line may be homologous to the dorsal trunk line of lampreys, and thus to the dorsal accessory line of gnathostomes, whereas the lateral longitudinal line has no homologue in lampreys.

Little is known regarding ventral lines in osteostracans, as the oralobranchial chamber was covered by a mosaic of small dermal elements that are rarely preserved in the same detail as the dorsal shield. However, Janvier (1974b) noted that *Tremataspis* exhibits traces of a ventral sensory line, ventrally adjacent to the gill slits, and that this line continued onto the trunk as far caudally as the cloaca. He suggested that the segment of the line ventral to the gill slits is comparable to the ventral line in lampreys. This trunk segment of the ventral line in osteostracans may, however, be homologous to the ventral accessory trunk line in gnathostomes.

The outer layers of the dermal skeleton on both the head and trunk of osteostracans exhibit a unique series of pores opening to the exterior of the dermal armor and interconnected by deeper canals, which, in turn, connect with the shallow grooves of the lateral line rows (Stensiö, 1927, 1932; Denison, 1947). This dermal network, frequently termed cosmine, has also been called the pore-canal system, and Stensiö suggested that it housed mucous glands and canals. More recently, Thomson (1977) noted the similarity of the size of the pore opening and the depth of the vertical canals to the morphology of gnathostomes ampullary organs and suggested that the pore-canal system was an extensive series of electroreceptors. In reconstructing the otic region of *Procephalaspis*, Janvier (1974b) illustrated a ramus lateralis communicans interconnecting the ganglia of the anterior and posterior lateral line nerves. Such a ramus is diagnostic of electroreceptive species that possess trunk electroreceptors innervated by the anterior lateral line nerve (Ronan and Northcutt, 1982), and its presence supports Thomson's hypothesis that osteostracans were electroreceptive.

The dermal armor of heterostracans (Fig. 2A, B) reveals a well developed lateral line system (White, 1935; Denison, 1964). In *Pteraspis* the lateral line system formed true canals that ran in the cancellous layer of the dermal skeleton and opened periodically as a series of pores, as in most gnathostomes. Three main longitudinal canals, two located on the dorsal shield (Fig. 2A) and one located on the ventral shield (Fig. 2B), ran the length of the head and continued on the trunk (White, 1935). The course of these lateral line canals is so very general that, in the absence of information on their innervation, due to the lack of a fossilized endocranium, it is almost impossible to predict their homologues in other craniates. One can use only superficial landmarks, such as the mouth, orbit, pineal foramen, and otic impressions, as relative landmarks in assessing possible homologies. As noted by Holmgren and Pehrson (1949), it is possible to derive the lateral line system of any known craniate from the heterostracan pattern.

Heterostracans also appear to have possessed a pore-canal system. Short canals radiate at right angles from the main lateral line canals and open into intercostal grooves (mucous grooves of Stensiö, 1932). The intercostal grooves run superficially in the dermal armor and are usually 30-50 μm in diameter with a depth of 60-70 μ m (Denison, 1964). In some taxa the grooves are open, whereas in others they form canals opening to the surface as narrow slits (23-30 μ m wide) between adjacent dentine ridges. The presence of a pore-canal system in heterostracans, as in osteostracans, suggests that this group was electroreceptive.

Lateral line canals in *Eptatretus* have been described as short grooves or canals in front of and behind the eye (Ayers and Worthington, 1907). On examining *Eptatretus stouti*, it is possible to discern four short longitudinal lines running parallel to each other, rostral to the eye, and three similarly running short lines immediately caudal to the eye, as well as three additional lines running at right angles to these postorbital lines. These lines are easily seen in live specimens, as they lack pigmented cells and appear as pale lines against the darker epidermis. Histological examination reveals no true canal organization as initially described by Ayers and Worthington; rather, these lines consist of shallow open grooves. Ayers and Worthington claimed that spindle-shaped neuromasts occur at the base of the lateral line grooves. However, ultrastructural observations by Fernholm (this volume) have not confirmed this earlier report. Similar lines do not appear to occur in *Myxine*.

There is similar confusion concerning the possible existence of lateral line nerves in myxinoids. A buccal nerve emerges from the medulla, immediately anterior and dorsal to the utricular nerve (Fig. 3), and can be traced into the skin as well as seen to join with branches of the ophthalmic nerve (Peters, 1963). It has been unclear whether the buccal nerve should be considered part of the trigeminal or facial nerves. In transverse serial sections of *Eptatretus* it is clear that dorsally running branches of the buccal nerve ramify in the skin in the vicinity of the postorbital lines. The preorbital lines may be innervated by branches of buccal nerve, but neuroanatomical tracing techniques must be applied, as it is also possible that these more rostral lines are innervated by other rami. Experimental tracing of horseradish peroxidase applied to the proximal cut end of the buccal nerve in *Eptatretus* indicates that the axons of this nerve terminate in a dorsal portion of the octavolateralis column that is comparable to the medial nucleus in gnathostomes

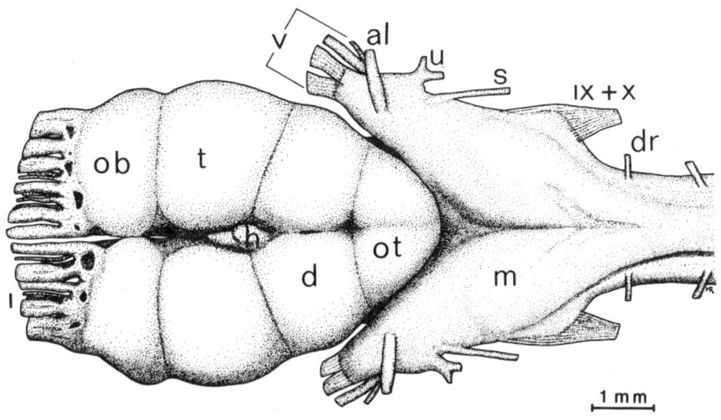

Fig. 3. Dorsal view of the brain of the Pacific hagfish, *Eptatretus stouti*. *al*, anterior lateral line (buccal) nerve; *d*, diencephalon; *dr*, dorsal root of spinal nerve; *h*, habenular nuclei; *m*, medulla oblongata; *ob* olfactory bulb; *ot*, optic tectum; *s*, saccular nerve; *t*, telencephalon; *u*, utricular nerve; *I*, olfactory nerve; *V*, trigeminal nerve; *IX* and *X*, glossopharyngeal and vagal nerves.

(Ronan and Northcutt, unpublished observations). These observations strongly support the interpretation that the buccal nerve of myxinoids is homologous to the anterior lateral line nerve of gnathostomes, and that the pre- and postorbital lines of *Eptatretus* are, in fact, lateralis lines. A posterior lateral line nerve or nervus acusticus b (Worthington, 1906) has been described in *Eptatretus*. However, horseradish peroxidase experiments on the glossopharyngeal-vagal complex in *Eptatretus* have not revealed a posterior lateral line nerve projection to the octavolateralis column.

Analysis of the variation of lateral line receptors and their distribution suggests that the ancestral vertebrates possessed at least three longitudinal lines or canals housing mechanoreceptive neuromasts and that these lines continued onto the trunk as dorsal, main, and ventral lines. It is also likely that these earliest vertebrates also possessed pit lines (free neuromast lines), but additional studies are needed to determine their exact number and topography. Similarly, the presence of a pore-canal system in both heterostracans and cephalaspidomorphs suggests that the earliest vertebrates possessed electroreceptors distributed on both the head and trunk.

Two hypotheses should be considered concerning the nature of the lateralis system of the earliest craniates. If the condition in myxinoids is plesiomorphic, the earliest craniates would be considered to have possessed a rudimentary lateral line system, restricted to the head and innervated only by an anterior lateral line nerve. The receptors of this system would have been limited to mechanoreceptors similar to neuromasts, and electroreception would be considered to have arisen with vertebrates. Alternately, if the condition in myxinoids is considered degenerate (apomorphic), then the heterostracan pattern is considered plesiomorphic for craniates, and myxinoids can be viewed as having evolved from early armored craniates that lost their dermal armor and much of their lateral line system in adapting to a burrowing existence. Again, in the absence of a relevant out-group for these characters, a decision must rest on arguments considering form-function suits and probabilities.

Gustatory organs

Anamniotic gnathostomes are characterized by at least two chemosensory systems in addition to the olfactory complex: a common chemical sense and a taste system mediated by specialized receptors, termed taste buds, and innervated by the facial, glossopharyngeal, and vagal cranial nerves (Finger, 1983). The common chemical sense is poorly understood, but is well developed on the pectoral fin rays of many teleost fishes and is mediated by nerves that end in small encapsulated endings, rather than on specialized chemoreceptors comparable to taste buds. Taste buds are generally found within various portions of the pharynx, as well as on the skin surface of the head and even the trunk in many jawed fishes. However, their distribution is poorly known, particularly for cartilaginous fishes, and it is presently impossible to determine the plesiomorphic condition for gnathostomes, *i.e.* whether taste buds were restricted to the pharynx primitively, or whether they occurred on the skin surface as well.

Taste buds initially occur on the inner surfaces of the pharyngeal bars in ammocoetes and are reported to occur secondarily in the skin of adults (Johnston, 1902, 1905). However, the receptors that Johnston described and termed end buds are known to be electroreceptors (Ronan and Bodznick, 1984). Microscopic examination of transverse sections through the heads of recently transformed *Petromyzon marinus* and adult *Ichthyomyzon unicuspis* do not reveal external taste buds. However, in *Lampetra*, Whitear and Lane (1983b) recently described isolated cells in the epidermis, which they termed oligovillous cells, that are suspected chemosensory receptors. These cells occur on both the head and trunk of ammocoetes, as well as adults, and are characterized by apical microvilli and a basal synapse constituted by a spur-like process of the neurite that indents the basal membrane of the oligovillous cell. These cells are suspected to be chemosensory, based on their similarity to teleost sensory cells. Thus it is possible that lampreys do not possess external taste buds but do possess chemoreceptors comparable to the common chemical sense of anamniotic gnathostomes.

There is little information on the distribution of taste buds in myxinoids. Histological sections of the head of *Eptatretus stouti* reveal taste buds distributed on the oral tentacles, on the skin at the base of the tentacles, in the epithelium of the opening of the prenasal duct, and, in particularly high densities, in the epidermis surrounding the mouth. Taste buds have been described on the tentacles of *Myxine* (Georgieva *et al.*, 1979). These buds consist of receptor cells with apical stereocilia and support cells bearing microvilli similar to the taste buds of other anamniotes. The pharyngeal surfaces have not been examined for the distribution of internal taste buds.

Taste buds clearly occur in representatives of all living groups of craniates and probably arose with the origin of craniates. At present it is impossible to decide whether they were restricted originally to the pharynx or whether they also occurred in the ectoderm. Although the skin of myxinoids has not been examined for the presence of single-celled chemoreceptors, it is likely that the earliest craniates possessed a common chemical sense.

Spinal and cranial nerves

The distribution of spinal and cranial nerves in lampreys has played a key role in speculations on the evolution of cranial nerves and head segmentation in craniates (Goodrich, 1930; Jarvik, 1980). Recent information from experimental neuroanatomical and embryological studies has forced a re-evaluation of a number of conclusions reached in earlier studies.

Spinal nerves

Gnathostomes are characterized by a single pair of spinal nerves per body segment. Each spinal nerve comprises a dorsal spinal root, bearing a sensory ganglion, and a ventral spinal root. These roots fuse peripherally and reiussue as a number of somatic and visceral rami. Traditionally, the spinal nerves of amniotes are believed to possess dorsal spinal roots composed solely of entering sensory neurites, whereas the ventral roots are believed to be composed solely of exiting motor axons. Recent studies (Willis and Coggeshall, 1978), however, have

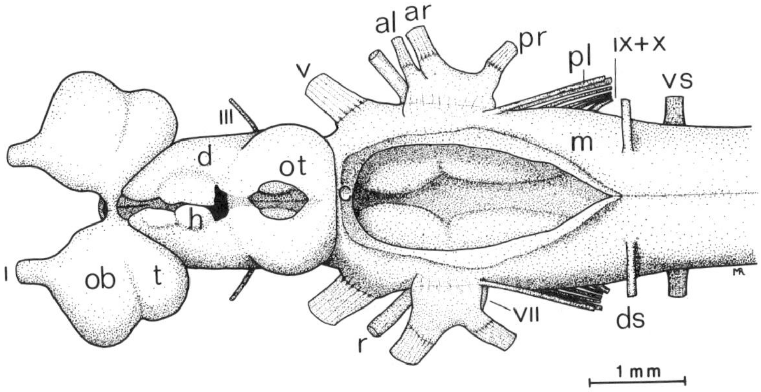

Fig. 4. Dorsal view of the brain of the silver lamprey, *Ichthyomyzon unicuspis*. *al*, anterior lateral line nerve; *ar*, anterior ramus of the otic nerve; *c*, cerebellum; *d*, diencephalon; *ds*, dorsal spinal nerve; *h*, habenular nuclei; *m*, medulla oblongata; *ob*, olfactory bulb; *ot* optic tectum; *pl*, posterior lateral line nerve; *pr*, posterior ramus of the otic nerve; *r*, ramus lateralis communicans; *t*, telencephalon; *vs*, ventral spinal nerve; *I*, olfactory nerve; *III*, oculomotor nerve; *V*, trigeminal nerve; *VII*, facial nerve; *IX* and *X*, glossopharyngeal and vagal nerves.

demonstrated that a total separation of sensory and motor fibers does not occur in mammals. Comparable information does not exist for nonmammalian gnathostomes, but the plesiomorphic pattern for gnathostomes is clearly a single pair of spinal nerves per body segment.

Lampreys differ from gnathostomes in possessing two pairs of spinal nerves per body segment. Dorsal and ventral nerves alternate (Fig. 4) and do not unite but course peripherally as totally distinct rami. The dorsal spinal nerve, like that in gnathostomes, possesses a sensory ganglion. Traditionally, the dorsal spinal nerve in lampreys is believed to comprise somatic and visceral sensory fibers, as well as all visceral motor axons, whereas the ventral spinal nerves are said to consist only of somatic motor axons (Johnston, 1902). Visceral fibers have been reported in the ventral spinal nerves, however (Healey, 1972).

Myxinoids possess a single pair of spinal nerves per segment (Peters, 1963). Although symmetry of the spinal nerves is not precise, in that dorsal and ventral spinal roots alternate, these roots fuse peripherally to form a single nerve. Goodrich (1937) concluded that fusion of the spinal roots in myxinoids parallels that in gnathostomes, based on the relationship of segmental arteries to these roots and on embryological evidence derived from *Eptatretus*.

Although the components of the spinal nerves in myxinoids have not been determined experimentally, it is possible that the dorsal and ventral roots consist predominantly of sensory and motor fibers, respectively (Peters, 1963).

There is little information regarding the spinal nerves in osteostracans and heterostracans. Stensiö (1927) noted that the foramina for the spinal nerves in the occipital region of the osteostracan shield alternate dorsally and ventrally, and he concluded that osteostracans, like lampreys, possessed separate dorsal and ventral spinal nerves. However, fusion of dorsal and ventral roots in both myxinoids (Peters, 1963) and gnathostomes occurs lateral to the chordal sheath, and thus it is impossible to determine what pattern existed in osteostracans. Similarly, neither a calcified neurocranium nor a chordal sheath occurred in heterostracans, so nothing is known regarding the distribution of spinal nerves.

Given the difference in the pattern of dorsal and ventral spinal root fusion in myxinoids and gnathostomes, it is probable that the earliest craniates possessed separate dorsal and ventral spinal nerves, as do living lampreys.

Cranial nerves

The cranial, or cephalic, nerves of craniates have traditionally been grouped into three phylogenetic categories: 1) ventral cranial nerves (III, IV, VI, and XII) that are serially homologous to the ventral spinal nerves of lampreys; 2) dorsal cranial nerves (V_1, V_2, VII, IX, and X) that are serially homologous to the dorsal spinal nerves in lampreys; and 3) special sensory cranial nerves (O, I, II, and VIII and the lateral line nerves) that arise embryonically from neurogenic placodal tissue (see Goodrich, 1930 and Jarvik, 1980 for reviews of the earlier literature). The optic "nerve" is usually removed from consideration, as it is not a true nerve but a neural tract formed by evagination of a part of the wall of the neural tube.

The special sensory cranial nerves have already been discussed and few details need be added. It is likely that the terminal nerve (o) arose with gnathostomes; it is probably a special sensory nerve and should not be interpreted as evidence of an additional head segment anterior to a premandibular segment. Gustation is usually considered to be mediated by special visceral sensory fibers of the facial, glossopharyngeal, and vagal nerves, which are serially homologous to visceral sensory components of the dorsal spinal nerves of lampreys. However, the glossopharyngeal and vagal nerves possess separate dorsal and ventral ganglia that arise from neural crest and epibranchial placodes, respectively (D'Amico-Martel and Noden, 1983). Although the facial nerve possesses a single ganglion, it also arises from neural crest and epibranchial placodal tissues. If taste buds are innervated by ganglion cells that arise from epibranchial placodes, as has been proposed (Landacre, 1910), there is no basis for comparing the gustatory nerves to spinal nerves. Rather, these nerves should be viewed as a special series of cephalic nerves, like lateral line nerves, that have no trunk equivalent.

Dorsal and ventral cranial nerve series have been recognized on the basis that these nerves, like those in the trunk of lampreys, innervate myotomal and hypomeric (lateral plate mesoderm) derivatives, respectively. However, recent experimental embryological studies reveal that the head branchiomeres arise from paraxial mesoderm rather than lateral plate mesoderm (Noden, 1983). Thus the branchiomeric motor column of the brain stem must be considered a special somatic motor column rather than a special visceral motor column (Gans and Northcutt, 1985). Thus, dorsal cranial nerves in lampreys are characterized by a sizeable somatic motor component that innervates striated branchiomeric muscles. A similar pattern of organization exists in the cephalic dorsal nerves of *Branchiostoma* (Bone, 1961) which suggests that this is a plesiomorphic pattern for cephalochordates and craniates. This suggests that head and trunk "myotomal" innervation differs fundamentally in all craniates.

There are additional problems with viewing the ventral cranial nerves as serially homologous to lamprey ventral spinal nerves, beyond the fact that all somatic motor fibers are not restricted to the ventral cranial nerves. Both the hypobranchial head muscles and the extrinsic eye muscles are said to arise from head somites. Although experimental evidence indicates that this is true of the hypobranchial muscles, a recent experimental study claims that the extrinsic eye muscles of birds arise from the prechordal plate (Wachtler *et al.*, 1984) rather than paraxial mesoderm. This observation, in conjunction with the dorsal rather than ventral course of the trochlear nerve, suggests that the pro-otic region of the craniate head may be organized in a profoundly different manner than the postotic region (Gans and Northcutt, 1983).

In this context, there is considerable debate in the literature regarding the original components comprising the nervus profundus (V_1 or the deep ophthalmic nerve) of craniates. Stensiö (1927) in his reconstruction of the head organization of osteostracans, suggested that the nervus profundus innervated a fully formed premandibular pouch. Subsequently, Whiting (1972) questioned Stensiö's interpretation and reinterpreted the head organization of osteostracans to be similar to modern lampreys. Given these conflicting interpretations of canals in fossil neurocrania, it seems preferable to accept the condition in myxinoids and lampreys as plesiomorphic, *i.e.* that the mandibular branchiomere is the most rostral pharyngeal segment, and the nervus profundus is not serially homologous to more dorsal cephalic nerves.

Reinterpretation of head segmentation theory in the context of new information suggests that the earliest craniates possessed dorsal spinal nerves with external ganglia and ventral spinal nerves, as in lampreys. In the earliest craniates, the head was characterized by a series of dorsal cephalic nerves that included somatic motor axons innervating branchiomeres, as well as a series of special sensory nerves that included a number of gustatory and lateral line nerves. The caudal region of the head exhibited a series of ventral cephalic nerves that innervated postotic muscles derived from myotomes. It is unclear, however, whether these myotomes developed *in situ* or migrated, in part, to form a hypobranchial series. Similarly, it is impossible to determine whether pro- otic "myotomal" muscles even existed in association with the rostral head skeleton or whether they were modified as extrinsic eye muscles. It is possible that these eye muscles developed with the origin of myopterygians.

Brain

In all craniates the brain arises embryonically from a neural plate that transforms into a hollow tube by either invagination or delamination. Similarly, in all living craniates the neural tube subsequently divides into a hind-, mid-, and forebrain by differential growth of the tube. The similarities in the embryology and cytology of these subdivisions support the view that the brains of the earliest craniates must have been similarly divided.

In gnathostomes further development of the brain is characterized by rapid growth of the side-walls and rostral roof (rhombic lip) of the hindbrain that results in the medulla oblongata and cerebellum, respectively. In contrast, a large portion of the hindbrain roof does not thicken but forms the thin roof (tela choroidea) of the fourth ventricle. In lampreys the hindbrain (Fig. 4) exhibits an expansive fourth ventricle but has a poorly developed rhombic lip that has traditionally been identified as a cerebellum (Johnston, 1902). This "cerebellum", however, is not organized into the same layers in lampreys, nor does it exhibit the same classes of neurons as does the cerebellum of gnathostomes (Larsell, 1967). This brain division in lampreys may be comparable only to the eminentia granularis, a closely related cellular population that also arises from the rhombic lip in gnathostomes. This hypothesis can be tested by examining the efferent pathways of this cell group in lampreys, as the eminentia granularis and cerebellum in gnathostomes possess very different efferent connections.

The brain of one osteostracan, *Kiaeraspis*, has been reconstructed (Stensiö, 1927, 1963) to show a cerebellum as large, proportionally, as the optic tectum in lampreys (Fig. 4). The endocranial cast of *Kiaeraspis* is expanded in the region that would correspond to a cerebellum, but the neurocranium of lampreys is similarly expanded and houses a greatly enlarged tela choroidea of the fourth ventricle. Thus the rhombic lip of osteostracans may have been no better developed than that of lampreys.

In myxinoids, the hindbrain (Fig. 3) is foreshortened in comparison to that of other craniates, and the fourth ventricle is extremely small. The reduced ventricular system is known to be derived, as in early embryonic stages the brain of *Myxine* exhibits a well developed ventricular system (Holmgren, 1946). The absence of much of the ventricular system and the rather uniform development of the more rostral lobes of the brain has complicated the recognition of homologies with brain divisions in other craniates (Worthington, 1906; Holmgren, 1919; Jansen, 1930; Bone, 1963). The lobes immediately rostral to the fourth ventricle (Fig. 3) have been interpreted as a cerebellum (Worthington, 1906; Holmgren, 1919) and as the midbrain roof (Jansen, 1930). Recent experimental neuroanatomical studies of *Eptatretus* (Amemiya, 1983; Kusunoki and Amemiya, 1983) clearly demonstrate that this division is homologous to the midbrain roof and that a cerebellum does not exist in myxinoids.

Interpretations of the hindbrain of heterostracans, based on impressions on the inner surface of the dorsal shield suggest that a cerebellum, if present, must have been relatively small, as in lampreys (Whiting and Tarlo, 1965).

These observations suggest that the hindbrain of the earliest craniates was relatively thin-walled with a large fourth ventricle, as in lampreys. A small cerebellum may have existed, or the rhombic lip may have consisted only of an eminentia granularis, and the cerebellum may have arisen with the origin of gnathostomes.

In all craniates the midbrain comprises a roof, or optic tectum, and a floor, or tegmentum (Figs. 3, 4). The optic tectum is usually bilobed and is a major target of the optic tracts. The optic tectum of lampreys, unlike that of gnathostomes, is characterized by a tela choroidea (Fig. 4). Myxinoids do not possess such a midbrain tela and have only a very reduced midbrain ventricle (Jansen, 1930). The neural impressions on the shield of heterostracans, however, suggest that these taxa possessed an optic tectum and a tela choroidea comparable to those in lampreys (Whiting and Tarlo, 1965). Thus a bilobed optic tectum with a well developed tela choroidea is likely the plesiomorphic condition for craniates.

The forebrain in all living craniates is subdivided into a caudal diencephalon and a more rostral telencephalon. The telencephalon forms telencephalic hemispheres by evagination, except in ray-finned fishes where the hemispheres form by eversion (Northcutt, 1981). In all craniates the hemispheres form rostral evaginations termed the olfactory bulbs (Figs. 3, 4). These similarities suggest that the earliest craniates also possessed paired hemispheres and olfactory bulbs that formed by evagination.

The forebrain of post-embryonic myxinoids exhibits only traces of the ventricular system (Jansen, 1930). Conel (1929) believed this reduction was due to embryonic growth within the supposed rigidity of an enclosing egg shell. However, recent studies (Platel and Delfini, 1981; Ebinger *et al.*, 1983) have demonstrated that the brain of myxinoids is several times larger than that of lampreys of comparable body weight. Not only are most brain regions larger in hagfishes than in lampreys of comparable size, many of these neural regions also possess more migrated and differentiated cell populations (Northcutt, 1981; Ronan, 1983). Thus the ventricular reduction in hagfishes is more likely related to expansion and differentiation of the walls of the neural tube than to external mechanical restraints on the embryo. In this context, it is probable that the relatively large telencephalon and medulla of hagfishes are related to well developed olfactory and tactile modalities and may be autapomorphic characters of myxinoids. Only the relatively small size of the optic tectum and octavolateralis column, as well as the absence of a cerebellum and motor nuclei for the innervation of extrinsic eye muscles, should be viewed as plesiomorphic or autapomorphic (degenerative) neural characters.

A description of the individual cell populations in the brains of hagfishes (Jansen, 1930; Bone, 1963) and lampreys (Johnston, 1902; Heier, 1948; Schober, 1964; Nieuwenhuys, 1977) and their interconnections is beyond the scope of this paper. Many, if not most, of the cell populations identified in the brains of gnathostomes can be recognized in hagfishes and lampreys. Unfortunately, there is little experimental information on the connections of these cell groups. In hagfishes, there are experimental neuroanatomical studies of the primary retinal efferents (Kusunoki and Amemiya, 1983) and the ascending and descending spinal pathways (Ronan, 1983). In lampreys, experimental data exist for the primary retinal efferents (Kennedy and Rubinson, 1977; Vesselkin *et al.*, 1980), the locations and laterality of the motor nuclei that innervate extrinsic eye muscles (Finger and Rovainen, 1978), the primary projections of the trigeminal nerve (Northcutt, 1979a) and the octaval nerve (Northcutt, 1979b), and the ascending and descending spinal pathways (Ronan, 1983). The extensive literature on the neurophysiology of lampreys has been recently reviewed (Rovainen, 1979, 1982). In the absence of extensive experimental studies of the interconnections of the cell populations in the brains of hagfishes and lampreys, it is impossible to make any meaningful statements regarding the origin and subsequent phylogeny of neural pathways in craniates.

Conclusions

As noted in the introduction, a reconstruction of a morphotype for the sense organs and brain of the earliest craniates requires that the polarity of neural characters in living craniates be established, and the conclusions drawn from such an analysis of polarity are themselves affected by the possible hypotheses of phyletic relationships. The present survey suggests that cephalaspidomorphs constitute a monophyletic group based on the following synapomorphies: 1) dorsocaudal naso-hypophyseal duct; 2) a reduced or absent supraorbital head lateral line; and 3) a ramus lateralis communicans. However, the ramus lateralis communicans may be a synapomorphy of vertebrates, as the presence of a pore-canal system (possibly indicative of electroreceptors) on the trunk of heterostracans raises the possibility that these receptors also may have been innervated by a recurrent branch of the anterior lateral line nerve. In fact, trunk electroreceptors innervated by a recurrent ramus could be a plesiomorphic character of craniates if the lateral line system of myxinoids is interpreted as degenerate.

The only neural characters possibly linking petromyzontids and gnathostomes are cathodal electroreceptors and their associated central pathways and an eminentia granularis. This assumes that the absence of these characters in myxinoids is a primitive condition. If the lateral line system of myxinoids is considered degenerate, these characters may be assumed to be primitive for craniates.

Janvier's (1981) hypothesis that heterostracans are the sister group of myopterygians involves two proposed synapomorphic neural characters: two vertical semicircular canals and a well developed lateral line system. Although it is true that myxinoids appear to possess only a single semicircular canal, they do possess anterior and posterior vertical cristae. Thus, neurologically, there is really no difference between hagfishes and lampreys with respect to this character. Interpretation of the lateral line system as a synapomorphy of vertebrates requires that the condition in hagfishes be considered primitive and not degenerate.

It is difficult, if not impossible, to determine the primitive state of many of the characters that would constitute a morphotype of the sense organs and brain of the earliest craniates, as many characters in myxinoids are different from those in petromyzontids and gnathostomes. Therefore it is impossible to decide whether these myxinoid characters are primitive or derived in the absence of a relevant outgroup for these characters or ontogenetic information on the characters. For this reason, ontogenetic studies of myxinoids are critically needed.

Many of the character differences between myxinoids and other craniates (poorly organized lateral line system, presumed absence of electroreceptors, absence of pineal and parapineal eyes, poorly organized lateral eyes and absence of extrinsic eye muscles, absence of mineralized dermal skeleton, and absence of arcual elements) can be interpreted as characterizing primitive craniates, or they may be derived (degenerative) characters of myxinoids, perhaps resulting from ancestral myxinoids adopting a burrowing niche (Hardisty, 1979).

Although a degenerate condition due to burrowing might be a reasonable hypothesis to account for the presumed loss of dermal armor, elongation of the prenasal ducts and body, and reduction of the lateral line system and vision, it is a *post hoc* conclusion and is useful only if the hypothesis can be tested. It should be possible to test this hypothesis by first listing the myxinoid characters that are suspected to have undergone degeneration in relation to burrowing and comparing these characters to those in other taxonomic groups, particularly marine burrowers. For example, do teleost or apodan burrowers exhibit similar reductions? Similarly, myxinoids are characterized by large and complex olfactory and trigeminal systems, as well as an extensive external chemosensory system, which may be derived specializations for burrowing. Do other craniate taxa exhibit similar sensory specializations associated with burrowing?

Excluding the neural characters that differ in myxinoids from those in other craniates, because we can not presently determine their polarity, it is possible to argue that the earliest craniates must have possessed paired olfactory organs, lateral eyes, paired otic organs with at least a single macula communis and two vertical semicircular cristae, and pharyngeal taste buds. They probably also possessed a common chemical sense and, possibly, simple skin photoreceptors. Similarly, they probably possessed a lateral line system, but it is presently impossible to conclude whether it was restricted to the head or extended onto the trunk, and whether it comprised both mechanoreceptors and electroreceptors or only one or the other.

If the unique neural characters of myxinoids are concluded to be apomorphic and associated with burrowing, then the earliest craniates were also likely characterized by pineal and parapineal eyes, otic organs that included a macula neglecta, and head and trunk lateral line systems that included electro- and mechanoreceptors.

The earliest craniates probably possessed separate dorsal and ventral spinal nerves like those of lampreys. The cephalic nerves probably consisted of dorsal and ventral nerves. The dorsal nerves would have innervated branchiomeric derivatives as well as ectodermal and endodermal sense organs, with the exception of lateral line receptors and taste buds. These receptors would have been innervated by special lateral line and gustatory cephalic nerves, respectively. The nervus profundus initially may have been a member of the dorsal series, or it may have been an additional special sensory nerve. The ventral cephalic nerves occurred post-otically and innervated epibranchial and hypobranchial head muscles. It is uncertain whether or not ventral cephalic nerves originally occurred rostral to the otic capsule.

The brain to body weight ratio of the earliest craniates was probably similar to that of modern lampreys, and the brain was divided into a hind-, mid- and forebrain. The hindbrain was characterized by an extensive fourth ventricle, and the rhombic lip was poorly developed and possibly consisted of only an eminentia granularis. The midbrain roof was formed by paired optic tecta, partially divided by a tela choroidea, and the forebrain was divided into a rostral telencephalon and a caudal diencephalon. The telencephalon comprised paired hemispheres and olfactory bulbs, both of which developed ontogenetically by evagination. It is probable that the internal organization of the brain of the earliest craniates was most similar to that of lampreys among living taxa.

Acknowledgements

I would like to thank Richard L. Puzdrowski and Dr. Mario Wullimann for critically reading the manuscript and offering many helpful suggestions. Dr. Mark C. Ronan kindly gave me permission to use two of his drawings in Figs. 3 and 4. In retrieving references for this work, Pat Kay displayed amazing persistence, for which I am very grateful. Mary Sue Northcutt has assisted in many phases of my own research and in the preparation of the manuscript. This work was supported in part by NIH Research Grants NS11006 and EY02485.

Literature Cited

AMEMIYA, F. 1983. Afferent connections to the tectum mesencephali in the hagfish, *Eptatretus burgeri*: an HRP study. J. Hirnforsch. **24**: 225-236.

ARIËNS KAPPERS, C.U. 1929. The evolution of the nervous system. Bohn, Haarlem.

AYERS, H. 1892. Vertebrate cephalogenesis. II. A contribution to the morphology of the vertebrate ear, with a reconsideration of its function. J. Morph. **6**: 1-360.

AYERS, H., and J. WORTHINGTON. 1907. The skin end-organs of the trigeminus and lateralis nerves of *Bdellostoma dombeyi*. Amer. J. Anat. **7**: 327-336.

BARRY, M.A., and R.L. BOORD. 1984. The spiracular organ of sharks and skates: anatomical evidence indicating a mechanoreceptive role. Science **226**: 990-992.

BJERRING, H.C. 1984. Major anatomical steps toward craniotedness: a heterodox view based largely on embryological data. J. Vert. Paleontol. **4**: 17-29.

BODZNICK, D., and R.G. NORTHCUTT. 1981. Electroreception in lampreys: evidence that the earliest vertebrates were electroreceptive. Science **212**: 465-467.

BODZNICK, D., and D.G. PRESTON. 1983. Physiological characterization of electroreceptors in the lampreys *Ichthyomyzon unicuspis* and *Petromyzon marinus* J. comp. Physiol. **152**: 209-217.

BONE, Q. 1961. The organization of the atrial nervous system of amphioxus (*Branchiostoma lanceolatum* Pallas.). Phil. Trans. R. Soc. (Lond.) **24B**: 241-269.

BONE, Q. 1963. The central nervous system. pp. 50-91 *In* Brodal, A., and R. Fänge [eds.] The biology of *Myxine*. Universitetsforlaget, Oslo.

BULLOCK, T.H., D.A. BODZNICK, and R.G. NORTHCUTT. 1983. The phylogenetic distribution of electroreception: evidence for convergent evolution of a primitive vertebrate sense modality. Brain Res. Rev. **6**: 25-46.

COLLIN, J.P. 1969. La cupule sensorielle de l'organe pineal de la lamproie de planer. Archs. Anat. Microsc. Morph. Exp. **58**: 145-182.

CONEL, J.L. 1929. The development of the brain of *Bdellostoma stouti*, I. External growth changes. J. comp. Neurol. **47**: 343-403.

CONEL, J.L. 1931. The development of the brain of *Bdellostoma stouti*, II. Internal growth changes. J. comp. Neurol. **52**: 365-501.

CRIM, J.W., A. URANO, and A. GORBMAN. 1979. Immunocytochemical studies of luteinizing hormone-releasing hormone in brains of agnathan fishes. I. Comparisons of adult Pacific lamprey (*Entosphenus tridentata*) and the Pacific hagfish (*Eptatretus stouti*). Gen. comp. Endocrinol. *37*: 294-305.

DAMAS, H. 1944. Recherches sur le développement de *Lampetra fluviatilis* L. Arch de Biol. **55**: 1-284.

D'AMICO-MARTEL, A., and D.M. NODEN. 1983. Contributions of placodal and neural crest cells to avian cranial peripheral ganglia. Amer. J. Anat. **166**: 445-468.

DEMSKI, L.S. 1984. The evolution of neuroanatomic substrates of reproductive behaviour: sex steroid and LHRH-specific pathways including the terminal nerve. Amer. Zool. **24**: 809-830.

DEMSKI, L.S., and R.G. NORTHCUTT. 1983. The terminal nerve: a new chemosensory system in vertebrates? Science **220**: 435-437.

DENISON, R.H. 1947. The exoskeleton of *Tremataspis*. Amer. J. Sci. **254**: 337-365.

DENISON, R.H. 1964. The cyathaspididae. Fieldiana. **13**: 309-473.

DOHRN, A. 1883. Studien zur Urgeschichte des Wirbeltierekörpers. III. Die Entstehung und Bedeutung der Hypophysis bei *Petromyzon planeri*. Pubbl. Staz. zool. Napoli **4**: 172-189.

EAKIN, R.M. 1973. The third eye. University of California Press, Berkeley.

EBINGER, P., K. WÄCHTLER, and S. STÄHLER. 1983. Allometrical studies in the brain of cyclostomes. J. Hirnforsch. **24**: 545-550.

EDDY, J.M.P. 1969. Metamorphosis and the pineal complex in the brook lamprey, *Lampetra planeri*. J. Endocrinol. **44**: 451-452.

EDDY, J.M.P. 1970. The structure and function of the pineal complex of *Lampetra* spp. Ph.D. Thesis. University of Wales.

EDDY, J.M.P. 1972. The pineal complex. pp. 91-103 *In* Hardisty, M.W., and I.C.

Potter [eds.] The biology of lampreys, vol. 2. Academic Press, New York.
EDDY, J.M.P., and R. STRAHAN. 1968. The role of the pineal complex in the pigmentary effector system of the lampreys, *Mordacia mordax* (Richardson) and *Geotria australis* Gray. Gen. comp. Endocrinol. **11**: 528-534.
ELDREDGE, N., and J. CRACRAFT. 1980. Phylogenetic patterns and the evolutionary process. Columbia University Press, New York.
FERNHOLM, B., and K. HOLMBERG. 1975. The eyes in three genera of hagfish (*Eptatretus, Paramyxine* and *Myxine*)--a case of degenerative evolution. Vision Res. **15**: 253-259.
FINGER, T.E. 1983. The gustatory system in teleost fish. pp. 285-309 *In* Northcutt, F.G., and R.E. Davis [eds.] Fish neurobiology, vol. 1. University of Michigan Press, Ann Arbor.
FINGER, T.E., and C.M. ROVAINEN. 1978. Retrograde HRP labeling of the oculomotoneurons in adult lampreys. Brain Res. **154**: 123-127.
FRITZSCH, B., M.D. CAPRON DE CAPRONA, K. WÄCHTLER, and K.H. KÖRTJE. 1984. Neuroanatomical evidence for electroreception in lampreys. Z. Naturforsch. **39**: 856-858.
FÜRBRINGER, M. 1897. Über die spino-occipitalen Nerven der Selachier und Holocephalen und ihre vergleichende Morphologie. Festschrift zum 70sten Geburtstage von Carl Gegenbauer. **3**: 349-788.
GANS, C., and R.G. NORTHCUTT. 1983. Neural crest and the origin of vertebrates: a new head. Science **220**: 268-274.
GANS, C., and R.G. NORTHCUTT. 1985. Neural crest: the implications for comparative anatomy. *In* Duncker, H.R., and G. Fleischer [eds.] Functional morphology of vertebrates. Gustav Fischer Verlag, Stuttgart (in press).
GEORGIEVA, V., R.A. PATZNER, and H. ADAM. 1979. Transmissions- und rasterelektronen- mikroskopische Untersuchung an den Sinnesknospen der Tentakeln von *Myxine glutinosa* L. (Cyclostomata). Zoologica Scripta **8**: 61-67.
GOODRICH, E.S. 1930. Studies on the structure and development of vertebrates. Macmillan, London.
GOODRICH, E.S. 1937. On the spinal nerves of the myxinoidea. Quart. J. Microsc. Sci. **80**: 153-158.
HALSTEAD, L.B. 1973. The heterostracan fishes. Biol. Rev. **48**: 279-332.
HARDISTY, M.W. 1979. Biology of the cyclostomes. Chapman and Hall, London.
HEALEY, E.G. 1972. The central nervous system. pp. 307-372 *In* Hardisty, M.W., and I.C. Potter [eds.] The biology of lampreys, vol. 2. Academic Press, New York.
HEIER, P. 1948. Fundamental principles in the structure of the brain. A study of the brain of *Petromyzon fluviatilis!. Acta Anat.* **5**: 1-213.
HOLMGREN, N. 1919. Zur Anatomie des Gehirns von *Myxine*. Kungl. Svenska vet. Akad. Handl. **60**: 1-96.
HOLMGREN, N. 1942. General morphology of the lateral sensory line system of the head in fish. Kungl. Svenska vet. Akad. Handl. **20**: 1-46.
HOLMGREN, N. 1946. On two embryos of *Myxine glutinosa.* Acta Zool. (Stockh.) **27**: 1-90.
HOLMGREN, N., and T. PEHRSON. 1949. Some remarks on the ontogenetical development of the sensory lines on the cheek in fishes and amphibians. Acta Zool. (Stockh.) **30**: 249-314.
JANSEN, J. 1930. The brain of *Myxine glutinosa.* J. comp. Neurol. **49**: 359-507.

JANVIER, P. 1974a. The structure of the naso-hypophysial complex and the mouth in fossil and extant cyclostomes, with remarks on amphiaspiforms. Zoologica Scripta **3**: 193-200.

JANVIER, P. 1974b. The sensory line system and its innervation in the Osteostraci (Agnatha, Cephalaspidomorphi). Zoologica Scripta **3**: 91-99.

JANVIER, P. 1978. Les negeoires paires des Ostéostracés et la position systématique des Céphalaspidomorphes. Ann. de Paléontol. (Vertébres). **64**: 113-142.

JANVIER, P. 1981. The phylogeny of the craniata, with particular reference to the significance of fossil "agnathans". J. Vert. Paleontol. **1**: 121-159.

JANVIER, P., and A. BLIECK. 1979. New data on the internal anatomy of the Heterostraci (Agnatha), with general remarks on the phylogeny of the Craniota. Zoologica Scripta **8**: 287-296.

JARVIK, E. 1965. Die Raspelzunge der Cyclostomen und die pentadactyle extremität als Beweis für monophyletische Herkunft. Zool. Anz. **175**: 8-143.

JARVIK, E. 1980. Basic structure and evolution of vertebrates. 2 vols. Academic Press, London.

JOHNSTON, J.B. 1902. The brain of *Petromyzon* J. comp. Neurol. **12**: 1-86.

JOHNSTON, J.B. 1905. The cranial nerve components of *Petromyzon*. Morph. Jb. **34**: 149-203.

KENNEDY, M.C., and K. RUBINSON. 1977. Retinal projections in larval, transforming and adult sea lamprey, *Petromyzon marinus*. J. comp. Neurol. **171**: 465-480.

KIAER, J. 1930. *Ctenaspis*, a new genus of cyathaspidian fishes. Skr. Svalb. Ishavet. **33**: 1-7.

KLEEREKOPER, H. 1969. Olfaction in fishes. Indiana University Press, Bloomington.

KLEEREKOPER, H. 1972. The sense organs. pp. 373-404 *In* Hardisty, M.W., and I.C. Potter [eds.] The biology of lampreys, vol. 2. Academic Press, New York.

KUSUNOKI, T., and F. AMEMIYA. 1983. Retinal projections in the hagfish, *Eptatretus burgeri*. Brain Res. **262**: 295-298.

LANDACRE, F.L. 1910. The origin of the cranial ganglia in *Ameiurus*. J. comp. Neurol. **20**: 309-411.

LARSELL, O. 1967. The comparative anatomy and histology of the cerebellum from myxinoids through birds. University of Minnesota Press, Minneapolis.

LOCY, W.A. 1905a. On a newly recognized nerve connected with the forebrain of selachians. Anat. Anz. **26**: 33-63.

LOCY, W.A. 1905b. A footnote to the ancestral history of the vertebrate brain. Science **22**: 180-183.

LØVTRUP, S. 1977. The phylogeny of vertebrata. Wiley, London.

LOWENSTEIN, O., M.P. OSBORNE, and R.A. THORNHILL. 1968. The anatomy and ultrastructure of the labyrinth of the lamprey (*Lampetra fluviatilis* L.). Proc. Roy. Soc. (Lond.) **170B**: 113-134.

LOWENSTEIN, O., and R.A. THORNHILL. 1970. The labyrinth of *Myxine*: anatomy, ultrastructure and electrophysiology. Proc. R. Soc. (Lond.) **176B**: 21-42.

MARINELLI, W., and A. STRENGER. 1954. Vergleichende Anatomie und Morphologie der Wirbeltiere. 1: *Lampetra fluviatilis* L. Franz Deuticke, Vienna.

McCORMICK, C.A. 1982. The organization of the octavolateralis area in actinopterygian fishes: a new interpretation. J. Morph. **171**: 159-181.

McCREADY, P.J., and R.L. BOORD. 1976. The topography of the superficial roots and ganglia of the anterior lateral line nerve of the smooth dogfish, *Mustelus canis*. J. Morph. **150**: 527-538.

MEREDITH, G.E., and A. BUTLER. 1983. Organization of eighth nerve afferent projections from individual endorgans of the inner ear in the teleost, *Astronotus ocellatus*. J. comp. Neurol. **220**: 44-62.

MUNZ, H., W.E. STUMPF, and L. JENNES. 1981. LHRH systems in the brain of the platyfish. Brain Res. **221**: 1-13.

NEWTH, D.R., and D.M. ROSS. 1955. On the reaction to light of *Myxine glutinosa*. J. exp. Biol. **32**: 4-21.

NIEUWENHUYS, R. 1977. The brain of the lamprey in a comparative perspective. Ann. N. Y. Acad. Sci. **299**: 97-145.

NODEN, D.M. 1983. The embryonic origins of avian cephalic and cervical muscles and associated connective tissues. Amer. J. Anat. **168**: 257-276.

NORTHCUTT, R.G. 1979a. Experimental determination of the primary trigeminal projections in lampreys. Brain Res. **163**: 323-327.

NORTHCUTT, R.G. 1979b. Central projections of the eighth cranial nerve in lampreys. Brain Res. **167**: 163-167.

NORTHCUTT, R.G. 1981. Evolution of the telencephalon in nonmammals. Ann. Rev. Neurosci. **4**: 301-350.

NORTHCUTT, R.G. 1985. Electroreception in non-teleost bony fishes. *In* Bullock, T.H., and W. Heiligenberg [eds.] Electroreception. Wiley, New York, (in press).

NORTHCUTT, R.G., and C. GANS. 1983. The genesis of neural crest and epidermal placodes: a reinterpretation of vertebrate origins. Quart Rev. Biol. **58**: 1-28.

PATTERSON, C. 1982. Morphological characters and homology. pp. 21-74 *In* Joysey, K.A., and A.E. Friday [eds.] Problems of phylogenetic reconstruction. Academic Press, New York. Systematics Association Special Volume No. 21.

PEHRSON, T. 1949. The ontogeny of the lateral line system in the head of dipnoans. Acta Zool. (Stockh.) **30**: 153-182.

PETERS, A. 1963. The peripheral nervous system. pp. 92-123 *In* Brodal, A., and R. Fänge [eds.] The biology of *Myxine*. Universitetsforlaget, Oslo.

PLATE, L. 1924. Allgemeine Zoologie und Abstammungslehre. Vol. II. Die Sinesorgane der Tiere. G. Fischer, Jena.

PLATEL, R., and C. DELFINI. 1981. L'éncephalisation chez la myxine (*Myxine glutinosa* L.). Analyse quantifiée des principales subdivisions encéphaliques. Cah. Biol. Mar. **22**: 407-430.

POPPER, A.N., and R.G. NORTHCUTT. 1983. Structure and innervation of the inner ear of the bowfin, *Amia calva*. J. comp. Neurol. **213**: 279-286.

RONAN, M.C. 1983. Ascending and descending spinal projections in petromyzontid and myxinoid agnathans. Ph.D. thesis, University of Michigan.

RONAN, M.C., and D. BODZNICK. 1984. Identification of electroreceptors in lampreys. Soc. Neurosci. **10**: 853 (abst.).

RONAN, M.C., and R.G. NORTHCUTT. 1982. Primary projections of the lateral line nerves in the northern silver lamprey. Soc. Neurosci. **8**: 764 (abst.).

ROVAINEN, C.M. 1979. Neurobiology of lampreys. Physiol. Revs. **59**: 1007-1077.

ROVAINEN, C.M. 1982. Neurophysiology. pp. 1-136 *In* Hardisty, M.W. and I.C. Potter [eds.] The biology of lampreys, vol. 4A. Academic Press, London.

RUBEL, E.W. 1978. Ontogeny of structure and function in vertebrates auditory system. pp. 135-237 *In* Jacobson, M. [ed.] Handbook of sensory physiology, vol. 9. Development of Sensory Systems. Springer-Verlag, New York.

SCHOBER, W. 1964. Vergleichend-anatomische Untersuchungen am Gehirn der Larven und adulten Tiere von *Lampetra fluviatilis* (Linné, 1758) und *Lampetra planeri* (Bloch, 1784). J. Hirnforsch. **7**: 107-209.

SEYDEL, O. 1895. Über die Nasenhöhle und das Jacobson'sche Organ der Amphibien. Eine vergleichend-anatomische Untersuchung. Morph. Jb. **23**: 453-543.

SPRINGER, A.D. 1983. Centrifugal innervation of goldfish retina from ganglion cells of the nervus terminalis. J. comp. Neurol. **214**: 404-415.

STAHL, B.J. 1977. Early and recent primitive brain forms. Ann. N. Y. Acad. Sci. **299**: 87-96.

STENSIÖ, E.A. 1927. The Downtonian and Devonian vertebrates of Spitsbergen. 1. Family Cephalaspidae. Skr. Svalb. Ishavet. **12**: 1-391.

STENSIÖ, E.A. 1932. The Cephalaspids of Great Britain. The British Museum, London.

STENSIÖ, E.A. 1947. The sensory lines and dermal bones of the cheek in fishes and amphibians. Kungl. Svenska vet. Akad. Handl. **24**: 1-195.

STENSIÖ, E.A. 1963. The brain and cranial nerves in fossil, lower craniate vertebrates. Skrifter utgitt av Det Norske Videnskaps-Akademi. I. Mat. - Naturv. Klasse. Ny Serie. No. **13**: 1-120.

STENSIÖ, E.A. 1968. The cyclostomes with special reference to the diphyletic origin of the Petromyzontida and Myxinoidea. pp. 13-71 *In* Ørvig, T. [ed.] Current problems of lower vertebrate phylogeny. Proceedings of the Fourth Nobel Symposium. Wiley, New York.

THOMSON, K.S. 1977. On the individual history of cosmine and possible electroreceptive function of the pore-canal system in fossil fishes. pp. 247-270 *In* Andrews, S.M., R.S. Miles, and A.D. Walker. [eds.] Problems in vertebrate evolution. Linn. Soc. Symp. Ser. 4.

THORNHILL, R.A. 1972. The development of the labyrinth of the lamprey (*Lampetra fluviatilis* Linn. 1758). Proc. R. Soc. (Lond.) **181B**: 175-198.

VESSELKIN, N.P., T.V. ERMAKOVA, J. REPÉRANT. A.A. KOSAREVA, and N.B. KENIGFEST. 1980. The retinofugal and retinopetal systems in *Lampetra fluviatilis*. An experimental study using radioautographic and HRP methods. Brain Res. **195**: 453-460.

VON KUPFFER, C. 1894. Über Monorhinie and Amphirhinie. Sitzber. Math.-physik. Classe. Akad. Wiss. München. **24**: 51-60.

WACHTLER, F., H.J. JACOB. M. JACOB, and B. CHRIST. 1984. The extrinsic ocular muscles in birds are derived from the prechordal plate. Naturwissen. **71**: 379-380.

WHITE, E.I. 1935. The ostracoderm *Pteraspis* Kner and the relationships of the agnathous vertebrates. Phil. Trans. R. Soc. (Lond.) **225B**: 381-457.

WHITEAR, M., and E.B. LANE. 1983a. Multivillous cells: epidermal sensory cells of unknown function in lamprey skin. J. Zool. (Lond.) **201**: 259-272.

WHITEAR, M., and E.B. LANE. 1983b. Oligovillous cells of the epidermis: sensory elements of lamprey skin. J. Zool. (Lond.) **199**: 359-384.

WHITING, H.P. 1972. Cranial anatomy of the ostracoderms in relation to the organization of larval lampreys. pp. 1-20 *In* Joysey, K.A., and T.S. Kemp [eds.] Studies in vertebrate evolution. Winchester Press, New York.

WHITING, H.P., and L.B.H. TARLO. 1965. The brain of the Heterostraci (Agnatha). Nature **207**: 829-831.

WILEY, E.O. 1981. Phylogenetics. Wiley, New York.

WILLIS, W.D., and R.E. COGGESHALL. 1978. Sensory mechanisms of the spinal cord. Plenum, New York.

WILSON, H.V., and J.E. MATTOCKS. 1897. The lateral sensory anlage in the salmon. Anat. Anz. **13**: 658-660.

WORTHINGTON, J. 1906. The descriptive anatomy of the brain and cranial nerves of *Bdellostoma dombeyi*. Quart. J. Microsc. Sci. **49**: 137-181.

YNTEMA, C.L. 1937. An experimental study of the origin of the cells which constitute the VIIth and VIIIth ganglia and nerves in the embryo of *Amblystoma punctatum*. J. exp. Zool. **75**: 75-101.

YOUNG, J.Z. 1935a. The photoreceptors of lampreys. I. Light-sensitive fibres in the lateral line nerves. J. exp. Biol. **12**: 229-238.

YOUNG, J.Z. 1935b. The photoreceptors of lampreys. II. The function of the pineal complex. J. exp. Biol. **12**: 254-270.

THE LATERAL LINE SYSTEM OF CYCLOSTOMES

Bo Fernholm

Department of Vertebrate Zoology
Swedish Museum of Natural History
Stockholm, Sweden

Introduction

In 1907, Ayers and Worthington reported that they found "fully formed and functional" lateral line grooves in *Eptatretus stouti* (*Bdellostoma dombeyi*). Earlier scientists had not been able to find lateral line grooves in hagfish and the report of Ayers and Worthington has not been generally accepted in the textbooks (Hardisty, 1979, p. 10; Starck, 1982, p. 518).

There has been a tendency for European authors not to accept Ayers and Worthington's observation. The reason for this, it will be shown, is the generic difference between the hagfish species on the European Atlantic coast and in the Pacific.

On the other hand, the lamprey lateral line system was described by Maurer in 1895. It is aberrant (Holmgren, 1942), but clearly recognizable, although with some primitive characteristics (Yamada, 1973).

Materials and methods

Specimens of *Myxine glutinosa, Paramyxine atami, Eptatretus stouti, E. deani, E. burgeri* and *E. cirrhatus* were studied, by use of the dissecting microscope, for the presence of lateral lines on the head skin.

Only specimens of *E. stouti* and *E. burgeri*, with a total length of 205-510 mm, were studied by light and electron (SEM and TEM) microscopy.

For light microscopy, head skin samples were fixed in Bouin's fluid, embedded in paraffin, sectioned, and stained with iron haematoxylin/eosin.

Head skin biopsies were taken after anaesthesia in MS 222, fixed for SEM in 2% glutaraldehyde in diluted seawater (Holland and Jespersen, 1973), dehydrated in ethanol, dried by use of the Freon critical point method and mounted on specimen stubs covered with Scotch double-stick tape. The specimens were rotary coated with gold and viewed in Stereoscan S4 or Hitachi HHS-2R scanning electron microscopes.

For TEM, head skin biopsies were fixed in 3% glutaraldehyde in O.2 M phosphate buffer, pH 7.1, in 0.45 M sucrose. Postfixation was in 1% OsO_4 in the same buffer and, after dehydration in ethanol, specimens were embedded in Epon. Specimens of *Petromyzon fluviatilis* were studied macroscopically and under the dissecting microscope.

Results

The pit lines of lampreys are well known and were not studied in any detail. For comparison they are figured together with the lateral line system of *E. stouti* (Fig. 1). It is obvious from the first glance that the system is more elaborate in the lamprey and that the only similarity to be found at this level of observation is the localization on the head rostral and caudal to the eye.

It was not possible to find the lateral line system in *Myxine glutinosa*. In all species of *Eptatretus* and *Paramyxine*, however, it could be observed.

Macroscopically, the lines found on the head of *E. burgeri* or *E. stouti* could easily be distinguished on live or clean-fixed specimens. In fixed specimens there is frequently a layer of slime covering the whole animal, giving it a greyish appearance. If the slime is scraped off, the line can be found in the darker underlying skin. Species differences were not studied, but it appears that the main pattern is similar for all *Eptatretus* studied. Considerable individual variation was noted in *E. burgeri* and *E. stouti* in the number of grooves in the different locations. In the rostral line group the variation was from 2 to 5 parallel lines. In the caudal line group a similar variation could be noted in both the horizontal and vertical lines. In *Paramyxine* and *E. cirrhatus* the grooves in front of the eyes seemed to be missing.

In the light microscope (Fig. 2), cross-sectioned grooves appear as epithelial invaginations covered with cells having the same staining reaction as the rest of the epithelium surface cells. These cells are the small mucous cells (Blackstad 1963) with a characteristic dark staining (Fig. 2). Except for these cells the epidermis is composed of large mucous cells, thread cells and undifferentiated cells. The epidermis is about 200 μm (10 cell layers) thick. In the dermis beneath the groove, a concavity can be observed indicating the presence in the dermis of another groove corresponding to the epidermal one. In no case could any trace of a covered epidermal canal be found.

The scanning electron microscope clearly demonstrates the presence of an open, 10-30 μm wide groove (Fig. 3) and also reveals a certain surface specialization of the epidermal cells in the groove. The microvilli generally found on the epidermal

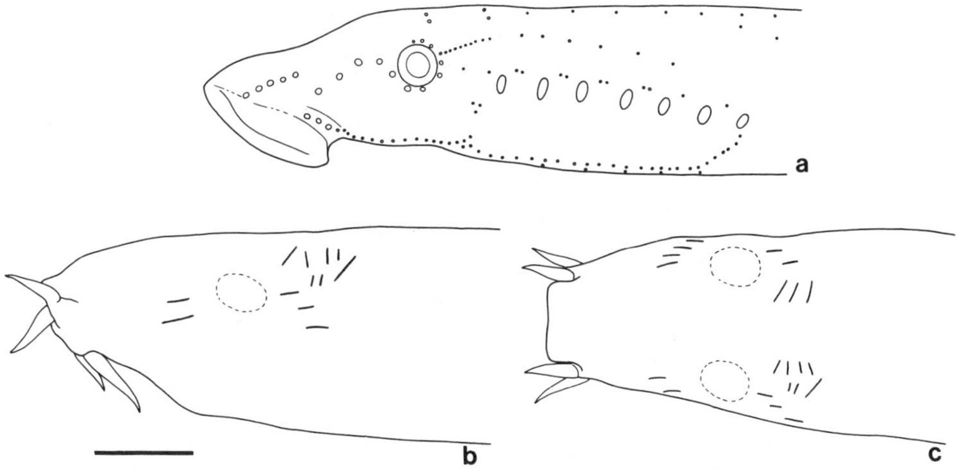

Fig. 1. Lateral line system of lamprey and hagfish. a) Head of *Petromyzon fluviatilis* (after Holmgren, 1942); b) head of 216 mm long specimen of *E. stouti*, from the left; c) from above. Eye spots indicated by dashed line in hagfish. Scale 10 mm.

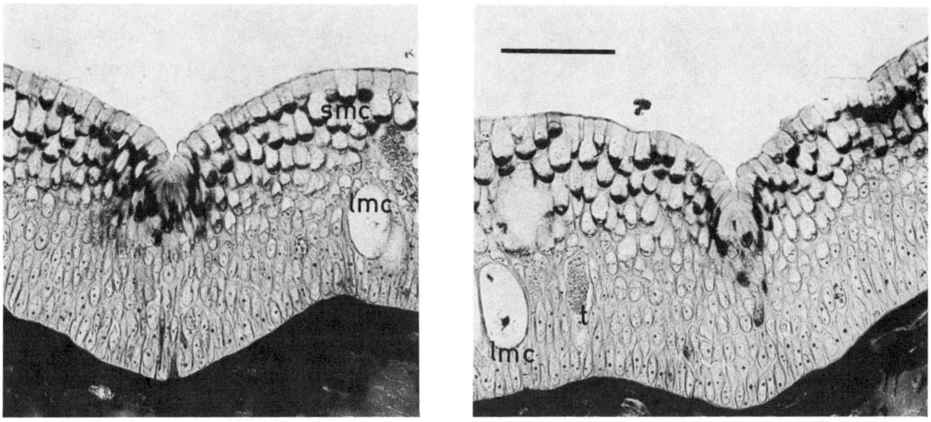

Fig. 2. Cross-sectioned grooves in the skin from the head of a 330 mm long specimen of *E. stouti*. Two parallel grooves from the same section are figured. *lmc*, large mucus cell; *smc*, small mucus cell; *t*, thread cell. LM. Scale 100 μm.

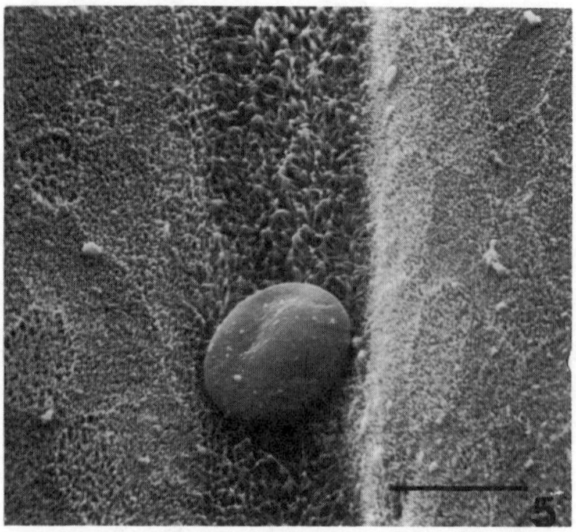

Fig. 5. Groove with one erythrocyte from 216 mm long specimen of *E. stouti*. Epidermal cell borders are seen except in the groove where the pattern is obscured by the longer microvilli. SEM, scale 10 μm.

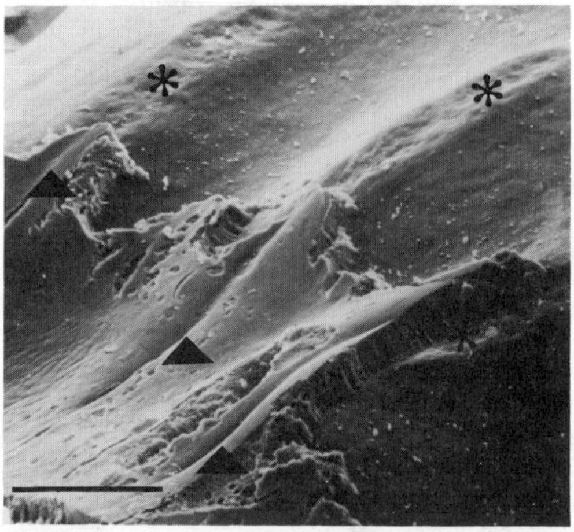

Fig. 6. Low magnification of same specimen as in Fig. 5. Epidermis partly removed. Top of triangles point at three parallel epidermal grooves and asterisks indicate corresponding grooves in underlying dermis. SEM, scale 400 μm.

surface are longer on the cells in the groove (Fig. 4 and 5). In some specimens more slime appears to be retained in the grooves than on the surrounding skin (Figs. 3,4). The SEM technique, in a specimen where the epidermis has been partly removed, is

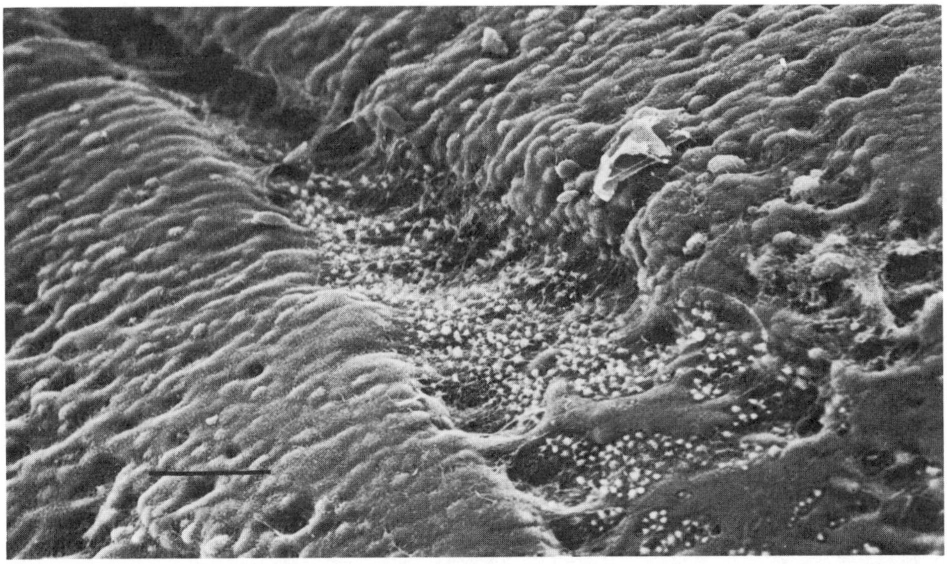

Fig. 3. Groove on head of 350 mm long specimen of *E. stouti*. SEM, scale 20 μ m.

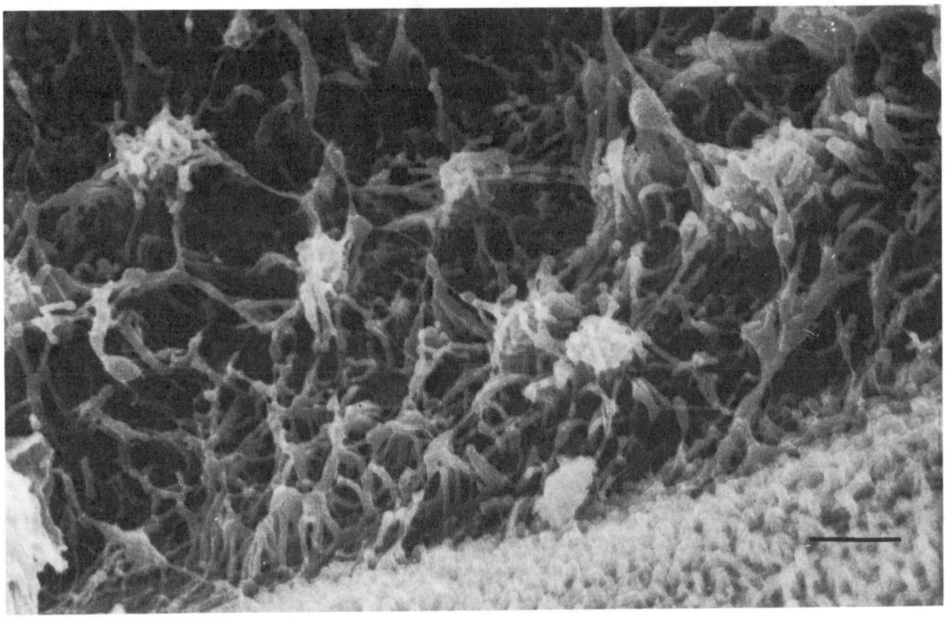

Fig. 4. Increased magnification of groove shown in Fig. 3. Borderline between "normal" epidermal cells (below) and groove or lateral line epidermal cells (above) with longer microvilli stuck together by remaining mucus. SEM, 1 μm.

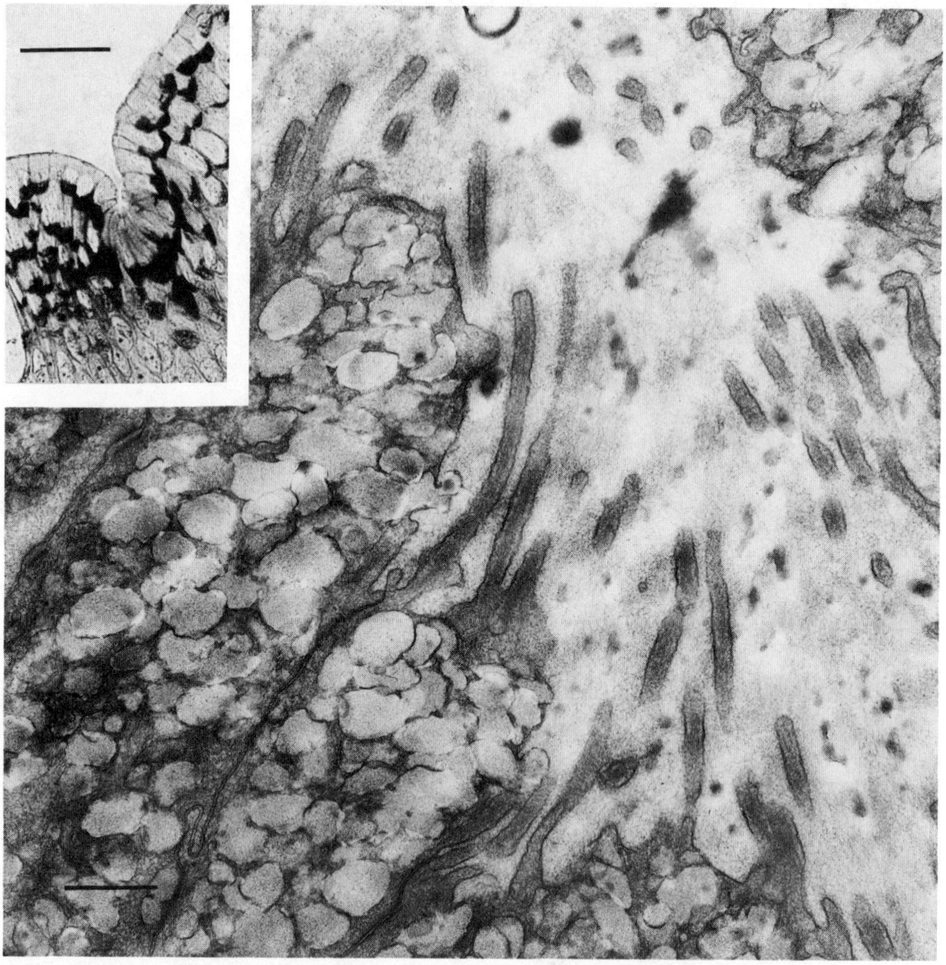

Fig. 7. Bottom of groove from head of 390 mm long specimen of *E. burgeri* showing the apical cytoplasm with light granuales and long microvilli. TEM, scale 0.5 μm. Inset. Third parallel groove from same section as in Fig. 2 to show staining reaction of cells in the groove. LM, scale 50 μm.

helpful in elucidating the dermal surface corresponding to the epidermal grooves (Fig. 6). Some cells had a projection bridging the narrow (10 μm wide) groove.

Studies of skin sections by transmission electron microscopy confirm that the cells in the grooves have the same general appearance as the other small mucous cells in the epidermal surface (Figs. 7 and 8). These cells have a basally situated nucleus surrounded by Golgi apparatus and basally fibrous material. It is this perinuclear

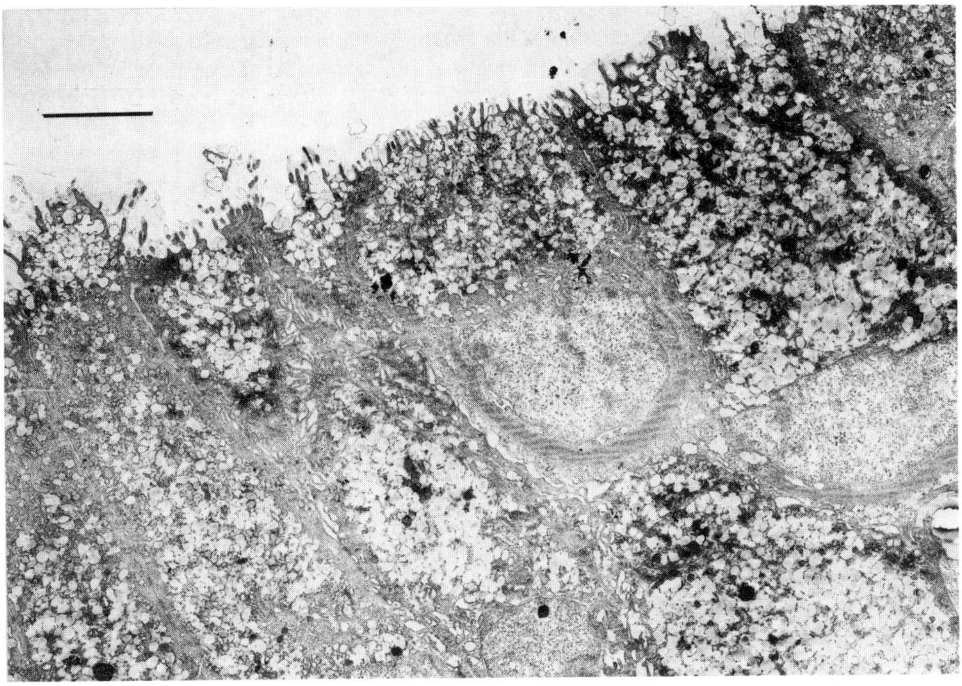

Fig. 8. Epidermis outside the groove from the same specimen of *E. burgeri* as in Fig. 7. Note cells of similar appearance as in the groove with light granules and microvilli. TEM, scale 50 μ m.

area that stains dark in light microscopy (Fig. 7 inset). The apical surface of the cells is covered with microvilli. The microvilli are about 0.1 μ m in diameter and about 1 μm long except in the grooves where they are about 2 μ m long. Most of the cell cytoplasm apical to the nucleus is filled with light granules, which are interpreted as secretory mucous granules. No cilia or innervation were observed.

It can thus be summarized that the cells found in the open grooves of the lateral line system seem to be slightly modified small mucous cells, the only observed difference being that the microvilli are longer and the cells are frequently more slender in the grooves.

Discussion

Part of the discrepancy in opinion over whether or not hagfish have a lateral line system can now be explained by the observed generic differences. A system of skin grooves was found in *Eptatretus* species from around the Pacific, while it was missing in *Myxine* of the Atlantic. Recently, McMillan and Wisner (1984) studied Pacific *Eptatretus* species and found that only two out of four species had the system. Wisner (personal communication) was also unable to find the system in two Pacific species of *Myxine*.

One important question, of course, is whether the organ that we can observe in *Eptatretus* is part of the octavo-lateralis system. With no ciliated cells, and no innervation found, it can certainly be argued otherwise. In the case of lampreys there can be no doubt. Specialized neuromast cells with cilia and innervation (Yamada, 1973) prove that it is an octavo-lateralis organ.

It is difficult to imagine how, and for what purpose, the observed "system" might function in *Eptatretus*. In *Petromyzon* the system is involved in electroreception (Bodznick and Northcutt, 1981). No electroreceptory capacity could be detected in *Eptatretus stouti* (Bullock *et al.*, 1982, and personal communication). If the organ had some sensory function it might logically be found in *Eptatretus* that is said to spend much time on the surface of the sea bottom (Worthington, 1905), and not in *Myxine*, that spends most of its time dug down into a muddy bottom.

One could argue that the hagfish organ might have a chemoreceptor function. However, that function is probably fulfilled by the taste buds found on the peri-oral tentacles, and sparsely in the skin at other locations (Georgieva *et al.*, 1979).

Boeke (1934) cites Plate (1924), and agrees that the closed canals observed in the epidermis by Ayers and Worthington (1907) are to be considered as artifacts. All figures of Ayers and Worthington (1907) seem to be from one and the same 11 inch long specimen, and I also believe that the closed canals are ruptures in the epidermis caused during the histological preparation. Two other misunderstandings seem to occur in Ayers and Worthington. They state that the same kind of "club-shaped bundles of spindle cells" that they find in the open grooves, also occur outside the grooves in the epidermis, and that nerve bundles run into them. Since, in most of these figures, nerves are from the tentacles (that is where taste buds are most easily observed) they may not have noted the difference between the cells of the open grooves and the innervated receptor cells of the taste buds. Secondly, since they do not show the thread cells of the epidermis, I suspect that they are interpreted as single sensory cells (Fig. 10, Ayers and Worthington, 1907).

Plate (1924) argues that the absence of the lateral line organ in *Myxine* is due to a secondary reduction coupled to their semi-parasitic way of life and that the reduction in *Eptatretus* has not proceeded so far, in that only the phylogenetically younger parts, *i.e.* the lateral lines on the body, have been lost (Plate, 1924, p. 90-91). However, Dean (1899, p. 273) observed that: "There is also no obvious evidence that an embryonic series of end-organs are present, comparable to a distinct lateral line." That may be taken as an indication that the system was never present laterally on the body.

As usual, when studying a primitive, but also obviously degenerate animal, we find it difficult to distinguish, for any one organ system, between what is degenerate and what is primitive.

The function of the so-called lateral line system of *Eptatretus* without ciliated receptor cells and without innervation cannot be important. Furthermore, another genus of hagfish, *Myxine*, obviously does quite well without it. Therefore, it seems to me most logical to support the idea that the line system found in *Eptatretus* is a degenerate, and not a functioning lateral line system. This assumption is further strengthened by the observation of the variability of the system found among hagfish genera and species (McMillan and Wisner, 1984), as well as the observed lateral variation within the same specimen.

The difference between the lamprey and hagfish lateral line systems pertains not only to the degree of degeneration of the organ in hagfish but also to the morphological type of organ. The lateral line system assumes three distinct and different morphological forms, *viz.* pit lines, sensory grooves and sensory canals. Generally the pit lines are considered to be more or less reduced canals or grooves (Holmgren, 1942). As has been noted, lampreys have a well developed pit line system while hagfish have a degenerate system with open grooves. The uncertainty about the degree of degeneration in hagfish makes it of doubtful significance to state functional lateral line systems as a synapomorphy for lampreys and gnathostomes (*cf.* Hardisty, 1979, p. 10). On the other hand the systems in hagfish and lampreys are so different that they in no way can be used to indicate a closer relationship between the two groups traditionally classified together as cyclostomes.

Acknowledgements

Thanks are due to Professor Kinoshita of the Misaki Marine Biological Station, Tokyo University, for supplying *E. burgeri* and working space, to R. McConnaughey, UCSD, for supplying *E. stouti* and *E. deani* and to N. Holland, UCSD, for supplying working space and help with electron microscopy at Scripps Institution of Oceanography.

The work was supported by grant B-BU 3501-100 from the Swedish Natural Science Research Council.

Literature Cited

AYERS, H., and J. WORTHINGTON. 1907. The skin end-organs of the trigeminus and lateralis nerves of *Bdellostoma dombeyi*. Amer. J. Anat. 7: 327.

BLACKSTAD, T.W. 1963. The Skin and the slime glands. *In* Brodal, A., and R. Fänge [eds.] The biology of *Myxine*. Oslo.

BODZNICK, D.A., and R.G. NORTHCUTT. 1981. Electroreception in lampreys: evidence that the earliest vertebrates were electroreceptive. Science **212**: 465-467.

BOEKE, J. 1934. Organe mit Endknospen und Endhugeln nebst eingesenkten Organen. pp. 949-988 *In* Bolck, L., E. Göbbert, E. Kallius, and W. Lubosch [eds.] Handbuch der vergleichenden Anatomie der Wirbeltiere. Urban & Scwarzenberg, Berlin.

BULLOCK, T.H., R.G. NORTHCUTT, and D.A. BODZNICK. 1982. Evolution of electroreception. Trends in Neuroscience. **5**: 50-53.

DEAN, B. 1899. On the embryology of *Bdellostoma stouti*. pp. 221-276 *In* Festschrift Carl v. Kuppfer. Jena.

GEORGIEVA, V., R.A. PATZNER, and H. ADAM. 1979. Transmissions- und raster-elektronenmikroskopische Untersuchung an den Sinnesknospen der

Tentaklen von *Myxine glutinosa* L. (Cyclostomata). Zool. Scripta. **8**: 61-67.
HARDISTY, M.V. 1979. Biology of the cyclostomes. Chapman and Hall, London.
HOLLAND, N.D., and A. JESPERSEN. 1973. The fine structure of the fertilization membrane of the feather star *Comanthus japonica* (Echinodermata: Crinoidea). Tissue & Cell **5**: 209-214.
HOLMGREN, N. 1942. General morphology of the lateral sensory line system of the head in fish. KVA Handl. **20**: 1-46.
MAURER, F. 1895. Die Epidermis und ihre Abkömmlinge. Verlag von Wilhelm Engelmann, Leipzig.
McMILLAN, C.B., and R.L. WISNER. 1984. Three new species of seven-gilled hagfishes (Myxinidae, *Eptatretus*) from the Pacific Ocean. Proc. Calif. Acad. Sci. **43**: 249.
PLATE, L. 1924. Die Sinnesorgane der Tiere. *In* Allgemeine Zoologie und Abstammungslehre. Teil II. Jena.
STARCK, D. 1982. Vergleichende Anatomie der Wirbeltiere auf evolutionsbiologischer Grundlage. Band III. Springer Verlag, Berlin.
YAMADA, Y. 1973. Fine structure of the ordinary lateral line organ. 1. The neuromast of lamprey, *Entosphenus japonicus*. J. Ultrastruct. Res. **43**: 1-17.
WORTHINGTON, J. 1905. Contribution to our knowledge of the myxinoids. Amer. Nat. **39**: 625-663.

FRESHWATER PARASITIC LAMPREY ON VANCOUVER ISLAND AND A THEORY OF THE EVOLUTION OF THE FRESHWATER PARASITIC AND NONPARASITIC LIFE HISTORY TYPES

Richard J. Beamish

Department of Fisheries and Oceans
Pacific Biological Station
Nanaimo, British Columbia, V9R 5K6, CANADA

Introduction

Lamprey (Petromyzonidae) are one of the oldest and most successful families of living fishes. Modern lampreys still resemble fossil lampreys which may be as old as 300 million years (Janvier and Lund, 1983). For any family of animals to survive as long as lamprey have, they must possess an extraordinary level of adaptability. One of the major adaptive features of lamprey has been their ability to be anadromous and parasitic, to be parasitic in freshwater and to develop nonparasitic species in freshwater. The least abundant of the three life history types are those with a freshwater parasitic life history. Of the 18 parasitic species, 8 are confined to freshwater (Table I) and 10 are anadromous. Three of the anadromous species are also parasitic in freshwater, only one is considered to be abundant (Table I). In contrast, most of the anadromous species and many of the 22 nonanadromous, nonparasitic species are considered to be relatively common.

In British Columbia, there are 4 known species of lamprey. The nonanadromous *L. richardsoni* is commonly found in most rivers and streams. The anadromous parasitic *L. tridentata* also is commonly found in many coastal rivers and streams. The anadromous parasitic *L. ayresi* is very abundant in the Fraser River, but to date has been reported in only a few other rivers (Beamish and Youson, unpubl. manuscript). A freshwater parasitic species, *L. macrostoma*, occurs in only one drainage basin and while common in this basin, it is rare in British Columbia (Beamish, 1982). A second form that is distinct and rare, is parasitic in freshwater in the laboratory. This form will be described for the first time in this report. The biology of these two freshwater parasitic forms and other species on the west coast of North America is compared to develop a theory for the evolution of freshwater parasitic and nonparasitic life history types.

Table I. Species of lamprey considered to be parasitic in freshwater.

Species	Estimated relative abundance	Reference[1]
Ichthyomyzon unicuspis	not common	1,2,3,4
Ichthyomyzon castaneus	not common	1,4,5
Ichthyomyzon bdellium	not common	2,3
Tetrapleurodon spadeceus	probably not abundant because of restricted distribution	6
Eudontomyzon danfordi	probably not abundant because of restricted distribution	7
Petromyzon marinus freshwater form	abundant	8
Lampetra fluviatilis freshwater form	not abundant	9
Lampetra japonica freshwater form	not abundant	9,10.11
Lampetra minima	rare	12
Lampetra macrostoma	not abundant	13
Lampetra similis	not abundant because of restricted distribution	14,15

[1] 1) Hubley, 1961; 2) Lee *et al.*, 1980; 3) Trautman, 1982; 4) Becker, 1983; 5) Scott and Crossman, 1973; 6) Hubbs and Potter, 1971; 7) Vladykov and Kott, 1979a; 8) Smith, 1971; 9) Maitland, 1980; 10) Heard, 1966; 11) McPhail and Lindsey, 1970; 12) Bond and Kan, 1973; 13) Beamish, 1982; 14) Moyle, 1976; Vladykov and Kott, 1979b.

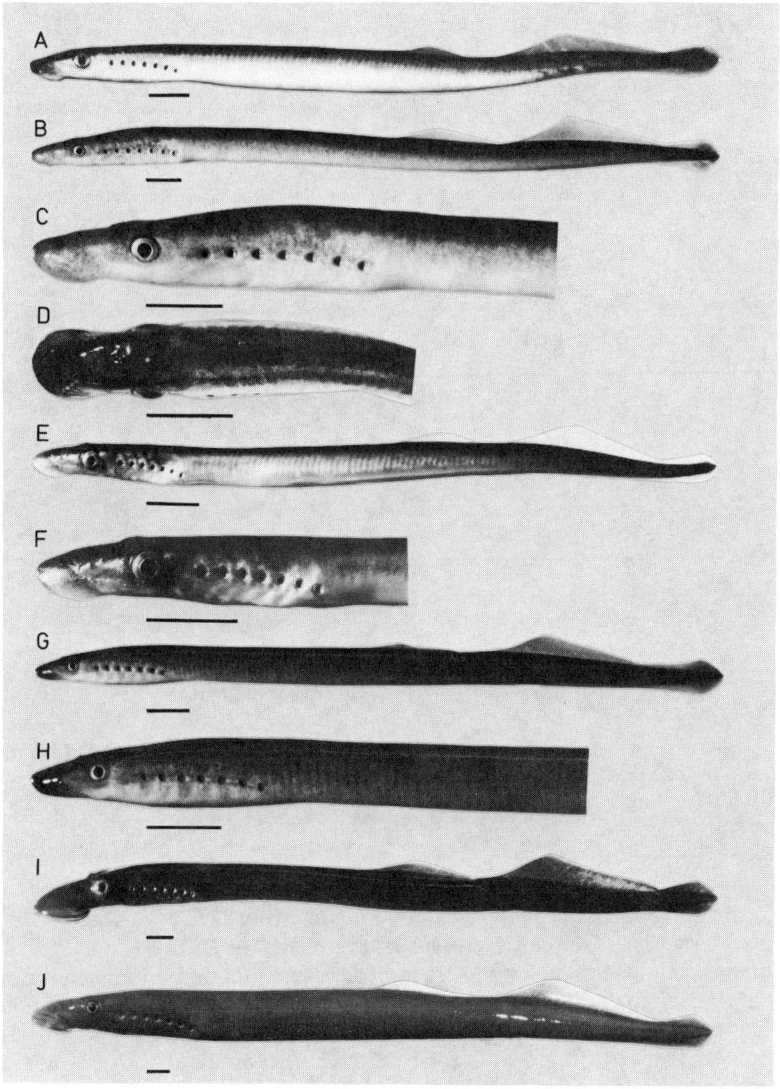

Fig. 1. British Columbia lamprey. A) Morrison Creek form, July 1980, showing silver colour and darkly pigmented tail. B) Morrison Creek form, October, 1982, showing loss of silver colour. C) Head region of above. D) Dorsal view of feeding Morrison Creek form showing pigmentation lines on each side of the dorsal. E) *L. ayresi* feeding in saltwater. F) Head region of above. G) *L. richardsoni*, October 1982. H) Head region of above. I) *L. macrostoma* feeding in freshwater. J) *L. tridentata* feeding in saltwater. Bar represents 1 cm.

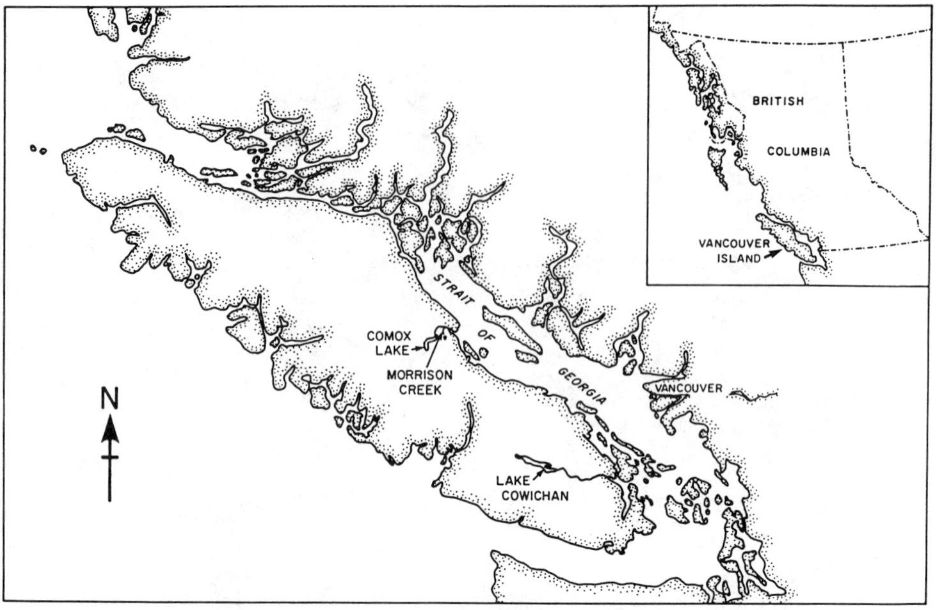

Fig. 2. Location of known freshwater parasitic lamprey on Vancouver Island, British Columbia.

Review of biology and relationships

L. macrostoma Beamish, 1982 (Fig. 1)

A freshwater parasitic lamprey was known from Lake Cowichan and the connecting Mesachie Lake on Vancouver Island (Carl, 1953; Beamish, 1982; Fig. 2). Initially it was believed to be a dwarf race of *L. tridentata* that either spent one year in freshwater prior to going to sea or was landlocked. In 1982, I described this form as a distinct species, *L. macrostoma*, because it was parasitic in freshwater for the duration of its feeding period and relative to *L. tridentata* it had a larger disc, a longer prebranchial length and a larger eye (Fig. 1). It was a close relative of *L. tridentata* and appeared to be a closer relative of *L. tridentata* than other related species (Table II).

L. macrostoma ranges in size from 18 to 27 cm for adult males and 18 to 26 cm for adult females. The average adult size of 20.8 cm is smaller than *L. tridentata* (*cf.* Beamish, 1982). The average size of 80 recently metamorphosed *L. macrostoma* collected in 1981 and 1982 was 11.7 cm (9.7 to 15.8). Since adults are larger, growth must occur after metamorphosis indicating that this species is an obligatory parasite or predator or both. *L. macrostoma* spawns later in the year than *L. tridentata* and in lakes rather than in rivers. Field observations and laboratory spawning studies

Table II. Species derived from *Lampetra tridentata.*

Species (reference)	Principal characteristics
Lampetra minima (Bond and Kan, 1973)	- parasitic - shorter length at maturity, 72-129 mm compared to 205-581 mm. - lower number of myomeres in adult, 60-65 compared to 15-21. - larger eye 0.024 compared to 0.015-0.016 - longer prebranchial 0.148 compared to 0.115-0.117 - paler and simpler colouration
Lampetra similis (Vladykov and Kott, 1979b)	- parasitic - lower number of myomeres, 61.5 (58-65) compared to 67.8 (62-71) - dentition more robust, more anterials - morphology of velar tentacles, shorter 7-9 and no "wings" - disc length larger 0.090-0.093 compared to 0.062-0.070 - smaller eye 0.020-0.024 compared to 0.018-0.037
Lampetra macrostoma (Beamish, 1982)	- parasitic - larger disc 0.10 (0.065-0.117) compared to 0.073 (0.064-0.082) - longer prebranchial 0.159 (0.152-0.172) compared to 0.131 (0.124-0.139) - larger eye, 0.028 (0.024-0.035) compared to 0.022 (0.019-0.026) - weakly pigmented velar tentacles - ability to remain in freshwater
Lampetra lethophaga (Hubbs, 1971)	- nonparasitic - small size at maturity, < 170 mm - small mouth - median cusp of supraoral, weak, or absent - cusps on circumorals often reduced by 1 - posterior circumorals reduced 9-15 - reduced number of anterials
Lampetra folletti (Vladykov and Kott, 1979b)	- nonparasitic - length of adult 186-211 mm - larger disc 0.072 (0.066-.078) compared to 0.062 (0.050-0.074) - stronger dentition - morphology of velar tentacles; 8-9 long slender - darker colouration
Lampetra hubbsi (Beamish, 1982)	- nonparasitic - small size of adults 117-142 - reduced distribution - lower number of myomeres 54-57 - reduced dentition - 3 velar tentacles compared to 5

indicate that *L. tridentata* requires or prefers (or both) to spawn in stronger currents than *L. macrostoma* (Beamish, unpubl. data). *L. macrostoma* is able to remain and feed in freshwater as an adult, while all attempts to keep *L. tridentata* in freshwater in the laboratory have been unsuccessful (Beamish, 1982; Beamish and Clarke, unpubl. manuscript). The spawning size, time, location and behaviour of *L. macrostoma* are sufficiently different from those of *L. tridentata* that it is unlikely that interbreeding occurs. Thus it fulfills all the criteria of biological species (Mayr, 1963).

L. macrostoma presently is not landlocked as there is no barrier between the lakes and sea capable of preventing access to the lake. The presence of anadromous salmon in the lake (Carl, 1953) clearly indicates the lakes are accessible to anadromous fishes.

Feeding juvenile adults readily attack resident fishes. Up to 50% of fish collected in the lake had been attacked by lamprey (Beamish, 1982). Some smaller fish were killed by the attacks; however, larger fish appeared to survive as indicated by the high percentage of scarred fish and the multiple scarring (Beamish, 1982).

A second freshwater parasitic lamprey from Vancouver Island

A second freshwater parasitic lamprey occurs in Morrison Creek on Vancouver Island (Fig. 2). It is related to *L. ayresi* or *L. richardsoni* and is not a derivative of *L. tridentata.* At this time, it is uncertain if this lamprey is a distinct species, a natural hybrid of *L. ayresi* and *L. richardsoni*, or a parasitic form of *L. richardsoni.* Morrison Creek originates from a series of springs and rivers, most of which flow underground from a small lake. The creek varies in width, but averages about 3-4 m. It is approximately 35 km long and it flows into the Puntledge River, a few kilometres upstream of the ocean.

The lamprey has been captured each year since 1977 when it was first observed in a collection of preserved lamprey that were caught in salmon fry traps. Trapping, specifically for this lamprey, started in 1978 and continued until 1984. It is not possible to compare catch per unit effort among years because trapping sites, effort, and the duration of trapping varied in an attempt to study the biology of this form. While direct comparisions can not be made among years, it was noted that total catches were rather constant, suggesting that the population was not undergoing substantial fluctuations in numbers (1980, 85 lampreys; 1981, 85 lampreys; 1982, 73 lampreys; 1983, 64 lampreys; 1984, 97 lampreys).

The lamprey was readily identified by its silver colour (Fig. 1) and the well developed and cornified teeth. Other lamprey that had degenerate teeth, no silver colour and were in spawning condition were easily distinguished from the "silver" lamprey and were considered to be *L. richardsoni* even though some could be the "silver" form in spawning condition. Numerous collections of ammocoetes were made throughout the stream and all ammocoetes were identified as either *L. tridentata* or *L. richardsoni* using the criteria of Richards *et al.* (1982). No *L. ayresi* ammocoetes were found.

On February 21, 1971, 18 metamorphosed lampreys were collected using electroshockers and kept alive in the laboratory. None was silver in colour. On March 16-17, it was noticed that two were silver. The remaining lamprey that were not silver spawned and died, while the two "silver" lamprey survived in freshwater. One was allowed to feed and the other died during an attempt to convert it to full strength salt water. Therefore it appears that the silver colour develops in February and March.

The "silver" form, or more properly called, the Morrison Creek form, was trapped as it moved within the river, primarily at night. Catches have been made as early as mid-March and as late as the end of August. However, most catches occur from mid-June until the end of August. Peak catches occur during the last week in June and the first week in July (Beamish, unpubl. data). The Morrision Creek form has not been caught in the stream after mid-August.

The Morrison Creek form ranges in size from 10 to 15 cm. There was no indication of growth in the population in the Creek from May 31 until August 5 as mean sizes among sampling dates were similar (Fig. 3).

Experiments carried out over a number of years indicated that the Morrison Creek lamprey could not acclimate to full strength Strait of Georgia seawater (Fig. 4; Table III). During many of the experiments the lamprey fed and other lamprey in freshwater holding tanks fed at the same time, indicating that the foregut was open, and the failure to osmoregulate in salt water was not related to delayed completion of metamorphosis. The analysis of blood ion levels clearly showed that the animals could not regulate blood ions in salt water (Table IV).

In 1982, it was possible to provide control experiments, in which one half of a sample was kept in freshwater and fed while the other half was subjected to gradually increasing concentrations of salt water and fed. Once again, no animals could be acclimated to full strength salt water (Fig. 4). The high blood sodium levels in salt water stressed animals, and the absolute inability to obtain survival in full strength salt water clearly indicates that this form is not able to osmoregulate in full strength salt water or in prolonged concentrations of diluted salt water, and therefore is not anadromous.

Examinations in late July of the gut contents of a small sample of lampreys (n=6) showed that some were empty but some had up to 2 ml of brown, mucus- like material. Thus, it appears that some feeding occurs, although it may be minimal. However, no lampreys larger than those in Fig. 3, other than a few spawning *L. tridentata*, have been found in Morrison Creek. The inability to demonstrate growth and the minimal amount of feeding suggests that this form increases in length very little after metamorphosis.

Feeding does occur in laboratory conditions. Morrision Creek lamprey fed on a variety of living and dead species but preferred live herring (*Clupea harengus pallasi*). They fed on live and dead coho salmon (*Oncorhynchus kisutch*), live and dead sockeye salmon (*Oncorhynchus nerka*), other dead lamprey of a variety of species, and dead herring. When feeding on dead lamprey, it appeared that the Morrison Creek form was removing mucus and often flesh was not consumed.

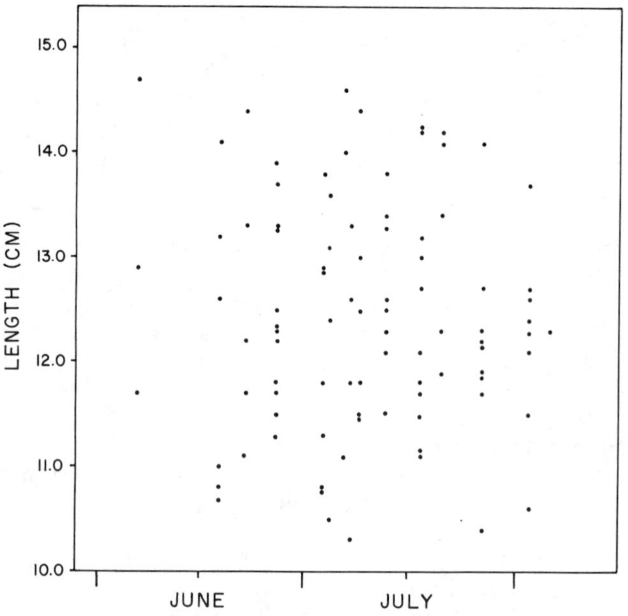

Fig. 3. Total lengths of the Morrison Creek form collected in 1984.

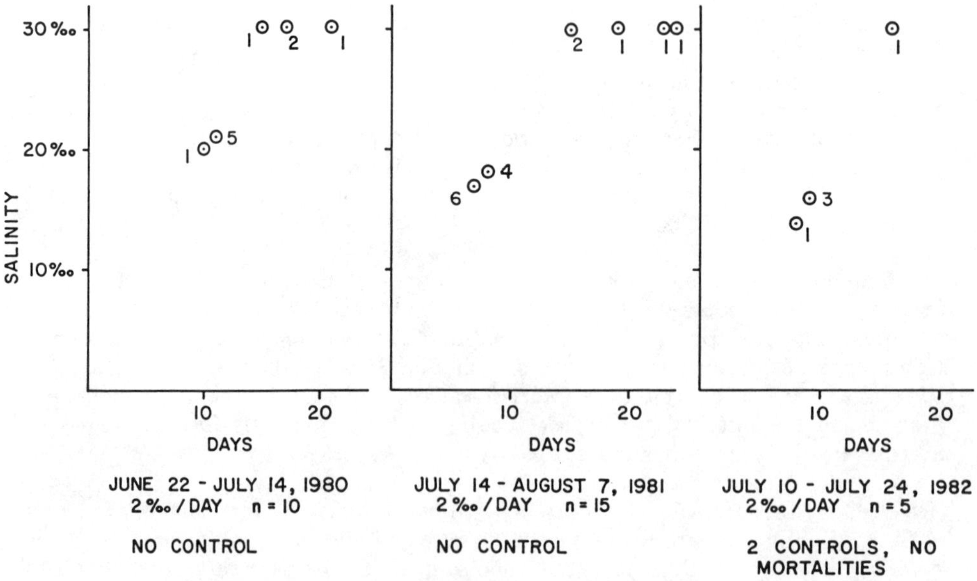

Fig. 4. Mortalities of the Morrison Creek form in increasing concentrations of saltwater. Points indicate when mortalities occurred. Numbers of deaths are indicated adjacent to points.

Table III. Attempts to acclimate Morrison Creek lamprey to salt water[1]

Date	Salinity change in concentration	n	Results
May 17, 1979	10 $^{o}/oo$/day	1	all died
June 12, 1979	10 $^{o}/oo$/day	1	all died
June 21-30, 1979	constant 15 $^{o}/oo$	6	all died
June 2, 1980	constant 11 $^{o}/oo$	1	all died
June 27, 1980	constant 11 $^{o}/oo$	2	all died
June 30, 1980	constant 11 $^{o}/oo$	3	all died
June 10, 1980	10 $^{o}/oo$/day	3	all died
June 14, 1980	10 $^{o}/oo$/day	5	all died
July 10, 1980	2 $^{o}/oo$/day	5	all died
July 19, 1980	2 $^{o}/oo$/day	6	all died
August 1, 1980	5 $^{o}/oo$/day	1	all died
August 25, 1980	2 $^{o}/oo$/day	2	all died

[1]Does not include experiments in Fig. 4

Table IV. Blood ion concentrations for Morrison Creek lamprey held in freshwater and dilute seawater.

Date	Salt water concentration	n	Na^{+}	K^{+}
July 24, 1981	freshwater	1	90	10.9
July 24, 1981	15-17 $^{o}/oo$	2	164	5.6
August 19, 1982	16 $^{o}/oo$	2	163.6 ± 16.3	5.7 ± 1.2
August 19, 1982	freshwater	2	115.3 ± 5.6	7.0 ± 0.4

When they attacked live coho salmon they made small wounds in the body and remained attached at this site. On one occasion 4 lamprey attacked one live coho salmon. After live herring were added to freshwater, actively feeding lamprey would attack and feed on the fish before it died. Lamprey would continue to feed on herring after death. When feeding on dead material, a lamprey won occasion would pull the material into rock crevices.

The preference for herring was interesting as *L. ayresi* prefers to feed on herring (Beamish, 1980). Since the Morrison Creek form cannot osmoregulate in salt water, it obviously cannot feed on this species outside the laboratory.

Feeding in the laboratory started in July, was most active during September and declined in October. In 1982 and 1983 a few fish fed until mid-November, however, most had stopped feeding by mid-October. The size of 24 laboratory-fed animals at the time of cessation of feeding was 18.7 cm (range 10.1-20.6) and 9.2 g (range 0.8-12.0). The mean size of lampreys in Fig. 3, was 12.4 cm and if lengths in 1982 were similar to 1984, lamprey grew an average of approximately 6.3 cm.

Morrison Creek lamprey were difficult to keep alive in the laboratory. They readily developed severe fungus infections that usually were fatal. Most success was obtained by keeping them separate or in smaller groups in large tanks. While no single handling and rearing technique was totally successful, it was better to reduce handling, and to keep the animals well fed. It is possible that poorly fed animals attacked each other and removed mucus in the same manner as was observed when they attacked dead lamprey. It is also possible that the physiological condition of the animals reduced resistance to disease. In general the majority of animals brought into the laboratory could not be kept alive. In contrast, there has been little difficulty maintaining and feeding all other species of British Columbia lamprey. If lamprey lived through to November, very little mortality occurred until after the spawning period in the following year.

The sex ratio was examined for smaller groups of samples collected since 1980. In all samples there has been an excess of males. From 10 to 24% of the fish that were captured were females. In 1984, 24 fish were examined for sex and 79% were males and 21% females. All males when captured had gonads that appeared mature, however, no males had any evidence of secondary sexual changes. Histological examination confirmed that the gonads contained mature sperm (Youson and Beamish, unpubl. manuscript). All females were immature when captured or were just beginning to mature.

On June 12, 1984, one female spawned in captivity with 4 males after being held in the laboratory for one year. The eggs developed and hatched but were not reared beyond hatching.

The Morrison Creek lamprey is morphologically different from *L. richardsoni* and *L. ayresi* (Beamish and Withler, unpubl. manuscript, fig. 1). It differs from *L. ayresi* in the number of cusps on some teeth, some aspects of the its morphology and in colour. Morrison Creek lamprey have an average length of 7.9 cm (range 5-11) cusps on the longitudinal lingual lamina and 9.7 cm (range 6-14) cusps on the transverse lingual lamina. *L. ayresi* has significantly (t test $P<0.001$) more cusps on the transverse lingual lamina, 13.7 (range 11-18). A small sample of ten *L. richardsoni* from other streams had 8 cusps on the longitudinal lingual lamina and 12.1 (10-15) on the transverse lingual lamina.

Morphological comparisons among *L. ayresi, L. richardsoni* and the Morrison Creek form indicate that the prebranchial lengths for *L. ayresi* and the Morrison Creek form are similar, but are longer than those for *L. richardsoni*. The eye of the *L. ayresi* is wider than *L. richardsoni* and the Morrison Creek form. The post orbital length for *L. ayresi* is equal or smaller than its eye width, while the post orbital length is longer than the eye width for *L. richardsoni* and the Morrison Creek form. The distance from the anterior of the eye to the anterior tip of the animal (sometimes called snout length, but it may be better to call this length the pre-orbital length) is similar in the Morrison Creek form and *L. ayresi* and both are longer than *L. richardsoni*.

The "silver" form of the Morrison Creek lamprey is much darker in the tail region than *L. ayresi* and the dorsal pigmentation extends further ventrally resulting in less silver colour (Fig. 1). When feeding in the laboratory there is a dorsal band with a greenish appearance that extends the length of the body on each side of the fish (Fig. 1). Lamprey that fed and grew in the laboratory lost their silver colour and became uniformly grey by the end of September.

At this time it is not possible to determine if the Morrison Creek lamprey is a new species, a natural hybrid or is a form of *L. richardsoni*. It is possible to say that based on conventional lamprey taxonomy, the Morrison Creek lamprey is not *L. richardsoni* and it is not *L. ayresi*. Whatever the form turns out to be, biologically it is more closely related to the nonparasitic *L. richardsoni* than to the parasitic *L. ayresi*.

Other L. tridentata derivatives..

Presently there are two other parasitic derivatives of *L. tridentata* and three nonparasitic derivatives (Table II).

L. similis is restricted to the Klamath River drainage of northern California and southern Oregon (Vladykov and Kott, 1979b). this lamprey is similar in size to *L. macrostoma* and smaller than *L. tridentata*. Vladykov and Kott provide very little life history information but from the information in Moyle (1976) and from its distribution it is possible that this species is parasitic in freshwater. The reduced number of velar tentacles suggests that this species is a more distant relative of *L. tridentata* than *L. macrostoma*.

L. minima is a dwarfed parasitic derivative of *L. tridentata* from the same drainage but known only from Miller Lake (Bond and Kan, 1973). The species is now believed to be extinct. Feeding occurred on a variety of species including other alive and dead lamprey and other dead fish. The spawning adult is actually smaller than the late larval stage (Kan and Bond, 1981) indicating that the parasitic phase must be short. Kan and Bond (1981) suggested that feeding could occur for only few weeks and Hubbs (1971) suggested that parasitism by this species was not obligatory. Kan and Bond (1981) suggest that this species evolved from a probable landlocked *L. tridentata* type that became geographically isolated as a result of volcanic eruptions 6,000 years ago.

There are three nonparasitic derivatives of *L. tridentata*. *L. lethophaga* and *L. folletti* are found in the same drainage as *L. similis* and *L. minima*. *L. hubbsi* is found to the south in the San Joaquin River basin in central California.

Theory of the evolution of the freshwater parasitic and nonparasitic life history types

At present, no other parasitic lampreys in British Columbia have been found to be resident in freshwater for the duration of their feeding phase. Clearly, the existence of freshwater parasitic forms in British Columbia are rare.

The rare occurrence of freshwater parasitic lampreys, relative to other life history types, suggests that anadromous parasitic lamprey do not readily develop into freshwater parasitic forms. Since some freshwater parasitic derivatives develop, they can only remain rare if the life history type is less successful than other types or it is less stable. If it is less stable then it is possible that freshwater parasitic forms eventually produce nonparasitic forms.

A possible evolutionary pathway for the establishment of freshwater parasitic and nonparasitic forms appears to start with the ability to osmoregulate in freshwater during feeding. Initially, only a few individuals would be able to accomplish this, but eventually there could be selection for large numbers of lamprey that do not to feed in full strength salt water. There would have to be an associated loss of instinct to migrate into full strength seawater and a decline in size. It is possible that these changes develop when a population is subjected to gradual changes in salinity, possibly during periods of glaciation. The population could remain in dilute salt water and eventually remain in freshwater or the population could develop in freshwater. The ability to osmoregulate in salt water could be lost in freshwater, and the parasitic habit eventually would no longer be obligatory. Precocious development would shorten the length of life of the metamorphosed individual to about one year. It is possible that males may shorten their life span first. Eventually totally nonparasitic forms are produced.

Support for this theory can be found from the biology of the Morrison Creek form, *L. macrostoma* and the various derivatives of *L. tridentata* that are found on the west coast of the United States. *L. macrostoma* is very similar to *L. tridentata.* However, it is smaller, feeds in freshwater as a juvenile adult and apparently does not migrate to sea even though it can osmoregulate in salt water and there are no obstructions in the short route the animal would have to take to the sea. Since *L. macrostoma* can osmoregulate in salt water as a feeding adult, it is possible that it only recently evolved into a freshwater parasitic species, indicating that the ability to osmoregulate in freshwater is the first major evolutionary change. Beamish *et al.* (1978) have shown that the landlocked sea lamprey has lost much of its capacity for osmoregulation in salt water, suggesting that the loss of the ability to osmoregulate in salt water occurs after freshwater colonization.

L. similis, while morphologically different from *L. macrostoma*, could be similar in its biology. Vladykov and Kott (1979b) do not provide any life history information, however, Moyle (1976) suggests that this species feeds in freswater.

L. minima was much closer to a nonparasitic life history type than *L. macrostoma* or *L. similis*. It was not known if it could osmoregulate in salt water, however, if the observations of Mathers and Beamish (1974) apply to this form, then the small size would indicate that the animal probably could not osmoregulate in full strength salt water. Mathers and Beamish (1974), Hardisty (1956) and others believed that the differentiation of the freshwater parasitic form of *Petromyzon marinus* involved a selection of adults for smaller size and reduced osmoregulatory performance in high salinities. Potter *et al.* (1980) felt that it was significant that the smaller individuals of several anadromous parasitic lamprey were least able to tolerate high salinities. Smith (1971) assumed that *P. marinus* invaded Lake Ontario after the Wisconsin glacial ice receded. Mathers and Beamish (1974) concluded that differentiation of the landlocked *P. marinus* could have resulted from gradual habitat selection as suggested by Hardisty (1954), in which feeding individuals of smaller size and perhaps not physiologically well suited for a marine existence, tended to remain in freshwater. Thus, there is evidence that the development of freshwater parasitic forms begins with the development of an ability to osmoregulate in freshwater as a feeding adult and an associated decrease in size.

The ability for anadromous forms to feed in freshwater is not common, as shown by the inability to hold juvenile adults of *L. tridentata* and *P. marinus* in freshwater (Potter and Beamish, 1977; Beamish, 1980, 1982; Beamish and Clark, unpubl. manuscript; Youson, pers. comm.; F.W.H. Beamish, pers. comm.). I have maintained an extremely small percentage of *L. ayresi* in freshwater throughout their trophic phase but most juvenile adult *L. ayresi* were unable to survive (Beamish and Youson, unpubl. manuscript).

The ability to osmoregulate in freshwater as a feeding juvenile adult may be more common in some species than others. The ability for all individuals in a population to remain nonanadromous could develop in freshwater from the few individuals that have this ability or it could evolve in dilute salt water as a population is subjected to a major environmental change. Periods of glaciation may produce conditions where it is advantageous for lamprey to feed in less saline waters in preference to migrating longer distances into full strength seawater. The connection between glaciation and the development of nonparasitic lampreys has been proposed by others (Loman, 1912; Enequist, 1937; Zhukov, 1965; 1968), however, the development of all freshwater resident lamprey can not be explained by glaciation (Hardisty and Potter, 1971b; Kan and Bond, 1981).

On Vancouver Island, Lake Cowichan was the site of a large glacial lake that formed as a result of an ice dam at the location of the present outlet (Alley and Chatwin, 1979). The glacial lake drained southwest into the Pacific Ocean. The drainage eventually changed after the valley became ice-free about 10,000 years ago. Lake Cowichan, the present lake, drains eastward into the Strait of Georgia. It is probable that the presence of *L. macrostoma* in Lake Cowichan is directly related to the glacial history of this lake.

Little is known about the glacial history of Morrison Creek. However, it is such a small creek that it is doubtful that there was a direct effect of glaciation on it. The creek is found near the end of a long valley that undoubtedly carried glacial melt water to the Pacific Ocean as the glaciers retreated up the valley. The creek is, however, not typical of smaller creeks on Vancouver Island, because its spring-fed source maintains rather constant flows and temperatures. At present there is little that would indicate why such an unusual form is present in Morrison Creek.

The Morrison Creek form and *L. minima* have reduced the length of the feeding period and *L. minima* has reduced the duration of the adult phase. Therefore, except for the brief parasitic phase which may not have been obligatory (Hubbs, 1971), the biology of *L. minima* is very close to a nonparasitic form. While it is correct to describe *L. minima* as a dwarf parasitic species, it also could be considered to be very close to a nonparasitic species. Kan and Bond (1981) showed that *L. minima* had the lowest absolute fecundity of all lamprey, but the relative fecundity was among the highest. They suggested that most of the lipid reserves were used to produce gonadal products, a feature that is common to nonparasitic forms.

Hubbs (1971) describes another form of *L. tridentata* from Goose Lake (another area close to the location of *L. minima*) in the Pit River system in which the males did not show signs of being parasitic while the females resembled the normal parasitic form. Thus, the male was more closely related to the nonparasitic brook lamprey than the female.

The three known nonparasitic derivatives of *L. tridentata* (Table II) occur in the same general area as *L. minima* and *L. similis*. Thus, it is possible that *L. minima* and some of the forms described by Hubbs (1971) were in the process of evolving into a nonparasitic form that was either similar to one of the nonparasitic species in TAble II or perhaps a distinct species.

The Morrison Creek form while not a *L. tridentata* derivative, was not able to osmoregulate in salt water and in the stream it does not appear to increase in size as a juvenile adult. If feeding occurred in the stream it may be for only a short period and probably on food items other than live fishes. A scavenging habit, similar to *L. minima*, was observed in the laboratory. The presence of precocious males that would feed in the laboratory even when mature sperm were present in the gonad at the same time that immature females existed in the population is similar to the form of *L. tridentata* described by Hubbs (1971) from Goose Lake. The Morrison Creek form, unlike *L. minima* has not shortened the length of the period after metamorphosis to less than one year.

Thus there is evidence that some populations of anadromous parasitic lamprey have produced freshwater parasitic derivatives. There is evidence of selection for smaller size and the loss of an ability to osmoregulate in full strength salt water. Some forms have reduced the desire to feed to the extent that spawning adults are similar in length to metamorphosing ammocoetes. There has been precocious development and a shortening of the post metamorphic stage to less than one year. Precocious development seems to occur in males first. While all these changes can be found, there is a difference in the degree of change that can be found in any particular species. However, the pattern of change still appears to be to: develop an ability to osmoregulate in freshwater; select for this character and build up a population with this ability ; select for smaller size; lose the instinct to migrate and remain in freshwater; lose the ability to osmoregulate in salt water; reduce the length of post metamorphic period to less than one year, possibly through precocious development and possibly occurring in males first; reduce and ultimately eliminate feeding resulting in a nonparasitic form.

My theory that nonparasitic forms evolved in the more traditional manner differs from the belief that nonparasitic species can develop directly when the ammocoete stage of an anadromous or freshwater parasitic form is extended, resulting in a longer feeding period as an ammocoete and a reduced post-metamorphic period without feeding (Hardisty and Potter, 1971a, 1971b; Bird and Potter, 1979; Vladykov and Kott, 1979a; Potter, 1980). While there is some evidence to support this "one step" process, I believe that it is unlikely that all the changes that need to occur to become nonanadromous and nonparasitic can occur by a simple extension of the larval period of an anadromous parasitic lamprey. The need to develop an ability to osmoregulate in freshwater, decrease the growth rate, lose the migratory instinct, lose the ability to osmoregulate in salt water, shorten the post-metamorphic period and lose the instinct to feed represent such major changes that it is probable that they occur in sequence. The relatively rare occurrence of freshwater parasitic forms worldwide and the occurrence of forms that are almost "intermediate" between freshwater parasitic and nonanadromous nonparasitic on the west coast of North America indicate that some nonparasitic forms evolve gradually from freshwater parasitic forms. The evolution of nonparasitic species from freshwater parasitic species also was suggested by Hubbs and Trautman (1937) for some nonparasitic species from central North America.

The rare occurrence of freshwater parasitic and freshwater nonparasitic derivatives of *L. tridentata* suggests that the rate of development of these forms is relatively slow. The absence, to date, of any nonparasitic derivatives of *L. tridentata* in British Columbia may indicate that there has not been sufficient time since the last glaciation for nonparasitic derivatives to develop. However, considering that nonparasitic forms exist to the south, it is possible that *L. macrostoma* could produce a nonparasitic form.

In contrast, nonparasitic derivatives of the *L. ayresi* type are not rare in British Columbia or on the west coast of North America. However, the occurrence of freshwater parasitic derivatives of this species remains rare. This could indicate that nonparasitic forms evolve directly from anadromous parasitic forms. However, as stated, I believe the many changes that must occur are too major to occur simultaneously during an extension of the larval period.

Instead, I propose that the rate of development of freshwater parasitic forms, and ultimately freshwater nonparasitic forms, may be faster for some species groups and specifically the *L. ayresi* group. The nonparasitic derivatives of this group probably have distributed themselves in the same manner as other freshwater fishes, accounting for the relative abundance of the *L. richardsoni* type on the west coast of North America. It is also possible that some of the *L. richardsoni* populations evolved separately from parasitic ancestors. Hubbs and Trautman (1937) also believed nonparasitic lamprey could have polyphyletic origins. Thus, there is no reason to believe that all existing freshwater populations of *L. richardsoni* resulted exclusively from colonizations following periods of glaciation. At present, it is not possible to estimate the length of time required for these nonparasitic forms to develop. It may be that some nonparasitic populations have evolved after the period of isostatic rebound, about 13,000 years BP (before present) that followed the retreat of the glaciers (Mathews *et al.*, 1970).

The Morrison Creek form may be the key to understanding the rate of development of freshwater parasitic and freshwater nonparasitic forms in the *L. ayresi* group. If the Morrison Creek form is a distinct species, then, except for the extended post-metamorphic period and the ability to be parasitic, its biology is very similar to *L. richardsoni*. If it is a natural hybrid, it shows that there still is a very close relationship between these two species, despite morphological and physiological differences.

It is important to remember that *L. ayresi* have not been found in Morrison Creek or in any river in the drainage basin. Thus, there is the possibility that *L. richardsoni* and the Morrison Creek form, tentatively called *L. richardsoni marifuga*, are a species complex. If this is true, then it not only demonstrates the very close and previously unknown relationship between the two life history types, but allows a variety of speculations to be made about the relationship of parasitic and nonparasitic forms. If subsequent studies confirm that this is the correct relationship for the Morrison Creek form, or that it is a distinct species, then the inability to osmoregulate in salt water, the scavenging habit in the stream, the precocious development in males, and the absence of net growth as adults indicates it is intermediate between a parasitic and a nonparasitic form. An intermediate position at the post-metamorphic stage supports the concept that the evolution of nonparasitic forms has occurred as a result of changes that occur after metamorphosis and not exclusively at the ammocoete stage.

Literature cited

ALLEY, N.F., and S.C. CHATWIN. 1979. Late Pleistocene history and geomorphology, southwestern Vancouver Island, British Columbia. Can. J. Earth Sci. **16**: 1645-1657.

BEAMISH, R.J. 1980. Adult biology of the river lamprey (*Lampetra ayresi*) and the Pacific lamprey (*Lampetra tridentata*) from the Pacific coast of Canada. Can. J. Fish. Aquat. Sci. **37**: 1906-1923.

BEAMISH, R.J. 1982. *Lampetra macrostoma*, a new species of freshwater parasitic lamprey from the west coast of Canada. Can. J. Fish. Aquat. Sci. **37**: 736-747.

BEAMISH, F.W.H., P.D. STRACHAN, and E. THOMAS. 1978. Osmotic and ionic performance of the anadromous sea lamprey, *Petromyzon marinus*. Comp. Biochem. Phyiol. **60A**: 435-443.

BECKER, G.C. 1983. Fishes of Wisconsin. University of Wisconsin Press, Madison, 1052 p.

BIRD, D.J. and I.C. POTTER. 1979. Metamorphosis in the paired species of lampreys, *Lampetra fluviatilis* (L.) and *Lampetra planeri* (Block). 1. A description of the timing and stages. J. Linn. Soc. (Lond.) Zool. **65**: 127-143.

BOND, C.E. and T.T. KAN. 1973. *Lampetra (Entosphenus) minima* n. sp., a dwarfed parasitic lamprey from Oregon. Copeia **1973**: 568-574.

CARL, G.C. 1953. Limnobiology of Cowichan Lake, British Columbia. J. Fish. Res. Board Can. **9**: 417-449.

ENEQUIST, P. 1937. Das Bachneunauge als ökologische Modifikation des Flussneunauges. Über die Flussneunaugen und Bachneunaugen Schwedens. Ark. Zool. **29**: 1-22.

HARDISTY, M.W. 1954. Sex ratio in spawning populations of *Lampetra planeri*.

Nature (Lond.) **173**: 874-875.

HARDISTY, M.W. 1956. Some aspects of osmotic regulation in lampreys. J. exp. Biol. **33**: 531-447.

HARDISTY, M.W., and I.C. POTTER. 1971a. The general biology of adult lampreys. pp. 127-206 *In* Hardisty, M.W., and I.C. Potter [eds.] The biology of lampreys, vol. 1. Academic Press, London.

HARDISTY, M.W., and I.C. POTTER. 1971b. Paired species. pp. 249-277 *In* Hardisty, M.W., and I.C. Potter [eds.] The biology of lampreys, vol. 1. Academic Press, London.

HEARD, W.R. 1966. Observations on lampreys in the Naknek River system of southwest Alaska. Copeia **1966**: 332-339.

HUBBS, C.L. 1971. *Lampetra (Entosphenus) lethophaga*, new species, the nonparasitic derivative of the Pacific lamprey. Trans. San Diego Soc. Nat. Hist. **16**: 125-164.

HUBBS, C.L., and I.C. POTTER. 1971. Distribution, phylogeny and taxonomy. pp. 1-65 *In* Hardisty, M.W., and I.C. Potter [eds.] The biology of lampreys, vol. 1. Academic Press, London.

HUBBS, C.L., and M.B. TRAUTMAN. 1937. A revision of the lamprey genus *Ichthyomyzon*. Univ. Mich. Mus. Zool. Misc. Publ. **35**, 109 p.

HUBLEY, R.C. 1961. Incidence of scarring on fish in the upper Mississippi River. Trans. Amer. Fish. Soc. **90**: 83-85.

JANVIER, P., and R. LUND. 1983. *Hardistiella montanensis* n. gen. et sp. (Petromyzonitida) from the lower carboniferous of Montana, with remarks on the affinities of the lampreys. J. Vert. Paleontol. **2**: 407-413.

KAN, T.T., and C.E. BOND. 1981. Notes on the biology of the Miller Lake lamprey *Lampetra (Entosphenus) minima*. *Northwest Sci*. **55**: 70-74.

LEE, D.S., C.R. GILBERT, C.H. HOCUTT, R.E. JENKINS, D.E. McALLISTER, and J.R. STAUFFER, Jr. 1980. Atlas of North American freshwater fishes. North Carolina Biol. Survey Publ. 1980-12. 867 pp.

LOMAN, J.C.C. 1912. Über die Naturgeschichte des Bachneunauges *Lampetra planeri*. Zool. Jb. (suppl.) **15**: 243-270.

MAITLAND, P.S. 1980. Scarring of whitefish (*Coregonus lavaretus*) by European river lamprey (*Lampetra fluviatilis*) in Loch Lomond, Scotland. Can. J. Fish. Aquat. Sci. 37: 1981-1988.

MATHERS, J.S., and F.W.H. BEAMISH. 1974. Changes in serum osmotic and ionic concentrations in landlocked *Petromyzon marinus*. Comp. Biochem. Physiol. **49A**: 677-688.

MATHEWS, W.H., J.G. FYLES, and H.W. NASMITH. 1970. Postglacial crustal movements in southwestern British Columbia and adjacent Washington State. Can. J. Earth Sci. **5**: 1409-1415.

MAYR, E. 1963. Animal species and evolution. Harvard University Press (Belknap Press), Cambridge, 797 p.

McPHAIL, J.D., and C.C. LINDSEY. 1970. Freshwater fishes of northwestern Canada and Alaska. Fish. Res. Board Can. Bull. 173, 381 p.

MOYLE, P.B. 1976. Inland fishes of California. University of California Press, Berkeley, 405 p.

POTTER, I.C. 1980. The Petromyzoniformes with particular reference to paired species. Can. J. Fish. Aquat. Sci. **37**: 1595-1615.

POTTER, I.C., and F.W.H. BEAMISH. 1977. The freshwater biology of adult anadromous sea lampreys *Petromyzon marinus*. J. Zool. (Lond.) **181**: 113-130.

POTTER, I.C., R.W. HILLARD, and D.J. BIRD. 1980. Metamorphosis in the southern hemisphere lamprey, *Geotria australis*. J. Zool. (Lond.) **190**: 405-430.

RICHARDS, J.E., R.J. BEAMISH, and F.W.H. BEAMISH. 1982. Descriptions and keys for ammocoetes of lamprey from British Columbia, Canada. Can. J. Fish. Aquat. Sci. **39**: 1484-1495.

SCOTT, W.B., and E.J. CROSSMAN. 1973. Freshwater fishes of Canada. Fish. Res. Board Can. Bull. 184, 966 p.

SMITH, B.R. 1971. Sea lampreys in the Great Lakes of North America. *In* Hardisty, M.W., and I.C. Potter [eds.] The biology of lampreys, vol. 1. Academic Press, London.

TRAUTMAN, M.B. 1982. The fishes of Ohio, 2nd ed. State University Press, Columbus, 793 p.

VLADYKOV, V.D., and E. KOTT. 1976a. A second nonparasitic species of *Entosphenus* Gill, 1862 (Petromyzonidae) from Klamath River system, California. Can. J. Zool. **54**: 974-989.

VLADYKOV, V.D., and E. KOTT. 1976b. A new nonparasitic species of lamprey of the genus *Entosphenus* Gill, 1862 (Petromyzonidae) from south central California. Bull. S. Calif. Acad. Sci. **75**: 60-67.

VLADYKOV, V.D., and E. KOTT. 1979a. Satellite species among the holarctic lampreys. Can. J. Zool. **57**: 860-870.

VLADYKOV, V.D., and E. KOTT. 1979b. A new parasitic species of the holarctic lamprey genus *Entosphenus* Gill, 1862 (Petromyzonidae) from Klamath River, in California and Oregon. Can. J. Zool. **57**: 808-823.

ZHUKOV, P.I. 1965. [Distribution and evolution of freshwater lampreys in the waters of the Belorussion Soviet Republic.] Vopr. Ikhtiol. **5**: 240-244 (in Russian).

ZHUKOV, P.I. 1968. [Routes of penetration of Ponto-Caspian ichthofauna into the rivers of the Baltic Sea Basin.] Zool. Zh. **47**: 1417-1419 (in Russian).

ORGAN DEVELOPMENT AND SPECIALIZATION IN LAMPREY SPECIES

John H. Youson

Department of Zoology
University of Toronto
Toronto, Ontario

Introduction

The term development has many meanings, but basically it can be divided into ontogenetic and phylogenetic types (Balinsky, 1970). In vertebrates, ontogenesis begins with the maturation of the gametes, extends through fertilization and differentiation of organ systems, and ends with the death of the individual. Phylogenetic development follows the modification of a species or a group of species through an extended period of time. Due to their lowly postion on the taxonomic scale of vertebrates, and the fact that they can claim as their ancestors the primitive ostracoderms, lampreys have been of interest for those studying both ontogenetic and phylogenetic development. During their evolutionary history, lampreys have modified their ancestral ostracoderm form through loss of certain characters and development of new specialized features. As a result, extant lampreys are considered as highly specialized vertebrates (Hubbs and Potter, 1971) with few links to extinct agnathans, to hagfishes or to any invertebrate line (Hardisty, 1982). Despite their history and dissemblance to any other living vertebrate, lampreys have provided insight into the possible evolution of many organ systems. This information has been a consequence of the nature of the lamprey life cycle which, through an extended larval period and a phase of metamorphosis, has provided an ideal opportunity to study ontogenetic development. An examination of ontogenesis reflects some of the trends of regression and specialization that may have taken place during the evolution of the organs of higher vertebrates. On the other hand, some of the ontogenetic processes have been shown to be unique to lampreys and have resulted in specialized organs which have undoubtedly contributed to the survival of lampreys over at least 280 million years. During this time they have shown a conservative evolution (Bardack and Zangerl, 1971). The following is a review of some of the features of lamprey organ "development" in the digestive and excretory systems which have contributed to both specialization of this vertebrate and their value as a source of information on the evolution of these organ systems in vertebrates. Although the more traditional phylogenetic considerations of morphology are primarily utilized,the author is in support of the view (Løvtrup, 1977) that physiological and biochemical considerations are also important in any phylogenetic evaluation.

Stages of lamprey ontogenesis

Lampreys pass through up to seven stages of development during their life cycle. These include, in order of their appearance: gametogenesis, embryogenesis, a larval phase, metamorphosis, adult growth (parasitic species only), sexual maturation, and senescence (aging). All lampreys reproduce through external fertilization with gametes which mature only several weeks before their release into the aquatic environment at the nest site. The maturation and release of these gametes is undoubtedly hormonally controlled (Larsen, 1980; Hardisty and Baker, 1982). The fertilized telolecithal eggs undergo holoblastic cleavage and after 13-15 days the larval (ammocoete) form is apparent (Piavis, 1971). It is during this period that many of the organs show signs of differentiation from organ rudiments which have appeared from subdivision of the germinal layers. At a size of 7.5-9.0 mm. the ammocoetes leave the nest site and burrow in the muddy substrate of their natal stream, but many of their organs are still in rudimentary form. There is interspecific variation in the time spent as an ammocoete (Hardisty and Potter, 1971a; Potter, 1980) but in all lampreys it will last a minimum of 2 years, with 5-7 years quite common. During the larval phase, growth of most organs is slow, while other organs (*e.g.* kidneys) show a progessive change through several generations of structures. In addition, many adult organs remain as primordia in ammocoetes.

The larval phase is terminated by the beginning of metamorphosis, the period when the ammocoete takes on adult characters. Hardisty (1982) calls this interval, "the long delayed completion of an interrupted embryonic development". Over the next 3 to 4 months organs either disappear, to be replaced by new ones, or are transformed. Clearly defined stages of metamorphosis based on external characteristics are now universal (Potter *et al.*, 1982a) and are partly responsible for the increased use of lampreys for studying a variety of parameters in developmental biology. During metamorphosis, all lamprey species follow one of two possible lines of development. In non-parasitic species, development of organs of digestion and excretion reach a partial degree of differentiation which reflect their nontrophic activity in a freshwater environment. In contrast, parasitic species generally show a more advanced stage of differentiation of these same organs by the end of metamorphosis. This is best illustrated in anadromous parasitic species (Hardisty and Potter, 1971b). During the parasitic adult phase growth is rapid (Beamish, 1980a).

A further stage of ontogenesis occurs in adults of all species as sexual maturation is approached. This phase is marked by the ripening of gonads, but organ regression and development of secondary sex characteristics are also featured. The final stage of development may be equated with aging, the ultimate stage of development of any vertebrate and, like many developmental events, hormones play a significant role (Larsen, 1980).

Digestive system

Mouth

The stomodaeum first appears in 6-8 day embryos and the lips of the oral hood by days 15-17. Oral cirrhi are present prior to burrowing of the larva and form a ring around the oral aperture which leads into the oral cavity. The efficiency of this mechanism for straining food has been emphasized (Mallatt, 1981) and there is speculation that it may have been present in ancestral agnathans (Whiting, 1972). The mouth (buccal and oral cavities) undergoes a dramatic transformation to the oral disc and buccal and oral cavities of the adult. Specialized features developing at this time are teeth (Manion and Piavis, 1977; Yoshie and Honma, 1979; Youson, 1980, 1981a; Lethbridge and Potter, 1981), fimbriae (Youson, 1980; Lethbridge and Potter, 1979), buccal glands (Gibbs, 1956), and a tongue-like piston (Johnels, 1948). They all show characteristic patterns of development either from, or in close relation to, larval strucures but also from primordial tissue which likely has been in a resting state since early embryogenesis. For example, the piston cartilage develops from primitive connective tissues, mucocartilage (Wright and Youson, 1982), whose cells seem to dedifferentiate before forming the adult cartilage (Johnels, 1948).

Oesophagus

The oesophagus of larval lampreys extends from the pharynx and ends near the tip of the liver, where it unites with the anterior intestine (Fig. 1). This straight tube has 3 or 4 longitudinal folds and develops in the fashion typical of holoblastic vertebrates (Piavis, 1971). The ciliated and mucous cells of the oesophagus reflect the need for movement and lubrication of ingested food particles as they pass to the intestine (Hansen and Youson, 1978). Changes in feeding habits and/or use of the oral disc in attachment in adults requires a new oesophagus (Hardisty *et al.*, 1970) independent of the pharynx which is involved in tidal ventilation (Randall, 1972). The adult oesophagus develops at metamorphosis in all species from a ridge of epithelial cells which evaginate from the dorsal wall of the pharynx (Weissenberg, 1925, 1926; Hardisty *et al.*, 1970). A cord of cells eventually acquires a continuous lumen throughout its length, but the timing of the final patenting of this lumen is essential for saltwater osmoregulation in anadromous species (Richards and Beamish, 1981) and shows individual variation (Hardisty *et al.*, 1970). Unlike the larval counterpart, the adult oesophagus possesses numerous longitudinal folds, which are particularly pronounced in parasitic species (Youson, 1981a). The larval oesophagus undergoes some regressive change before redifferentiation into part of the adult anterior intestine (Elliott and Youson, unpublished).

Intestine

Both larval and adult intestines have increased surface area for absorption, due to the presence of a typhlosole. This longitudinal fold shows interspecific variation in size and in the degree to which it spirals and twists towards the cloaca (Battle and Hayashida, 1965). The typhlosole is much smaller in Geotriidae than in all other lamprey species so far examined (Hilliard *et al.*, 1983). The submucosal tissue of

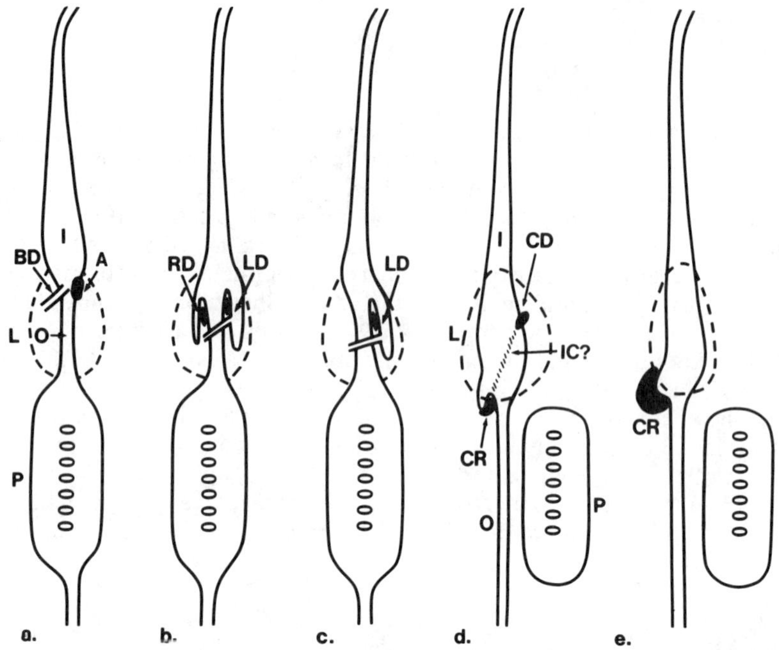

Fig. 1. Diagrammatic representation of the pharynx, *P*; liver, *L*; bile duct, *BD*; oesophagus, *O*; pancreas, *A*; and intestine, *I*; in larva of *P. marinus* (a), *G. australis* (b), and *M. mordax* (c). The latter species have either one (*LD*) or two (*RD, LD*) diverticula. Adult *P. marinus* (d) has a cranial (*CR*) and caudal (*CD*) pancreas while adult *G. australis* (e) has a single cranial pancreas. Adults have no bile duct and a new oesophagus (*O*) separate from the pharynx (*P*). *IC*, intermediate cord of cells.

the larval typhlosole serves as a site of haemopoiesis but in the adult this tissue is transferred to the fat column (Percy and Potter, 1977; Potter *et al.*, 1982b). Southern Hemisphere lampreys possess intestinal diverticula (Fig. 1), but whereas *Geotria australis* possesses left and right diverticula (Maskell, 1930; Hilliard *et al.*, 1983), *Mordacia mordax* has a single structure (Strahan and Maclean, 1969). The intestinal epithelium of the larval anterior intestine of holarctic lampreys is primarily specialized for absorption and secretion of digestive enzymes (Ermisch, 1966; Barrington, 1972; Hansen and Youson, 1978) and the posterior intestine for absorption only. The secretory cells of the diverticula of *M. mordax* and *G. australis* are equivalent to pancreatic exocrine cells of higher vertebrates (Maskell, 1930; Strahan and Maclean, 1969) and are a site for high activity of amylase and lipase but not trypsin (Strahan and Maclean, 1969). The latter is present in the anterior intestine of these species and in holarctic lampreys (Barrington, 1936).

The entire mucosal surface of the adult intestine possesses many smaller longitudinal folds, including over the typhlosole. The number and degree of elaboration of these folds varies in anterior and posterior regions of the intestine and also between species (Youson, 1981a; Hilliard *et al.*, 1983). In general, nonparasitic species show fewer folds than parasitic species in the immediately postmetamorphic stage (Hilliard *et al.*, 1983). Despite these variations, development of folds is a characteristic event of metamorphosis and follows a morphogenetic pattern equated with villi and fold development in the intestines of vertebrate embryos (Youson and Connelly, 1978). Development of the lamprey intestine at metamorphosis also provides insight into tissue regression, dedifferentiation, and differentiation of a specialized intestinal epithelium (Youson and Horbert, 1982) which does not become fully differentiated until the onset of feeding (Langille and Youson, 1984a, b). Like the intestine of stomachless teleosts, the intestine of parasitic adult lampreys is separated into regions specialized for either protein and/or lipid absorption (Fig. 2). However, the large diameter anterior intestine is also important in marine osmoregulation, where swallowed salt water is held and where cells with the efficiency and appearance of gill chloride cells (Langille and Youson, 1984a) take up sodium and chloride ions and permit the passive transport of water (Pickering and Morris, 1973). Besides being a site of protein absorption (Langille and Youson, 1984b), the epithelium of the posterior intestine and hindgut likely eliminate the bile pigment, biliverdin (Langille and Youson, 1983).

The intestine undergoes a marked atrophy during sexual maturation of all lamprey species. Extirpation of gonads and hypophysectomy have illustrated that this event is under hormonal control (Larsen, 1980). Intestinal regression is initiated much earlier in nonparasitic species (Hilliard *et al.*, 1983), and in anadromous parasitic species results in loss of marine osmoregulation (Morris, 1972; Beamish, 1980b) and perhaps a site for the elimination of biliverdin (Langille and Youson, 1983).

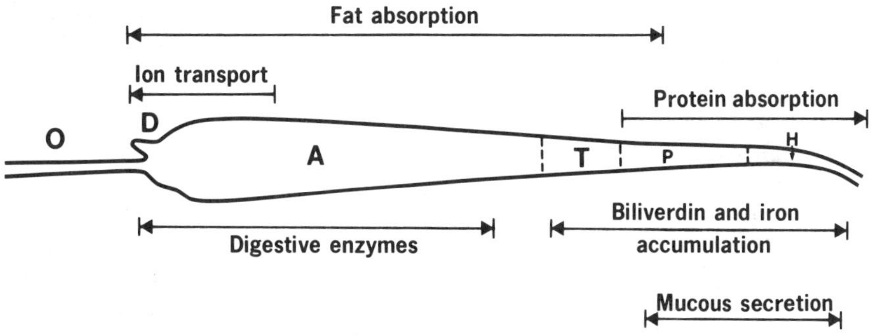

Fig. 2. Functions of various portions of the alimentary canal in adult *P. marinus*. *A*, anterior intestine; *D*, diverticulum; *H*, hindgut; *O*, oesophagus; *P*, posterior intestine; *T*, transition zone.

Liver

A greenish tinge to the developing gut (Piavis, 1971) marks the appearance of the liver primordium (hepatic pedicle) when the 3.0-5.0 mm (10-13 day) lamprey embryos demonstrate a ramified tubular liver (Brachet, 1897), which is characteristic of the ammocoete and mirrors the embryonic liver of higher forms (Sidon and Youson, 1983a). The lumina (canaliculi) of the parenchyma communicate with a network of bile ducts which ultimately deliver bile to the intrahepatic gall bladder and a common bile duct. The latter unites with the intestine at the oesophagal-intestinal junction in holarctic species (Youson, 1981b) or at a diverticulum in Southern Hemisphere species (Maskell, 1930; Strahan and Maclean, 1969). The exocrine (ductular) component of the liver in all lamprey species is lost at metamorphosis when the gall bladder, bile canaliculi, and bile ducts disappear (Youson, 1981b). These structures pass through a regression which parallels the events of human biliary atresia (Youson and Sidon, 1978; Sidon and Youson, 1983a). The morphology of the remaining hepatocytes reflects bile stasis (Sidon and Youson, 1983b) and loading with iron (Macey *et al.*, 1982; Youson *et al.*, 1983a, b). Following the loss of bile canaliculi, the hepatocytes seem to have the unique potential of transporting bile across the lateral cell membranes (Sidon and Youson, 1984). The method of transport of bile to a site of elimination is not known, but blood is expected to be the vehicle (Youson, 1981b). Extensive alterations to the hepatic vasculature take place at metamorphosis and primarily involve the hepatic portal and arterial vessels (Minelli and Rossini, 1961).

In spite of the potential bile stasis resulting from biliary atresia, the adult liver shows only minor colour change from the larval condition, *i.e.*, brown to reddish orange, with the latter reflecting the accumulation of some bilirubin (Kott, 1970). Battle and Hayashida (1965) indicate no colour differences in recently metamorphosed nonparasitic (*Ichthyomyzon fossor* and *Lampetra lamottenii*) and parasitic (*Petromyzon marinus*) species. However, sexual maturation is marked by a pronounced colour change in livers of all lamprey species. The colour is related to sex but shows interspecific variability. For example, pale leaf-green livers of male *P. marinus* compare to colour of livers in females of *Lampetra fluviatilis* while dark green livers are typical of females of *P. marinus* and males of *L. fluviatilis* (Lanzing, 1959; Kott, 1970; Larsen, 1973). Pickering (1976) shows that testosterone has a greater effect than oestradiol on liver colouration in *L. fluviatilis* while Kott (1970) indicates that the colour is due to the accumulation of biliverdin. It is noteworthy that this bile pigment begins to concentrate in the liver as the intestine commences to atrophy.

Endocrine pancreas

Although many cells of the gastro-entero-pancreatic system or amine precursor uptake and decarboxylation series were earlier claimed to originate from the neural crest (Pearse and Polak, 1971; Hardisty and Baker, 1982), more recent views favour an endodermal origin of these cells (Rutter, 1980; Andrew, 1984). In this context, it is of interest that cells of the endocrine pancreas of ammocoetes can only be traced to the epithelium of the oesophagus, bile duct, and intestine (Barrington, 1972). In fact, cells arise throughout larval life as buds of epithelial cells from the alimentary canal and eventually from follicles and islets in the submucosal connective tissue

(Ermisch, 1966; Morris and Islam, 1969). These groups of cells at the oesphageal-bile duct-intestinal junction (Fig. 1) in Northern Hemisphere species (Barrington, 1972) and between the oesophagus and inner edge of the two large diverticula (Fig. 1) in the Southern Hemisphere species, *G. australis* (Maskell, 1930; Hilliard *et al.*, 1985), are equivalent to the islets of Langerhans in the pancreatic tissue of other vertebrates (Barrington, 1972). However, only insulin- immunoreactive cells are present in the larval islet tissue of *L. fluviatilis* and *L. planeri* (Van Noorden *et al.*, 1972) and *P. marinus* (Elliott and Youson, unpublished data).

At metamorphosis the junction of the oesophagus and intestine, which in larvae is situated near the caudal tip of the liver, becomes positioned at the cephalic end of the liver near the heart (Fig. 1). In some species a small intestinal diverticulum is present at this junction (Youson, 1981a). In holarctic species, a cephalic pancreas appears in the submucosal connective tissue at this junction while a more caudal pancreas forms in the connective tissue connecting the transforming intestine to the liver at about its midpoint. The degree to which this caudal pancreatic tissue is embedded in the liver is variable among species (Barrington, 1972; Youson, unpublished). Furthermore, an intermediate cord of cells may connect the two larger masses of pancreatic tissue (Fig. 1). In contrast, the adults of Southern Hemisphere species, *G. australis* (Maskell, 1931; Hilliard *et al.*, 1985) and probably *M. mordax* (Strahan and Maclean, 1969), possess only a single mass of pancreatic tissue at the oesophageal-intestinal junction (Fig. 1) which corresponds to the cephalic pancreas of adult Petromyzontidae. The volume of the single mass in *G. australis* approximates the total volume of the three regions of pancreatic tissue in holarctic species (Hilliard *et al.*, 1985).

The method of formation of the adult pancreatic tissue during metamorphosis has never been definitively documented, but present evidence indicates that there is a marked difference in Northern and Southern Hemisphere species (Barrington, 1972; Hilliard *et al.*, 1985). The descriptive studies of Boenig (1927, 1929) on *L. planeri* convinced Barrington (1972) of the certain involvement of larval islet tissue in holarctic species in the formation of the adult cranial pancreas, while the caudal pancreas forms from cells of the degenerating intrahepatic and extrahepatic bile ducts. Recently, Hilliard *et al.* (1985) studied serial sections of metamorphosing *G. australis* and describe proliferating larval islet tissue as it remains alongside the most anterior region of the intestine during its progressive forward movement. According to these authors, the absence of caudal and intermediate pancreatic tissue is due to the lack of involvement of the bile duct in pancreatic morphogenesis during metamorphosis. The position of the bile duct in ammocoetes of both *G. australis* and *M. mordax* precludes its participation in development of any caudal pancreatic tissue.

Differential staining and immunocytochemical techniques have demonstrated that at least two cell types are present in the endocrine pancreatic tissue of adult lampreys. Immunofluorescence of islet tissue in adult *L. fluviatilis* reveals that a B-cell population is reactive to insulin antisera while a D-cell population is immunoreactive to mammalian somatostatin (Van Noorden and Pearse, 1974; Falkmer *et al.*, 1977; Van Noorden *et al.*, 1977). A similar situation has been demonstrated in adults of *P. marinus* using the peroxidase-anti-peroxidase technique (Elliott and Youson, in preparation). Brinn and Epple (1976) and Epple and Brinn (1975) have used differential staining in *P. marinus* to describe B cells and four types of acidophils (P cells). Adults of *G. australis* possess B cells and one type of P cell (Hilliard *et al.*, 1985).

Ontogenetic and phylogenetic considerations

We have little definitive information on the mode of feeding and on the digestive system of vertebrates considered to be ancestral to lampreys. The anaspids seem to be the most closely related group to modern-day petromyzonids,and suggestions for their adult feeding habits vary from detritus filter-feeding (Whiting, 1972) to the presence of a rasping tongue and parasitism (Stensiö, 1958). Fossils of the more recent *Mayomyzon* show that it was likely an adult or a transforming animal with a tongue-like piston, but we have no idea of the type of food (if any) that it ingested. Data on larval stages is lacking but the size of fossil *Mayomyzon* (Bardack and Zangerl, 1971) suggests that if it had a larval phase, it was of short duration (Hardisty, 1982). This is consistent with the view that the larval phase has been gradually extended during the evolutionary history of lampreys in order to take advantage of the increasing food supply in the freshwater environment (Hardisty, 1979). It is also a good example of "ontogenetic hypertrophy" (Smith, 1960), that is, that developmental sequences tend to become longer or more complex in evolution. An increase in free-living developmental longevity was tolerable to evolving ancestral lampreys because they were able to cope with the main problem of lengthening development, *i.e.*, providing an adequate food supply. They had inherited an efficient system of filtering food, perhaps from their anaspid ancestors (Whiting, 1972).

The issue of the origin of parasitic and nonparasitic species is always a further consideration when dealing with the phylogenetic development of the digestive system, and fossilized *Mayomyzon* provides no answer to this question. Its lanceolate-shaped liver and straight digestive tube are consistent features of modern-day lampreys, but the absence of teeth in *Mayomyzon* is a curiosity (Bardack and Zangerl, 1968). If parasitic species preceded nonparasitic species in lamprey evolution (Hardisty, 1979), this earliest of lampreys might have been expected to be equipped with teeth.

The straight tube of the alimentary canal of all lamprey species is a feature which is considered a primitive vertebrate character mainly due to a similar structure in protochordates (Smith, 1960). The anatomic integration of the respiratory and the digestive systems in ammocoetes is no doubt a reflection of both phylogenetic and ontogenetic development but an oesophagus separate from the pharynx was necessitated by macrophagous feeding and oral attachment in adults. The significance of ammocoete filter-feeding to their successful survival and the phylogenetic significance of this feeding device to protochordate and chordate relationships has been discussed extensively (Mallatt, 1981). The development of this new oesophagus during lamprey evolution and the disparate fashion of gill ventilation in hagfishes and lampreys serves as just one of several classic examples of the long separation of these two agnathan groups. The phylogenetic significance of the intestinal diverticula in lampreys has received wide attention (Strahan and Maclean, 1969; Barrington, 1972; Hardisty, 1979). Their absence in larvae of holarctic lampreys and large size in Southern Hemisphere species has led to the question of which is the more primitive lamprey group (Strahan and Maclean, 1969). The "protopancreas" of *M. mordax* may be the forerunner of the pancreas of gnathostomes. A more advanced situation in *M. mordax* may be illustrated by the greater quantities of digestive enzymes in the diverticulum compared to the intestinal epithelium (Strahan and Maclean, 1969). It would follow that holarctic species are more closely related to the "primitive" hagfish condition where secretory cells are located along a large part of the intestine and no diverticulum is present (Adam, 1963).

The "primitive" nature of the alimentary canal of lampreys is further illustrated by the absence of a true stomach which likely first evolved in vertebrates as a storage organ (Smith, 1960). It is of interest that the anterior intestine of parasitic adult lampreys expands during feeding (Youson and Connelly, 1978; Langille and Youson, 1984a), for this region of the alimentary canal may provide us with a view of an early step in the evolution of the vertebrate stomach. The presence of enzyme-secreting cells at this site is perhaps further support for this hypothesis. However, an ability for ion transport in osmoregulation and for lipid absorption (Fig. 2) is not a specialization usually equated with the vertebrate stomach. The involvement of the intestine in marine osmoregulation is a feature which equates lampreys with teleosts but which separates them from hagfishes (Morris, 1965). Protein absorption, as demonstrated in the posterior intestine of adult lampreys, is performed by the intestinal epithelium of many fishes (Noaillac-Depeyre and Gas, 1973; 1983) but it is particularly prevalent in stomachless fish (Stroband and Van Der Veen, 1981). This is illustrative of parallel evolutionary development of a mechanism in two distinctly different vertebrate groups for perhaps different purposes. The apparent ability of lampreys to excrete biliverdin, and perhaps other bile products, into the hindgut region in a retrograde fashion (Langille and Youson, 1983) has no known parallel among the vertebrates. This unique capability was acquired as a specialization following the loss of biliary connection between the liver and the alimentary canal. The atrophy of the intestine at sexual maturity is a feature characteristic of many anadromous fishes.

The transformation of the liver during lamprey metamorphosis from an exocrine and "endocrine" gland in ammocoetes to an entirely "endocrine" gland in adults has no equal in vertebrates. We also do not know whether the absence of bile ducts reflects the primitive origins of lampreys or whether it is a specialization of modern forms. Moreover, there is no firm evidence of the adaptive value of this atresia (Youson, 1981b). One could appreciate that adult lampreys feeding on blood and body fluids might not require bile acids and salts for absorption of lipids (Langille and Youson, 1984a), but bile ducts are also absent in those lamprey species which feed on body tissue (Youson, 1981b). Perhaps the absence of bile ducts is supportive of the view that extant lampreys evolved from entirely marine ancestors where water conservation was an important consideration. The fact that lampreys can survive following extirpation of up to 95% of the liver (Larsen, 1978) and that this organ has limited involvement in glucose metabolism (Larsen, 1980), are sufficient data to question the importance of the organ to adults up to the period immediately preceding sexual maturity. It may serve principally as a storage organ (bile products and iron) in the period commencing with metamorphosis and up to the beginning of sexual maturation, when in the female the synthesis of vitellogenin is performed, and in the male lipid is stored. If parasitic species evolved from nonparasitic species, this period of storage was extended in the former and the stored material became less of a hindrance to other liver functions (*e.g.*, synthesis of serum proteins) as the liver enlarged and had greater storage capacity. Hence, this may explain the presence of smaller amounts of iron and fewer biliary vacuoles in livers of sexually mature compared to recently metamorphosed individuals of the same parasitic species (Youson and Sargent, unpublished data). If one adopts the more widely accepted view that nonparasitic species evolved from parasitic species (Hardisty, 1979; Potter, 1980; Hardisty, 1982), then it has to be interpreted that the absence of bile ducts has not been an obstacle to the survival of feeding adult lampreys and perhaps it has an important adaptive significance.

The phylogenetic relationship of lamprey pancreatic endocrine tissue has been discussed extensively (Cotronei, 1927; Boenig, 1929; Barrington, 1945, 1972; Hardisty, 1979, 1982; Hardisty and Baker, 1982) and there is no doubt of its homology to the islets of Langerhans of gnathostomes. The existence of at least two cell types in islet tissue of adult lampreys and hagfishes attests to this specialization, but poor vascularization, follicular and cyst-like arrangement of cells, and the absence of glucagon-secreting A cells reflect its primitiveness (Hardisty and Baker, 1982). In addition, ammocoetes show a continuous production of follicles from the epithelium of the alimentary canal in a manner which likely reflects the ontogenesis and phylogenesis of the vertebrate pancreas. A further deviation from the typical vertebrate scheme is development of the large number of somatostatin-immunoreactive (D) cells in adults of holarctic lamprey species, when similar immunoreactivity is absent in islet tissue of the larval stage. It is of great interest that D cells appear only after loss of the bile duct at metamorphosis. Perhaps this is a further explanation for the adaptive significance of atresia of bile ducts in lampreys, that is, the need for an expansion and specialization of the endocrine pancreatic tissue. It follows that the smaller number of D cells in hagfishes (Van Noorden *et al.*, 1977) may be accounted for by the persistence of the bile duct from which much of the islet tissue originates (Falkmer *et al.*, 1974). Moreover, the presence of only one P cell in the single (cephalic) pancreas of *G. australis* may be due to the lack of involvement of the bile duct in formation of this tissue at metamorphosis (Hilliard *et al.*, 1985). Future studies should be directed towards the origin and functional significance of D cells in adult lampreys.

Excretory system

Pronephros

Nephrogenic tissue arises from lateral mesoderm of early lamprey embryos and probably extends the length of the coelomic cavity. The most anterior of the nephrotomes differentiate first, and the paired pronephroi each appear with 3 to 8 tubules just behind the posterior end of the branchial region (Wheeler, 1899) at the time of hatching (Youson, 1981c). Torrey (1938) has shown that the pronephroi of large ammocoetes function to take up fluid through their ciliated nephrostomes, so undoubtedly the pronephroi of young ammocoetes are capable of some urine production. The fine structure of the cells of both the glomus and tubules reflect this potential (Youson, 1981c). The elements of pronephros undergo some regression during larval life (Bowen, 1969) and apparently connection with the excretory duct is lost. Contrary to earlier opinion, the organ never completely disappears. It is present in varying degrees of elaboration within the pericardial cavity (which separates from the coelom at metamorphosis) at sexual maturity in all lamprey species so far examined (Youson, 1981c).

Larval opisthonephros

Paired opisthonephroi are concomitant with the pronephroi in larval lampreys. They begin to differentiate from nephrogenic tissue immediately posterior to the pronephroi at the time prolarvae leave the nest, and they become the primary larval kidneys. Growth of these kidneys is rapid during the first three years of larval life in *P. marinus* but it is slower over the next 3 to 5 years (Ooi and Youson, 1976). Development is continuous throughout the larval life and takes place through the addition of tubules and renal corpuscles at the posterior end. There is some question whether posterior development is accompanied by anterior regression (Ooi and Youson, 1976) resulting in a backward progression of the kidney tissue (Wheeler, 1899). These nephrons are similar to those in other vertebrate kidneys in that they are composed of both renal corpuscle and tubular portions. However, they differ in that the renal corpuscles are compound, sausage-shaped and placed end to end. They are also longer in the more posterior regions (most recently developed) of the kidneys (Fig. 3). The fine structure of the renal corpuscle reveals a typical vertebrate filtration apparatus (Youson and McMillan, 1970a). The tubule shows a regional specialization, with the most proximal end (neck segment) resembling a ciliated nephrostome, a proximal segment involved in absorption (Youson and McMillan, 1970b) and a distal segment with cells reflecting involvement in ion transport and glycogen storage (Youson and McMillan, 1971a). As in many gnathostome fishes, the larval kidney is also a haemopoietic organ (Potter *et al.*, 1982b). The larval opisthonephroi undergo an abrupt degeneration during metamorphosis (Ooi and Youson, 1979). The events of this regression are similar to those seen in the pronephros during larval life and during the ontogeny of the excretory systems of most vertebrates. The timing of this regression is correlated with the development of the definitive adult kidney (Ooi and Youson, 1977) in order to prevent proteinuria.

Adult opisthonephros

The remaining portion of the nephrogenic tissue is located behind the larval opisthonephroi in paired nephric folds (Fig. 3) and it differentiates into the definitive adult kidneys at metamorphosis. Nephrons develop simultaneously in each kidney from this nephrogenic cord which extends to the cloaca. The proximal end of each nephron becomes a nephric capsule and extends between capillaries (Youson and Ooi, 1979) while the remainder differentiates into a tubule with regional specialization (Ooi and Youson, 1977; Youson, 1984). Unlike the situation in gnathostomes, the nephric capsules (not a true Bowman's capsule) of each nephron become apposed to one another and form a single, sausage-shaped renal corpuscle that extends the length of the kidney (Fig. 3). This compound renal corpuscle contains many fused glomeruli, *i.e.* a glomus, which is surrounded by epithelium from many capsules. Each capsule is continuous, with a single renal tubule which extends towards the ventral tip of the kidney, where a common

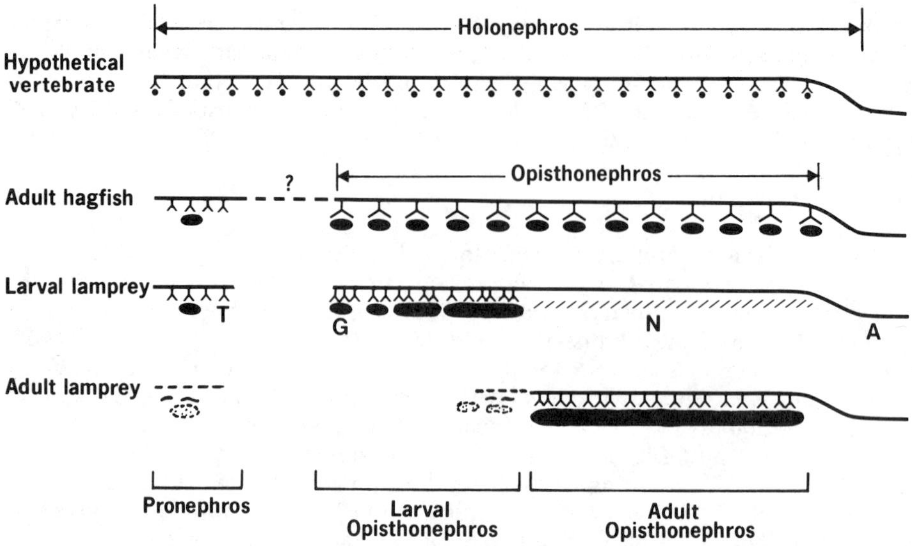

Fig. 3. Schematic interpretation of the relationship of the kidneys of hagfishes, and larval and adult lampreys to one another and to the kidney of a hypothetical vertebrate. See the text for description. *A*, archinephric duct; *G*, glomus; *N*, nephrogenic tissue; *T*, tubule.

collecting duct is shared and is continuous with the archinephric (excretory) duct. The degree of elaboration of the kidneys is variable among lamprey species with respect to the size and location of the renal corpuscle, the arrangement of the tubules, and the size of the archinephric duct (Youson, 1981c). In general, the definitive kidney of nonparasitic species show similarities to the ammocoete kidney. On the other hand, the kidneys of anadromous species show a high degree of specialization which has been equated with their ability to osmoregulate in salt- and freshwater (Beamish, 1980b; Logan *et al.*, 1980a, b; Youson, 1982a, b.). Features of the kidney which are important to this mechanism are the chloride-like cells of the distal tubule (Miyoshi, 1970; Youson and McMillan, 1971b), the extensive vascular surface of the glomus, and perhaps, the parallel arrangement and looping of the tubules in the ventral part of the kidney (Youson, 1981c). In contrast to other vertebrates below Class Aves, lampreys have no renal portal system (Youson and McMillan, 1971c). Unlike the opisthonephroi of larval lampreys and many gnathostome fishes, the opisthonephroi of adult lampreys are not a storage site for haemopoietic tissue. However, cells lining the sinusoids play a major role in erythrophagocytosis (Youson, 1971; Youson and McMillan, 1971c) while others are a storage site for vitamin A (Wake, 1982).

Adrenocortical homologue

Hardisty (1972) has provided an in-depth review of the embryological development of the adrenocortical homologue (AH cells, interrenal tissue) in lampreys which, according to Poll (1904) and Sterba (1955), follows the typical vertebrate pattern, that is, from a mesodermal blastema in conjunction with the developing kidneys. In young larvae (> 9 mm) AH cells have been reported to develop from coelomic epithelium of the pronephric region (Sterba, 1955) and they may develop in this manner throughout the body cavity in association to both the larval and adult opisthonephroi and the posterior cardinal veins.

The most densely concentrated population of AH cells is in the pronephros (Hardisty and Baines, 1971; Hardisty, 1972) but it is now clear that they are diffusely scattered along the walls of the posterior cardinal veins and in the larval and adult opisthonephroi (Youson, 1972, 1973a; Seiler and Seiler, 1973). In the larval and adult opisthonephroi they show an intimate relationship to the arterial circulation and may be located within the renal corpuscle (Youson, 1972). Attempts to identify the enzyme Δ^{5}-^{3}ß-hydroxysteroid dehydrogenase (3ß-HSD) through histochemistry in AH cells of ammocoetes have met with failure in all species (Seiler *et al.*, 1970; Hardisty and Baines, 1971; Youson, 1972). However, following an increase in size and in cytoplasmic/nuclear volume ratio of AH cells with the commencement of metamorphosis (Sterba, 1955), 3ß-HSD is detectable (Seiler *et al.*, 1981) and therefore indicates a greater activity of the enzyme in transformation of pregnenolone to progesterone at this phase of the life cycle. The presence of the 3ß-HSD has been detected only in adults in extracts of presumptive adrenocortical tissue using spectrophotometric techniques (Weisbart *et al.*, 1978).

The eventual fate of the AH cells of the larval opisthonephroi following the complete regression of the kidneys is not known, but their viability when adjacent renal tissue is degenerating has been noted (Youson, 1980). It is possible that AH cells persist in the rudiment of the larval opisthonephroi just as they do in the rudiments of the pronephroi. AH cells are not prominent in the kidneys of parasitic adult lampreys of *P. marinus* but they are conspicuous during the upstream migration (Youson, 1972). Therefore AH cells must continue to differentiate from coelomic cells and/or they proliferate during development and growth of the adult opisthonephroi.

Morphology of the AH cells in larval *L. planeri* (Hardisty and Baines, 1971; Hardisty, 1972; Seiler *et al.*, 1973) and both larval and adult *P. marinus* (Youson, 1972, 1973b; Weisbart *et al.*, 1978) demonstrate their capability for steroidogenesis. Furthermore, incubated AH tissue is able to convert radioactive steroid precursors to detectable levels of compounds such as 11-deoxycortisol and androstenedione (Weisbart and Youson, 1975). Despite morphological and *in vitro* biochemical information, the homology of AH tissue in lampreys to adrenocortical tissue in higher vertebrates is questionable (Hardisty and Baker, 1982).

Ontogenetic and phylogenetic considerations

The ontogenetic history of renal excretory tissue during the lamprey life cycle follows the pattern known for almost every vertebrate group (Torrey, 1965). That is, there are three generations of kidneys which follow each other during successive events of ontogeny. However, there are two features which combine to make the lamprey situation unique. First, ontogeny is prolonged due to an extended larval phase and secondly, two or more generations of kidneys may function at the same time. Although we have no factual information, it is possible that vertebrates ancestral to lampreys had a maximum of two generations of kidneys. This view is supported by the representation of co-existing functional pronephroi (Holmgren, 1950) and opisthonephroi (Heath-Eves and McMillan, 1974) in adult hagfishes. Despite being far removed from one another in terms of their phylogenetic development (Hardisty, 1979, 1982), hagfishes and lampreys are still both agnathans and may have shared some common features in their earlier history. The appearance of three generations of kidneys in extant lampreys is probably due to the extension of the larval phase during the course of lamprey phylogeny. Originally, nephrogenic tissue behind the pronephroi and extending to the cloaca might have been used entirely for development of the adult kidneys. This would have made the pronephroi the excretory organs during a short larval phase. However, an extension of the larval phase and the accompanying increase in body size would have put pressure on the excretory system, resulting in utilization of some of the nephrogenic tissue for a second generation kidney. This second kidney (larval opisthonephros) proved to be highly efficient, resulting in a tendency for a premature degeneration of the pronephros before metamorphosis. Replacement of the larval opisthonephros was ultimately necessitated by demands of marine osmoregulation, which may have been acquired later in lamprey phylogeny (Lutz, 1975; Hardisty, 1979).

The ontogeny of lamprey renal tissue into three generations also has some significance to the view of the existence of a holonephric or archinephric kidney in a hypothetical vertebrate ancestor. This theory contends that paired segmentally-arranged nephrons were present throughout the length of the coelom in a vertebrate ancestor (Torrey, 1965). It has been suggested that the renal tissue of hagfishes most closely resembles this arrangement in extant vertebrates (Hardisty, 1979; Youson, 1981c), yet lampreys have at least parts of three generations of kidneys co-existing at certain periods of the life cycle. Furthermore, there are many similarities to each of the three kidneys, particularly in their tubules and in the distribution, shape, and compound nature of their renal corpuscles. Similarity in shape and distribution is also shared between young ammocoetes and adult hagfishes. In fact, one can visualize a progression from the holonephros through hagfishes and larval lampreys to the adult lamprey kidneys (Fig. 3). This progression is based on the gradual fusion of holonephric glomeruli to form segmentally-arranged small glomera, as present in hagfish pronephroi and opisthonephroi. These small glomera are also found in ammocoete pronephroi and at the anterior end of their opisthonephroi. The opisthonephroi of adult lampreys each have a single large glomus, which may have resulted from the union of smaller glomera. That fusion of glomera is possible, is supported by the presence of longer glomera at the posterior ends of the larval opisthonephroi. The existence of the longer glomera in this position in the larval opisthonephroi is consistent with the view expressed earlier that extension of the larval phase during lamprey phylogeny resulted in utilization of nephrogenic tissue which may have formally developed into the adult kidney. Proof for the above may be provided following the examination of the glomera in opisthonephroi from larval lamprey species such as *Geotria* and *Mordacia*, which spend a relatively short time as ammocoetes compared

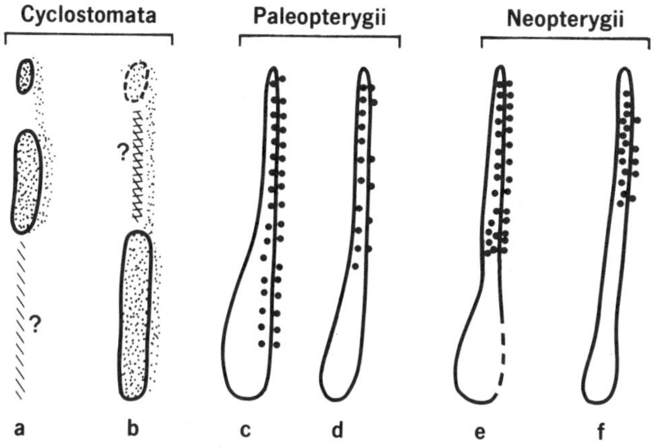

Fig. 4. Distribution of adrenocortical tissue as diffusely scattered islets (dots) in the kidneys and around dorsal vessels in larval (a) and adult (b) lampreys is compared with adrenocortical tissue in corpuscles (dark circles) in *Acipenser* (c), *Polypterus* (d), *Amia* (e), and *Lepisosteus* (f). Note the progressive anterior accumulation from c to f.

to many holarctic species (Potter, 1980). The adaptive significance of the absence of a renal portal system in larval and adult lampreys is not clear. Due to the absence of this system in the mammalian kidney it is tempting to suggest that, in addition to illustrating parallel evolution, it is also a further indication of the specialization of the lamprey kidney.

There is little doubt that the agnathan "presumptive" adrenocortical homologue (AH) represents the most primitive vertebrate condition (Hardisty, 1972, 1979; Hardisty and Baker, 1982). The tendency among vertebrates for a more anterior concentration of this tissue within the coelomic cavity or within kidneys has long been reported (Chester Jones *et al.*, 1962). Among the more primitive gnathostome fishes, the distribution of AH reflects the position of the animal on the taxonomic scale (Fig. 4). The distribution, and in fact the existence, of the AH in hagfishes is a matter of debate, but there is some evidence to indicate that it is confined to the pronephric region (Chester Jones and Phillips, 1960; Idler and Burton, 1976) and is similar to the position of AH in higher fishes. On the other hand, the diffuse distribution of small islets of AH cells throughout the nephric folds in the pronephric, larval opisthonephric, and adult opisthonephric kidneys of lampreys does not have a parallel in vertebrates. Even the most primitive Osteichthyes have their numerous AH cells aggregated into yellow corpuscles which, although nonencapsulated, are isolated from renal and haemopoietic tissues (for review see Youson and Butler, 1985). Lampreys may closely resemble an original vertebrate condition which was believed to be the co-existence of AH cells with kidney tubules (Chester Jones and Phillips, 1960). Even though the intimacy of AH cells and the arterial circulation in lampreys is unique, the association of these cells to the posterior cardinal veins is a feature consistent with the Osteichthyes.

Summary and conclusions

The digestive system has many examples which illustrate that lampreys are a specialized vertebrate group but at the same time reflect on their primitive origins. Thus, in the adult the suctoral mouth and an oesophagus independent of a pharynx are specialized features, whereas the intestine, endocrine pancreas and liver would seem, at first glance, to represent stages in the ontogenetic and phylogenetic development of these organs. However, this straight (primitive) intestine shows regional specialization of function both comparable and unique to vertebrates. Although isolated from the alimentary canal through the absence of bile ducts, the liver of adult lampreys cannot be considered primitive. The existence of bile ducts in larvae and their programmed atresia at metamorphosis is an indication that a liver without bile ducts may have evolved in lampreys as either a specialization in function (*e.g.* storage), a requirement of ontogenesis (caudal endocrine pancreas), or due to a lack of need (gut excretion of bile). The endocrine pancreas seems to represent a simple collection of islet tissue with only some of the secretory properties of the islets of Langerhans of higher vertebrates and only marginal association with an exocrine pancreas. A feature for future study is the relationship between the atretic bile ducts and the development of somatostatin (D) cells, for it may provide insight into the ontogeny and functional significance of this cell type among the vertebrates.

The excretory system of lampreys is both a unique and a highly specialized organ system. Morphogenesis of the renal tissue during the extended ontogenetic phases of larval life and metamorphosis provides an opportunity to examine various developmental parameters through three generations of kidneys. It also provides some clue to the possible evolution of the excretory system in lampreys, and the structure of the kidney in organisms considered to be ancestral to all vertebrates. Despite these connotations of primitiveness, the adult lamprey has a highly evolved, unique, and specialized kidney which is characterized by the presence of a single renal corpuscle, regional differentiation of the tubules, and the absence of a renal portal system. The diffuse distribution of presumptive adrenocortical tissue within all three generations of kidneys is likely representative of the most primitive vertebrate condition. This is in keeping with present physiological and biochemical evidence on the corticosteroidogenic activity of this tissue.

Acknowledgements

This study was supported by grants from Medical Research Council and the Natural Sciences and Engineering Research Council of Canada.

Literature Cited

ADAM, H. 1963. Structure and histochemistry of the alimentary canal. pp. 256-288 *In* Brodal, A., and R. Fänge [eds.] The biology of *Myxine*. Universitetsforlaget, Oslo.

ANDREW, A. 1984. The development of the gastro-entero-pancreatic neuro-endocrine system in birds. pp. 91-109 *In* Falkmer, S., R. Hakanson, and F.

Sundler [eds.] Evolution and tumor pathology of the neuroendocrine system. Elsevier, Amsterdam.

BALINSKY, B.I. 1970. An introduction to embryology. Saunders, Philadelphia, 725 pp.

BARDACK, D., and R. ZANGERL. 1968. First fossil lamprey: a record from the Pennsylvanian of Illinois. Science **162**: 1265-1267.

BARDACK, D., and R. ZANGERL. 1971. Lampreys in the fossil record. pp. 67-84 *In* Hardisty, M.W., and I.C. Potter [eds.] The biology of lampreys, vol. 1. Academic Press, London.

BARRINGTON, F.J.W. 1936. Proteolytic digestion and the problem of the pancreas in the ammocoete larva of *Lampetra planeri*. Proc. R. Soc. (Lond.). **121B**: 221-232.

BARRINGTON, F.J.W. 1945. The supposed pancreatic organs of *Petromyzon fluviatilis* and *Myxine glutinosa*. Q. J. Microsc. Sci. **85**: 391-417.

BARRINGTON, F.J.W. 1972. The pancreas and intestine. pp.135-169. *In* Hardisty, M.W., and I.C. Potter [eds.] The biology of lampreys, vol. 2. Academic Press, London.

BATTLE, H.I., and K. HAYASHIDA. 1965. Comparative study of the intraperitoneal alimentary tract of parasitic and nonparasitic lampreys from the Great Lakes region. J. Fish. Res. Bd. Can. **22**: 289-306.

BEAMISH, F.W.H. 1980a. Biology of the North American anadromous sea lamprey, *Petromyzon marinus*. Can. J. Fish. Aquat. Sci. **37**: 1924-1943.

BEAMISH, F.W.H. 1980b. Osmoregulation in juvenile and adult lampreys. Can. J. Fish. Aquat. Sci. **37**: 1739-1750.

BOENIG, H. 1927. Studien zur Morphologie und Entwicklungsgeschichte des Pankreas beim Bachneunauge [*Lampetra (Petromyzon) planeri*]. I. Teil. Z. mikrosdk. - anat. Forsch. **8**: 489-511.

BOENIG, H. 1929. Studien zur Morphologie und Entwicklungsgeschichte des Pankreas beim Bachneunauge *Lampetra (Petromyzon) planeri*. III. Die Histologie und Histogenese des Pankreas. Z. Mikrosk. - anat. Forsch. **17**: 125-184.

BOWEN, P.C. 1969. The cytology of the pronephros of lampreys. Ph.D. Dissertation. University of Oxford, Oxford, U.K.

BRACHET, A. 1897. Sur le developpement du foie et sur le pancreas de l'Ammocoetes. Anat. Anz. **13**: 621-636.

BRINN, J.E., and A. EPPLE. 1976. New types of islet cells in a cyclostome, *Petromyzon marinus* L. Cell Tiss. Res. **171**: 317-329.

CHESTER JONES, I., and J.G. PHILLIPS. 1960. Adrenocorticosteroids in fish. Symp. Zool. Soc. (Lond.) **1**: 17-32.

CHESTER JONES, I., J.G. PHILLIPS, and D. BELLAMY. 1962. The adrenal cortex throughout the vertebrates. Br. Med. Bull. **18**: 110-114.

COTRONEI, G. 1927. L'organo insulare di *Petromyzon marinus* (Nuovo richerche sui Petromyzonti). Pubbl. Staz. zool. Napoli. **8**: 71-127.

EPPLE, A., and J.E. BRINN. 1975. Islet histophysiology: evolutionary correlations. Gen. comp. Endocrinol. **27**: 320-349.

EPPLE, A., and J.E. BRINN. 1976. New perspectives in comparative islet research. pp. 83-95 *In* Grillo, T.A.I., L. Leibson, and A. Epple [eds.] The evolution of pancreatic islets. Pergamon Press, New York.

ERMISCH, A. 1966. Beitrage zur Histologie und Topochemie des Inselsystems der Neunaugen unter naturlichen und experimentellen Bedingungen. Zool. Jb. **83**: 52-106.

FALKMER, S., N.W. THOMAS, and I. BOQUIST. 1974. Endocrinology of the Cyclostomata. pp. 195-257 *In* Florkin, M., and B.Y. Scheer [eds.] Chemical zoology, vol. 8. Academic Press, London.

FALKMER, S., R.P. ELDE, C. HELLERSTROM, B. PETERSSON, S. EFENDIC, J. FOHLMAN, and J.B. SILJEVALL. 1977. Some phylogenetic aspects of the occurrence of somatostatin in the gastro-entero-pancreatic system. A histological and immunocytochemical study combined with quantitative radio-immunological assays of tissue extracts. Arch. Histol. Jpn. **40**: 99-117.

GIBBS, S.P. 1956. The anatomy and development of the buccal glands of the lake lamprey (*Petromyzon marinus* L.) and the histochemistry of their secretion. J. Morph. **98**: 429-470.

GORBMAN, A., and H.A. BERN. 1962. A textbook of comparative endocrinology. Wiley, New York, 468 pp.

HANSEN, S.J., and J.H. YOUSON. 1978. Morphology of the epithelium in the alimentary tract of the larval lamprey, *Petromyzon marinus* L. J. Morph. **155**: 193-217.

HARDISTY, M.W. 1972. The interrenal. pp. 171-192 *In* Hardisty, M.W., and I.C. Potter [eds.] The biology of lampreys, vol. 2. Academic Press, London.

HARDISTY, M.W. 1979. Biology of the cyclostomes. Chapman and Hall, London, 428 pp.

HARDISTY, M.W. 1982. Lampreys and hagfishes: analysis of cyclostome relationships. pp. 165-260 *In* Hardisty, M.W., and I.C. Potter [eds.] The biology of lampreys, vol. 4B. Academic Press, London.

HARDISTY, M.W., and M. BAINES. 1971. The ultrastructure of the interrenal tissue of the lamprey. Experientia **27**: 1072-1075.

HARDISTY, M.W., and B.I. BAKER. 1982. Endocrinology. pp. 1-115 *In* Hardisty, M.W., and I.C. Potter [eds.] The biology of lampreys, vol. 4B. Academic Press, London.

HARDISTY, M.W., and I.C. POTTER. 1971a. The behaviour, ecology and growth of larval lampreys. pp. 85-125 *In* Hardisty, M.W., and I.C. Potter [eds.] The biology of lampreys, vol. 1. Academic Press, London.

HARDISTY, M.W., and I.C. POTTER. 1971b. The general biology of adult lampreys. pp. 127-206 *In* Hardisty, M.W., and I.C. Potter. [eds.] The biology of lampreys, vol. 1. Academic Press, London.

HARDISTY, M.W., I.C. POTTER, and E.R. STURGE. 1970. A comparison of the metamorphosing and macrophthalmic stages of the lampreys *Lampetra fluviatilis* and *Lampetra planeri*. J. Zool. (Lond.) **162**: 383-400.

HEATH-EVES, M.J., and D.B. McMILLAN. 1974. The morphology of the kidney of the Atlantic hagfish, *Myxine glutinosa* L. Amer. J. Anat. **139**: 309-334.

HILLIARD, R.W., D.J. BIRD, and I.C. POTTER. 1983. Metamorphic changes in the intestine of three species of lampreys. J. Morph. **176**: 181-196.

HILLIARD, R.W., A. EPPLE, and I.C. POTTER. 1985. The morphology and histology of the endocrine pancreas of the Southern Hemisphere lamprey, *Geotria australis* Gray. J. Morph. (in press).

HOLMGREN, N. 1950. On the pronephros and the blood in *Myxine glutinosa*. Acta Zool. (Stockh.) **31**: 233-348.

HUBBS, C.I., and I.C. POTTER. 1971. Distribution, phylogeny and taxonomy. pp. 1-65 *In* Hardisty, M.W., and I.C. Potter [eds.] The biology of lampreys, vol. 1. Academic Press, London.

IDLER, D.R., and M.D.M. BURTON. 1976. The pronephroi as the site of presumptive interrenal cells in the hagfish, *Myxine glutinosa* L. Comp. Biochem. Physiol. **53A**: 73-77.

JOHNELS, A.G. 1948. On the development and morphology of the skeleton of the head of *Petromyzon*. Acta Zool. (Stockh.) **29**: 139-279.

KOTT, E. 1970. Differences between the livers of spawning male and female sea lamprey (*Petromyzon marinus*). Can. J. Zool. **48**: 745-750.

LANGILLE, R.M., and J.H. YOUSON. 1983. Biliverdin accumulation in the caudal intestinal segment of juvenile adult lampreys, *Petromyzon marinus* L. Can. J. Zool. **61**: 1824-1834.

LANGILLE, R.M., and J.H. YOUSON. 1984a. Morphology of the intestine of prefeeding and feeding adult lampreys, *Petromyzon marinus* L.: the mucosa of the diverticulum, anterior intestine, and the transition zone. J. Morph. **182**: 39-61.

LANGILLE, R.M, and J.H. YOUSON. 1984b. Morphology of the intestine of prefeeding and feeding adult lampreys, *Petromyzon marinus* L.: the mucosa of the posterior intestine and hindgut. J. Morph. **182**: 137-152.

LANZING, W.J.R. 1959. Studies on the river lamprey *Lampetra fluviatilis* during its anadromous migration. Uitsgeversmaatschappij, Neerlandia. Utrecht.

LARSEN, L.O. 1973. Development in adult, freshwater river lampreys and its hormonal control. Starvation, sexual maturation and natural death. Thesis, University of Copenhagen.

LARSEN, L.O. 1978. Subtotal hepatectomy in intact or hypophysectomized river lampreys (*Lampetra fluviatilis* L.): effects on regeneration, blood glucose regulation, and vitellogenesis. Gen. comp. Endocrinol. **35**: 197-204.

LARSEN, L.O. 1980. The physiology of adult lampreys, with special reference to natural starvation, reproduction, and death after spawning. Can. J. Fish. Aquat. Sci. **37**: 1762-1779.

LETHBRIDGE, R.C., and I.C. POTTER. 1979. The oral fimbriae of the lamprey *Geotria australis*. J. Zool. (Lond.) **188**: 267-277.

LETHBRIDGE, R.C., and I.C. POTTER. 1981. The development of teeth and associated feeding structures during the metamorphosis of the lamprey, *Geotria australis*. Acta Zool (Stockh.) **62**: 201-227.

LOGAN, A.G., R.J. MORIARTY, and J.C. RANKIN. 1980a. A micropuncture study of kidney function in the river lamprey, *Lampetra fluviatilis*, adapted to fresh water. J. exp. Biol. **85**: 137-147.

LOGAN, A.G., R. MORRIS, and J.C. RANKIN. 1980b. A micropuncture study of kidney function in the river lamprey, *Lampetra fluviatilis* adapted to sea water. J. exp. Biol. **88**: 239-247.

LØVTRUP, S. 1977. The phylogeny of vertebrata. Wiley, London, 330 pp.

LUTZ, P.L. 1975. Adaptive and evolutionary aspects of the ionic content of fishes. *Copeia* **1975**: 369-373.

MACEY, D.J., J. WEBB, and I.C. POTTER. 1982. Distribution of iron-containing granules in lampreys, with particular reference to the Southern Hemisphere lamprey *Geotria australis* Gray. Acta Zool. (Stockh.) **63**: 91-99.

MALLATT, J. 1981. The suspension feeding mechanism of the larval lamprey *Petromyzon marinus*. J. Zool. (Lond.) **194**: 103-142.

MANION, P.J., and G.W. PIAVIS. 1977. Dentition throughout the life history of the landlocked sea lamprey, *Petromyzon marinus*. Copeia **1977**: 762-766.

MASKELL, F.G. 1930. On the New Zealand lamprey, *Geotria australis* Gray. Part

II. On the mid-gut diverticula, the bile-duct, and the problem of the pancreas in the ammocoetes stage. Trans. N.Z. Inst. **61**: 478-498.

MASKELL, F.G. 1931. On the New Zealand lamprey, *Geotria australis* Gray. Part III. The loss of the mid-gut diverticula of the ammocoetes stage at metamorphosis. Trans. N.Z. Inst. **62**: 120-128.

MINELLI, G.L., and M.C. ROSSINI. 1961. Structura e rapporti vascolari del fegato nello larva e nell'adulto di Lampreda (*Lampetra planeri*). Arch. Stal. Anat. Embriol. **66**: 385-406.

MIYOSHI, M. 1970. The fine structure of the mesonephros of the lamprey *Entosphenus japonicus* Mertens. Z. Zellforsch-mikrosk. Anat. **104**: 213-230.

MORRIS, R. 1965. Studies on salt and water balance in *Myxine glutinosa* L. J. exp. Biol. **42**: 359-371.

MORRIS, R. 1972. Osmoregulation. pp. 193-239 *In* Hardisty, M.W., and I.C. Potter [eds.] The biology of lampreys, vol. 2. Academic Press, London.

MORRIS, R., and D.S. ISLAM. 1969. The effect of hormones and hormone inhibitors on blood sugar regulation and the follicles of Langerhans in ammocoete larvae. Gen. comp. Endocrinol. **12**: 81-90.

NOAILLAC-DEPEYRE, J., and N. GAS. 1973. Absorption of protein macromolecules by the enterocytes of the carp (*Cyprinus carpio* Y.). Z. Zellforsch. mikrosk. Anat. **146**: 525-541.

NOAILLAC-DEPEYRE, J., and N. GAS. 1983. Étude cytophysiologique de l'epithelium intestinal du poisson-chat (*Ameiurus nebulosus* L.). Can. J. Zool. **61**: 2556-2573.

VAN NOORDEN, S., and A.G.E. PEARSE. 1974. Immunoreactive polypeptide hormones in the pancreas and gut of the lamprey. Gen. comp. Endocrinol. **23**: 311-324.

VAN NOORDEN, S., J. GREENBERG, and A.G.E. PEARSE. 1972. Cytochemical and immunofluorescence investigations on polypeptide hormone localization in the pancreas and gut of the larval lamprey. Gen comp. Endocrinol. **19**: 192-199.

VAN NOORDEN, S., Y. OSTBERG, and A.G.E. PEARSE. 1977. Localization of somatostatin-like immunoreactivity in the pancreatic islets of the hagfish, *Myxine glutinosa* and the lamprey, *Lampetra fluviatilis*. Cell Tiss. Res. **177**: 281-285.

OOI, E.C., and J.H. YOUSON. 1976. Growth of the opisthonephric kidney during larval life in the anadromous sea lamprey, *Petromyzon marinus* L. Can. J. Zool. **54**: 1449-1458.

OOI, E.C., and J.H. YOUSON. 1977. Morphogenesis and growth of the definitive opisthonephros during metamorphosis of the anadromous sea lamprey, *Petromyzon marinus* L. J. Embryol. exp. Morph. **42**: 219-235.

OOI, E.C., and J.H. YOUSON. 1979. Regression of the larval opisthonephros during metamorphosis of the sea lamprey, *Petromyzon marinus* L. Amer. J. Anat. **154**: 57-79.

PEARSE, A.G.E., and J.M. POLAK. 1971. Neural crest origin of the endocrine polypeptide (APUD) cells of the gastrointestinal tract and pancreas. Gut **12**: 783-788.

PERCY, R., and I.C. POTTER. 1977. Changes in haemopoietic sites during the metamorphosis of the lampreys, *Lampetra fluviatilis* and *Lampetra planeri*. J. Zool. (Lond.) **183**: 111-123.

PIAVIS, G.W. 1971. Embryology. pp. 361-400 *In* Hardisty, M.W., and I.C. Potter [eds.] The biology of lampreys, vol. 1. Academic Press, London.

PICKERING, A.D. 1976. Stimulation of intestinal degeneration by oestradiol and testosterone implantation in the migrating river lamprey, *Lampetra fluviatilis* L. Gen. comp. Endocrinol. **30**: 340-346.

PICKERING, A.D., and R. MORRIS. 1973. Localisation of ion transport in the intestine of the migrating river lamprey *Lampetra fluviatilis* L. J. exp. Biol. **58**: 165-176.

POLL, H. 1904. Allemeines zur Entwickelungsgeschichte der Zwischenniere. Anat. Anz. **25**: 16-25.

POTTER, I.C. 1980. Ecology, growth, and duration of larval life in lampreys. Can. J. Fish. Aquat. Sci. **37**: 1641-1657.

POTTER, I.C., R.W. HILLIARD, and D.J. BIRD. 1982a. Stages in metamorphosis. pp. 137-164 *In* Hardisty, M.W., and I.C. Potter [eds.] The biology of lampreys, vol. 4B. Academic Press, London.

POTTER, I.C., R. PERCY, D.L. BARBER, and D.J. MACEY. 1982b. The morphology, development and physiology of blood cells. pp. 234-292 *In* Hardisty, M.W., and I.C. Potter [eds.] The biology of lampreys, vol. 4A. Academic Press, London.

RANDALL, D.J. 1972. Respiration. pp. 287-306 *In* Hardisty, M.W., and I.C. Potter [eds.] The biology of lampreys, vol. 2. Academic Press, London.

RICHARDS, J.E., and F.W.H. BEAMISH. 1981. Initiation of feeding and salinity tolerance in the Pacific lamprey, *Lampetra tridentata*. Mar. Biol. **63**: 73-78.

RUTTER, W.J. 1980. The development of the endocrine and exocrine pancreas. pp. 30-38 *In* Fitzgerald, P.J., and A.M. Morrison [eds.] The pancreas. Williams and Wilkins, Baltimore.

SEILER, K., and R. SEILER. 1973. Zur Topographie des Interrenal-und-Adrenal-Systems des Bachneunauges (*Lampetra planeri* Bloch). Gegenbaurs morph. Jb (Leipzig). **119**: 796-808.

SEILER, K., R. SEILER, and R. CLAUS. 1981. Histochemical and spectrophotometric demonstration of hydroxysteroid dehydrogenase activity in the presumed steroid producing cells of the brook lamprey (*Lampetra planeri* Bloch) during metamorphosis. Endokrinologie. **78**: 297-300.

SEILER, K., R. SEILER, and G. HOHEISEL. 1973. Zur Cytologie des Interrenal Systems beim Bachneunauge (*Lampetra planeri* Bloch). Gegenbaurs morph. Jb. (Leipzig). **119**: 823-856.

SEILER, K., R. SEILER, and G. STERBA. 1970. Histochemische Untersuchungen am Interrenalsystem des Bachneunauges (*Lampetra planeri* Bloch). Acta Biol. Med. Ger. **24**: 553-554.

SIDON, E.W., and J.H. YOUSON. 1983a. Morphological changes in the liver of the sea lamprey, *Petromyzon marinus* L., during metamorphosis: I. Atresia of the bile ducts. J. Morph. **177**: 109-124.

SIDON, E.W., and J.H. YOUSON. 1983b. Morphological changes in the liver of the sea lamprey, *Petromyzon marinus* L., during metamorphosis: II. Canalicular degeneration and transformation of the hepatocytes. J. Morph. **178**: 225-246.

SIDON, E.W., and J.H. YOUSON. 1984. Relocalization of membrane enzymes accompanies biliary atresia in lamprey liver. Cell Tiss. Res. **236**: 81-86.

SMITH, H.M. 1960. Evolution of chordate structure. Holt, Rinehart and Winston. New York, 529 pp.

STENSIÖ, E.A. 1958. Les cyclostomes fossiles ou ostracoderms. pp. 171-425 *In* Grasse, P.P. [ed.] Traite de Zoologies Anatomie, Systematique, Biologie. Vol. 13. Masson, Paris.

STERBA, G. 1955. Das Adrenal-und Interrenalsystem in Lebensablauf von *Petromyzon planeri* Bloch. I. Morphologie und Histologie einschliebliche Histogenese. Zool. Anz. **155**: 151-168.

STRAHAN, R., and J.L. MACLEAN. 1969. A pancreas-like organ in the larva of the lamprey *Mordacia mordax*. Aust. J. Sci. **32**: 54-55.

STROBAND, A.W.J., and E. H. VAN DER VEEN. 1981. Localization of protein absorption during transport of food in the intestine of the grasscarp, *Ctenopharyhgodon idella* (VAL.). J. Exp. Zoology **218**: 149-156.

TORREY, T.W. 1938. The absorption of colloidal carbon from body cavity of ammocoetes. A study of the structure and function of the larval kidneys and blood forming tissues. J. Morph. **63**: 163-179.

TORREY, T.W. 1965. Morphogenesis of the vertebrate kidney. pp. 559-579 *In* Detlann, R.K., and H. Ursprung [eds.] Organogenesis. Holt, Rinehart and Winston, New York.

WAKE, K. 1982. The Sternzellen of Von Kupffer - after 106 years. pp. 1-12 *In* Knook, D.L., and E. Wisse [eds.] Sinusoidal liver cells. Elsevier, Amsterdam.

WEISBART, M., and J.H. YOUSON. 1975. Steroid formation in the larval and parasitic adult sea lamprey, (*Petromyzon marinus* L.). Gen. comp. Endocrinol. **27**: 517-526.

WEISBART, M., J.H. YOUSON, and J.P. WEIBE. 1978. Biochemical, histochemical, and ultrastructural analyses of presumed steroid-producing tissues in the sexually mature sea lamprey, *Petromyzon marinus* L. Gen. comp. Endocrinol. **34**: 26-37.

WEISSENBERG, R. 1925. Fluss-und Bachneunauge (*Lampetra fluviatilis* L. und *Lampetra planeri* Bloch.) ein morphologisch-biologischer Vergleich. Zool. Anz. **63**: 293-306.

WEISSENBERG, R. 1926. Beitrage zur Kenntnis der Biologie und Morphologie der Neunaugen. I. Vorderdarm und Mundbewaffnung bei *Lampetra fluviatilis* und *planeri*. Z. mikrosk.-anat. Forsch. **5**: 153-184.

WHEELER, M.W. 1899. The development of the urogenital organs of the lamprey. Zool. Jahrb. Abt. Anat. Ontog. Tiere. **13**: 1-88.

WHITING, H.P. 1972. Cranial anatomy of the ostracoderms in relation to the organization of larval lampreys. pp. 1-19 *In* Joysey, K.A., and T.S. Kemp [eds.] Studies in vertebrate evolution. Oliver and Boyd, Edinburgh.

WRIGHT, G.M., and J.H. YOUSON. 1982. Ultrastructure of mucocartilage in the larval anadromous sea lamprey, *Petromyzon marinus*. Amer. J. Anat. **165**: 39-51.

YOSHIE, S., and Y. HONMA. 1979. Scanning electron microscopy of the buccal funnel of the Arctic lamprey, *Lampetra japonica*, during its metamorphosis, with special reference to tooth formation. Jap. J. Ichthyol. **26**: 181-191.

YOUSON, J.H. 1971. Blood cell destruction in the opisthonephric kidney of the sea lamprey, *Petromyzon marinus* L. Can. J. Zool. **49**: 962-963.

YOUSON, J.H. 1972. Structure and distribution of interstitial cells (presumptive interrenal cells) in the opisthonephric kidneys of larval and adult sea lamprey, *Petromyzon marinus* L. Gen. comp. Endocrinol. **19**: 56-68.

YOUSON, J.H. 1973a. A comparison of presumptive interrenal tissue in the opisthonephric kidney and dorsal vessel region of the larval sea lamprey, *Petromyzon marinus* L. Can. J. Zool. **51**: 796-799.

YOUSON, J.H. 1973b. Effects of mammalian corticotrophin on the ultrastucture of presumptive interrenal cells in the opisthonephros of the lamprey, *Petromyzon marinus* L. Amer. J. Anat. **138**: 235-252.

YOUSON, J.H. 1980. The morphology and physiology of lamprey metamorphosis. Can. J. Fish. Aquat. Sci. **37**: 1687-1710.

YOUSON, J.H. 1981a. The alimentary canal. pp. 95-189 *In* Hardisty, M.W., and I.C. Potter [eds.] The biology of lampreys, vol. 3. Academic Press, London.

YOUSON, J.H. 1981b. The liver. pp. 263-332 *In* Hardisty, M.W., and I.C. Potter. [eds.] The biology of lampreys, vol. 3. Academic Press, London.

YOUSON, J.H. 1981c. The kidneys. pp. 191-261 *In* Hardisty, M.W., and I.C. Potter [eds.] The biology of lampreys, vol. 3. Academic Press, London.

YOUSON, J.H. 1982a. The morphology of the kidney in young adult anadromous sea lampreys, *Petromyzon marinus* L., adapted to seawater. I. General morphology and fine structure of the renal corpuscle and the proximal segments. Can. J. Zool. **60**: 2351-2366.

YOUSON, J.H. 1982b. The morphology of the kidney in young adult anadromous sea lampreys, *Petromyzon marinus* L., adapted to seawater. II. Distal and collecting segments, the archinephric duct, and the intertubular tissue and blood vessels. Can. J. Zool. **60**: 2367-2381.

YOUSON, J.H. 1984. Differentiation of the segmented tubular nephron and excretory duct during lamprey metamorphosis. Anat. Embryol. **169**: 275-292.

YOUSON, J.H., and D.G. BUTLER. 1985. Distribution and structure of the adrenocortical homolog in *Polypterus palmas* Ayres. Acta Zool (Stockh.) (in press).

YOUSON, J.H., and K.L. CONNELLY. 1978. Development of longitudinal mucosal folds in the intestine of the anadromous sea lamprey, *Petromyzon marinus* L., during metamorphosis. Can. J. Zool. **56**: 2364-2371.

YOUSON, J.H., and W.R. HORBERT. 1982. Transformation of the intestinal epithelium of the larval anadromous sea lamprey, *Petromyzon marinus* L. during metamorphosis. J. Morph. **171**: 89-117.

YOUSON, J.H., and D.B. McMILLAN. 1970a. The opisthonephric kidney of the sea lamprey of the Great Lakes, *Petromyzon marinus* L. I. The renal corpuscle. Am. J. Anat. **127**: 207-232.

YOUSON, J.H., and D.B. McMILLAN. 1970b. The opisthonephric kidney of the sea lamprey of the Great Lakes, *Petromyzon marinus* L. II. Neck and proximal segments of the tubular nephron. Am. J. Anat. **127**: 233-258.

YOUSON, J.H., and D.B. McMILLAN. 1971a. The opisthonephric kidney of the sea lamprey of the Great Lakes, *Petromyzon marinus* L. III. Intermediate, distal, and collecting segments of the ammocoete. Amer. J. Anat. **130**: 55-72.

YOUSON, J.H., and D.B. McMILLAN. 1971b. The opisthonephric kidney of the sea lamprey of the Great Lakes, *Petromyzon marinus* L. IV. Intermediate, distal, and collecting segments of the adult. Amer. J. Anat. **130**: 281-304.

YOUSON, J.H., and D.B. McMILLAN. 1971c. Intertubular circulation in the opisthonephric kidneys of adult and larval sea lamprey, *Petromyzon marinus* L. Anat. Rec. **170**: 401-412.

YOUSON, J.H., and E.C. OOI. 1979. Development of the renal corpuscle during metamorphosis in the lamprey. Amer. J. Anat. **155**: 201-222.

YOUSON, J.H., and E.W. SIDON. 1978. Lamprey biliary atresia: first model system for the human condition? Experientia. **34**: 1084-1086.

YOUSON, J.H., P.A. SARGENT, and E.W. SIDON. 1983a. Iron loading in the liver of parasitic adult lampreys, *Petromyzon marinus* L. Amer. J. Anat. **168**: 37-49.

YOUSON, J.H., P.A. SARGENT, and E.W. SIDON. 1983b. Iron loading in the livers of metamorphosing lampreys, *Petromyzon marinus* L. Cell Tissue Res. **234**: 109-124.

ZANANDREA, G. 1959. *Lampetra fluviatilis* culturata in mare nel Golfo di Gaeta. Pubbl. Staz. zool. Napoli **31**: 265-307.

EARLY DEVELOPMENT OF ORAL, OLFACTORY AND ADENOHYPOPHYSEAL STRUCTURES OF AGNATHANS AND ITS EVOLUTIONARY IMPLICATIONS

Aubrey Gorbman[1] and Arnold Tamarin[2]

Department of Zoology[1]
Department of Biological Structure[2]
Department of Oral Biology[2]
University of Washington, Seattle, WA

Ideas concerning the earliest evolution of the vertebrate head must be based on paleontological evidence as well as on adult and embryonic morphology of present day agnathans. Unfortunately, paleontological evidence for evolution of certain soft structures of the head is not really available, so that embryonic development of such structures is often the basis for speculation in this field (*e.g*. Stensiö, 1968). Here, we would like to address one phase of this problem; the formation of the agnathan adenohypophysis and some contiguous structures from the nasopharyngeal canal, and the presumed homology of the nasopharyngeal canal with the adenohypophyseal anlage, or Rathke's pouch, of higher vertebrates.

It is useful at the outset to review, at least briefly, the history of research on development of the nasopharyngeal (=nasohypophyseal) canal and adenohypophysis of the Agnatha. Single papers published by C. von Kupffer on head development of lampreys (1894) and hagfish (1899) have been the primary and frequently cited sources of information for almost all later workers and reviewers. This is understandable for the hagfishes because for a century the embryos of *Eptatretus stouti* collected about 1896 by Bashford Dean at Monterey, California have been almost the exclusive source for studies of myxinoid head development. These embryos were the basis of von Kupffer's 1899 study, as well as for studies by Stockard (1906a,b) on thyroid and mouth development and Conel (1929, 1931) on brain development. Three developing *Myxine* embryos collected from fishermen's nets in Sweden (two in a poor state of preservation) yielded papers by Holmgren (1946) on general development, and by Fernholm (1969) on pituitary development. Fernholm's *Myxine* embryo was 4.5 cm in length and cannot be taken to represent early development. The reason for the scarcity of hagfish embryo material rests on the fact that eggs are laid under unknown circumstances in the sea bottom; generally more than 100 meters below the surface.

Since large numbers of lamprey embryos can be obtained readily from eggs fertilized in the laboratory, their scarcity cannot be the basis for the dearth of information about development in these species. Yet, von Kupffer's 1894 imprecise drawings have been repeated in papers and reviews for almost a century; a recent example is in Leach's (1951) publication on nasopharyngeal development in *Petromyzon*.

The penalty we have paid for lack of more modern information is that reviewers since von Kupffer's time have based their thinking and interpretations on von Kupffer's fairly crude drawings, which are in effect merely diagrams. When interpretively copied by reviewers, these diagrams of the development of hagfish head structures have become more and more stylized (Figs. 1, 2); in some instances erroneous details have been introduced and, consequently, misinterpretations have been perpetuated.

Recently, Sholdice and McMillan (1985) have described the later development of the adenohypophysis in *Petromyzon* and, according to their evidence, it is not correct to consider the nasopharyngeal duct to be equivalent to the adenohypophysis, as von Kupffer and his reviewers have done. They noted that the original 2-layered nasopharyngeal duct eventually loses its lumen and in ammocoete larvae it remains for several years as a solid cord of cells extending from the olfactory structures to a position below, and in contact with, the infundibulum. In the final year of larval life the nasopharyngeal lumen is re-established. In the limited part of the length of nasopharyngeal duct, where it contacts the infundibulum (neurohypophysis) dorsally, the adenohypophysis forms by budding of many follicular groups of cells (Fig. 3). The layer of follicles so formed between the dorsal layer of the nasopharyngeal duct and the neurohypophysis is the definitive adenohypophysis. Thus, in lamprey development, there is never a Rathke's pouch-like nor solid cylindrical rudiment in the formation of the definitive adenohypophysis. Furthermore, it is clearly improper to consider the entire nasopharyngeal duct to be the homologue or the developmental equivalent of the adenohypophysis.

Early development of the nasopharyngeal canal of lampreys

According to von Kupffer (1894), folds of tissue on the lamprey head approach each other and gradually cover over an area of ectoderm that is already in contact with the forebrain (Fig. 4). The olfactory organ forms from the antero-dorsal part of this covered-over ectoderm while the posterior part extends further posteriorly to form the nasopharyngeal (=nasohypophyseal) duct. In lampreys, this duct ends blindly and never opens into the pharynx as it does in hagfishes. According to von Kupffer's interpretation, the entire lamprey nasopharyngeal duct is the rudiment of the adenohypophysis and therefore, in most subsequent reviews of the subject, it is labelled "hypophysis" (v. Kupffer, 1906; Pasteels, 1958; Stensiö, 1968) or "adenohypophysis" (Hardisty, 1979).

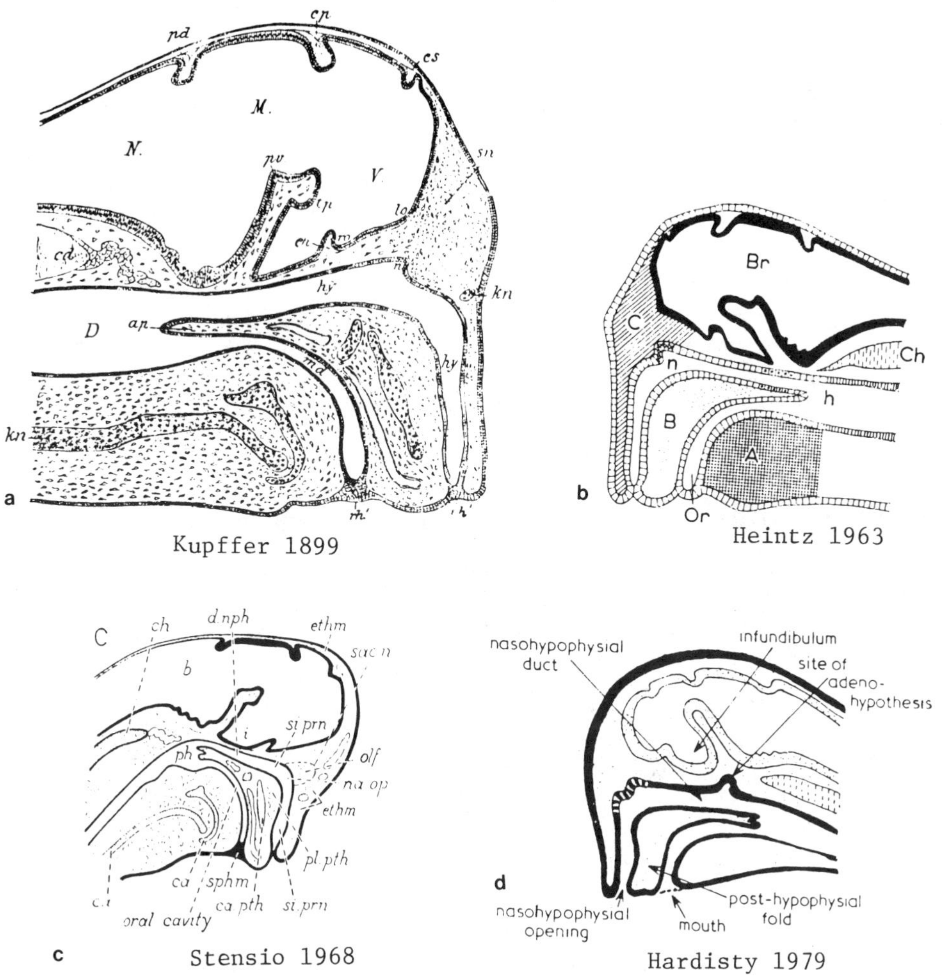

Fig. 1. *a* The original von Kupffer (1899) illustration of a sagittal section of the oldest hagfish embryo he described. *b*, *c*, and *d* are reproductions of this same figure in later reviews, variously modified. Note that in the most recent version (Hardisty, 1979) important changes have been introduced: the nasohypophyseal and mouth closure membranes have been removed and a Rathke's pouch-like diverticulum of the nasohypophyseal duct has been added! Key to some of von Kupffer's labels: *ch*, optic chiasma; *D*, pharynx (Darm); *hy*, nasohypophyseal duct; *md*, mouth (Mund); *n*, olfactory area of hy; *V*, *M*, and *N* fore-, mid- and hindbrain. *a*. from von Kupffer (1899); *b*. from Heintz (1963); *c*. from Stensiö (1968); *d*. from Hardisty (1979).

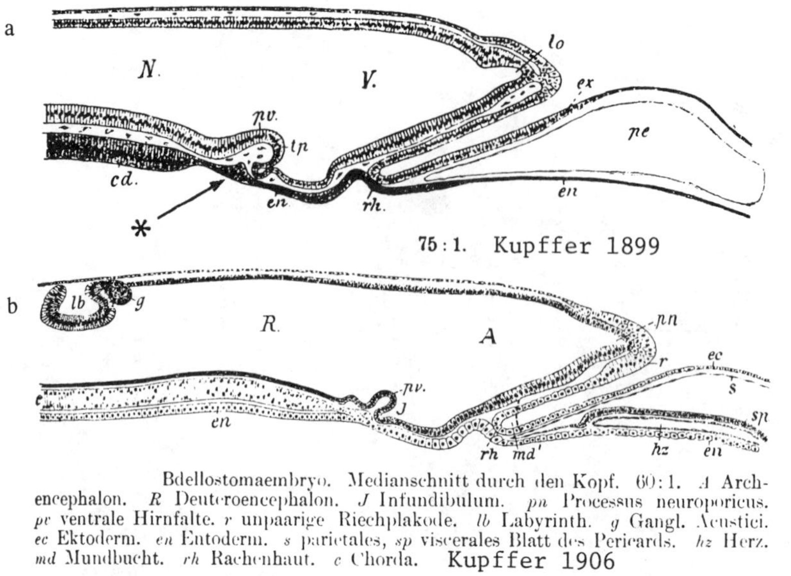

Fig. 2. *a* The original figure from von Kupffer (1899) of a sagittal section of an earlier (than Fig. 1) hagfish embryo and *b* a version of this figure published in a subsequent review (von Kupffer, 1906), together with its German caption. In *a* we have added an arrow and asterisk to indicate what we would now consider to be the adenohypophyseal rudiment. This is eliminated in *b*. Also, note that in *b*, though the caption indicates it is a median section, a lateral structure, the otic vesicle has been *added* to it! From von Kupffer (1899 and 1906).

Much of the early development of the nasohypophyseal structures in lampreys is visible on the surface of the head. Recent scanning electron micrography of lamprey larvae clearly illustrates the sequence of events in early formation of the nasopharyngeal duct (Gorbman and Tamarin, 1985). This was done with laboratory-fertilized eggs of *Petromyzon marinus* which were incubated at 21°C and fixed at development stages as defined by Piavis (1971). In stage 13 embryos there is no indication of formation of nasal nor adenohypophyseal structure (Fig. 5). By stage 14 (Figs. 6, 7) a superficial fold of tissue appears on the head surface; the future dorsal lip of the mouth. As this first fold grows antero-dorsally it covers the ectoderm which contacts the forebrain with a second ectodermal layer, a small lumen remaining between them. It is of interest that part of the epithelium being covered by the dorsal lip is ciliated and clearly differentiated from the rest of the head ectoderm (Fig. 8). The ciliated cells are the presumptive olfactory epithelium and cover a broad area of the head surface. The more posterior cells covered by the dorsal lip form a cylindrical structure, the nasopharyngeal duct. Its tubular character is apparent at its anterior end (Fig. 8).

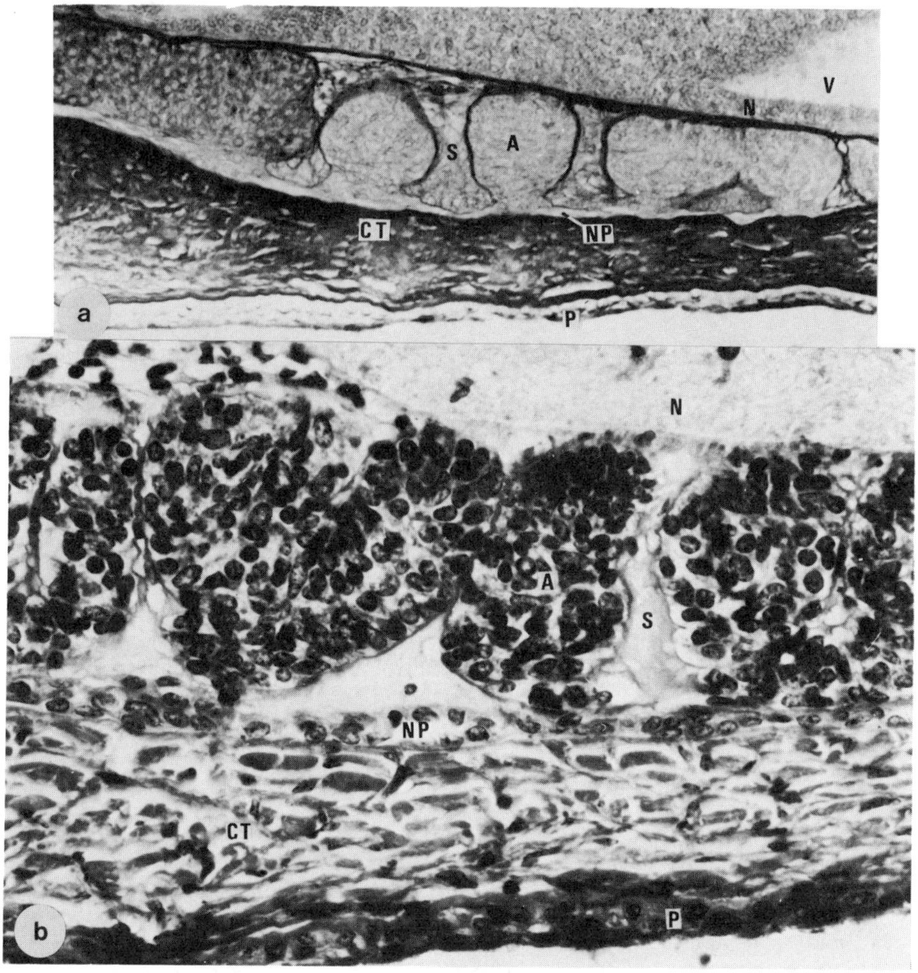

Fig. 3*a*. Sagittal section of developing adenohypophysis of 5-year ammocoete of *Petromyzon marinus*. Follicles of adenohypophysial tissue (*A*) are still connected ventrally to the narrow nasopharyngeal (= nasohypophyseal) duct (*NP*). Other labels: *N*, neurohypophysis and, *V*, third ventricle above it; *S*, connective tissue septum that contains vascular supply and separates adenohypophyseal follicles from each other; *CT*, connective tissue lamina between nasopharyngeal duct and pharynx below; *P*, dorsal pharyngeal epithelium. x 200. *b*. Sagittal section of developing adenohypophysis of year 5-6 ammocoete. Adenohypophyseal follicles, *A*, are here almost completely separated from the nasopharyngeal duct *NP* epithelium below. The two layers of the nasopharyngeal duct are visible and separated by a lumen. The label, *NP*, is placed within this small lumen. Other labels are as in 3*a*. x 275. Photographs provided by J. Sholdice and D. B. McMillan. See Sholdice and McMillan (1985).

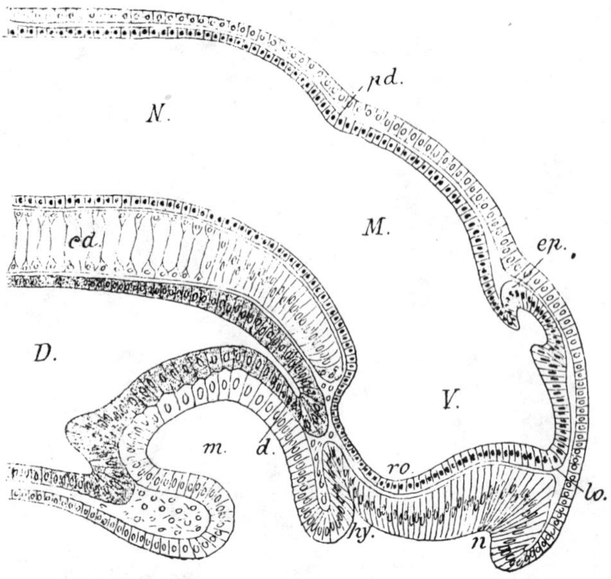

Fig. 4. Diagram of a sagittal section of the head of an approximately stage 14 lamprey embryo from von Kupffer 1899. This diagram has often been copied in later reviews. Key to some of the abbreviations: *d*, preoral gut; *D*, pharynx; *ep*, epiphysis; *hy*, "hypophysial" diverticulum; *m*, mouth; *n*, olfactory area; *V*, *M*, and *N* fore-, mid-, and hindbrain.

Two more head folds develop. The second fold to form becomes the ventral margin of the mouth, while the third is the most anterior and forms rostral to the first fold. The third fold is arc-shaped and is joined to the dorsal lip (first fold) at both sides thus enclosing the olfactory epithelium anteriorly and laterally (Figs. 9, 10).

Further development of the nasopharyngeal canal involves its lengthening (Fig. 10) and eventual loss of its lumen. Reestablishment of the lumen and final differentiation of the adenohypophysis from a small part of the dorsal epithelium of the canal are delayed for a period of years (Sholdice and McMillan, 1985). It is most remarkable that the ammocoete larva conducts its free living existence for so long a period apparently without a differentiated pars distalis or pars intermedia. Under certain circumstances *Petromyzon marinus* ammocoetes may delay entry into the metamorphic process, and the accompanying presumptive completion of adenohypophyseal differentiation, for as long as 18 years (Purvis, 1980).

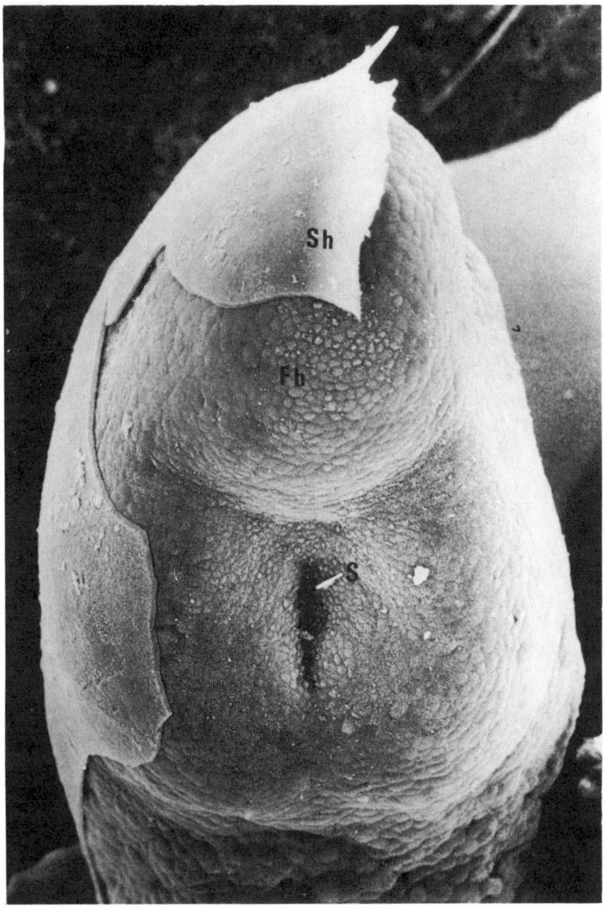

Fig. 5. Scanning electron micrograph; ventral view of the head of a Piavis stage 13 embryo of *Petromyzon marinus*, before any of the superficial folds on the head have appeared. *Fb*, superficial bulge of the forebrain area; *S*, stomodeal area; *Sh*, partly removed egg shell.

Early development of the nasopharyngeal canal of hagfish

Von Kupffer's (1899) preliminary report on California hagfish embryos has been the only source of facts on which zoologists during the last century have based their speculations about early vertebrate evolution. For this reason it is worth examining his data more critically than reviewers have done in the recent past. The original report was clearly not intended to be definitive since it was delivered as a "Sitzungsbericht" (meeting report) of the Gesellschaft für Morphologie und

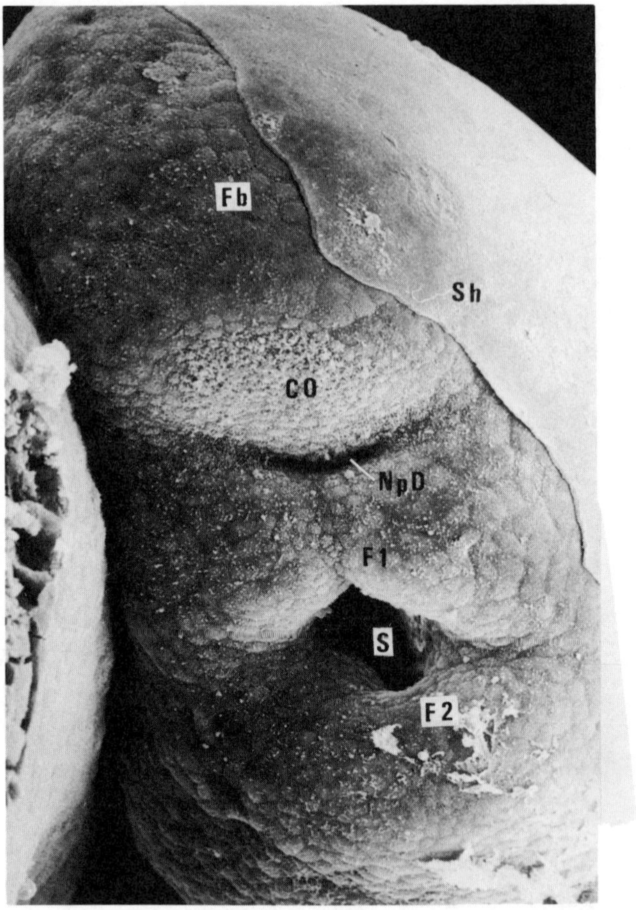

Fig. 6. Scanning electron micrograph; ventral view of the head of a stage 14 embryo. A transverse fold of tissue (*F1*) has begun to grow anterior to the stomodeal (*S*) area. *F1* is the future dorsal lip. As it grows anteriorly it covers the head ectoderm, which forms the nasopharyngeal duct, *NpD*. The second, less prominent superficial fold (*F2*) forms the ventral lip. Still to be covered by the growing *F1* is an area of superficial ectoderm, labeled *CO*, the ciliated olfactory epithelium.

Physiologie in Munich in 1899. The drawings are not precise depictions, but diagrams with a minimum of detail (Figs. 1, 2a). In von Kupffer's 1906 review he repeats one of the diagrams of the 1899 report (Fig. 2b), but with modification and further simplification. The structure in the 1899 sketch, which we now identify as the initial adenohypophyseal thickening, is eliminated in the 1906 version. Furthermore, in the 1906 drawing, which is labeled "Bdellostoma Embryo Medianschnitt durch den Kopf" (Bdellostoma embryo, median section through the head. Fig. 2b) an otic vesicle, a lateral structure, is incomprehensibly added!

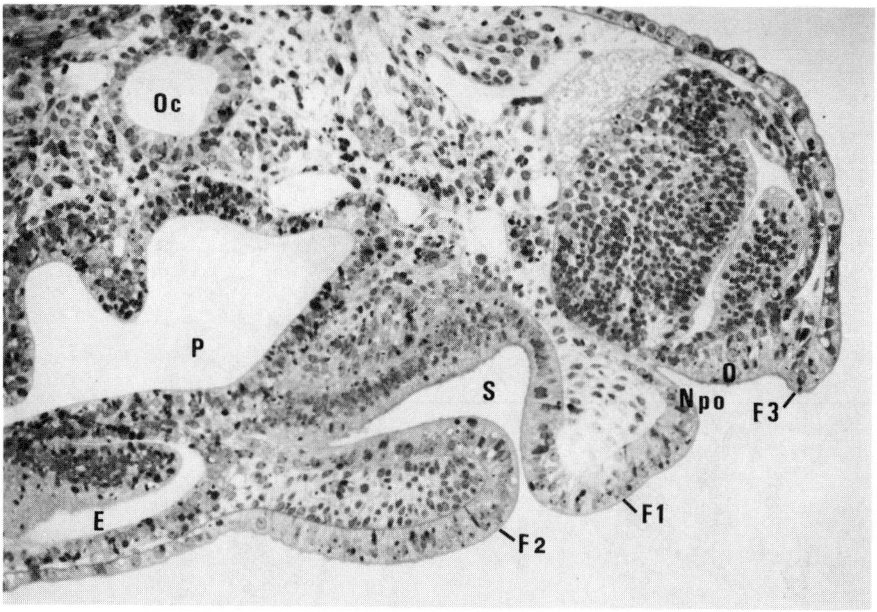

Fig. 7. Sagittal section of the head of a stage 14-15 *Petromyzon marinus* embryo. Labels: *E*, subpharyngeal gland, or endostyle; *F1, F2, F3* three superficial folds that define the oral and nasopharyngeal structures; *Npo*, nasopharyngeal opening. Nasohypophyseal duct extends posteriorly from the *Npo*. *O*, olfactory epithelium (ciliated) defined anteriorly by head fold *F3*; *Oc*, otic capsule; *P*, pharynx; *S*, stomodeum.

Considerable space in von Kupffer's 1899 report is devoted to discussion of the technical difficulties encountered due to poor preservation. For example, he says (in our translation), "Unfortunately I must reveal that the degree of preservation of the eggs was not thorough, and this made it difficult to prepare useful serial sections or to isolate intact embryos. Older embryos are well preserved; the eggs in younger stages of development are mostly unusable." Further, he says, "The fixative only partially penetrated. Thus, a large part of the younger embryos was macerated; another part was flattened, and only a few are usable. These few my assistant, Dr. Neumayer, isolated after painstaking and prolonged effort." Stockard (1906) also was impressed by these difficulties encountered by Dean and von Kupffer. He refers to von Kupffer's 1899 report by saying, "Von Kupffer had in 1900 [sic] published the results of a similar study which he made on scant and defective material, as is repeatedly mentioned throughout his paper." The problems with von Kupffer's sectioned embryos, and their interpretation, are raised here because some of von Kupffer's conclusions probably are based on artefacts, and will be discussed further on.

Von Kupffer (1899) opens his descriptions with a discussion of his oldest embryo (Fig. 1). He notes that there are at this stage two cavities in the head, a

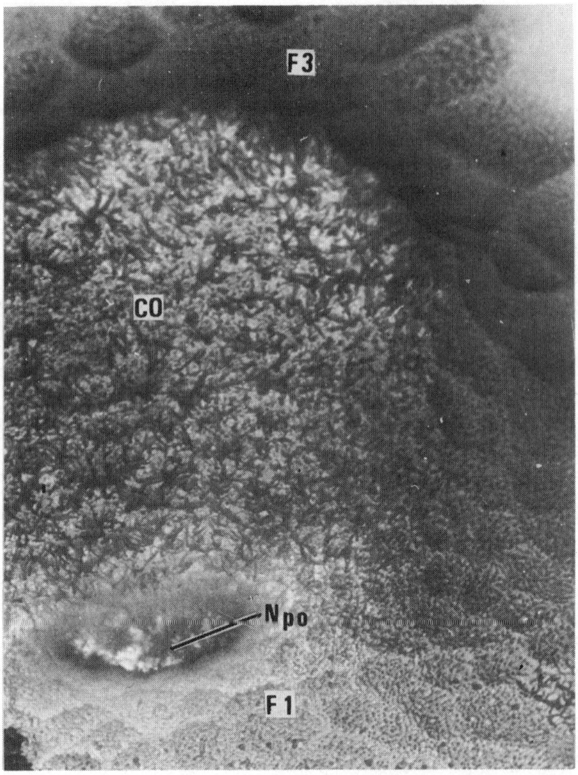

Fig. 8. Scanning electron micrograph of the nasopharyngeal opening of a stage 14-15 lamprey embryo, at about the same stage as that of Fig. 7. The anterior fold, *F3*, is visible, limiting the anterior distribution of the ciliated presumptive olfactory epithelium, *C0*. The label *Npo* points to the posterior opening of the nasopharyngeal duct which lies antero-dorsal to the first fold, *F1*.

more dorsal one, the nasohypophyseal (nasopharyngeal) canal, and a more ventral one, the stomodeum. Both open into the pharynx posteriorly and end anteriorly in a closing membrane that separates them from the outside surface. Here von Kupffer draws an interesting conclusion (cited in translation):

> "From this fact several different questions arise. The first is whether the epithelial plates, by which both canals are closed from the exterior, are primary structures, or whether we are dealing here with a secondary closure of an earlier opening. In the first case the closure plate for the mouth cavity would be blocked off by pharyngeal epithelium, and for the hypophyseal canal there would be a comparable arrangement. In that case the epithelium of both canals would be endodermal, and this yields the paradoxical conclusion that the nasal epithelium is formed only from endoderm. It would be much simpler to accept an interpretation of the meaning of these relationships that both canals were closed secondarily."

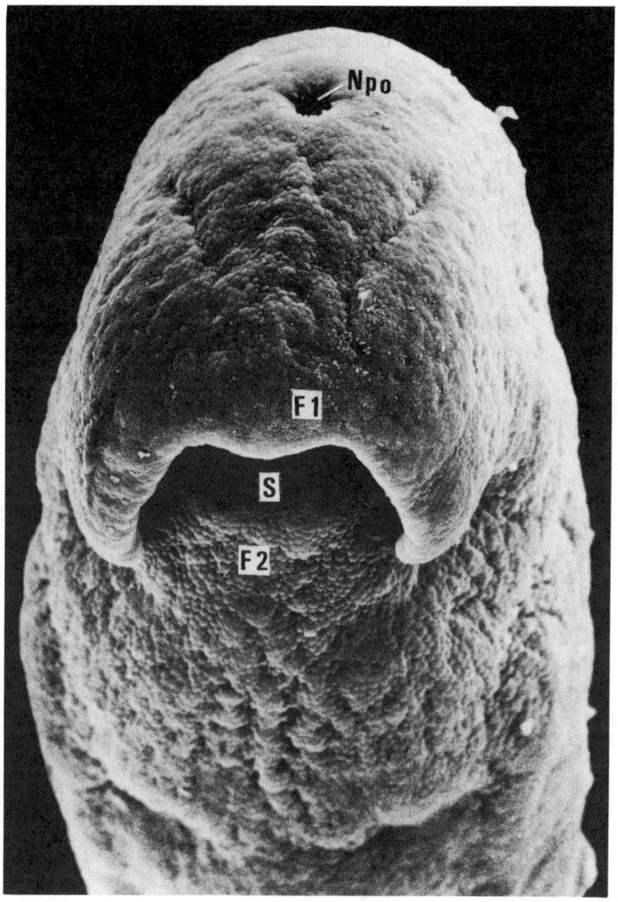

Fig. 9. Scanning electron micrograph; ventral view of a stage 17 lamprey embryo. Due to growth of the dorsal lip (*F1*) the nasopharyngeal opening (*Npo*) now is directed anteriorly rather than ventrally as in Figs. 6 and 7. *F2*, ventral lip of mouth; *S*, stomodeum.

In essence, what von Kupffer is saying here is that the stomodeum and nasopharyngeal canals are at first closed off from the exterior of the embryo. They are then opened at an intermediate stage and then, at the later stage of his diagram, closed again by a "sekundäre Rachenhaut." Of course, in further development these reclosed openings must finally be opened again. This unlikely series of events is based on the fact that a single intermediate stage embryo is represented in an interpretive sketch (v. Kupffer, 1899. Fig. 15a, b) as having an opening between the single, undivided tubular gut and the exterior. Since the embryo had been dissected away from the yolk surface, as described by von Kupffer, any closure between the yolk sac surface and the embryonic head would have been ruptured in any case.

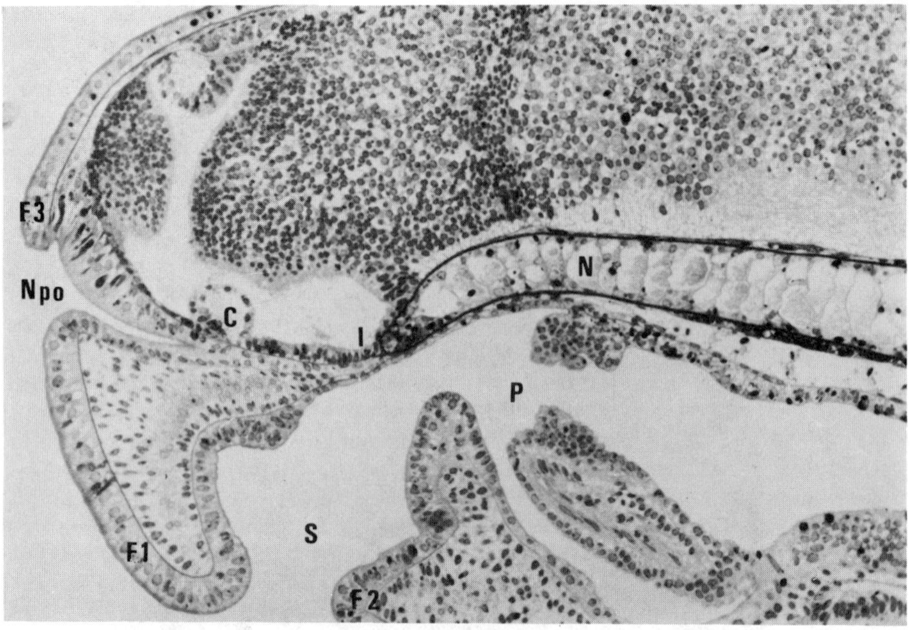

Fig. 10. Sagittal section of a stage 16 lamprey embryo. Growth of the dorsal lip (*F1*) has lengthened the nasopharyngeal duct (the wedge shaped structure extending posteriorly from the nasopharyngeal opening, *Npo*. Other labels: *F2*, lower lip; *F3*, anterior fold over the olfactory structures; *I*, infundibulum; *C*, optic chiasma; *N*, notochord; *P*, pharynx; and *S*, stomodeum.

Fig. 11. (Next page) Sagittal reconstructions of hagfish embryos, based on serial sections of *Eptatretus stouti* in the Dean-Conel collection (Gorbman, 1983). *a.* An early embryo in which the brain (coarse dots) is in direct contact with the notochord (vertical hatch) and yolk endoderm (fine stipple) below it. Yolk is indicated by an area of circles. In *b.* the infundibulum (*in*) of the forebrain has deepened and the endoderm below it has thickened (see also Fig. 12*a*). This thickened endoderm, by virtue of its location next to the infundibulum, can be traced and it becomes adenohypophysis. The first splitting of the endoderm is visible anterior to the adenohypophysis. In *c.* the infundibulum (*in*) is considerably larger. Splitting of the endoderm has formed a continous lumen from the head to the pharynx. A shelf of tissue, the oro-nasal shelf, begins to grow antero-ventrally, initiating the separation of a more dorsal space, the nasopharyngeal duct, and a more ventral one, the stomodeum. The stomodeum is already open posteriorly to the pharynx, *ph. hb*, hindbrain. In *d.* a deeper head fold has formed, bringing ectoderm to a point ventral to the head.

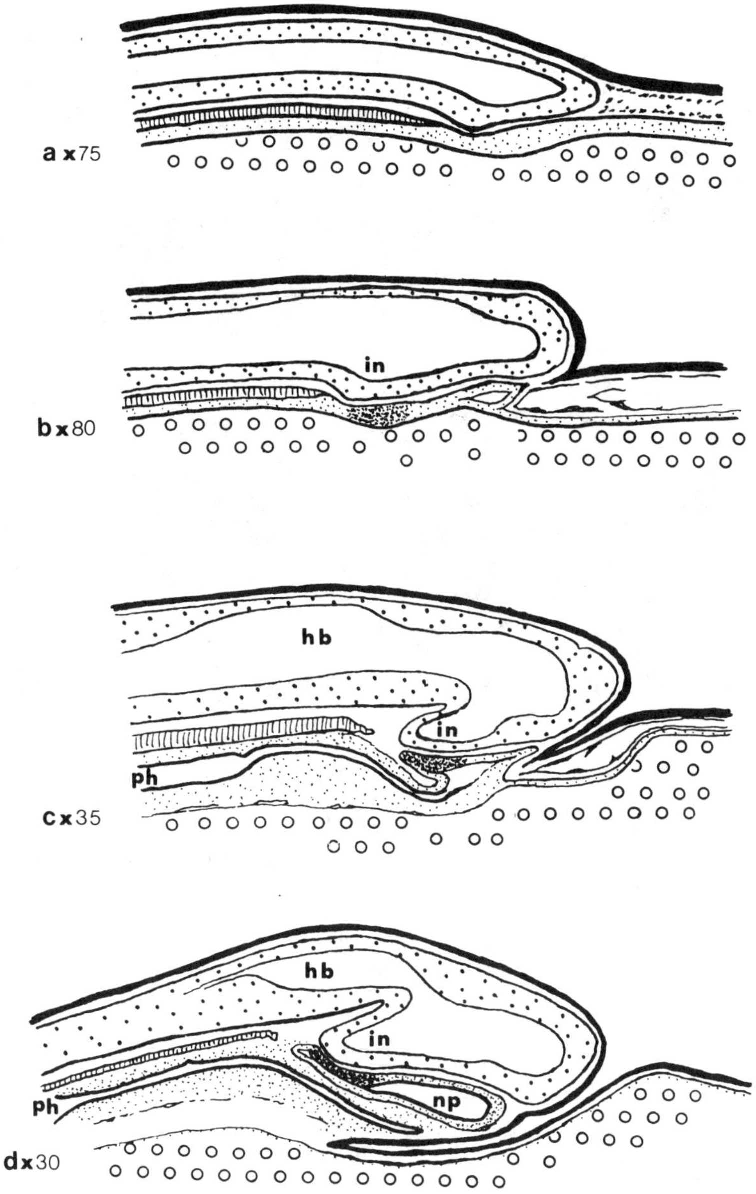

Fig. 11. (Continued) Separation of the nasopharyngeal from the narrow stomodeal cavity is completed. The nasopharyngeal duct (*np*) still bears a thickened area next to the infundibulum, the future adenohypophysis. Posteriorly, the nasopharyngeal duct ends blindly, but will soon open to the pharynx, as shown in Fig. 1 (adapted from Gorbman, 1983).

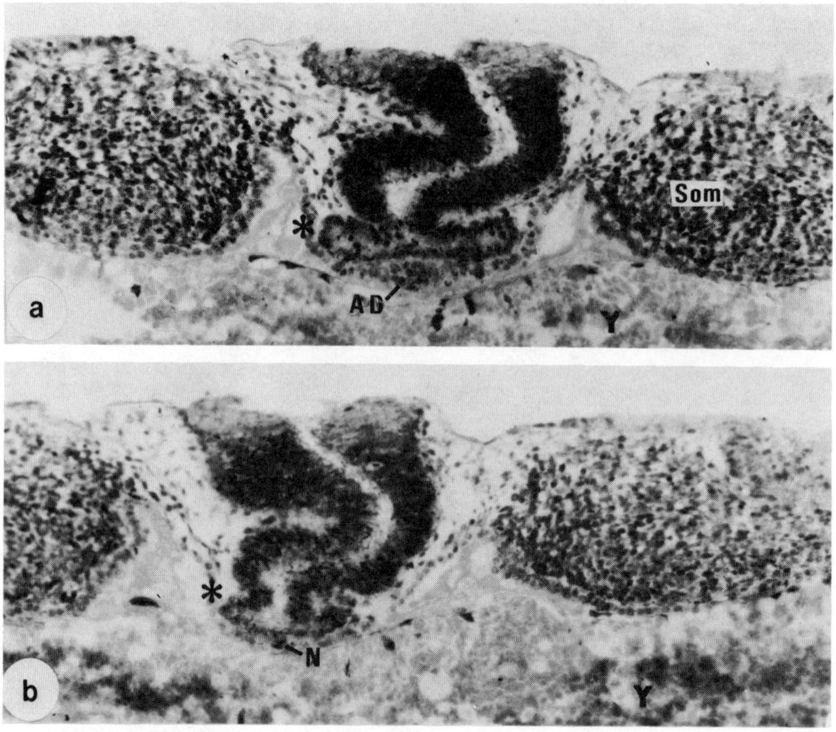

Fig. 12. *a* and *b* are cross sections of the same hagfish embryo at a stage like that in Fig. 11*b*. *a* is through the thickened adenohypophysial rudiment next to the infundibulum. Due to compression, the infundibulum just above the adenohypophysis is squeezed into a flattened shape and no lumen is visible. *b* is a section only about 50 μm posterior to *a*. The adenohypophyseal thickening is passed and the beginning of the notochord (*N*) is visible. *Y*, is yolk; the asterisk indicates the thin layer of endoderm lateral to the midline. (From Gorbman, 1983).

Since there appeared to be inconsistencies in von Kupffer's (1899) reasoning and conclusions, it seemed to be highly desirable to reexamine the question of the possible endodermal origin of the head spaces in the hagfish. Fortunately, serial sections of more than forty hagfish embryos of various degrees of development were found in the Anatomical Museum of Harvard University. They were deposited there by Professor J.L. Conel in *ca.* 1935 after he had completed his studies of brain development (Conel, 1929; 1931). The embryos had been collected originally by Bashford Dean in 1898. Thirty embryos were presented to Conel by Dean (Conel, 1929), and ten more were given to him by L. Neumayer, who had been given them by Dean earlier (Conel, 1931).

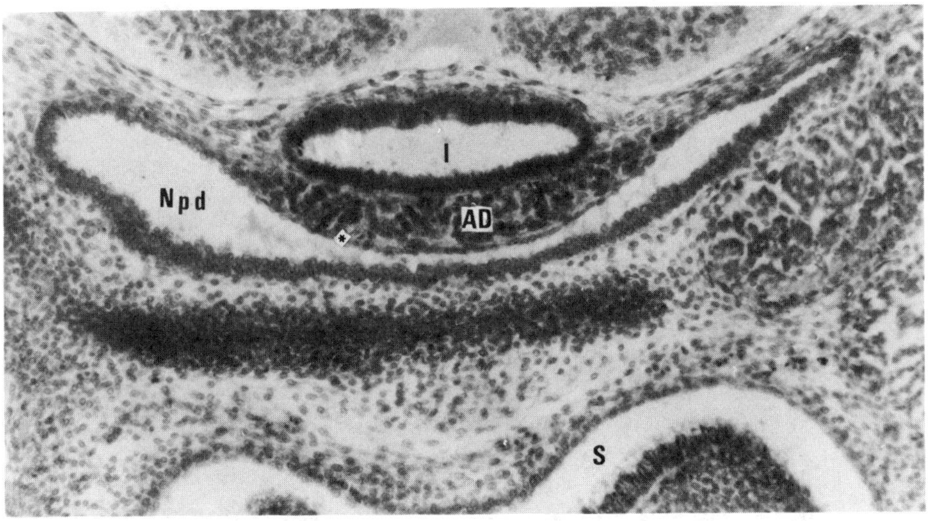

Fig. 13. Cross section in the adenohypophyseal region of a later hagfish embryo equivalent in development to the stage illustrated in Fig. 1. The adenohypophysis (*AD*) has proliferated from the dorsal epithelium of the broad nasopharyngeal duct (*Npd*). After budding of adenohypophyseal tissue from the dorsal nasopharyngeal epithelium, the remaining epithelium (marked by asterisk) is very thin. The broad oro-nasal shelf, already containing skeletal elements, separates the nasopharyngeal duct from the stomodeum (*S*). *I*, infundibulum. (From Gorbman, 1983).

These embryos were the subject of a recent study (Gorbman, 1983). Most were suitably fixed and almost all of them were dissected so as to leave a region of yolk beneath the embryo itself. This was fortunate, since it is probably because von Kupffer's specimens were dissected free of the yolk that the artefactual problems of interpretation of his material arose. All but three of the hagfish embryos of the Dean-Conel collection were cut transversely. Two are sagitally sectioned, and one, horizontally. Since the details of this study are published (Gorbman, 1983) only pertinent illustrations and discussion are repeated here in order to permit comparison with lampreys and to support speculation concerning evolutionary relationships of the nasopharyngeal duct.

One of the most unusual features of the early hagfish embryos, so far described by von Kupffer (1899) (Fig. 2) and by Gorbman (1983), is that most or all of the ventral surface of the forebrain, including the diencephalon, is in contact with yolk sac endoderm. This contact exists even before a lumen appears in the endoderm to form the archenteric cavity. This fact is especially clearly verifiable in the two youngest embryos in the Dean-Conel collection (embryos #2375 and #2331, both of which are younger than the earliest embryo diagrammed by von Kupffer) (von Kupffer, 1899; Fig. 3). The youngest embryo that we studied is younger than any

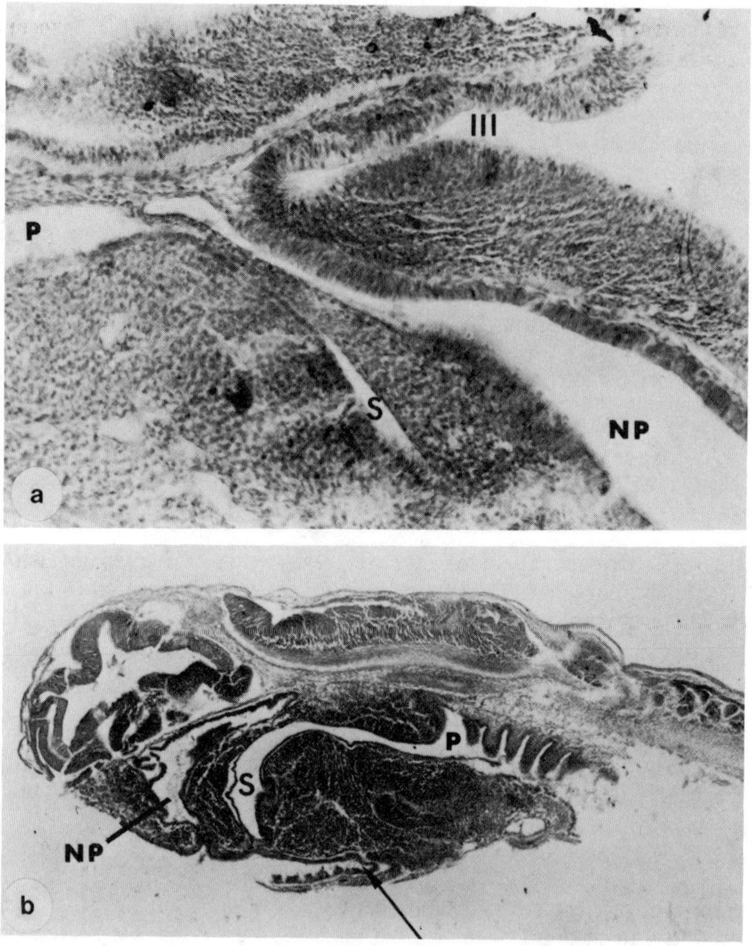

Fig. 14. *a* and *b* are sagittal sections of *Eptatretus* embryos slightly younger than that in Fig. 1. In *b* the separation of nasopharynx (*NP*) from stomodeum (*S*) by the oro-nasal shelf is shown. The dorsal layer of the nasopharyngeal duct is thickened near its blind posterior end. This is clearer in *a*, which is an enlargement of another similarly aged embryo (here, anterior is toward the right). In *a* the dorsal epithelium of the nasopharyngeal duct is thickened where it touches the infundibulum (lumen of infundibulum is labelled *III*). The nasopharyngeal duct, although it still ends blindly, has opened to the pharynx (*P*) posteriorly. (From Gorbman, 1983).

of von Kupffer's, and in it there is no indication of adenohypophysis formation in the epithelium contacting the shallow infundibulum (see Fig. 11a). However, in embryo #2331 (Fig. 12a), though the infundibulum is still shallow, the yolk

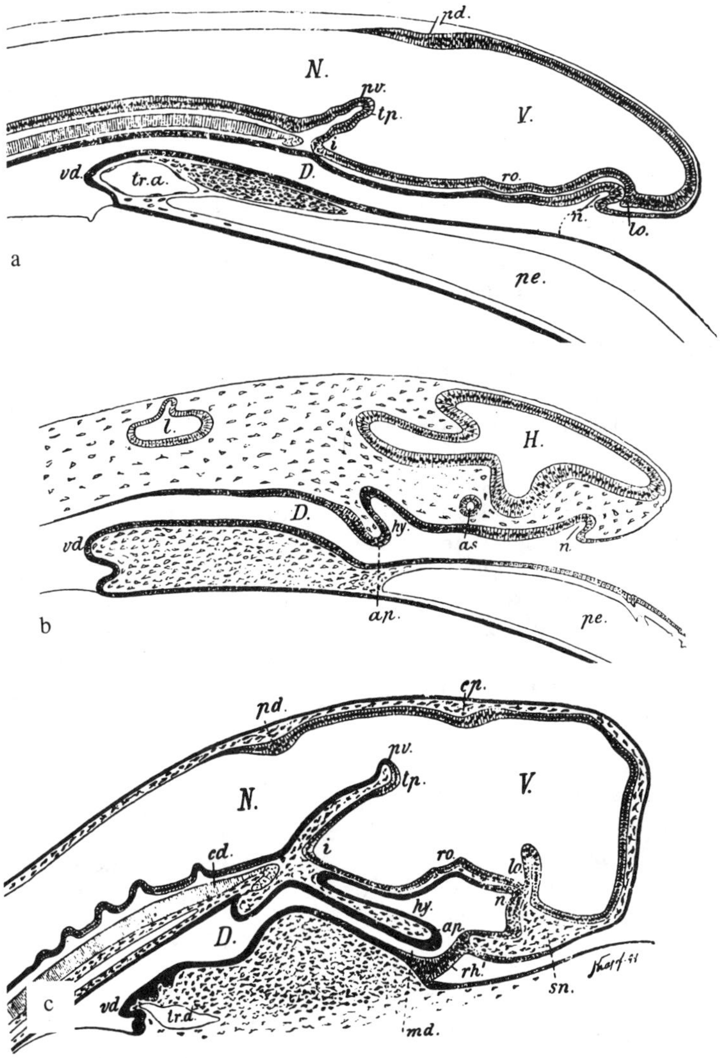

Fig. 15. Additional diagrams from von Kupffer (1899) indicating structure in hagfish embryos roughly equivalent to that in Fig. 11*c* and 11*d*. *a* and *b* represent sagittal sections of the same embryo, *a* being median and *b* being lateral. Of chief interest here is the "growth" of the lamina of tissue (oro-nasal shelf) that separates the nasopharyngeal cavity (*hy*) from the stomodeum (*md*). Note in *a* that von Kupffer indicates by means of a dotted line next to the label *n* where there may have been a closure of the space below the head. However, since this embryo probably had been dissected free of the yolk this could not be determined in any case from the embryo he studied. Other labels: *D*, pharynx; *i*, infundibulum; *l*, otocyst; *cd*, notochord; *n*, olfactory structures. Additional discussion of these figures in the text.

endoderm just below it is considerably thickened, being about 4 to 5 cells thick, in contrast to the endoderm continuous with it laterally, rostrally or caudally, where it is only one-cell thick. It is of especial interest that von Kupffer drew this feature into his 1899 diagram (Fig. 2a), without any remark about it and then eliminated it in his 1906 review (Fig. 2b). In later Dean-Conel embryos (Fig. 11b, c, d) this thickened layer remains in the same position below the infundibulum and it is thus easily identifiable as the same structure as it differentiates. Meanwhile the infundibulum in later embryos (exemplified by specimens #2336 and #2377: Fig. 13) grows large and saccular, reflecting its final sac-like shape in the adult. The original single archenteric space is divided into two by growth of a horizontal shelf of tissue from a level just posterior to the hypophysis to the antero-ventral extremity of the head (Fig. 11c), a distinct head-fold having also differentiated by this time (Figs. 11d, 14b, 15c). This horizontal septum thus forms two separate broad spaces in the head, both endoderm-lined. The dorsal space is the nasopharyngeal structure and the ventral one may be called the stomodeum (called "oral cavity" by Heintz, 1963 and by Stensiö, 1968).

The nasopharyngeal cavity is broad anteriorly, where it soon forms the large olfactory organ, and it narrows in the adenohypophyseal region. In Fig. 11d and Fig. 14 it ends blindly just posterior to the adenohypophysis, but it soon opens into the dorsal pharynx in slightly older embryos (Fig. 1). In hagfish embryos, where the nasopharyngeal duct opens into the pharynx, adenohypophyseal separation from the thickened juxtainfundibular is well advanced (Fig. 13). The process resembles that described in metamorphosing ammocete lampreys, *i.e.* multiple invaginations from the dorsal nasopharyngeal epithelium form a broad layer of epithelial follicles below the infundibulum.

It must be emphasized that in none of the 32 hagfish embryos studied, from the earliest to the latest in the series, was there an opening from the nasopharyngeal or oral cavities to the exterior. Thus, the "paradox" raised by von Kupffer (1899) has no resolution in the Dean-Conel series of embryos. We must conclude that, paradoxical or not, the entire nasopharyngeal and stomodeal spaces in the head of the hagfish embryo are endoderm-lined.

General discussion

Although there are some obvious differences in the modes of formation of the oral and nasopharyngeal spaces and structures in the heads of the developing hagfish and lamprey, there are also some interesting similarities. The lamprey's stomodeum and nasopharyngeal canal form on the exposed anterior surface of the head. The principal separation between the two is created by the growth of the dorsal lip. In the hagfish embryo the initial common oral-nasopharyngeal cavity is formed by a split of the endoderm while it is still in contact with the yolk below it. The shelf-like division between the nasopharyngeal and oral cavities is ultimately created by a growth of a tissue lamina that in many ways could correspond to the lamprey's dorsal lip, except that in hagfish it is completely covered by endoderm. We would like to propose the term "oro-nasal shelf" for this partitioning lamina in the hagfish and to point out that its role is analogous, if not homologous, to the palate in higher vertebrates; *i.e.* it separates the nasal space from the oral cavity. Growth of the dorsal lip in the lamprey and the oro-nasal shelf in the hagfish contribute the lower epithelial layer of their respective nasopharyngeal canals: however, in neither case does this layer contribute to the formation of the adenohypophysis.

Another similarity between the lamprey and hagfish modes of head development is in the pattern of differentiation of the adenohypophysis. In both species it forms by multiple budding of follicular cell groups arising from the dorsal layer of the nasopharyngeal canal. In both agnathans these follicles form a flattened layer of tissue in contact, and coextensive, with the neurohypophysis, the differentiated ventral extremity of the infundibulum. In neither agnathan is there a hollow cylinder of tissue that would correspond to a Rathke's pouch. Previous authors have quite uniformly considered the entire nasopharyngeal canal in the proximity of the infundibulum to be the hypophyseal precursor, and have labeled their diagrams and photographs of this structure to indicate this incorrect conviction.

How are we to interpret these apparent similarities and differences between the two agnathan types? In one, the oral, nasal and andenohypophyseal structures form from superficial folds of head ectoderm, while in the other they form from yolk endoderm and the spaces are created by splitting within this endoderm. Yet, once the initial pattern has been set, then the dorsal lip of the lamprey's head is homologous to the palate-like oro-nasal shelf that separates the nasopharyngeal from oral spaces in the hagfish. It should be noted that long ago C.R. Stockard (1906a), after a study of development of the hagfish mouth and gills, came to the conclusion that the "tongue", a massive structure in the floor of the oral cavity bearing the teeth of the developing hagfish, is homologous with the lower jaw of gnathostomes. There is nothing in our own study that would be incompatible with Stockard's proposal. Thus, to Stockard "the myxinoids . . . are gnathostomatous vertebrates, and therefore the name cyclostomes should no longer be used . . . ."

There are many questions that have been reopened by our study. How seriously are we to regard the different "germ layer" origins of the head structures in lampreys and hagfish? Are the apparent differences in early development and germ layer origin as profound as they appear to be? Are the differences in head development between the two agnathans profound enough so that we must favour a diphyletic theory of their origin from the vertebrate line?

The realization that the myxinoid alimentary canal-related head spaces and olfactory structures are completely lined by endoderm introduced the interesting question as to whether this is a primitive feature. At this point, given this one new fact, and given the strategic phylogenetic position of the myxinoids and their extinct evolutionary ancestors, a certain amount of speculation may be admissible. First, it should be noted that the association of the subneural gland with the cerebral ganglion in ascidians is probably the closest invertebrate homologue or analogue to the vertebrate neurohypophysis-adenohypophysis relationship (Barrington, 1975). The ascidian subneural gland is a pharyngeal derivative, and is presumably endodermal in nature. Thus, although its endodermal nature makes difficult the homology of the ascidian subneural gland with the vertebrate adenohypophysis in general, there is no such difficulty in homologising it with the myxinoid adenohypophysis on the basis of germ layer origin.

How are we to reconcile the similarity in the later patterns of development of the oral and nasopharyngeal structures of all agnathans with their very different early development and germ layer origins in lampreys and hagfish? The later similarities are reassuring restatements of the relatedness of the two agnathan groups to each other. The earlier developmental dissimilarities have two possible bases:

(1) a great difference in the amount of yolk and telolecithality in the eggs of the two groups and/or
(2) more basic differences due to greater phylogenetic ancientness or specialization of one of the two groups.

The first possibility can be dismissed because the highly telolecithal eggs of selachians, birds and reptiles have not materially affected the relatively "orthodox" pattern of differentiation of their oral, olfactory and adenohypophyseal structures. We would like to propose here a simplistic interpretation of the "endodermalization" of the hagfish oral-nasopharyngeal structures as an expression of their primitiveness and relatedness to the protochordates. We can propose that there may have been a gradual need for greater cephalization and anterior brain development in early vertebrate evolution that lifted the head from the blastoderm. This lifting enables a more precocious and extensive development of the head fold and subcephalic pocket. According to this scenario, the early less cephalized vertebrate head structures developed while the differentiating central nervous system lay directly upon the yolk, as it now does in the hagfish embryo. With greater emphasis on olfactory and cerebral development, earlier growth of a larger brain raised the head fold above the yolk and blastoderm, and placed a layer of ectoderm below the brain as well as above it, as is the case in the lamprey and all other vertebrates. In the hagfish, the only epithelial source adjacent to the brain that is available for adenohypophyseal or olfactory organogenesis is endoderm; in the lamprey it is ectoderm. It would seem that for the induction of such structures by the adjacent brain it is immaterial whether the adenohypophyseal epithelium is endodermal or ectodermal! In this interpretation, the hagfish is much more primitive than the lamprey, and a diphyletic origin of the two agnathan groups is probably required to explain their fundamental differences. These proposals, at least, offer a new insight into the factors that may have influenced certain evolutionary directions in the agnathan groups. They deserve further study by modern procedures and from modern viewpoints.

Acknowledgements

We sincerely appreciate the contribution of Luella Parsons to the preparation of this manuscript.

Literature cited

BARRINGTON, E.J.W. 1975. General and comparative endocrinology. Oxford University Press. London. pp. 88.
CONEL, J.L. 1929. The development of the brain of *Bdellostoma stouti*. I. External growth changes. J. comp. Neurol. **47**: 343-403.

CONEL, J.L. 1931. The development of the brain of *Bdellostoma stouti*. II. Internal growth changes. J. comp. Neurol. **47**: 343-403.

FERNHOLM, B. 1969. A third embryo of *Myxine*. Consideration on hypophysial ontogeny and phylogeny. Acta Zool. **50**: 169-177.

GORBMAN, A. 1983. Early development of the hagfish pituitary gland: evidence for the endodermal origin of the adenohypophysis. Amer. Zool. **23**: 639-654.

GORBMAN, A. and A. TAMARIN. 1985. Head development in relation to hypophysial development in a myxinoid, *Eptatretus* and a petromyzontid, *Petromyzon*. *In* Yoshimura, F., and A. Gorbman [eds.] The pars distalis: structure, function and regulation. Elsevier, Amsterdam.

HARDISTY, M.W. 1979. Biology of the cyclostomes. Chapman and Hall, London.

HEINTZ, A. 1963. Phylogenetic aspects of myxinoids. *In* Brodal, A., and R. Fänge [eds.] The biology of Myxine. Universitetsforlaget, Oslo.

HOLMGREN, N. 1946. On two embryos of *Myxine glutinosa*. Acta Zool. **27**: 1-90.

KUPFFER, C. VON. 1894. Studien zur vergleichenden Entwicklungsgeschichte des Kopfes der Kranioten. II. Die Entwicklung des Kopfes von *Petromyzon planeri*. Munchen und Leipzig.

KUPFFER, C. VON. 1899. Zur Kopfentwicklung von *Bdellostoma*. Sitzungsber. Gesellsch. Morph. Physiol. (München) **15**: 21-35.

KUPFFER, C. VON. 1906. Die Morphogenie des Centralnervensystems. *In* Handb. verg. exper. Entwicklungslehre Wirbeltiere. Bd. 2. Oskar Hertwig, Jena.

LEACH, W.J. 1951. The hypophysis of lampreys in relation to the nasal apparatus. J. Morph. **89**: 217-246.

PASTEELS, J. 1958. Developpement des Agnathes. pp. 106-144 *In* Grasse, M. [ed.] Traité de Zoologie, vol. 13. Masson, Paris.

PIAVIS, G.W. 1971. Embryology. *In* Hardisty, M.W., and I.C. Potter [eds.] The biology of lampreys. Academic Press, New York.

PURVIS, H.A. 1980. Effects of temperature on metamorphosis and the age and length at metamorphosis in Sea Lamprey (*Petromyzon marinus*) in the Great Lakes. Can. J. Fish. Aquat. Sci. **37**: 1827-1834.

SHOLDICE, J.A. ,and D.B. McMILLAN. 1985. Pituitary cysts in the sea lamprey of the Great Lakes, *Petromyzon marinus*. Gen. comp. Endocrinol. **57**: 135-149.

STENSIÖ, E. 1968. The cyclostomes with special reference to the diphyletic origin of the Petromyzontidae and Myxinoidea. *In* Ørvig, T. [ed.] Current problems of lower vertebrate phylogeny. Almquist and Wiksell, Stockholm.

STOCKARD, C.R. 1906a. The development of the mouth and gills of *Bdellostoma stouti*. Amer. J. Anat. **5**: 481-517.

STOCKARD, C.R. 1906b. The development of the thyroid gland in *Bdellostoma stouti*. Anat. Anz. **29**: 91-99.

IMMUNOLOGIC RELATIONS AMONG FISH GROUPS

Ger T. Rijkers**

Dept. of Immunology
University Hospital for Children and Youth
Utrecht, The Netherlands

Introduction

In order to survive, each organism has to maintain its internal integrity, which means that invading micro-organisms have to be successfully combatted. During evolution a number of ways to achieve this goal have evolved, culminating in a highly complex and integrated immune system in mammals. Phylogenetic studies have shown that non-specific defence mechanisms, like phagocytosis, are already present in invertebrates. Specific immunity is only observed in vertebrates. In this respect, fishes have a special position because they are the first group of animals in which an immune system, characterized by the presence of specific antibodies, occurs.

This overview will deal with several aspects of immunity in fish. The current knowledge about non-specific humoral defence, non-specific cellular defence, humoral immunity and cellular immunity will be presented and (where possible) different classes of fish will be compared.

Non-Specific Humoral Defence

In higher vertebrates, a number of components have been described with a potent anti-bacterial and/or anti-viral activity which function in a non-specific way. Although some components act totally independently of the immune system, others are activated by antibody (*e.g.* complement).

** Original research reported was performed in collaboration with Willem B. van Muiswinkel at the Department of Experimental Animal Morphology and Cell Biology, Agricultural University, Wageningen, Netherlands.

Lysozyme, C-reactive protein and interferon have all been described in fish (Rijkers, 1982). Their biological significance and their relation to the specific defence system are largely unknown at present.

Natural agglutinins are 60-300 kD glycoproteins with an activity directed against carbohydrate moieties on surface membranes of xenogeneic erythrocytes. These natural agglutinins have been found in representatives from all classes of fish (Rijkers, 1982). Their role in defence systems is suggested by their opsonic activity (Acton and Weinheimer, 1974).

Complement has been demonstrated by functional criteria in all classes of fish. Activation can occur via either classical (antigen-antibody complexes) or alternative (bacterial cell wall components) pathways. The structural and biochemical studies performed up to now indicate that both complexity and regulation of complement activation are similar in fish and mammals.

The complement cascade can only be activated when the antibody molecules (in antigen-antibody complexes) and complement components are from the same or a closely related species. This phenomenon can be used to study (by an immunological technique) relations between fishes. Although this approach seems promising (see Table I), it has no general applicability because in a comparable system using *Barbus conchonius* antibodies only isologous complements are effective, while closely related species such as *B. nigrofasciatus*, *B. filamentosus* and *B. lateristriga* are not (Rijkers and Van Muiswinker, 1977).

Non-specific cellular defence

Phagocytosis, the cellular uptake and digestion of particulate material, functions as a means of food acquisition in protozoans. In multicellular organisms this process serves to engulf invading microorganisms. In invertebrates, phagocytosis is one of the major defence mechanisms.

In vertebrates, phagocytosis is mediated through cells of the monocyte/macrophage lineage and granulocytes. Here phagoctyes not only function in the efferent phase of the immune response, that is removal of opsonized or non-opsonized material, but also play a pivotal role as antigen-presenting cells. After cellular uptake and partial digestion, antigen fragments are exposed at the cell membrane where these antigen fragments are presented to lymphocytes. In mammals these processes are most evident in the germinal centers of spleen and lymph nodes (Nieuwenhuis, 1981). In fish the melano-macrophage clusters in spleen and kidney seem to play a comparable role. In these clusters antigen is trapped and retained (Secombes *et al.*, 1982) while lateron plasma cells develop (Lamers and De Haas, in press).

The relative contribution of phagocytosis in overall defence at low temperatures merits special attention. While proper deficiency models are not available, it is not possible to weight the importance of phagcytosis as such in total defence. It has been demonstrated, however, that lowering the ambient temperature dramatically delays the antibody response of fishes (Rijkers *et al.*, 1980a; Rijkers *et al.*, 1981).

Table I. Complement activation* in cyprinoid fish.

Complement source	Activation	Comment
carp (*Cyprinus carpio*)	+	positive control
bream (*Abramis brama*)	+	55/58 positive
chub (*Leuciscus cephalus*)	+	5/8
nase (*Chondrostoma nasus*)	+	2/2
barbel (*Barbus barbus*)	+	2/4
rosybarb (*Barbus conchonius*)	-	pooled sera
goldfish (*Carassius auratus*)	-	0/7
grasscarp (*Ctenopharyngodon idella*)	-	0/4
roach (*Rutilus rutilus*)	-	0/4
bleak (*Alburnus alburnus*)	-	0/3
rainbow trout (*Salmo gairdneri*)	-	pooled sera
catfish (*Clarias lazera*)	-	0/5
mammals	-	rabbit, guinea pig
birds	-	chicken
amphibia	-	axolotl
invertebrates	-	earthworm, snail

* Complement activation was assessed by the ability of fresh sera to visualize plaque-forming cells in cell suspensions of pronephros of carp immunized with sheep red blood cells. Data from Rijkers *et al.* (1980).

Simultaneously, the number of polymorph nuclears in lymphoid organs increases. Because it also has been demonstrated that at low temperatures cellular immunity is depressed (Hildemann and Cooper, 1963), these data suggest that at low temperatures phagocytosis outweighs specific immunity.

Humoral immunity

There is an overwhelming amount of evidence demonstrating the capacity of all classes of fish to mount a specific humoral immune response as measured by the appearance of specific antibodies in serum following proper antigenic stimulation. In Agnatha, generally poor antibody responses can be elicited towards a limited number of antigens. Repeated immunizations are needed to obtain only moderate antibody titres (Thoenes and Hildemann, 1969). Chondrichthyes are capable of producing antibodies against a variety of soluble, particulate and bacterial antigens. The latent period is relatively long and maximum titres are obtained after 40-60 days. The capacity to develop immunological memory (*i.e.* a heightened and accelerated secondary antibody response) is questionable in this class of animals.

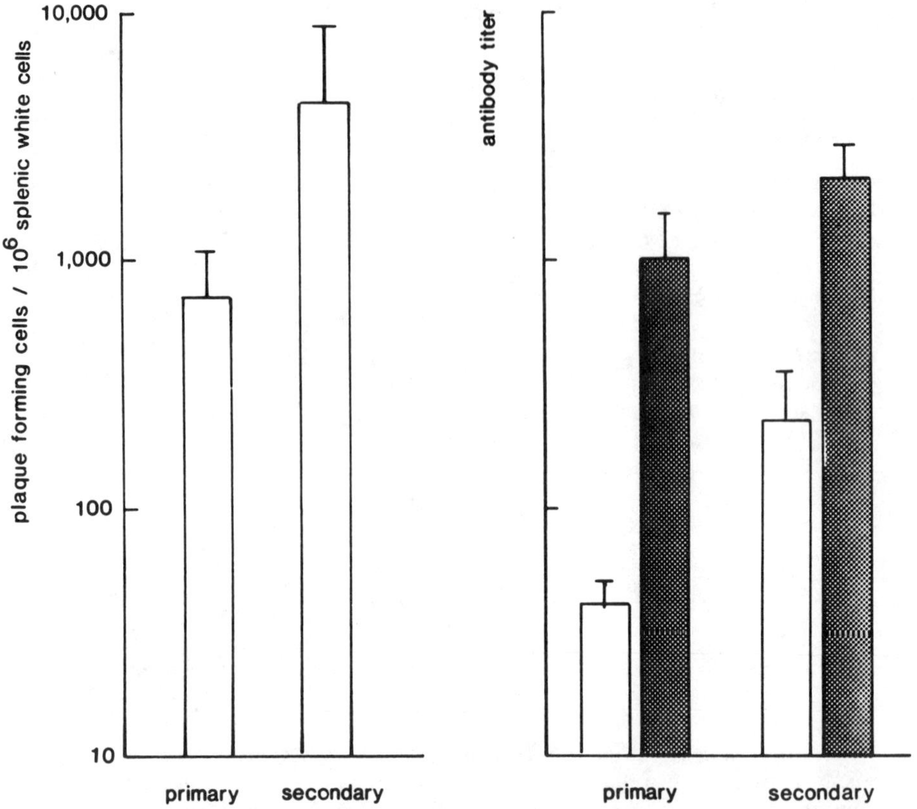

Fig. 1. Humoral immune responses of *Barbus conchonius*. A primary immune response was induced by an intramuscular injection of 10^8 sheep red blood cells; a secondary response by a second injection 30 days after the first. Peak plaque forming cell numbers (left panel) were reached on day 7 during a primary, on day 5 during a secondary response. Haemagglutinating (hatched bars) and haemolysing antibodies (open bars, right panel) reached maximum titres on day 14 during a primary, on day 5-8 during a secondary response. Mean values ± 1 S.E. depicted (n=4). Data from Rijkers and Van Muiswinkel, 1977.

Since the beginning of this century it has been demonstrated that teleost fish respond to antigenic stimulation by the production of specific antibodies. Both primary and secondary responses have been observed (Fig. 1). It appears that priming with low doses of antigen is optimal for memory formation, although in such cases it takes a certain time (3-6 months) to develop a high secondary response (Fig. 2). The immunological memory and the secondary response itself are specific for the priming antigen.

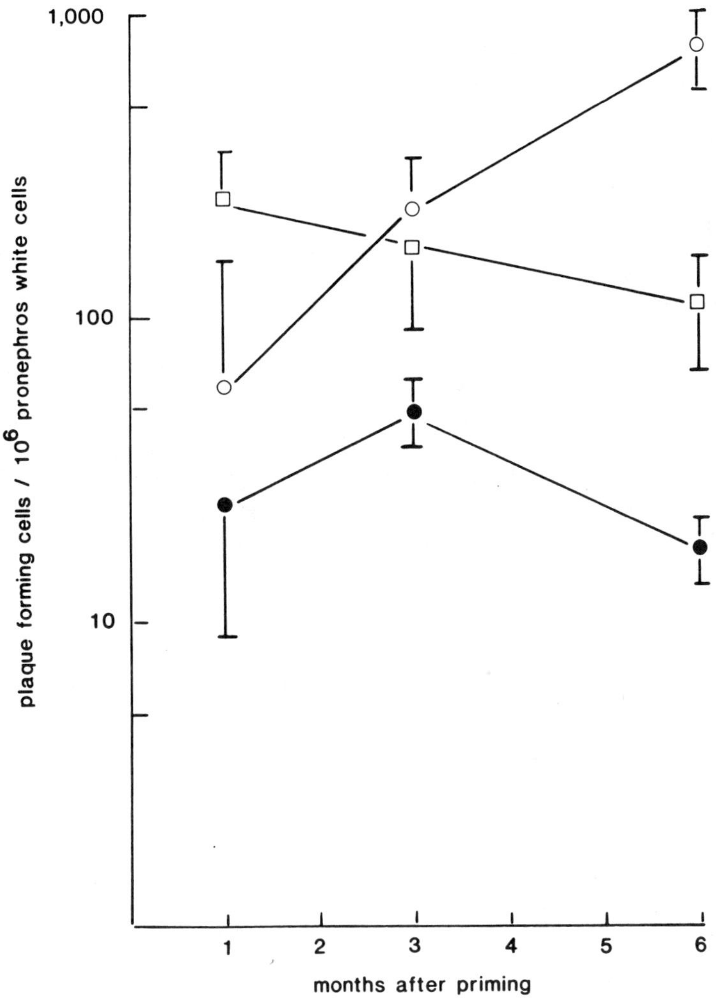

Fig. 2. Development of immunological memory in carp. Animals were primed with 10^5 (o), 10^9 (□) sheep red blood cells or with saline (●). At several intervals after priming 5 animals out of each group were challenged with 10^9 SRBC. The number of plaque-forming cells in pronephros was determined 14 days after challenge. Each point represents the arithmetic mean ± 1 S.E. (data from Rijkers *et al.*, 1980b).

For a number of species, the antibody-producing cells have been localized (Rijkers *et al.*, 1980a; Rijkers, 1980). Kidney (pronephros and mesonephros) appears to be the main source of antibody-producing cells, while spleen is of minor importance, at least in some species (Rijkers, 1980).

It can be concluded that, especially in bony fish, the capacity to mount a humoral immune response is well developed in terms of specificity and memory.

Immunoglobulins

From early studies it was concluded that fish lacked immunoglobulins because, upon eletrophoresis, γ-globulins were not detected in serum (*e.g.* Engle *et al.*, 1958). We now know that fish are capable of mounting specific antibody responses, and in this section the relevant data on the immunoglobulin nature of those antibodies will be presented.

Studies on immunoglobulins in Agnatha have resulted in conflicting conclusions regarding structural conformations. According to Marchalonis, lamprey (*Petromyzon marinus*) immunoglobulin is comprised of heavy and light chains (Marchalons and Edelman, 1968) while Litman suggests that the molecule contains identical subunits (Litman *et al.*, 1970). A possible explanation might be the nature of the antigens used for immunization. The immunoglobulins of Marchalonis were induced by viral protein antigens, while Litman may have characterized an inducible class of agglutinins to cell surface carbohydrates. Natural agglutinins to xenogeneic erythrocytes have been described for lower vertebrates (Rijkers, 1982). They can be functionally distinguished from immunoglobulins by their heat stability. A physiochemical comparison reveals that natural agglutinins in fish resemble invertebrate agglutinins more than vertebrate immunoglobulins (Rijkers, 1982).

In Chondrichthyes, antibody activity resides in 17S and 7S macroglobulin serum fractions. Based upon molecular weight of native immunoglobulin molecules and isolated heavy and light chains (Table II), it was shown that sharks possess both pentameric and monomeric immunoglobulin. Since heavy chains of both 17S and 7S immunoglobulin are indistinguishable by a variety of biochemical and immunological techniques, the 17S and 7S Ig are molecular forms of one immunoglobulin class.

In the majority of teleost fish only high molecular weight immunoglobulins are found. Using methodology similar to that described above, it was shown that in this class of fish immunoglobulins have a tetrameric configuration, which has been confirmed in electron microscope studies (Shelton and Smith, 1970; Acton *et al.*, 1971). Monomeric, next to tetrameric, Ig has been found in grouper and margrate (Clem, 1971).

Heavy chains of fish immunoglobulins are, because of their molecular weight, carbohydrate content and other physiochemical characteristics, comparable with mammalian μ chains. Recent studies using monoclonal antibodies against catfish Ig suggest the existence of κ and λ type light chains. J chains can be demonstrated in sharks and catfish but not in gar, paddlefish, pike and carp.

Table II. Physiochemical properties of fish immunoglobulin.

Class & species	Molecular weight ($x10^{-3}$) native	heavy chain	light chain	Formula	Serum level (g/l)	Ref.
Chondrichthyes						
lemon shark	850	71	23	$(L_{2}\mu_{2})_{5}$	4-5	1,2
	160	71	23	$L_{2}\mu_{2}$	7-8	1,2
Chondrosteans						
paddlefish	870	75	24	$(L_{2}\mu_{2})_{2}$	17	3
Holosteans						
gar	650	70	22	$(L_{2}\mu_{2})_{4}$		4
Teleosts						
carp	608	77	24	$(L_{2}\mu_{2})_{4}$	2	5
catfish	610	70	23	$(L_{2}\mu_{2})_{4}$		6
pike	645	60	23	$(L_{2}\mu_{2})_{4}$	2-5	7
mammals						
man IgM	950	70	23	$(L_{2}\mu_{2})_{5}$	1.3 ± 0.4	8,9
IgG	150	53	23	$L_{2}\gamma_{2}$	9.0 ± 2.2	8,9

1: Frommel *et al.* (1971); 2: Clem and Small (1967); 3: Pollara *et al.* (1968); 4: Bradshaw *et al.* (1971); 5: Andreas *et al.* (1975); 6: Hall *et al.* (1973); 7: Clerx *et al.* (1980); 8: Edelman (1973); 9: Zegers *et al.* (1975).

Serum levels, synthetic rate and metabolic turnover of fish immunoglobulin are comparable with mammals (Lobb and Clem, 1981, Table II). In addition, serum immunoglobulins can also be detected in intestinal and surface mucus and in bile (Lobb and Clem, 1981; Fletcher and Grant, 1969).

Cellular immunity

Cellular immunity involves all the specific immune reactions mediated by a combination of lymphoid cells and mononuclear phagocytes and their non-antibody effector molecules. *In vivo* cell-mediated immunity is manifested in delayed type hypersensitivity reactions and transplantation immunity. Assessment of cellular immune capacity in mammals largely depends on a number of *in vitro* assays: mixed leukocyte reactions (MLR) and cell-mediated lympholysis, antibody-dependent cellular cytotoxicity, *in vitro* production of lymphokines (interleukins, interferon, *etc.*), and proliferative lymphocyte response towards T cell mitogens.

Table III. Mitogen reactivity of fish lymphocytes.

Species	Lymphocyte source	Mitogen PHA	Con A	LPS
Pacific hagfish	peripheral blood	+		
Nurse shark	peripheral blood	-	-	
Rainbow trout	peripheral blood	+	+	+
	thymus		+	-/+
	pronephros		-/+	+
Blue gill	thymus	+	+	+
	pronephros	+	+	+
Salmon	peripheral blood	+	+	+
Catfish	peripheral blood		+	+
Carp	peripheral blood	+	+	+
	thymus	+	+	+
	pronephros	+	+	+

PHA = phytogaemagglutinin; Con A = Concanavalin A;
LPS = lypopolysaccharide

Lymphocytes of fish respond *in vitro* to mitogens by blast transformation (Table III). Quantitatively, the response is in most instances an order of magnitude lower than that observed in mammalian species. There is one exception (rainbow trout) to the general rule that cells from all lymphoid organs respond to both so-called T cell mitogens (such as Con A) as well as B cell mitogens (LPS). For trout, a differential response of thymocytes and pronephros cells to Con A and LPS was described (Etlinger *et al.*, 1976), but more recently those data have been challenged (Warr and Simon, 1983).

In mixed leucocyte reactions, for which both positive (Etlinger *et al.*, 1977; Cuchens and Clem, 1977) and negative (McKinney *et al.*, 1976) results have been reported, besides poor culture techniques, the lack of information on the genetic background of the experimental animals poses another complicating factor in interpreting these data.

Up to now no equivalents of antibody-dependent lympholysis, cell-mediated lympholysis or NK cells have been described in fish. The spontaneously occurring or mitogen-inducible cytotoxic cell in sharks appears to be a macrophage or a granulocyte (Petty and McKinney, 1981, 1983).

Among the interleukins identified, but far from characterized in fish, are an IL_2 activity present in supernatants of mitogen-stimulated lymphocytes (Grondel and Harmsen, 1984) and MIF produced by lymphocytes upon mitogenic or antigenic stimulation (Jayamaran *et al.*, 1979; McKinney *et al.*, 1981; Morrow and Harris, 1978).

The kinetics of cellular immune reactions have been extensively studied by transplantations of scales or skin. The transplantation technique itself can most easily be performed by exchanging scales between individual animals of the same species (allografts). The cellular reactions which occur at the site of grafting are, in essence, the same as those in mammals. Following transplantation, both autografts (transplanted from one site to another on the same individual) and allografts become revascularized. The time required for restoration of circulation varies from 1 day at 32°C to 12-15 days at 10°C (Hildemann, 1957; Sailendri, 1973). Allografts become overgrown with hyperplastic host tissues and elicit capillary leakage and vasodilation at the contact zone with the recipient tissue. Invading cells have been indentified as lymphocytes and mononuclear phagocytes (McKinney *et al.*, 1981; Finstad and Good, 1966; Borysenko and Hildemann, 1969). It has been shown that clearance of the dense hyperplastic tissue grown over the graft can be used as a criterion for the survival end point of the graft (Hildemann and Haas, 1960). The following immunological characteristics are in accordance with findings in mammals: second-set grafts are rejected more rapidly than first-set (see below); immunological memory is long-lived; memory is donor-specific (third party donor); xenografts (from a different species) are rejected faster than allografts; no isohaemagglutinating antibodies are involved in the rejection process; the antigen dose does not affect the median survival time (MST) of the grafts; only living tissue evokes immunological memory.

In jawless and cartilaginous fish, first-set allografts are rejected in a chronic way (MST > 30 days, Fig. 3). Advanced bony fish show an acute type of rejection (MST < 14 days). It is interesting that in bony fish kept at optimal temperatures allograft rejection proceeds even faster than in mammals. Holostean and chondrostean fish reject allografts in a chronic or sub-acute way. In all species studied thus far, accelerated second-set graft rejection is observed, *i.e.* MST of second-set grafts always lies in the acute/sub-acute range.

On the basis of data given in Figure 3, it is tempting to conclude that during phylogeny cellular immune capacity increases progressively. However, this conclusion may be premature for the following reasons: certain invertebrates show a subacute or even acute type of graft rejection (Cooper, 1976). In urodele amphibians allografts are rejected in a chronic way. Furthermore, virtually nothing is known about the genetics or the major histocompatibility complex (MCH) in lower vertebrates. Therefore, the relative slowness of allograft rejection does not necessarily reflect a primitive cellular immune system, but can also reflect the variability in MHC. Other (*in vitro*?) assays are needed to gain a more complete insight into the phylogeny of cell-mediated immunity.

Lymphocyte heterogeneity

In the preceding paragraphs it has been argued that, in fish, both cellular (rejection of transplanted allografts) and humoral (presence of specific antibodies) immune reactivity occurs. The question is whether these reactions are mediated by different lymphocyte populations or, in other words, whether fish possess, by analogy with mammals, T and B lymphocytes. Bearing on this question are data on

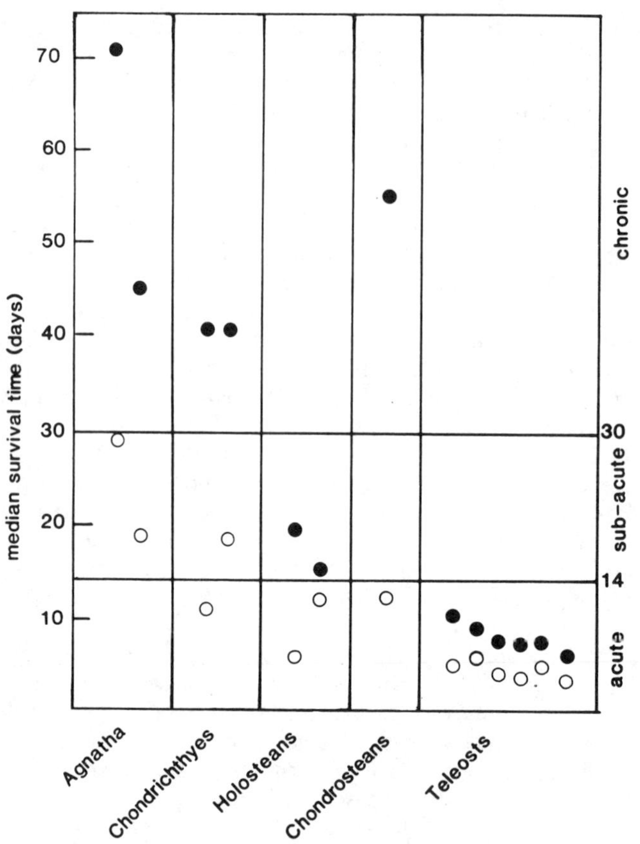

Fig. 3. Allograft rejection in fish. Median survival time of first-set (•) and second set (o) allografts in animals kept at optimal temperatures.

anatomic localization of fish lymphocytes, cell surface markers and functional ablation and hapten-carrier studies.

Since fish do not possess bone marrow, the lymphoid stem cell compartment must necessarily be a different organ from that in mammals (Rijkers, 1980). In all classes of fish a thymus, spleen and pronephros are found, providing the anatomical prerequisites for lymphocyte heterogeneity. A notable exception is the hagfish, a species mounting (admittedly low) specific antibody responses and rejecting allografts in the absence of a thymus or any other organized lymphoid tissue (Hildemann and Thoenes, 1969; Thoenes and Hildemann, 1969). Despite the presence of multiple lymphoid organs, difficulties have been met in demonstrating lymphocyte subpopulations based on differences in cell surface markers.

Mammalian lymphocytes can readily be divided into T and B lymphocytes by virtue of the lack of surface immunglobulin (sIg) on T cells; that is, T cells do not react with antisera against serum Ig. Using similar protocols, the vast majority of fish lymphocytes, including thymocytes, bear sIg (Table IV, see also Warr, 1980). Whereas it has been argued that the reactivity of (rabbit) anti-Ig antisera with rainbow trout thymocytes is due to cross-reactivity with carbohydrate moieties (Yamaga *et al.*, 1978), this certainly does not hold true for carp thymocytes (Fiebig and Ambrosius, 1976). Differences do exist, however, in the quantity and quality of sIg on lymphocytes from different lymphoid organs in most species. In carp, goldfish, skate and rainbow trout the amount of sIg per cell is lower in thymus than in spleen and peripheral blood (Fiebig *et al.*, 1977; Warr *et al.*, 1977; De Luca *et al.*, 1978; Ellis and Parkhouse, 1975; Yamaga *et al.*, 1977). Recent work from Abrosius' group indicates that sIg on thymocytes differs from sIg on pronephric cells and serum Ig. In carp, serum Ig exists in a tetrameric configuration $(H_2L_2)_4$. Pronephric lymphocytes can be divided into two groups, one where either monomeric Ig (H_2L_2) or half molecules (HL) are present on the cell surface and another group which carries the so-called thymocyte sIg. Thymocytes carry only H chain dimers, which differ from H chain in serum Ig and therefore are termed τ chains (Fiebig *et al.*, 1980a, b; H. Ambrosius, personal communication). Quite interestingly, this model suggested for carp is reasonably comparable with current models for mammalian T cell antigen receptors (Romain and Schlossman, 1984).

Table IV. Reactivity with fish lymphocytes of conventional antisera and monoclonal antibodies raised against serum immunoglobulin.

Species	antibody	Lymphocyte source PBL	spleen	head kidney	thymus	Ref.
catfish	conventional	99*	99	n.d.	n.d.	1
	monoclonal	33	10-20	n.d.	n.d.	1
trout	conventional	90	99	96	99	2
	monoclonal	n.d.	30	12	5	3
carp	conventional	30-58	25-45	30-58	65	4
	monoclonal IG^+T^+	n.d.	100	100	100	5
	monoclonal IG^+T^-	n.d.	40	40	1	5

*% politive cells; n.d. = not done; PBL = peripheral blood lymphocytes

1: Lobb and Clem (1982); 2: Etlinger *et al.* (1977); 3: DeLuca *et al.* (1983); 4: Emmrich *et al.* (1975); 5: Secombes *et al.* (1983).

At present, in three species, monoclonal antibodies (MoAb's) raised against serum Ig have been used in studies addressing the issue whether all lymphocytes carry surface Ig (Table IV). From the data it can be concluded that it is possible to generate MoAb's reactive with serum Ig (Ig^+) but unreactive with thymocytes (T^-). Furthermore, these MoAb's react with variable percentages of lymphoctyes in spleen and pronephros. On the other hand, MoAb's reactive with both serum Ig and thymocytes (Ig^+T^+) stain all lymphoctyes. These results indicate that probably all lymphocytes in fish carry sIg, but that heterogeneity exists in the part of the molecule exposed on the membrane.

Only negative results have been reported on the occurrence of 'mammalian type' cell surface markers on fish lymphocytes such as C3 and Fc receptors (Wrathmell and Parish, 1980), or the ability to rosette with heterologous erythrocytes (De Luca *et al.*, 1983). Based upon the observation that the murine Thy-1 antigen is present on both T cells and brain cells, Cuchens and Clem (1977) prepared a rabbit antiserum against bluegill brain tissue. In combination with complement the antiserum killed ± 70% of pronephros lymphocytes, thereby abrogating the PHA response without affecting LPS responsiveness. The results suggest that PHA-responsive lymphocytes carry cell surface antigens cross-reactive with brain tissue antigens.

Functional ablation studies addressing lymphocyte heterogeneity in fishes are scarce and the data are conflicting. Splenectomy affects the antibody response in some species while it has no effect in others (see also Rijkers and Van Muiswinkel, 1977). Thymectomy in fish is difficult to perform because the organ is hardly accessible and has a high regenerative capacity. The only report available dealing with neonatal thymectomy (Tx) shows that Tx abrogates allograft rejection as well as the anti-SRBC antibody response (Sailendri, 1973). Since no T cell-independent B cell functions were studied, no conclusions with respect to lymphocyte heterogeneity can be drawn from these studies.

Another functional approach in studying lymphoctye heterogeneity has been the use of hapten-carrier systems. In all species studied thus far, carrier priming enhances a subsequent anti-hapten response (Warr *et al.*, 1977; Stolen and Mäkelä, 1975; Ruben *et al.*, 1977; Ruben and Edwards, 1980; Weiss and Avtalion, 1977), with larval lampreys as a notable exception (Fujii *et al.*, 1979). In goldfish, it is even possible to physically separate hapten- reactive and carrier-reactive cells on nylon-wool columns (Warr *et al.*, 1977; Ruben and Edwards, 1980). These studies show that cellular cooperation does occur during a humoral immune response in fish but not that it is a cooperation between lymphoctyes belong to different lineages.

The data discussed above do not permit us to answer the question as to whether fish lymphoctyes can be divided into T and B cells. The two extreme possibilities are that all the lymphocytes are B cells (McKinney *et al.*, 1976) (by analogy with amphibians) or all lymphocytes are thymus-derived (Turpen *et al.*, 1973); these are probably oversimplifications. All functional studies performed thus far, and reviewed in this paper, show that in fish, immune reactions occur which in mammals are mediated by T and B cells. However, the physical separation of lymphocytes on the basis of membrane characteristics and the subsequent demonstration of different functional capacities have not, as yet, been accomplished. The recent description of monoclonal antibodies, reactive with non-Ig determinants on thymocytes (Table IV), should lead to important advances in this field.

Summary

Fishes are the first group of animals having an immune system characterized by the occurrence of specific antibodies. Only one class of immunoglobin (Ig) is found, comparable to IgM in mammals. In primitive fish (Chondrichthyes) Ig's have a pentameric configuration, the more advanced classes have tetrameric Ig. In terms of antigen specificity and serum levels, antibodies are comparable to mammals though the antibody repertoire probably is more limited. The major site of antibody production is the kidney (pro- and mesonephros).

Cellular immunity is well developed in fishes. In advanced fishes (teleosts) allograft rejection is completed in 7-8 days, which is even faster than in man. In primitive fish allografts are rejected over a longer time period. *In vitro* studies of cell-mediated immunity are more difficult to interpret, but cell-cell cooperation in antibody responses (hapten-carrier systems) and proliferative responses to (mammalian) T cell mitogens and allogenic cells are firmly established.

Controversy has existed about lymphocyte heterogeneity in fishes because the major discriminating phenotypic marker of B cells, namely the expression of surface Ig, was also found on thymocytes. However, immunochemical and molecular characterization of surface structures on thymocytes showed that, although there is cross-reactivity, clear differences do exist between T cell receptors and Ig.

In conclusion, both humoral and cellular immune responses are operative in all groups of fishes. Moreover, primitive classes also use a number of defense mechanisms which are otherwise mainly observed in invertebrates. Advanced classes, such as teleosts, have a more developed immune system which, although less refined, in its effectiveness is comparable with mammals.

Acknowledgements

Stimulating discussions with Prof. J. F. Jongkind (Erasmus University, Rotterdam) and Dr. W. B. van Muiswinkel (Agricultural University, Wageningen) during preparation of this manuscript are gratefully acknowledged. Original research referred to in this paper was made possible through technical assistance of Mrs. E. M. H. Frederix-Wolters and Mr. S. H. Leenstra, J. A. M. Wiegerinck, R. van Oosterom and J. Wijnen. Thanks also go to Mrs. H. van Moorsel for typing the manuscript.

Literature Cited

ACTON, R.T., P.F. WEINHEIMER, H.K. DUPREE, E.E. EVANS, and J.C. BENNET. 1971. Biochemistry. **10**: 2028-2036.

ACTON, R.T., and P.F. WEINHEIMER. 1974. Contemp. Topics Immunobiol. **4**: 271-282.

ANDREAS, E.M., R.F. RICHTER, D. HADGE, and H. AMBROSIUS. 1975. Acta Biol. Med. Germ. **34**: 1407-1415.

BORYSENKO, M., and W.H. HILDEMANN. 1969. Transplantation. **8**: 403-411.

BRADSHAW, C.M., L.W. CLEM, and M.M. SIGEL. 1971. J. Immunol. **106**: 1480-1487.

CLEM, L.W. 1971. J. biol. Chem. **246**: 9-18.

CLEM, L.W., and P.A. SMALL. 1967. J. exp. Med. **125**: 893-920.

CLERX, J.P.M., A. CASTEL, J.F. BOL, and G.J. GERWIG. 1980. Vet. Immunol. Immunopathol. **1**: 125-144.

COOPER, E.L. 1976. Comparative immunology. Englewood-Cliffs: Prentice-Hall. 388 pp.

CUCHENS, M.A., and L.W. CLEM. 1977. Cell. Immunol. **34**: 219-227.

DeLUCA, D., G.W. WARR, and J.J. MARCHALONIS. 1978. Eur. J. Immunol. **8**: 525-530.

DeLUCA, D., M. WILSON, and G.W. WARR. 1983. Eur. J. Immunol. **13**: 546-551.

EDELMAN, G.M. 1973. Science. **180**: 830-840.

ELLIS, A.E., and R.M.E. PARKHOUSE. 1975. Eur. J. Immunol. **5**: 726-728.

EMMRICH, F., R.F. RICHTER, and H. AMBROSIUS. 1975. Eur. J. Immunol. **5**: 76-78.

ENGLE, R.L., K.R. WOODS, E.C. PAULSEN, and J.H. PERT. 1958. Proc. Soc. exp. Biol. Med. **98**: 905-909.

ETLINGER, H.M., H.O. HODGINS, and J.M. CHILLER. 1976. J. Immunol. **116**: 1547-1553.

ETLINGER, H.M., H.O. HODGINS, and J.M. CHILLER. 1977. Eur. J. Immunol. **7**: 881-887.

FIEBIG, H., and H. AMBROSIUS. 1976. pp. 195-203 *In* Wright, R.K., and E.L. Cooper [eds.] Phylogeny of thymus and bone marrow-bursa cells. Elsevier/North-Holland Biomedical Press, Amsterdam.

FIEBIG, H., I. SCHERMBAUM, and H. AMBROSIUS. 1977. Acta Biol. Med. Germ. **36**: 1167-1177.

FIEBIG, H., I. SCHERMBAUM, and H. AMBROSIUS. 1980a. Mol. Immunol. **17**: 971-984.

FIEBIG, H., I. SCHERMBAUM, and H. AMBROSIUS. 1980b. Acta Biol. Med. Germ. **39**: 845-853.

FINSTAD, J., and R.A. GOOD. 1966. pp. 173-189 *In* Smith, R.T., P.A. Miescher, and R.A. Good. [eds.] Phylogeny of immunity. Gainesville: Univ. Florida Press.

FLETCHER, T.C., and P.T. GRANT. 1969. Biochem. J. **115**: 65P.

FROMMEL, D., G.W. LITMAN, J. FINSTAD, and R.A. GOOD. 1971. J. Immunol. **106**: 1234-1243.

FUJII, T., H. NAKAGAWA, and S. MURAKAWA. 1979. Dev. comp. Immunol. **3**: 609-620.

GRONDEL, J.L., and E.G.M. HARMSEN. 1984. Immunology. **52**: 477-482.

HALL, S.J., E.E. EVANS, H.K. DUPREE, R.T. ACTON, P.F. WEINHEIMER, and J.C. BENNETT. 1973. Comp. Biochem. Physiol. **46B**: 187-197.

HILDEMANN, W.H. 1957. Ann. N.Y. Acad. Sci. **64**: 775-791.

HILDEMANN, W.H., and R. HAAS. 1960. J. Cell comp. Physiol. **55**: 227-233.

HILDEMANN, W.H., and E.L. COOPER. 1963. Fed. Proc. **22**: 1145-1151.

HILDEMANN, W.H., and G.H. THOENES. 1969. Transplantation. **7**: 506-521.

JAYARAMAN, S., M. MOHAN, and V.R. MUTHUKKARUPPAN. 1979. Dev. comp. Immunol. **3**: 67-76.

LAMERS, C.H.J., and M.J.H. DE HAAS. Cell Tissue Res. (in press).

LITMAN, G.W., D. FROMMEL, J. FINSTAD, J. HOWELL, B.W. POLLARA, and R.A. GOOD. 1970. J. Immunol. **105**: 1278-1285.

LOBB, C.J., and L.W. CLEM. 1981. J. Immunol. **127**: 1525-1529.

LOBB, C.J., and L.W. CLEM. 1982. Dev. comp. Immunol. **6**: 473-579.

LOBB, C.J., M.O. OLSON, and L.W. CLEM. 1984. J. Immunol. **132**: 1917-1923.

McKINNEY, E.C., G. ORTIZ, J.C. LEE, M.M. SIGEL, D.M. LOPEZ, R.S. EPSTEIN, and T.F. McLEOD. 1976. pp. 73-82 *In* Wright, R.K., and E.L. Cooper [eds.] Phylogeny of thymus and bone marrow-bursa cells. Elsevier/North-Holland Biomedical Press, Amsterdam.

McKINNEY, E.C., T.F. McLEOD, and M.M SIGEL. 1981. Dev. comp. Immunol. **5**: 65-74.

MARCHALONIS, J.J., and G.M. EDELMAN. 1968. J. exp. Med. **127**: 891-914.

MORROW, W. J. M., and J. E. HARRIS. 1978. 4th Eur. Immunol. Meeting. Budapest. **31**.

NIEUWENHUIS, P. 1981. Immunol. Today. **2**: 104-110.

PETTY, C.L., and E.C. McKINNEY. 1981. Dev. comp. Immunol. **5**: 53-64.

PETTY, C.L., and E.C. McKINNEY. 1983. Eur. J. Immunol. **13**: 133-137.

POLLARA, B., A. SURAN, J. FINSTAD, and R.A. GOOD. 1968. Proc. Natl. Acad. Sci. U.S.A. **59**: 1307-1312.

RIJKERS, G.T. 1980. Thesis. Agricultural University. Wageningen, The Netherlands. 176 pp.

RIJKERS, G.T. 1982. Dev. comp. Immunol. **6**: 1-3.

RIJKERS, G.T., and W.B. VAN MUISWINKEL. 1977. pp. 233-240 *In* Solomon, J.B., and J.D. Horton [eds.] Developmental immunobiology. Elsevier/North Holland Biomedical Press, Amsterdam.

RIJKERS, G.T., E.M.H. FREDERIX-WOLTERS, and W.B. VAN MUISWINKEL. 1980a. Immunology. **41**: 91-97.

RIJKERS, G.T., E.M.H. FREDERIX-WOLTERS, and W.B. VAN MUISWINKEL. 1980b. pp. 93-102 *In*: Manning, M.J. [ed.] Phylogeny of immunological memory. Elsevier/North-Holland Biomedical Press, Amsterdam.

RIJKERS, G.T., E.M.H. FREDERIX-WOLTERS, and W.B. VAN MUISWINKEL. 1980c. J. Immunol. Methods. **33**: 79-86.

RIJKERS, G.T., J.A.M. WIEGERINCK, P. VAN OOSTEROM, and W.B. VAN MUISWINKEL. 1981. pp. 477-482 *In*: Solomon, J.B. [ed.] Aspects of developmental and comparative immunology, vol. I. Pergamon Press, Oxford.

ROMAIN, P.L., and S.F. SCHLOSSMAN. 1984. J. clin. Invest. **74**: 1559-1565.

RUBEN, L.N., G.W. WARR, J.M. DECKER, and J.J. MARCHALONIS. 1977. Cell. Immunol. **31**:266-283.

RUBEN, L.N., and B.F. EDWARDS. 1980. Contemp. Topics Immunobiol. **9**: 55-89.

SAILENDRI, K. 1973. Thesis. Madurai University. 106 pp.

SECOMBES, C.J., M.J. MANNING, and A.E. ELLIS. 1982. Immunology. **47**: 101-105.

SECOMBES, C.J., J.J. VAN GRONINGEN, and E. EGBERTS. 1983. Immunology. **48**: 165-175.

SHELTON, E., and M. SMITH. 1970. J. mol. Biol. **54**: 615-617.

STOLEN, J.S., and O. MÄKELÄ. 1975. Nature. **254**: 718-719.

THOENES, G.H., and W.H. HILDEMANN. 1969. pp. 711-722 *In* Sterzl, J., and J.

Rina [eds.] Developmental aspects of antibody formation and structure. Czechslovak Academy of Science, Prague.
TURPEN, J.B., E.B. VOLPE, and N. COHEN. 1973. Science. **182**: 931-933.
WARR, G.W. 1980. Contemp. Topics Immunobiol. **9**: 141-170.
WARR, G.W., D. DeLUCA, J.M. DECKER, J.J. MARCHALONIS, and L.N. RUBEN. 1977. pp. 241-248 *In*: Solomon J.B., and J.D. Horton [eds.] Developmental immunobiology. Elsevier/North-Holland Biomedical Press, Amsterdam.
WARR, G.W., and R.C. SIMON. 1983. Dev. comp. Immunol. **7**: 379-384.
WEISS, E., and R.R. AVTALION. 1977. Dev. comp. Immunol. **1**: 93-104.
WRATHMELL, A.B., and N.M. PARISH. 1980. pp. 143-153 *In* Manning, M.J. [ed.] Phylogeny of immunological memory. Elsevier/North-Holland Biomedical Press, Amsterdam.
YAMAGA, K., H.M. ETLINGER, and R.T. KUBO. 1977. pp. 297-304 *In* Sercarz, E.E., L.A. Herzenberg, and C.F. Fox [eds.] ICN-UCLA Symposia on molecular and cellular biology, Vol. 6. Immune system: genetics and regulation. Academic Press, New York.
YAMAGA, K.M., R. T. KUBO, and H. M. ETLINGER. 1978. J. Immunol. **120**: 2074-2079.
ZEGERS, B.J.M., J.W. STOOP, E.E. REERINK-BRONGERS, P.C. SANDER, R.C. AALBERSE, and R.E. BALLIEUX. 1975. Clin. Chim. Acta. **65**: 319.

EVOLUTION OF TEMPERATURE REGULATION AND OF CONSTANCY OF FUNCTION (HOMEOKINESIS) AT DIFFERENT TEMPERATURES

C. Ladd Prosser with contributions by Joseph Ayers*
Edward Green and Douglas Nelson

Department of Physiology and Biophyics
University of Illinois at Urbana-Champaign
Urbana, Illinois 61801

This paper diverges from the assigned topic of temperature regulation in primitive vertebrates to consider the evolution of temperature adaptation in general. Subsequently, some of the ways in which the general adaptations to temperature may apply to Agnatha and Chondrichthyes will be considered. All organisms, both prokaryotes and eukaryotes, have mechanisms for lessening the kinetic effects of cooling and warming.

Most organisms vary in temperature to conform with ambient temperature. Conformers have diverse ways of maintaining relative constancy of energy metabolism and activity when internal temperature varies. These adaptations provide thermal *homeokinesis*. Temperature regulation refers to maintenance of relatively constant body temperature over a range of environmental temperatures. These adaptations, behavioral or metabolic-insulative, constitute thermal *homeostasis*.

Homeokinesis appeared early in cellular evolution and reached a high degree of perfection in fishes that lived in regions of changing temperature. Whether fishes evolved in marine, brackish or freshwater environments, paleontological evidence tends to show that they appeared first in temperate climates, not in tropics, polar regions or deep sea. Primitive fishes would have been subject to diurnal, seasonal and geographic differences in temperature. The following is a listing of the known homeokinetic adaptations to temperature which are of general occurrence.

(1) One kind of genetically encoded homeokinetic adaptation of enzyme proteins results in some kinetic independence of temperature change. Primary structure of proteins is critical for activation energy. In general, the Q_{10} of

---

* Northwestern University Marine Laboratory, Nahant, MA

enzymes of homeotherms is larger than of poikilotherms. The energetics of enzymes of poikilotherms are less affected by temperature change. Other genetically encoded adaptations are in protein conformations by which enzymes vary in sensitivity to extremes of heat or cold. The genotype sets the limits within which a phenotype can vary. Some induced variations are capacity adaptations which allow for activity in an "equable" range of temperature; other variations, resistance adaptations, permit survival at extremes of heat or cold.

(2) Most poikilothermic organisms adapt to low temperature by increased activity and to high temperatures by decreased activities of critical enzymes. The net result is a tendency toward constancy of energy production. Many microorganisms change enzyme activities according to temperature of culture. These changes compensate for the normal Q_{10} effects and tend to maintenance of metabolic constancy over a tolerated temperature range (Christophersen, 1973). Enzyme compensation, acclimation, has been described for bacteria and yeast cells and probably evolved very early. The controlling feedback mechanisms are not well understood but they resemble enzyme induction to nutrients. Enzyme activities, compensatory for alterations in temperature, occur in varying degrees in all plants and animals. Acclimatization has been identified in many invertebrate animals from both high and low latitudes but laboratory acclimation of individual invertebrates has not been much studied. Most teleost fishes show positive acclimation for energy-yielding enzymes, and less acclimation for hydrolytic and degradative enzymes. No data are available for prochordates or cyclostomes; it is probable that they can show metabolic compensations for temperature.

(3) In teleost fishes the compensatory changes in enzyme activity result in part from selective synthesis and degradation of specific enzymes. Changes in amounts of cofactors have been suggested, but they are variable since most cofactors serve in several reactions. We have recently investigated whether the compensatory changes in activity of energy-yielding enzymes can occur in isolated cells as well as in intact fish. Catfish hepatocytes in primary culture show over a period of two weeks at low temperature a compensatory increase and at high temperatures a decrease in activity of cytochrome c oxidase, citrate synthase, glucose-6-P-dehydrogenase and NAD-cytchrome c reductase, and show less change in activity of lactate dehydrogenase. We conclude that temperature can act at the cellular level on synthesis and degradation of specific proteins.

(4) Another strategy of temperature compensation is synthesis and degradation of proteins in general, also changes in production of substrates such as glycogen and lipids. The net result in catfish liver and heart, possibly in other organs, is hypertrophy during cold acclimation. Protein content increases while DNA remains constant. Apparently general synthesis (as opposed to synthesis of specific enzymes) is increased by cold and reduced by warm acclimation. Changes in protein/DNA ratios were not observed in the cultured cells, hence the hypertrophy *in vivo* may have a hormonal basis. This mechanism of temperature compensation in fishes may have evolved very early; the effect is a net change in total enzyme activity available to the animal.

(5) Another way of coping with temperature change is change in the composition of phospholipids. Fatty acids which are incorporated into membrane -

plasma membranes and intracellular organelles - are more unsaturated and may be of longer chains when deposited at low rather than at high temperatures. Changes in lipid composition as an adaptive response to temperature probably evolved very early and has been well documented for bacteria, protozoa, plants and animals. The effect of these changes is to counteract increased fluidity at high temperatures and decreased fluidity in the cold. Changes in membrane fluidity alter permeability of cell membranes and the activity of membrane-bound enzymes. Fishes from the Bering Sea have more unsaturated fatty acids in their membrane phospholipids and more fluid membranes than fishes from warmer waters, when both are measured at intermediate temperatures (Cossins and Prosser, 1978). As primitive fishes extended their range from temperate to polar or deep oceanic water, they made increasing use of desaturases and other lipogenic enzymes for incorporating more unsaturated fatty acids into membranes.

(6) Another strategy used by fishes for coping with temperature extremes is reduction in metabolism, *i.e.* becoming lethargic. This strategy has been developed in ecological expansion, also in changes in life cycles of primitive fishes. Some modern teleosts such as small-mouth bass and flathead catfish are inactive during the winter in ice-covered ponds; large-mouth bass and channel catfish continue to feed at temperatures of 4° to 10°C. Lethargy conserves energy but limits activity. At high temperatures some lungfish enter a state of estivation in a cocoon of mud. A related adaptation is to use temperature as a trigger for events in life cycles. The migrations of lampreys are correlated with critical water temperature. In Connecticut, *Petromyzon marinus* spend as much as 7 years as larvae in freshwater; at maturity they metamorphose and when water temperature falls to 6°C (late summer) they go to sea, where adults feed for 2-3 years, then the fish return to streams and spawn at 12-15°C (Hardisty and Potter, 1971).

Metamorphosed river lampreys (*Lampetra fluviatilis*) in Sweden move downstream in March-May, adults migrate upstream in late summer or early fall, and spawning in May-June requires 10°C water (Sjoberg, 1980). Anadromous sea lampreys *Petromyzon marinus* of eastern U.S. migrate upstream for spawning from March to September according to local temperature. Migration occurs in March in North Carolina, in April in Maryland, in May in Massachusetts and in June in New Brunswick (Beamish, 1980). *Petromyzon marinus* of the Great Lakes begin upstream migration at 3-4°C, continue migration to higher than 18°C; embryos develop best in the range of 18-23°C (Morman *et al.*, 1980). Maximum growth rate of small lampreys is at 20°C, of large ones at 15°C (Farmer, 1980). It is concluded that temperature is an important trigger for different parts of the life cycle of lampreys.

(7) An adaptation much used by Arctic and Antarctic fishes for maintaining activity at temperatures approaching the freezing point of seawater is production of antifreeze compounds. Unrelated fishes in Antarctica and the Bering Sea have very similar glycoproteins which cause the freezing points to be significantly lower than the melting points; this is either an example of convergent evolution or of a descent from a common ancestor. Fishes of the North Atlantic have polypeptides which serve the same function as the glycoproteins of Antarctic fishes. Many insects use polyhydric alcohols such as glycerol as antifreezes. Other insects are adapted to

tolerate freezing of extracellular fluids, but intracellular freezing is reduced or absent because of small amounts of free water.

(8) At high but sublethal temperatures, heat shock proteins are induced. Heating of bacteria, yeast, *Drosophila*, or sunfish for a few hours to high temperatures -- 28-30°C -- induces heat shock proteins. Following the induction of heat shock proteins (hsps) further heating to a lethal temperature is reduced in effectiveness. How protection results is not known. We have found that the temperature for inducing hsps can be altered in green sunfish by temperature acclimation. The widespread distribution of specific hsps indicates conservatism in the evolution of the proteins.

(9) Adaptations that extend the limits of activity into either cold or warm temperatures permit extension of geographic range. Environmental temperatures, and consequently limiting temperatures, have changed during geological time since fishes evolved. Mechanisms of heat or cold tolerance (resistance adaptations) are different from those of capacity adaptations. The first sign of heat or cold stress is for cell membranes to become leaky. Potassium is lost and, depending on the medium, sodium is gained. Changes in ion permeability occur at temperature extremes in cells of all kinds of organisms and may determine the tolerated limits. One mechanism of control of permeability is change in fluidity of cell membranes, possibly caused by the effects of temperature on composition of phospholipids, which in turn affect channel properties. Another cause of limiting stress or mortality is inactivation of enzyme proteins. Functional binding of substrates and cofactors, catalytic reactions, depend on secondary and tertiary structures. Denaturation of proteins and melting of lipids result in enzyme inactivation. However, death usually occurs with less heating or cooling than is needed to denature proteins or to melt membrane lipids. Correlations exist between thermal resistance and enzyme inactivation in organisms from different environments. Why thermal resistance of enzymes evolved to temperatures never experienced by the animals that use them is not known. One hypothesis is that thermal limits for proteins are determined by higher-order conformations that depend on weak intramolecular bonds. The high-order conformation depends on primary structure that is inherited and sets the range within which higher conformations exist.

(10) In multicellular animals the nervous systems are the first organs to fail at temperature extremes. In fishes during progressive heating and cooling, the behavioral sequence is: hypermotility, hyperresponsiveness, motor incoordination, loss of equilibrium, respiratory coma (Freidlander *et al.*, 1976). Inhibitory synapses block before loss of spontaneous activity, then multisynaptic excitation, unisynaptic excitation and antidromic or axon conduction. Central nervous failures at high and low temperatures have also been observed in invertebrates - insects, crustaceans, and molluscs. The temperature for each function to fail can be altered by previous thermal history; genetic differences also occur. Resistance adaptations, both metabolic and neural, were undoubtedly present in primitive fishes.

(11) A metabolic adaptation to low temperature which approaches homeothermy is heat production and retention in specific regions of the body. Active tuna, lamnid sharks, swordfishes and others have complex retes which, by countercurrent heat exchange between arterial and venous blood flow, allow deep

core retention of heat. In some of these fish, heat is produced by lateral bands of muscle, in others (billfish) heat production is by a fat-rich organ beneath the brain. Among invertebrates, bees approach homeothermy in the hive; large insects cannot take off in flight before the nervous system is warmed by mesothoracic muscles. Some primitive fish may have been large enough for this mechanism to evolve for active swimming in cold water or in niche exploitation.

(12) Behavioral thermoregulation is widely used by fishes and takes many forms. In a thermal gradient, fishes initially settle at a selected temperature. This is related to their temperature of acclimation; fish from low temperatures select a lower temperature than warm-acclimated fish. When fish are left in a gradient for

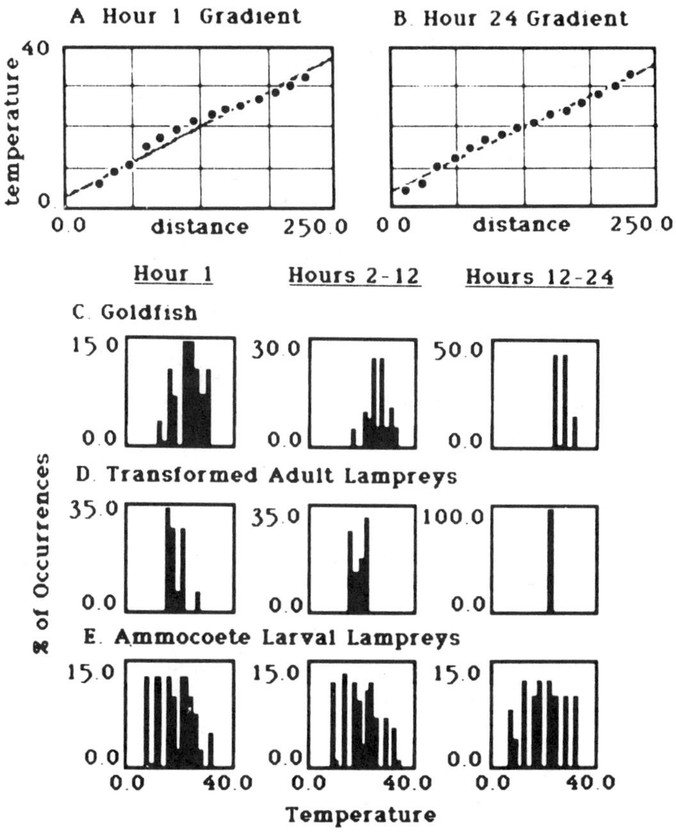

Fig. 1. Occurrence of fishes in a temperature gradient which was linear from 2°C to 37°C. Fish were acclimated to 10°C. Measurements of initial selection were made during first hour in gradient, later measurements in period 2 to 12 hours and final preferendum during 12 to 24 hours. Upper row of histograms for goldfish, middle row for adult lampreys and lower row for ammocoetes. Data obtained by Joseph Ayers.

a long time -- 12 to 14 hours -- they move to a final preferendum which appears to be independent of acclimation. The mechanism of this shift from initial selection to final preferendum is not known (Crawshaw, 1975; Crawshaw *et al.*, 1981). Figure 1 shows that postmetamorphic lampreys from the Connecticut River basin, acclimated to 8°C, select a temperature of 18.77°C whereas after 24 hours in the gradient they go to 22°C. Ammocoete larvae fail to show this behavior in a gradient; apparently some mechanism develops on metamorphosis that leads to ability to select temperature. Ammocoetes of *Petromyzon marinus* in freshwater are most active (as judged by number caught) at 10-14°C (Hardisty and Potter, 1971). These results differ from data on ammocoetes from Presque Isle which show a final preferendum of 13.6-14.5°C (Reynolds and Casblin, 1978). Adult lampreys from Minnesota showed initial selection (2 1/2 hours) of 14.5°C (McCauley *et al.*, 1977). It is possible that the differences in ammocoete behavior indicate genetically different races in New England and the Great Lakes.

Pacific lampreys showed a mean selected temperature of 16-17°C (Lemons and Crawshaw, 1978). The fact that lampreys can behaviorally regulate their body temperature by selection suggests the early appearance of this adaptation.

The adaptive value of temperature selection is to keep the fish in a temperature of "optimal" metabolic range. It also relates to spawning. Adult tautogs along the New Jersey coast migrate offshore in the fall and return in the spring; their migration depends on water temperature, not on photoperiod. Green sunfishes, after 1 to 2 hours in a gradient, selected the same temperatures to which they had been acclimated -- 25°C, 15°C and 5°C, Figure 2 (Nelson and Prosser, 1979).

(13) The most highly developed mechanism of temperature regulation is that of homeotherms -- birds and mammals. They achieve relative constancy of body temperature by (a) insulation by feathers and hair, (b) control of blood peripheral vasoconstriction and vasodilation, often in local body regions and (c) changes in metabolic range such that more heat is produced at low ambient temperatures than in the thermoneutral zone. Regulation at high temperature is by evaporative cooling. This method of temperature regulation -- circulatory and metabolic -- is not used by fishes except in the local production mentioned previously.

(14) The mechanisms of regulation -- behavioral and circulatory-metabolic -- have similar neural bases. The two types of regulation differ in their effectors, but may be similar in receptors and integrators. Temperature receptors exist at three

Fig. 2. (*Next page*) Behavioral thermoregulation by green sunfish (*Lepomis cyanellus*). Plots of initial temperature selection (1 to 2 hours). (a) selected temperature by normal 25°C acclimated fish, (b) distribution after preoptic lobe lesion, (c) selected temperature by 15° acclimated fish, (d) deep body temperature recorded while in gradient, (e) distribution of 15°C acclimated fish after brain lesion, (f) body temperature of lesioned fish, (g) distribution of 5°C acclimated fish, (h) lesioned 5°C acclimated fish. Modified from Nelson and Prosser, 1979.

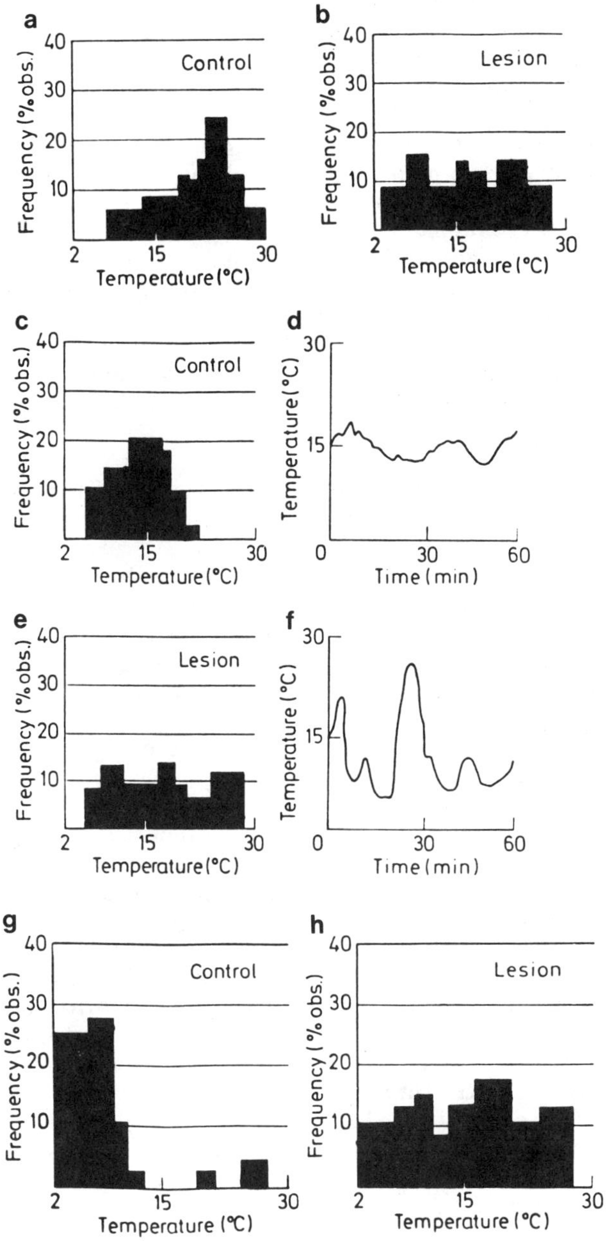
a
Control
Frequency (%obs.)
40
30
20
10
2
15
30
Temperature (°C)
b
Lesion
Frequency (%obs.)
40
30
20
10
2
15
30
Temperature (°C)
c
Control
Frequency (% obs.)
40
30
20
10
2
15
30
Temperature (°C)
d
Temperature (°C)
30
15
0
30
60
Time (min)
e
Lesion
Frequency (%obs.)
40
30
20
10
2
15
30
Temperature (°C)
f
Temperature (°C)
30
15
0
30
60
Time (min)
g
Control
Frequency (%obs.)
40
30
20
10
2
15
30
Temperature (°C)
h
Lesion
Frequency (% obs.)
40
30
20
10
2
15
30
Temperature (°C)

sites: (1) peripheral sense cells, (2) specific temperature-sensitive neurons in the spinal cord, and other parts of nervous systems, and (3) neurons in a temperature regulating center. The relative importance of temperature-sensitive neurons varies in different kinds of vertebrates. Some temperature-sensing endings may have multiple inputs, and temperature-regulating centers may have been derived from other functions such as respiration (Nelson *et al.*, 1984; Prosser and Nelson, 1981).

Peripheral thermoreceptors have not been studied in cyclostomes. However, thermokineses are a general property of animals and temperature sensing, apart from the metabolic responses, must have evolved very early. Ciliate protozoans select "optimal" temperatures and back away from hot or cold ends of a gradient. It is probable that the same sense cell in metazoans may serve several functions. The ampullae of Lorenzini of elasmobranchs may serve primarily as electroreceptors, but they are spontaneously active with maximum frequency at mid-temperature; firing decreases to zero at 2°C and at 34°C. Responses may occur to as little as 0.05°C change (Hensel, 1955). In the teleost *Leuciscus*, mechanoreceptors were maximally sensitive to touch at 18°C after 5°C acclimation, and at 22°C after 15°C acclimation (Spath, 1967). Responses by breathing rate and heart rate in Pacific lampreys occur faster than changes in body temperature, and faster than selection in a gradient, hence, peripheral receptors probably give the first signals of temperature (Lemons and Crawshaw, 1978). Multifunctional peripheral receptors may have given rise to the specific heat and cold receptors of homeotherms.

All neurons are sensitive to cooling or heating and the distinction between specific and non-specific temperature receptor neurons is not sharp. The following are criteria of specific thermoreceptor neurons: (1) A temperature threshold, either warm or cold, corresponding to behavioral temperature regulation. (2) Rate of firing showing a high slope of frequency as a function of temperature, that is, having a high Q_{10}. Values of Q_{10} of 4 have been recorded for specific receptor neurons as opposed to Q_{10}s of 2 for non-specific neurons. (3) Sensitivity high over a narrow range of temperature. (4) Rate of temperature changes, ΔT, may be as important as absolute temperature. (5) Cold receptors increasing frequency of firing as the temperature falls. Central temperature receptors are not restricted to temperature-regulating regions of the nervous system. Thermoregulatory neurons receive input from peripheral receptors and from distant regions of the CNS.

Frequency of firing as a function of temperature in Purkinje cells of slices of goldfish cerebellum is shown in Figure 3. Q_{10} values varied from 1.0 to 4.0. In addition to changes in frequency of spontaneous firing, changes in patterns were also observed. Temperature sensitive units in diencephalon of trout range in Q_{10}s from 4.6 to 15 (Greer and Gardner, 1974). Some cerebellar units fire in bursts, and as the temperature is raised firing becomes continuous; on recooling the bursting reappears (Friedlander *et al.*, 1976). These patterns of response of cerebellar neurons to temperature are non-specific but they probably have some influence on a thermoregulatory center.

Probably in all vertebrate animals a temperature-regulating center is present in the preoptic hypothalamus; other regions may also serve a regulatory function. A criterion of a regulatory center is its connection to effector structures. The medial

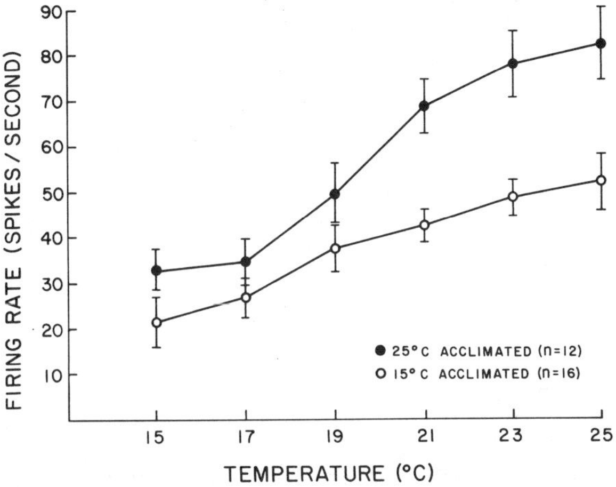

Fig. 3. Frequency of firing of two Purkinje neurons of cerebellum as a function of temperature. Brain slice preparation. Non-specific temperature effects are shown. Recorded by E. Green.

and lateral preoptic regions of the brain of sunfish (*Lepomis cyanellus*) and goldfish (*Carassius auratus*) apparently function as thermoregulatory centers. Normal fish select a given temperature in a gradient (Figure 2); after lesions in the preoptic areas behavioral thermoregulation is disrupted (Fig. 2); these lesions did not destroy normal exploratory behavior. Recordings from single units in the preoptic region showed several patterns of response to temperature (Fig. 4). Neurons responded to warming by increasing frequency in one of three ways: linear, exponential or hyperbolic (Nelson *et al.*, 1984). As the brain was cooled, other neurons increased in frequency. In addition to the responses to brain warming, some units increased firing either linearly or exponentially in response to rise in temperature of skin (Fig. 4). No cold-sensitive peripheral input to central neurons was observed. Intracellular recordings showed that some central neurons were synaptically driven, presumably from thermoreceptors elsewhere in the nervous system or from the periphery; such cells gave synaptic potentials. Other neurons gave no synaptic potentials and were presumably specific receptors. A neuronal model summarizing the intracellular recordings from preoptic neurons is shown in Figure 5 (Nelson *et al.*, 1984). Warmth-sensitive, endogenously active units (Rc) drive other neurons (W) by excitatory synapses; W cells receive input from either central warmth receptors (Rc) or peripheral warmth receptors (WREp). Cold-sensitive interneurons show both excitatory and inhibitory synaptic potentials and are not endogenously active; activity of C cells results from synaptic input from a postulated (not yet detected) excitatory input from peripheral cold receptors (CRp). Output from W and C cells presumably goes to motor centers which result in selection in a temperature gradient.

The nature of regulating circuitry in primitive fishes is unknown, but the model presented from a teleost provides a starting point for speculation.

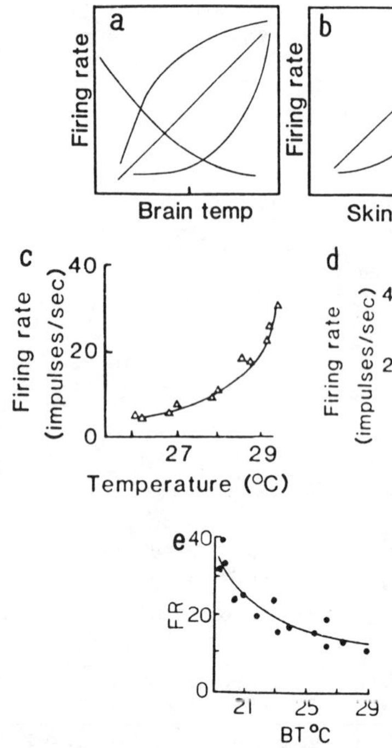

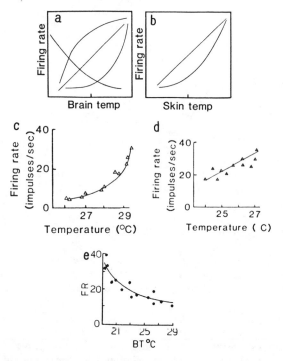

Fig. 4. Patterns of responses of single units in preoptic hypothalamus. (a) Four types of response to brain warming or cooling. (b) Two types of responses to warming skin of mouth or operculum. (c) Non-linear response of one unit to brain warming, (d) linear response, (e) response of a unit to cooling. From Nelson and Prosser, 1981; Nelson *et al.* 1984.

Fig. 5. (*Next page*) Schematic diagram of neuronal circuit derived largely from intracellular recordings from preoptic hypothalamus of green sunfish. Central warm-sensitive thermoreceptors (*Rc*) detect brain temperature. One subpopulation of these central receptors sends excitatory output to integrating neurons (*W*) which combine this input with signals from peripheral warm receptors (*WR*). Output from these (*W*) cells descends in brainstem to alter motor output and produce thermoregulatory behavior. Output from (*W*) cells presumably controls behavior on the warm side of thermodistribution curve in a gradient, thus protecting against elevations in body temperature. Control of behavior in cold temperatures arises from a different subset of warm-sensitive central thermoreceptors (*Rc*) which provide inhibitory input to cells receiving excitatory drive from central thermo-insensitive cells (*I*). This combination of inputs produces

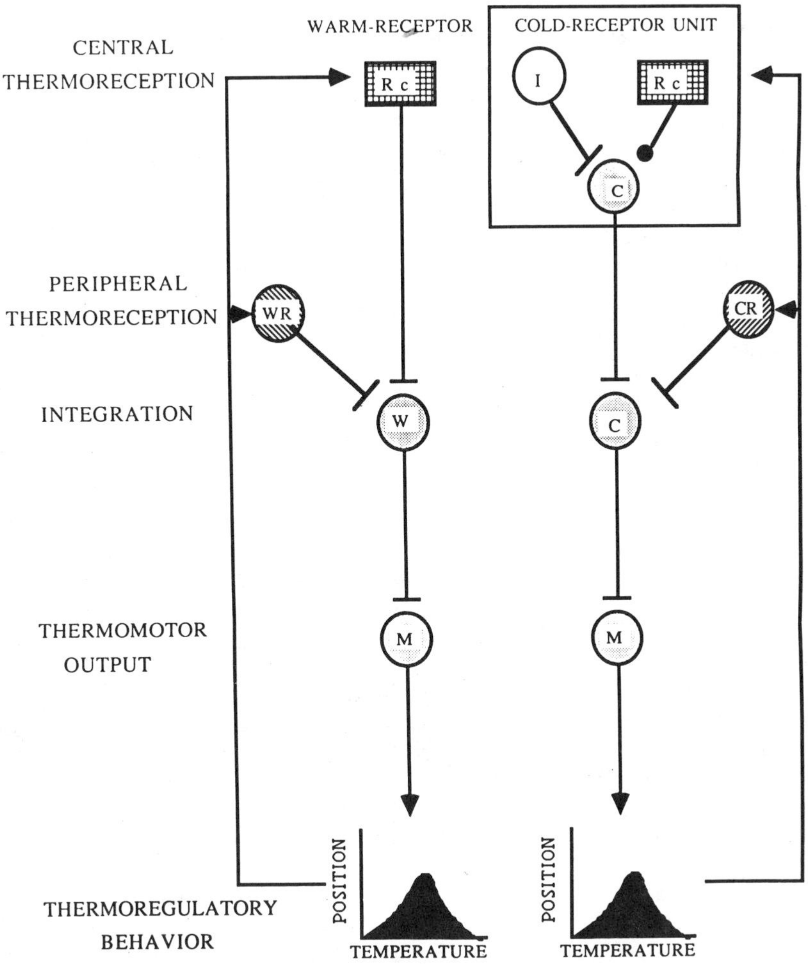

Fig. 5. (*Continued*) a neuron characterized by cold sensitivity (*C*). Excitatory output from these cells combines with excitatory input from peripheral cold thermoreceptors (*CR*) and results in descending thermomotor signals which protect against decreases in body temperature. According to this scheme only one class of true central thermoreceptor neurons exist (*Rc*). Evolution of this system is postulated to involve additional parallel pathways for different kinds of control. Additional complexity probably includes increased importance of peripheral receptors. Peripheral cold-receptor input to the hypothalamus was not identified in green sunfish.

Literature cited

BEAMISH, F.W.H. 1980. Biology of North American anadromous sea lamprey, *Petromyzon marinus*. Can. J. Fish. Aquat. Sci. **37**: 1924-1943.

CHRISTOPHERSEN, J. 1973. Basic aspects of temperature action on microorganisms. pp. 3-85 *In* Precht, H., J. Christophersen, H. Hensel,and W. Parcher [eds.] Temperature and life. Springer-Verlag, New York.

COSSINS, A., and C.L. PROSSER. 1978. Evolutionary adaptation of membranes to temperature. Proc. Natl. Acad. Sci. U.S.A. **75**: 2040-2043.

CRAWSHAW, L.D. 1975. Attainment of final thermal preferendum in brown bullheads acclimated to different temperatures. Comp. Biochem. Physiol. **52A**: 171-173.

CRAWSHAW, L.D., B. MOFFIT, D. LEMONS, and J. DOWNEY. 1981. Evolutionary development of vertebrate thermoregulation. Amer. Sci. **69**: 543-561.

FARMER, G.J. 1980. Biology and physiology of feeding in adult lampreys. Can. J. Fish. Aquat. Sci. **37**: 1751-1761.

FRIEDLANDER, M.J., N. KOTCHABHAKDI, and C.L. PROSSER. 1976. Effects of cold and heat on behavior and cerebellar function in goldfish. J. comp. Physiol. **112**: 19-45.

GREER, G.L., and D.R. GARDNER. 1974. Characterizations of responses from temperature-sensitive units in trout brain. Comp. Biochem. Physiol. **48A**: 189-203.

HARDISTY, M.W., and I.C. POTTER. 1971a. Behaviour, ecology and growth of larval lampreys. pp. 85-125 *In* Hardisty, M.W., and I.C. Potter [eds.] The biology of lampreys, vol. 1. Academic Press, New York.

HARDISTY, M.W., and I.C. POTTER. 1971b. General biology of adult lampreys. pp. 127-206 *In* Hardisty, M.W., and I.C.Potter [eds.] The biology of lampreys, vol. 1. Academic Press, New York.

HENSEL, H. 1955. Quantitative Beziehungen zwischen Temperaturereiz und Actionspotentialen der Lorenzinischen Ampullen. Z. vergl. Physiol. **37**: 509-526.

LEMONS, D.E., and L.I. CRAWSHAW. 1978. Temperature regulation in Pacific lamprey. Fed. Proc. **37**: 929.

McCAULEY, R.W. *et al.* 1977. Photokinesis and behavioural thermoregulation in adult sea lampreys. J. exp. Zool. 202: 431-437.

MORMAN, R.H., D.W. CUDDY, and D.C. RUGEN. 1980. Factors influencing distribution of sea lamprey (*Petromyzon marinus*) in Great Lakes. Can. J. Fish. Aquat. Sci. **37**: 1811-1826.

NELSON, D.O., and C.L. PROSSER. 1979. Effect of preoptic lesions on behavioural thermoregulation of green sunfish, *Lepomis cyanellus* and of goldfish, *Carassius auratus*. J. comp. Physiol. **129**: 193-197.

NELSON, D.O., and C.L. PROSSER. 1981. Intracellular recordings from thermosensitive preoptic neurons. Science **213**: 787-789.

NELSON, D.O., J.E. HEATH, and C.L. PROSSER. 1984. Evolution of temperature regulatory mechanisms. Amer. Zool. **24**: 791-809.

PROSSER, C.L., and D.O. NELSON. 1981. The role of nervous systems in temperature adaptation of poikilotherms. Ann. Rev. Physiol. **43**: 281-300.

REYNOLDS, U.U., and M. CASBLIN. 1978. Behavioral thermoregulation by ammocoete larvae of sea lamprey *Petromyzon marinus* in an electric shuttlebox. Hydrobiol. **61**: 145-147.

SJOBERG, K. 1980. Ecology of the European river lamprey (*Lampetra fluviatilis*) in northern Sweden. Can. J. Fish. Aquat. Sci. **37**: 1974-1980.
SPATH, M. 1967. Die Wirkung der Temperatur auf die Mechanoreceptoren des Knockenfisches, *Leuciscus rutilus* L. Z. vergl. Physiol. **56**: 431-462.

RESPIRATION IN PHYLETICALLY ANCIENT FISHES

Warren Burggren

Department of Zoology
University of Massachusetts
Amherst, MA

Kjell Johansen

Department of Zoophysiology
University of Aarhus
Aarhus, Denmark

Brian McMahon

Department of Biology
University of Calgary
Calgary, Alberta

Introduction

Physiologists studying evolutionary trends in fishes are restricted to examination of extant species. This makes the identification of 'primitive' *vs.* 'derived' physiological characters extremely difficult, particularly since physiological processes at the organismal level appear so labile in both ontogenetic and phylogenetic contexts. Unlike the extensive morphological knowledge based upon both the fossil record and dissection of extant species, there is but scant physiological information on respiratory processes in phyletically ancient fishes. We thus have interpreted 'primitive' rather broadly in order best to convey the tremendous diversity of early evolutionary trends in gas exchange mechanisms exhibited by fishes.

Respiratory gas exchange can be very generally (and somewhat arbitrarily) divided into a number of processes with their associated mechanisms and structures. 'Ventilation' entails the renewal of the respiratory medium (water and/or air) to which the respiratory membranes are exposed. 'Exchange' relates to the actual transfer of oxygen and carbon dioxide between blood and the respiratory medium. 'Transport' describes the mechanisms and pathways by which the respiratory gases are conveyed between the tissues and the gas exchange organs. The ensuing discussion describes evolutionary trends in respiratory gas exchange in primitive fishes on the basis of these functional divisions.

Evolution of ventilatory mechanisms

Like most aquatic organisms, phyletically ancient fishes possess multiple respiratory sites, either external (*e.g.* the general body surface or external gills) or enclosed (internal gills or air-sacs). Mechanisms for ventilation of these surfaces clearly must be considered separately.

Ventilation of external respiratory sites

Cutaneous gas exchange may have played a very important respiratory role in fish ancestors and many early fishes. This may apply in particular to larval stages which had to survive in hypoxic water during the development of more complete adult ventilatory mechanisms. Cutaneous ventilation in aquatic organisms is often viewed as a passive complement to locomotor or other movements (Feder and Burggren, 1985). However, active components can be important. In larval *Notopterus*, for example, an external ventilatory current running counter to the direction of blood flow in the majority of skin capillaries is produced by movements of temporary pectoral fins (Liem, 1982). In *Neoceratodus*, which shows the most primitive characteristics of any extant lungfish, the larva possesses cilia which develop respiratory currents across both the general body surface and inside the opercula within a week of hatching (Whiting and Bone, 1980). This ciliation is retained for at least six weeks of larval life. Unfortunately, quantitative information on cutaneous exchange relative to total gas exchange is known for only a few adult primitive fishes and almost no larval forms (see section on Gas Exchange, below).

External gills, either as extensions of the internal gills as in elasmobranchs, or true external gills (separate from the internal gills) as in the Polypterini and Dipnoi (Fig. 1), are also common in the larval stages of primitive jawed fishes. At least the true external gills of lung fishes are capable of sweeping movements resulting from contraction of their own intrinsic musculature, acting to break up stagnant boundary layers of water around the gill filaments. Most interestingly, the surface of the external gills of the newly hatched larvae of *Protopterus* are also ciliated, which should offer an obvious aid to water convection and increased diffusion of respiratory gases prior to development of a muscular apparatus for active movement of the gills or for water irrigation (Greenwood, 1958).

Ventilation of internal respiratory sites

Although ventilation of an internal surface resulting solely from locomotion (ram ventilation) is common during swimming in both elasmobranchs and teleosts, ventilation of an internal respiratory cavity in the quiescent state has required the evolution of specialized pumps. Initially, such ventilatory pumping systems

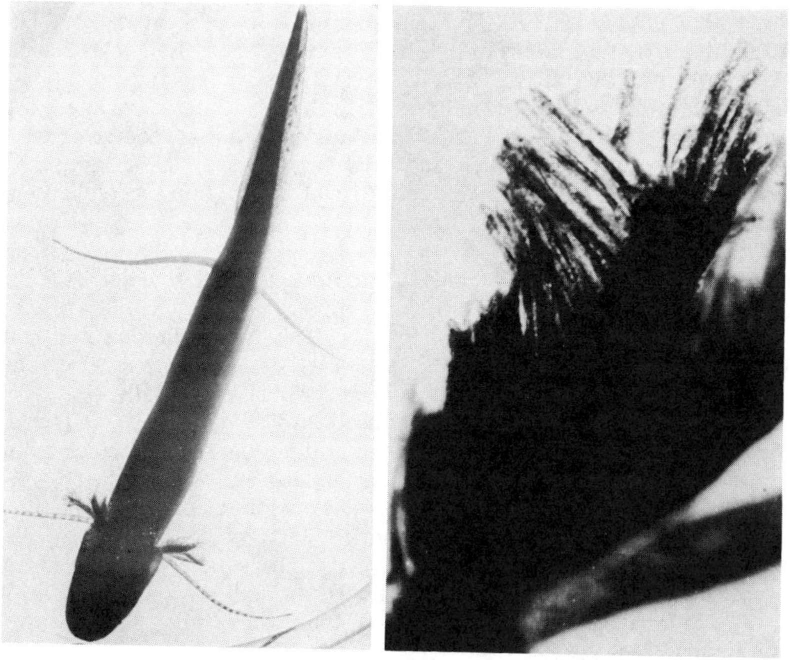

A B

Fig. 1. A. External gills in larval *Protopterus aethiopicus* of approx. 30 mm length. B. Higher magnification to show capillary loops in gill filaments.

probably arose from modification of an existing system serving some other function. In the ancestors of the phyletically ancient fishes, the initial system was almost certainly a branchial basket, perhaps similar to that seen in the cephalochordate *Branchiostoma (Amphioxus)*. Here the ventilatory water current is generated by a ciliary pump and the primary function is filter-feeding. The branchial basket, with its large surface area and extensive blood supply, could have taken over much of the respiratory function from external sites in the ancestors of the fishes. This could not only have allowed the evolution of larger, more active, proto-fishes than would be possible using cutaneous respiration alone, but also (by reducing the dependence on cutaneous gas exchange) might have allowed the development of the extensive body armor seen in some primitive fish fossils.

The ammocoete larva of the lamprey still exhibits a food gathering system based on filtration of an internal water current (Hardisty, 1979). Almost certainly this system supplements gas exchange. Ciliary pumping still functions in filter-feeding, as in the cephalochordates, but the feeding/ventilatory current of both larva and adult is facilitated by the actions of two 'new' pumps: the paired velar flaps located in the pharynx and the active contraction and passive elastic relaxation of the branchial apparatus itself. The ammocoete velum and its associated branchial musculature seem reasonably effective as a ventilatory pump, generating water flow of 0.6-3.0 ml g^{-1} min^{-1} (Rovainen and Schieber, 1975). The magnitude of this ventilatory flow is not too dissimilar from that of adult lampreys (Johansen *et al.*, 1973) or indeed from many teleosts (Shelton, 1970).

The pumping actions of both a velar apparatus and the branchial walls persist in adult myxinoids. In *Myxine*, inhalant water enters the velar chamber primarily *via* the nostril and nasopharyngeal ducts (Fig. 2). The velar pumping mechanism, as described by Johansen and Strahan (1963), involves several stages. The ventilatory cycle commences with the velar folds carried scrolled up dorsally (Fig. 3.1). The first phase involves a slow ventro-lateral unscrolling (Fig. 3.2, 3.3), followed by the main ventilatory pumping action, a rapid rescrolling movement which compresses the entrapped water posteriorly into the pharynx and across the gills (Fig. 3.4) and simultaneously draws freshwater into the velar chamber anteriorly *via* the nostril. The ventilatory action of the velum is aided both by contractions of the velar chamber itself, and by a 'peristaltic' contraction which progresses from the pharyngeal chamber into the afferent gill ducts, through the gill pouch and into the efferent ducts (Johansen and Strahan, 1963), thus contributing to both inspiratory and expiratory phases.

In adult lampreys, the velum is reduced to a small simple flap valve. The ventilatory current is now entirely generated by a compression of water in the branchial chambers produced by active contraction of the branchial basket musculature and subsequent passive relaxation of its contained elastic elements (see

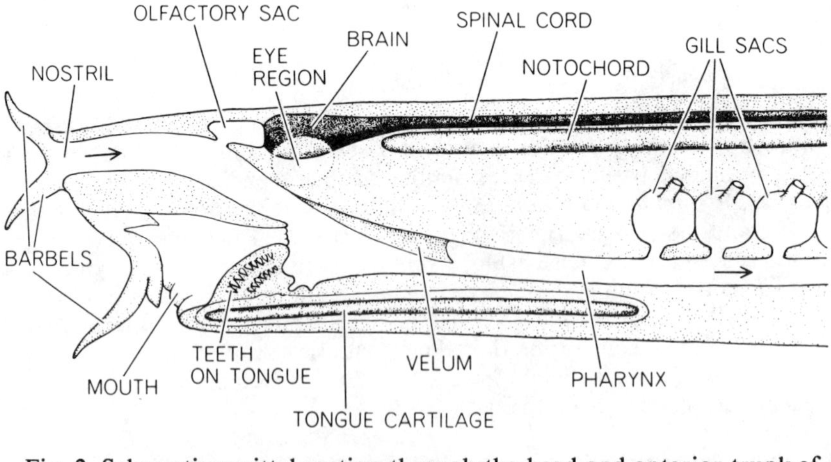

Fig. 2. Schematic sagittal section through the head and anterior trunk of the hagfish. Arrows indicate direction of water flow. From Jensen (1966).

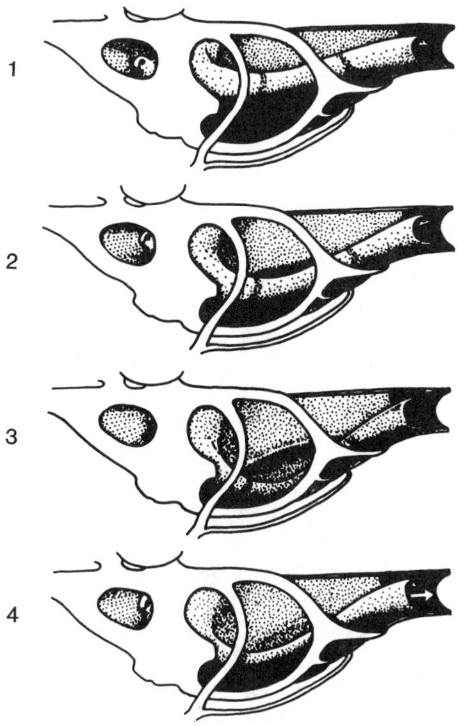

Fig. 3. Mechanism of velar pumping in myxinoids. Velar chamber is shown from left side with left pharyngeal wall removed. 1, resting; 2, velar scroll beginning to unroll; 3, velar scroll unrolled to full extent; 4, velar scroll beginning to move dorsally. Arrow shows direction of water flow. From Johansen and Strahan (1963), after Strahan (1958).

Randall, 1972). The normal pattern of water flow in the adult involves tidal ventilation, where water first enters and then leaves through the gill openings, although unidirectional water flow in through the mouth and out through the gill openings is possible. Tidal ventilation is clearly the only possible pattern in predatory lampreys when the head is immersed in the prey.

The velum may thus represent an ancient ventilatory structure, perhaps being originally the only pump in those primitive agnathans whose bone-encapsulated heads lacked movable parts within the pharyngeal apparatus. At least in living cyclostomes this bony armor has been lost, allowing the involvement of movements of branchial skeletal elements in the ventilatory processes of higher (jawed) fishes.

The specialization of several pairs of such movable branchial elements has allowed the development of a ventilatory mechanism which has persisted through the evolution of more advanced fishes and extends into higher vertebrates. In essence, this mechanism still involves the synchronous activity of two *separate* pumps - a compression pump located anterior to, and a suction pump located posterior to, the gill sieve (see Shelton, 1970). The anatomy and physiology are described most easily for teleosts where the musculo-skeletal elements surrounding the buccal cavity form the first, compression (buccal) pump while those of the opercular cavity behind the gill sieve form a second, suction (opercular) pump. The situation is actually slightly more complex for the more 'primitive' elasmobranchs, where individual gill slit openings are retained. Hughes and Ballintijn (1965) studied the ventilatory cycle in the dogfish *Scyliorhinus canicula* by means of simultaneous measurements of movements of jaws and gill slits, of pressures developed in the orobranchial and parabranchial cavities, and by electromyographic recordings of the activity of key muscles. The compression pump is formed by movements of the jaw and associated musculo-skeletal elements, particularly the floor of the orobranchial cavity (Fig. 4). The musculo-skeletal elements surrounding the individual parabranchial cavities behind each gill sieve function as suction pumps drawing water through that gill slit (Hughes and Ballintijn, 1965). The activity of each individual pump is represented (summated) as the parabranchial suction pump in Fig. 4B.

For ease of explanation, Hughes and Ballintijn (1965) divided each ventilatory pumping cycle into 4 phases (Fig. 4). In phase 1, the orobranchial cavity is expanding, drawing water in through the open mouth. In phase 2 the jaws close and coordinated contraction of several different muscles causes elevation of the orobranchial cavity floor, compressing water back towards and through the gill curtain. This compression peaks, and begins to decline, as shown by the pressure waveforms, in phase 3. In phase 4 the gills slits, which were open earlier to allow exhalation of water crossing the gills, close and expansion occurs in the parabranchial chambers behind each gill. Due to increasing volume these now develop sub-ambient (and particularly sub-orobranchial cavity) pressure, which

Fig. 4. (*Next page*) A. Diagram of a dogfish in side view (anteriorly) and horizontal section (posteriorly) showing the path of water current over the gills. Horizontal sections pass through the external gill slits and show changes in volume of the parabranchial and oro-branchial cavities. Pressures in these cavities are indicated with respect to zero pressure outside the fish. The movements of the mouth and branchial regions are shown with full line arrows, with thickness representing relative strength of contraction, from Hughes and Ballintijn (1965). B. Pressure in the orobranchial and parabranchial cavities and movements of the lower jaw and gill region of the dogfish. The main phases of activity in eight respiratory muscles are also shown. *Add md*, adductor mandibulae; *Lev pq*, levator palatoquadrati; *Lev hmd*, levator hyomandibulae; *Con hy*, constrictor hyoideus; *Con br*, constrictor branchiales; *Interarc dot*, interarcualis dorsalis; *Coraco-hy* coracohyoideus; *Coraco-br* coracobranchiales. From Shelton (1970) after Hughes and Ballintijn (1965).

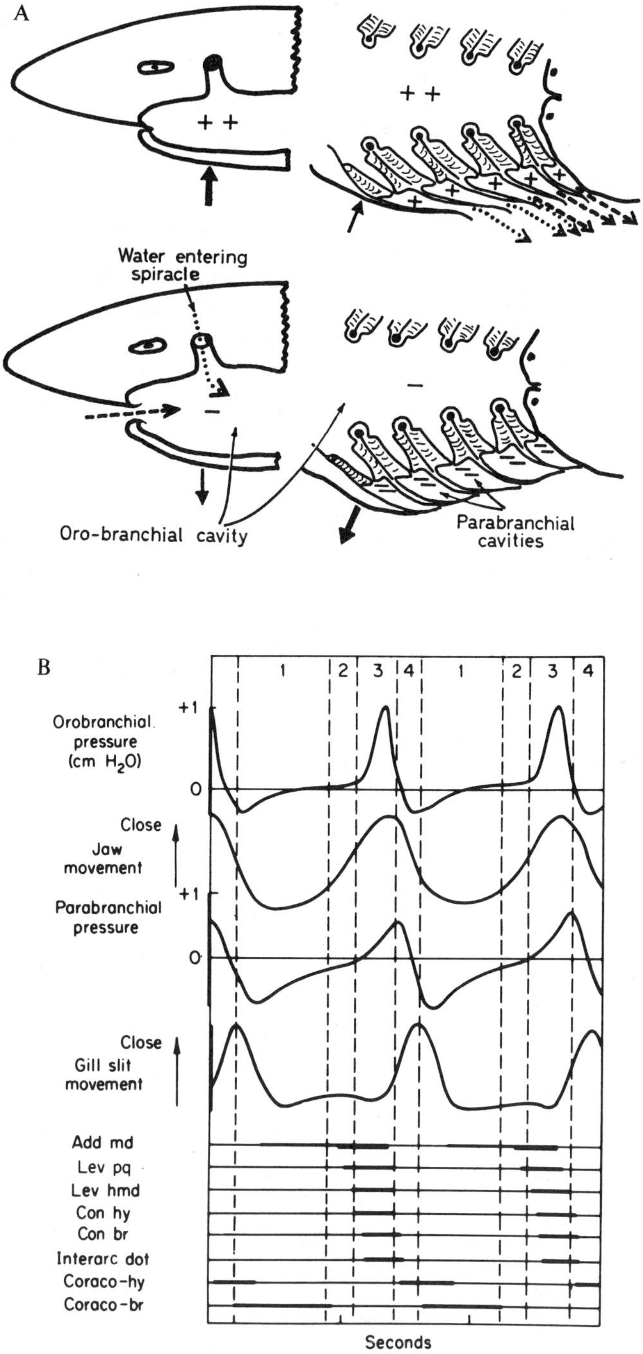
A
+ +
+ +
Water entering spiracle
−
−
Oro-branchial cavity
Parabranchial cavities
B
1
2
3
4
Orobranchial pressure (cm H_2O)
+1
0
Close
Jaw movement
+1
Parabranchial pressure
0
Close
Gill slit movement
Add md
Lev pq
Lev hmd
Con hy
Con br
Interarc dot
Coraco-hy
Coraco-br
Seconds

draws water across the gills. Note that this suction force is at its peak in phase 1, *i.e.* alternating in phase with the compression pump. In this way the two pumps generate a virtually continual flow of water across the gill surfaces. With the proviso that 1) in the Holocephali and in all bony fishes the gills are enclosed in a single opercular chamber, and 2) the structures involved may be greatly modified, an essentially similar mechanism powers water ventilation in all primitive or advanced jawed fishes (McMahon, 1969; Shelton, 1970).

One particularly relevant example of such a modification of this basic mechanism in a phyletically ancient fish group is evident in the sturgeon *Acipenser transmontanus*, and provides an interesting evolutionary parallel to the situation described for the parasitic lamprey above. The mouth of *Acipenser* is extensively modified as a protrusible suction tube used for feeding in muddy bottom sediments. When not actively feeding, the mouth is maintained above the sediments and the majority of the inhalant water stream enters the mouth and exits *via* the gills as in other gnathostome fishes (Burggren, 1978). However, when the mouth is buried beneath the surface (or surgically closed) the sturgeon can switch to unidirectional ventilation *via* the opercular opening (Fig. 5). During buccal and opercular expansion (phase 1) water passes into the opercular cavity *via* a permanent aperture at the upper margin of the operculum. This water then passes in a retrograde direction into the buccal cavity dorsally over the gill sieve, not passing over the gill lamellae. The water then returns posteriorly through the gill sieve with the buccal compression phase, flowing in the conventional direction through the gill lamellar spaces. Interestingly, the spiracle appears to account for very little water movement in *Acipenser* during either ventilatory pattern (Burggren, 1978). The aperture may

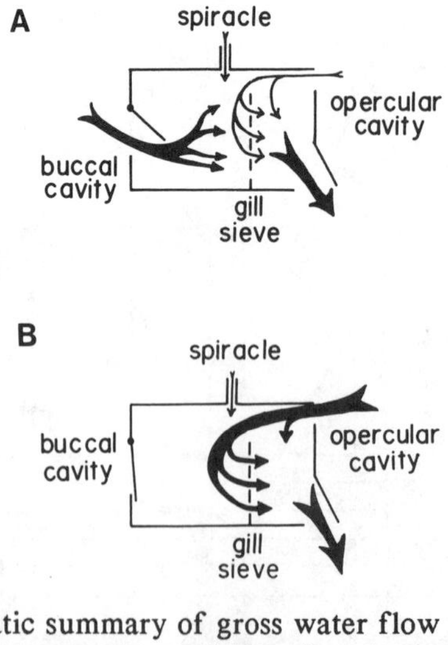

Fig. 5. Diagrammatic summary of gross water flow patterns through the buccal and opercular cavities of *Acipenser transmontanus* (A) during unrestrained buccal water intake and (B) when buccal water intake is eliminated. From Burggren (1978).

make a larger contribution in elasmobranchs, particularly in those forms living mostly buried in mud. Magid (1966) has postulated that significant water flow occurs through the spiracle of *Polypterus*, but more work is needed to understand fully its role in this fish.

Most studies of ventilatory mechanisms in other phyletically ancient fishes have concentrated on air breathing (see Gas Exchange, below). Aquatic ventilation has been poorly studied, but appears similar to that described above for elasmobranchs and teleosts.

The transition to air breathing

A surprisingly large number of the phyletically ancient fishes are either facultative or obligate air breathers. Clearly, the evolution of air-breathing came early in the evolution of fishes. The extant ancient air breathing fishes are presumably the remnants of a multitude of such fishes which evolved in the warm, hypoxic freshwater thought to have been typical of the later Devonian (Tappan, 1974). The Rhipidistian fishes (Crossopterygii), from which it is generally assumed that the terrestrial vertebrates evolved, were important members of this group. That the Crossopterygii are now effectively extinct, except for the highly modified and strictly aquatic coelacanth *Latimeria chalumnae*, leaves us with a distinct gap in our understanding of the evolution of respiratory processes in the vertebrates. This may explain the considerable interest which has always been devoted to air-breathing in other groups of phyletically ancient fish.

The structures utilized for aerial gas exchange in fishes are extremely diverse. They include the gills or, more often, extensions of them; diverticula of the buccal and opercular cavities; pharynx, oesophagus, stomach, and intestine; the swim-bladder and the skin (see reviews by Carter and Beadle, 1931; Johansen, 1970; Randall *et al.*, 1981a). Amongst the extant phyletically ancient fishes, however, structures commonly used for aerial gas exchange are restricted to invaginations of the pharyngeal region (*i.e.* lungs or air bladders). Jarvik (1980) summarizes the generally held view that lungs, as evident in the Dipnoi and polypterids, are of different origin embryologically from the air sacs found in the Holostei and primitive Teleostei. He considers only the former structures to be homologous with the lungs of the tetrapods.

Despite this significant difference in embryological derivation, the mechanisms for air ventilation of lungs and air bladders appear similar in all these fishes. In essence, the evolution of air-breathing in fish required the conversion of the existing water-pumping mechanism to serve a new function: aerial ventilation of an internal cavity, either air sac or lung. This transition involved relatively simple modification to the aquatic ventilatory mechanism of the primitive gnathostomes.

The most complete account of the physiological adjustments permitting this transition has been given for the lungfish *Protopterus aethiopicus* (McMahon, 1969). A combination of X-ray cinematography (Fig. 6), electromyography and pressure recording (Fig. 7) was used to study the mechanisms of both aquatic and aerial ventilation. Aquatic ventilation occurred by a process essentially similar to that of other bony fishes, except that the operculum of the lungfish is a soft and muscular

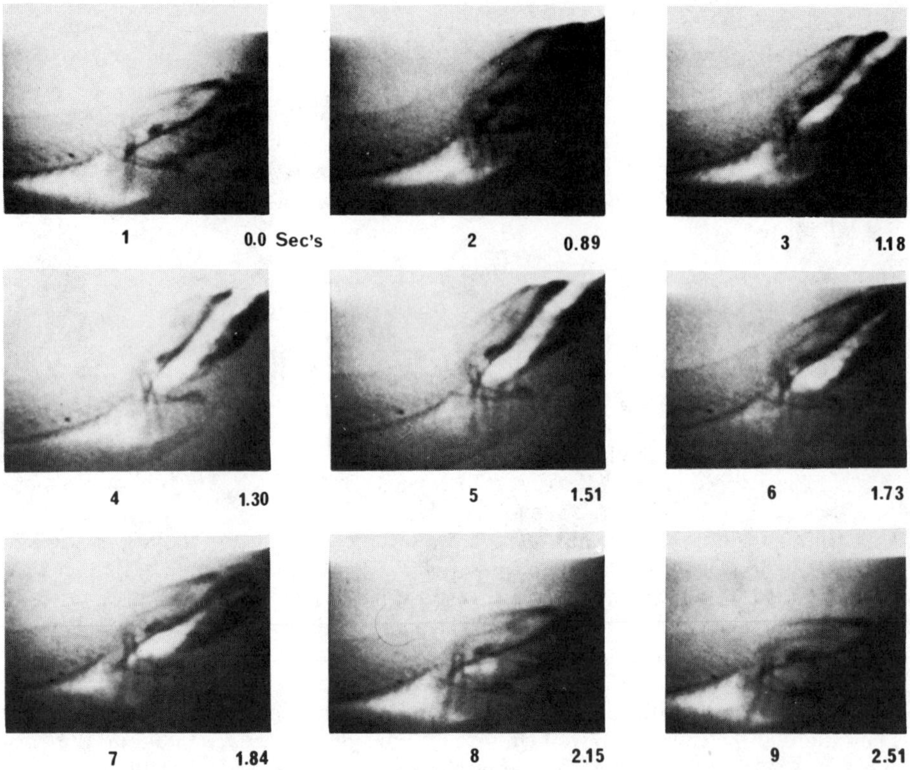

Fig. 6. Selected stills from a cineradiographic analysis of a single air ventilatory sequence in *Protopterus aethiopicus*. From McMahon (1969).

structure rather than a bony plate as in most teleost fishes. The operculum of lungfishes thus plays only a minor role in aquatic ventilation, leaving the buccal compression pump as the dominant force powering water flow across the gills. Fig. 7A details the participation of the muscle systems and pressures generated during aquatic ventilation in this species.

Aerial ventilation uses the same muscular and structural elements as are involved in aquatic ventilation, but with several physiological modifications made at the level of the central pattern generator controlling ventilatory movements. The first modification is that, although a single aerial ventilation involves only the equivalent of a single ventilatory cycle directly, modification of both the preceding and succeeding cycles is involved (Fig. 7B). The first modified cycle occurs as the animal is approaching the surface and serves to expel water from the buccal cavity preparatory to taking in air (Fig. 6.1). This cycle is modified in two ways. First, buccal compression is extended, forcing virtually all of the contained water out through the opercular valve. Secondly, activity in the constrictor hyoideus muscle,

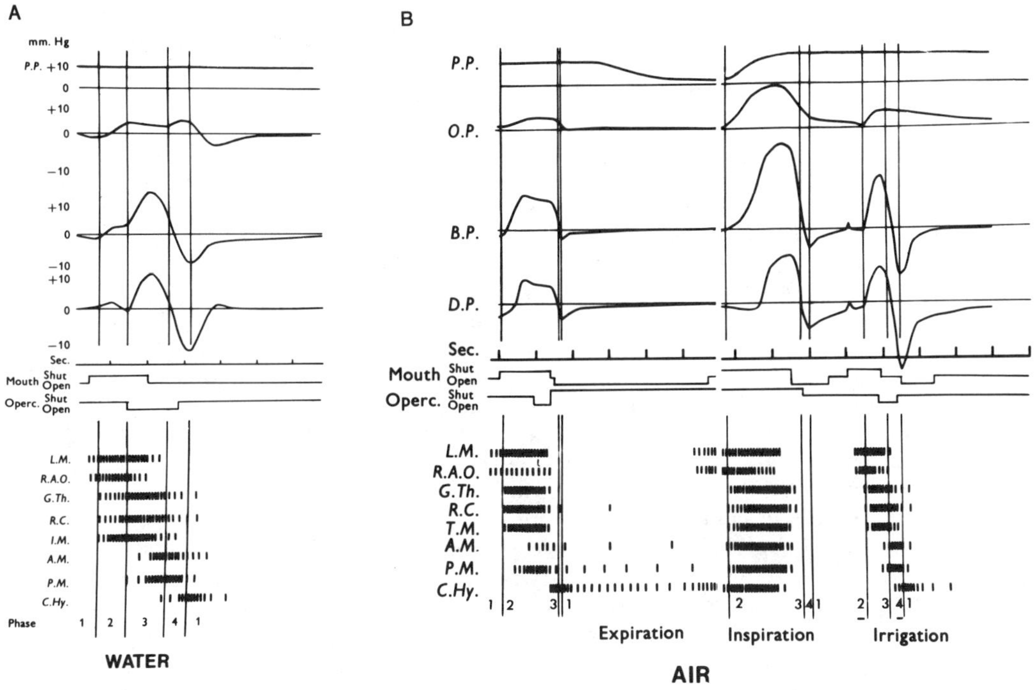

Fig. 7. Synchronized records from implanted pressure catheters, electromyographic electrodes and observations of mouth and opercular movements during: (A) a single aquatic ventilatory sequence and (B) a single air ventilatory sequence in *Protopterus aethiopicus*. *P.P.*, intrapulmonary pressure; *B.P.*, buccal cavity pressure; *O.P.*, opercular cavity pressure; *D.P.*, pressure differential recorded between buccal and opercular cavities. Diagrammatic representation of electrical activity recorded in: *L.M.*, levator mandibulae muscle; *R.A.O.*, retractor anguli oris muscle; *R.C.*, rectus cervicis muscle complex; *I.M.* intermandibularis muscle; *G.Th.*, geniothoracicus muscle; *C.Hy*, constrictor hyoideus muscle; *A.M.*, anterior and *P.M.* posterior muscles of the cranial rib. From McMahon (1969).

which normally closes the opercular flap in phase 4, occurs earlier, and more intensely, closing the operculum tightly and preventing reflux of water as the animal's snout breaks the surface and aerial ventilation commences.

The first phase (buccal and opercular expansion) of the true air ventilation cycle now takes place after the snout has penetrated into air (Fig. 6.2). The duration of this phase is greatly increased and the displacement of the buccal floor consequently increased so that the buccal cavity is much more distended than occurs in water ventilation. Early in this phase the glottis opens and pulmonary pressure falls as pulmonary gas escapes. In animals ascending vertically to the surface under natural conditions lung deflation occurs very rapidly, aided by the considerable hydrostatic pressure applied to the opened lung. Under the experimental conditions of a shallow water column used in the production of the data for Figs. 6 and 7, hydrostatic pressure assist was minimal and expiration presumably occurred largely by the action of the smooth muscle coating of the lung (Poll, 1962). Nonetheless, Fig. 6.4 shows that complete emptying of the lung occurs. Expansion of the buccal cavity continues during the following expiration, minimizing admixture of exhalant and inhalant gases, and thus ensuring high lung PO_2 following breathing (Lenfant and Johansen, 1968; McMahon, 1970). Further modification of this phase is seen in the extended (continued) activity of the constrictor hyoideus muscle, (Fig. 7A), which tightly closes the opercular opening, preventing water entry into the buccal cavity (and hence the lung) during the expiration/inspiration process. As this phase ends the jaws are closed and sealed and the animal's head is resubmerged (Fig. 6.5-6.6). In the buccal compression phase of the actual air breathing cycle the buccal floor elements rise, compressing the gas in the buccal cavity and driving it back through the open glottis and into the lung (Fig. 6.6-6.8). Air leakage is prevented by passive closure of the oral valves and active closure of the opercular valves, again resulting from intense premature activity in the constrictor hyoideus muscle which tightly closes the operculum as well as compressing the air in the opercular cavity. Pressures developed in the buccal cavity during air compression, approximating 20 mm Hg, exceed those developed in aquatic buccal compression. These high pressures may be needed to overcome possible hydrostatic pressure effects, lung air-way resistance and the stiffness of the abdominal walls and other structures. Almost all of the buccal gas is forced into the lungs. The buccal expansion phase of the subsequent cycle occurs under water and is of greater than usual amplitude. On compression, this water is forced explosively through the gill sieve removing trapped air which might interfere with subsequent aquatic exchange.

Protopterus normally fills the lung with a single air breathing sequence (Figs. 6 and 7), as do most air-breathing fishes under natural conditions. Under experimental conditions where the animal is confined in shallow water, occasional double (McMahon, 1969) or multiple (*Lepidosiren*, Bishop and Foxon, 1968) buccal pumping sequences result from the animal's inability to function correctly with the body flexed (rather than straight) and with reduced hydrostatic assist.

Lung ventilation occurs *via* essentially the same process in other Dipnoi (*Lepidosiren*, Bishop and Foxon, 1968; *Neoceratodus*, Grigg, 1965) and in *Protopterus aethiopicus* during estivation (Delaney and Fishman, 1977). Similar modification of the buccal compression phase powers ventilation of the air bladder in the Holostei (*Amia*, Johansen *et al.*, 1970, and *Lepisosteus*, Rahn *et al.*, 1971).

Despite this preponderance of buccal pumping in aerial ventilation of both fishes and amphibians, buccal filling and compression has several disadvantages (Randall *et al.*, 1981b) and has been replaced in higher vertebrates by systems which use an aspiratory or suction powered pump. According to Farrell and Randall (1978), an aspiratory suction mechanism is seen first in a 'primitive' air breathing teleost, the osteoglossid *Arapaima gigas*. These authors measured an internal aspiratory force (sub-ambient pressure) within the air bladder, perhaps resulting from an arching of the body with consequent lateral expansion of the ribs which they considered to assist buccal compression. This view, however, has recently been strongly criticized by Greenwood and Liem (1984) whose more detailed study utilized high speed X-ray cinematography to show that there is a time lapse of 60-90 msec between closure of the mouth and appearance of air in the air-bladder. Greenwood and Liem (1984) conclude that a sub-ambient pressure in the air sac (if actually occurring) could not supplement the volume pumped by the buccal force pump and argue that there is as yet no evidence for aspiratory air ventilation of the lung or gas bladder in fishes.

Patterns of respiratory gas exchange

The extant phyletically ancient fishes, though morphologically similar or even degenerate compared with their ancestors, are anything but primitive in their gas exchange capabilities.

The agnathans

Branchial gross structure in the agnathan fishes contrasts markedly with the independently-supported branchial arches of gnathostomes. The branchial respiratory surfaces of both lampreys and hagfishes are incorporated into rounded, sac-like "pouches" or "baskets" (Fig. 2), ventilated either unidirectionally (hagfishes) or tidally (adult lampreys) (see above). Lampreys universally have seven gill pouches, while this number varies from five to 14 in various species of hagfishes. The cartilaginous 'branchial skeleton' is quite extensive in the lampreys, but less well defined in myxinoids (Johansen, 1963). The anterior and posterior internal wall of each branchial pouch bears a hemibranch, differentiated into lamellae which dichotomise to form secondary lamellae. The distribution, spacing, fine structure and surface area of these secondary lamellae, at least in lampreys, are very similar to that in teleost fishes (Lewis and Potter, 1976; Lewis, 1976), a rather remarkable fact considering the evolutionary distance between these two groups (Hardisty, 1979). The afferent branchial arteries of both hagfish and lampreys divide to supply the anterior and posterior hemibranchs of adjacent gill pouches (Johansen and Strahan, 1963; Jensen, 1965; Nakao and Uchinomiya, 1978). As in the majority of more advanced fishes, the bulk flows of water and of blood through the gill pouches of the hagfish are countercurrent, an anatomical arrangement maximizing the potential for gas exchange. Counter-current flow has not been confirmed for the lamprey.

Relatively few quantitative data are available on the respiratory physiology of myxinoids, except on metabolic rate. Oxygen uptake in *Eptatretus stouti*, a hagfish inhabiting the outer Pacific sublittoral zone, has been reported at about 8-10 $\mu l\ O_2\ g^{-1}\ h^{-1}$ at 10°C (Munz and Morris, 1965). This value is very low compared with teleosts at similar temperatures (Shelton, 1970). A recent study of the hagfish, *Myxine glutinosa* L., has directly measured the branchial ventilation rates and volumes in addition to O_2 consumption (Steffensen *et al.*, 1984). At 7°C, a water temperature normally encountered by this species, the frequency of the velar pumping was 18 beats min^{-1}, generating a water flow of 0.019 ml $min^{-1}\ g^{-1}$. O_2 consumption at 7°C was 30-35 $\mu l\ O_2\ g^{-1}\ h^{-1}$ in normoxic water. These values are well within the range of metabolic rates reported for teleosts at similar temperatures (Shelton, 1970). Hardisty (1979), reviewing the data on metabolic rate in myxinoids, suggests that there may be pronounced species differences related to ecological factors, particularly water depth, and he predicts that the more lethargic life-style of deep water myxinoids would be reflected in a reduced metabolic rate. A systematic survey of metabolic rate in hagfishes has yet to be made, however.

Interestingly, Steffensen *et al* (1984) indicate that at least 80% of O_2 uptake by *Myxine glutinosa* can occur across the skin. Certainly, the very thin epidermis and dense sub-epidermal capillary network of the hagfish (Hans and Tabencka, 1938) will facilitate cutaneous gas exchange. A wide variety of fishes, both primitive and advanced, depend heavily upon cutaneous gas exchange (see Feder and Burggren, 1985, for review). In the case of the hagfish, cutaneous respiration may be of particular importance when inhalation through the anteriorly placed nostril is compromised during feeding.

Lampreys appear to possess a highly efficient gas exchange, in accordance with both their great tolerance of changing ambient conditions and their comparatively active life-style. The gill surface areas and epithelial thicknesses for both the ammocoete and adult of *Lampetra fluviatilis* are comparable to those of active teleost species (Lewis and Potter, 1976; Lewis, 1976). Consequently, the branchial O_2 diffusing capacity in *Lampetra planeri* and *Petromyzon marinus* (Lewis, 1976) is comparable to that of teleost fishes (Hughes and Morgan, 1973; Hughes, 1984). Oxygen uptake in lampreys, reported from 20-120 $\mu l\ O_2\ g^{-1}\ h^{-1}$, varies not only with species, but also with temperature, developmental stage and availability of substrata for burrowing (see Johansen *et al.*, 1973; Hardisty, 1979). However, oxygen uptake is generally higher than reported for myxinoids and compares favorably with many more advanced fishes. The respiratory role of the skin of adult lampreys has been estimated to be only 20% of total O_2 uptake (Korolewa, 1964). Cutaneous gas exchange declines in importance as metabolic rates rise in a wide variety of vertebrates (Feder and Burggren, 1985), perhaps explaining its diminished importance in adult lampreys relative to hagfish.

Lampreys are extremely tolerant of very low ambient oxygen levels, maintaining or even increasing their O_2 uptake at a PO_2 as low as 10 mm Hg even in comparatively warm water (Johansen *et al.*, 1973; Claridge and Potter, 1975). In resting normoxic *Entosphenus tridentata*, venous blood has a comparably high degree of O_2 saturation, since only about 10% of the O_2 available from circulating blood is extracted in passage through the tissues. During progressive hypoxia, venous PO_2 falls less rapidly than arterial PO_2, and O_2 utilization increases to nearly 30% when ambient PO_2 falls below 60 mm Hg. Utilization of the large venous O_2 reserve at rest during normoxia is clearly important in maintaining O_2 uptake when hypoxia is encountered.

During activity, lampreys (*L. fluviatilis*) can elevate O_2 uptake up to 7 times above resting levels. Beamish (1973) and Johansen *et al.* (1973) have shown that their large venous O_2 reserve is similarly tapped during exercise. Maintained O_2 consumption during hypoxia or increased O_2 consumption during exercise is also assisted by marked increases in branchial water flow and cardiac output. Mechanisms for adjustments of blood flow patterns within the secondary lamellae exist in lamprey gills (Youson and Freeman, 1976), and redistribution of regional blood flow patterns could also play a role during either hypoxia or exercise.

The Chondrichthyes

The elasmobranchs (in particular the dogfish) are among the 'white rats' of fish respiratory physiology, perhaps rivalled only by the salmonids in terms of large data base. It is beyond the scope of this paper to review these data, and the reader is referred to comprehensive reviews by Scheid and Piiper (1976) and Heisler (1984). At the other extreme, almost nothing is known of the respiratory physiology of the Holocephali. This dearth of information results in part from the comparatively rare occurrence and delicate nature of these animals. Because of the unavoidable imbalance in discussion of these two groups of Chondrichthyes, as well as the comparatively remote position of the Chondrichthyes from the main line of higher vertebrates evolution, we pass now to actinopterygian fishes.

The Chondrostei

Perhaps attesting to the selective advantage of aerial respiration in phyletically ancient fishes, only two closely related actinopterygian ancestors of the teleost, the sturgeon and the paddlefish, *Polyodon*, have retained a total dependency on aquatic gas exchange.

The sturgeon, like many teleosts, has four holobranchs receiving afferent blood from the dorsal aorta (Table I). Additionally, the sturgeon retains hyomandibular

Table I. Distribution of visceral and branchial arches in phyletically ancient fishes. From Hughes (1984).

Genus	Mandibular Arch	Spiracle	Hyoid Arch	Branchial Arches I	II	III	IV	V	VI	VII
Scyliorhinus	ps	+	ph	H	H	H	H			
Hexanchus	ps	+	ph	H	H	H	H	H		
Heptanchus	ps	+	ph	H	H	H	H	H	H	
Raia	ps	+	ph	H	H	H	H	.		
Chimaera	.	-	ph	H	H	H	ah	.		
Latimeria	.	-	ph	H	H	H	H	.		
Neoceratodus	.	-	ph	H	H	H	H	.		
Protopterus	.	-	ph	.	.	H	H	ah		
Acipenser	ps	+	ph	H	H	H	H	.		
Huso	ps	-	ph	H	H	H	H	.		
Lepisosteus	ps	-	ph	H	H	H	H	.		
Amia	ps	-	.	H	H	H	H	.		
Polypterus	.	+	.	H	H	H	ah	.		

Abbreviations: *ah*, anterior hemibranch; *H*, holobranch; *ph*, posterior hemibranch; *ps*, pseudobranch (external).

and hyoid arches that bear hemibranchs, and a patent but small spiracular opening as the remnant of the gill slit between the oromandibular and hyomandibular arches. As mentioned earlier, only limited water flow occurs through the spiracle. Moreover, approximately 98% of the total respiratory surface area resides on holobranchs of arches III-VI in *Acipenser transmontanus* (Burggren *et al.*, 1979). The gill septum in the sturgeon is much reduced compared to elasmobranchs, with about 50% of the gill filament attached to the septum arising from the branchial arch (Hughes, 1984). The gross organization of the secondary lamellae on the hemibranchs of the sturgeon is comparable to that of other craniate fishes (Byczkowska-Smyk, 1962; Burggren *et al.*, 1979). Weight-specific surface area is very low when compared with most teleost fishes (Hughes, 1984). Similarly, aerobic metabolic rate is only 50-60 μl O_2 g^{-1} h^{-1} at 15°C in resting sturgeon, and increases only 2-3 times at maximum swimming speed (Burggren and Randall, 1978). These values are far lower than for many teleost fishes at comparable sizes and temperatures (Shelton, 1970).

Basic parameters of ventilatory performance (frequency, volume, O_2 extraction, blood oxygenation) in *Acipenser transmontanus* in air-saturated water (Fig. 8) (Burggren, 1978; Burggren and Randall, 1978) show few qualitative differences from those in distantly related, highly derived teleost fishes. Blood in the dorsal aorta is fully oxygen-saturated, and its PO_2 is often 10-15 mm Hg higher than the PO_2 of expired water (Burggren and Randall, 1978), as generally found in teleosts (Randall, 1984). This is generally indicative of countercurrent flow of water and blood in the gills, but could also be explained by a cross-current arrangement as has been suggested for elasmobranchs (see Hughes, 1984; Piiper and Scheid, 1984).

Interestingly, *Acipenser transmontanus* is an 'O_2 conformer' with respect to aerobic metabolism and ambient O_2 availability (Burggren and Randall, 1978). Oxygen uptake begins to fall when ambient PO_2 decreases only slightly below air saturation, and at a PO_2 of about 40 mm Hg is only 5% of normoxic aerobic metabolic rate (Fig. 8). While some other fishes have been observed to allow O_2 uptake to fall at various degrees of non-lethal hypoxia, *Acipenser* is unusual in that, following return to air-saturated water, it does not show any compensatory increases in ventilation or O_2 uptake, nor does blood hydrogen ion concentration fall (Burggren and Randall, 1978). These data strongly suggest that no O_2 debt has been incurred during hypoxic exposure. There appears to be no shift to anaerobic metabolism during hypoxic exposure; the sturgeon simply shuts down tissue metabolism. *Acipenser transmontanus* is found frequently in deoxygenated benthic regions of lakes, in ice-covered waters and in stagnant regions of estuaries - environments that may be less easily occupied by more active fishes that must expend considerably more energy by maintaining O_2 uptake during hypoxia.

The bichir, *Polypterus*, and a close relative, the reedfish, *Calamoichthys*, share a common ancestry with the sturgeon, but are similarly highly derived from the ancestral outgroup. Few respiratory studies have been made of these animals, with most attention focusing on the fact that they use paired, regularly ventilated lungs for gas exchange (Purser, 1926; Magid, 1966; Sacca and Burggren, 1982). Gas exchange has been quantified in *Calamoichthys calabaricus* (Sacca and Burggren, 1982). When in oxygenated water, total O_2 uptake is achieved by contributions from the gills (28%), the skin (32%) and the lungs (40%). Interestingly, the reedfish

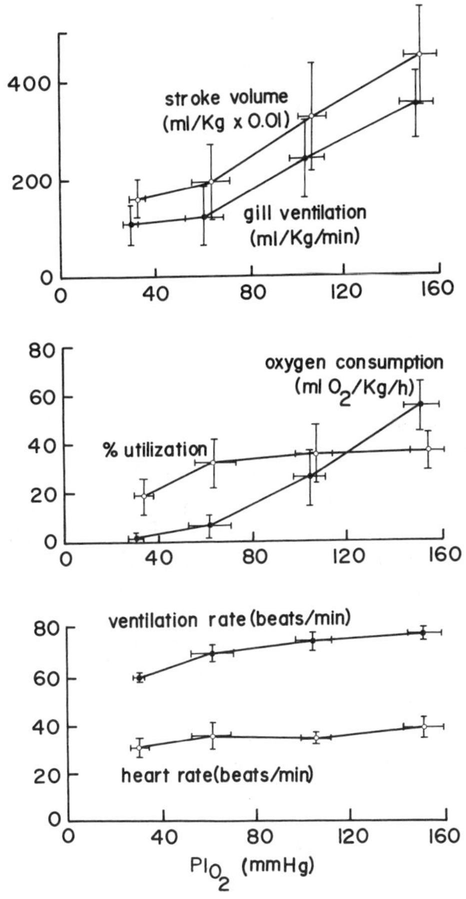

Fig. 8. Ventilatory parameters, O_2 consumption and heart rate in *Acipenser transmontanus* during normoxia and exposure to hypoxia. From Burggren and Randall (1978).

makes 5-10 daily terrestrial sojourns to forage. O_2 uptake more than doubles during these foraging trips, primarily resulting from increased pulmonary O_2 uptake.

Holostei

The extant holosteans - the bowfin (*Amia calva*) and the garfish (*Lepisosteus osseus*) - attract particular interest because they are facultative air breathers and because their natural habitat includes a large temperature range. In their northern-most areas of distribution (southern Ontario, Canada), they survive winters under ice cover. Respiratory gas exchange under these conditions is exclusively aquatic.

As temperature rises, both *Amia* and *Lepisosteus* become facultative air breathers, becoming increasingly dependent upon air breathing for their O_2 requirements (Johansen *et al.*, 1970; Rahn *et al.*, 1971; Randall *et al.*, 1981b;[2] Smatresk and Cameron, 1982). *Amia* has also been reported to estivate buried in mud in areas where water has receded during drought (Neill, 1950), but this interesting habit has not yet been studied from a respiratory point of view.

Both *Amia* and *Lepisosteus* have well-developed gills for aquatic gas exchange. In *Amia* the hyomandibular arch bears a pseudobranch, but the hyoid arch bears no hemibranch (Table I). There is no spiracle. *Lepisosteus* differs in having a posterior hemibranch on the hyoid arch. In both of these holosteans the interbranchial septum is well-developed proximally, but the distal one-third of the gill filaments are unsupported (Randall *et al.*, 1981b; Smatresk and Cameron, 1982). A unique morphological adaptation for air exposure is apparent in the gills of *Amia*, where the secondary lamellae are fused into a lattice work of rectangular pores, presumably to prevent their complete collapse in air (Daxboeck *et al.*, 1981; Laurent, 1984). The surface area of the gills of *Amia* matches that typical of purely aquatic teleost fish showing similar activity levels (Daxboeck *et al.*, 1981). Comparable data are not available for *Lepisosteus*. Aerial gas exchange in these holosteans is accomplished by intermittent ventilation of a vascularized swim bladder, which received blood that has first traversed the branchial arches (see section on Circulation, below).

At low water temperatures (*i.e.* 10°C) the gills of both *Amia* and *Lepisosteus* are the major sites for gas exchange (Fig. 9), but at 20-25°C the swim bladder accounts for 40-75% of O_2 uptake (Johansen *et al.*, 1970; Rahn *et al.*, 1971; Randall *et al.*, 1981b; Smatresk and Cameron, 1982). In *Amia*, O_2 uptake may reflect an increase in spontaneous activity level in addition to a direct temperature effect. Certainly, in active *Amia* at 20°C, the swim bladder PO_2 declined at twice the rate in active, compared to resting, fish (Johansen *et al.*, 1970).

At high water temperature, when aerial O_2 uptake predominates in both *Amia* and *Lepisosteus*, the gills and skin remain the most important route for CO_2 elimination, as reflected in gas exchange ratios (CO_2 elimination/O_2 uptake) in *Amia* of 0.21 for the swim bladder and 1.61 for the gills (Randall *et al.*, 1981b). Interestingly, the parenchyma of the swim bladder in *Amia*, as in many other air breathing fish, lacks carbonic anhydrase, and this may contribute to its relatively minor role in CO_2 elimination (Burggren and Haswell, 1979; Randall, 1984).

The Dipnoi

The Dipnoi have been extensively studied, primarily because of their perceived importance in understanding the evolution of early tetrapods. Additionally, their remarkable ability to withstand desiccation during estivation has attracted much attention. It is important to emphasize at the outset that the three extant genera of lungfishes show considerable differences in their respiratory physiology. The Australian *Neoceratodus forsteri* is an obligate water breather with well developed, efficient gills. The lungs play a role in gas exchange only in very hypoxic water or during vigorous activity. Species of *Protopterus*, the African lungfishes, are all obligate air breathers, and spend months or even years totally removed from water

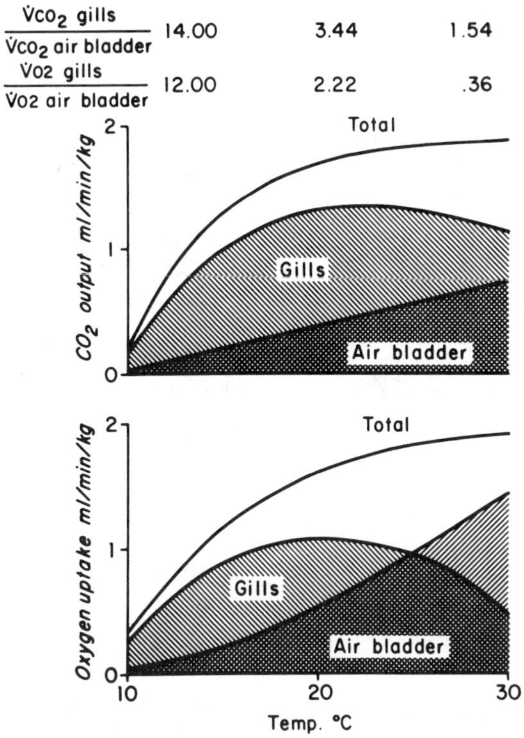

Fig. 9. CO_2 elimination (top graph) and O_2 uptake (bottom) by gills and swimbladder of *Amia clava* over the temperature range 10 - 30°C. From Johansen *et al.* (1970).

during estivation (Smith, 1931). *Lepidosiren paradoxa*, the South American lungfish, is also an obligate air breather, and undergoes short periods of estivation in some areas of its distribution (Johansen and Lenfant, 1967).

The relative contributions of aquatic and aerial gas exchange in three genera of lungfishes in aerated water at 20°C are shown in Fig. 10. *Neoceratodus* achieves nearly 100% of its O_2 uptake from water, while aquatic exchange accounts for only 12% and 6% of O_2 uptake in *Protopterus* and *Lepidosiren* respectively. CO_2 elimination is exclusively aquatic in *Neoceratodus*, whereas in *Lepidosiren* and *Protopterus* air breathing accounts for about 30% of CO_2 elimination.

Air exposure is a naturally occurring event during estivation in *Protopterus* and *Lepidosiren*, and has been a very useful experimental tool in studying the varying respiratory capabilities of the lungfishes to respond to a decline in O_2 uptake ability (Fig. 11). For example, the obligate air breathers, *Protopterus* and *Lepidosiren* respond to brief air exposure with a small but significant increase in systemic arterial O_2 saturation and a minimal reduction in O_2 uptake (Lenfant *et al.*, 1970).

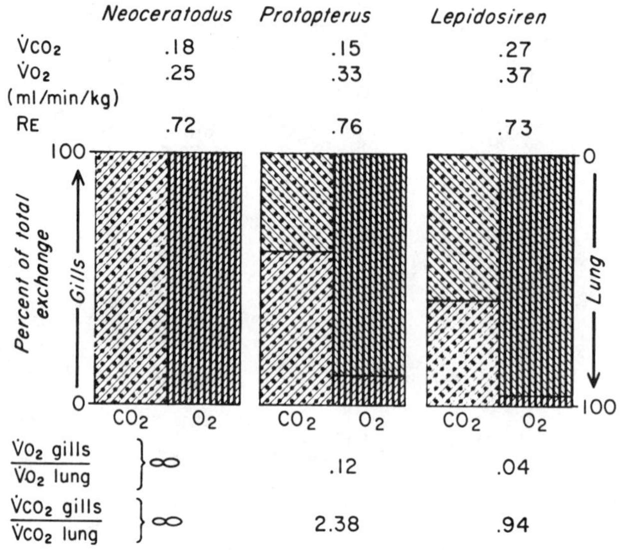

Fig. 10. Relative concentrations of aquatic and aerial breathing to total gas exchange at 20°C in the three species of lungfish. From Lenfant *et al.* (1970).

Neoceratodus, however, is unable to maintain a high systemic arterial O_2 saturation during air exposure, and O_2 uptake falls by 40%.

The Dipnoi are one of the few phyletically ancient gnathostome fishes in which developmental changes in respiration have been studied. The eggs of the lungfishes *Protopterus* and *Lepidosiren* develop in nests laid in water which on occasion may be severely hypoxic. Parental care for the eggs includes a stirring and agitation of the ambient water, and this may be very important for gas exchange of the eggs. The air breathing habit of lungfishes develops soon after hatching, with larvae only 25-30 mm in length having been observed to breathe air (Johnels and Svensson, 1954; Smith, 1931).

O_2 uptake from air and water as a function of development and body mass has been measured in *Protopterus amphibius* (Johansen *et al.*, 1976). The smallest fish studied (3.7 g) had total O_2 uptake from water and air (30°C) of 60 $\mu l\ O_2\ g^{-1}\ h^{-1}$ compared with 30 $\mu l\ g^{-1}\ h^{-1}$ in a 225 g specimen. While total O_2 uptake changed by a factor of two within the mass range studied, the O_2 uptake from the water *via* gills and skin changed 8-fold. Thus, fish in the immediate post-larval and juvenile states depend on aquatic gas exchange for 70% or more of the total O_2 requirement compared to values of 10-15% for adults of 300-500 g. In natural habitats with low water PO_2 the larger specimens would be nearly totally dependent on aerial O_2 uptake. Small juvenile specimens observed in the field in hypoxic water or subjected to hypoxic water in the laboratory always stayed close to the water surface, where the O_2 content is higher. This is a common strategy among both strictly aquatic and air breathing fish in hypoxic water (Burggren, 1982).

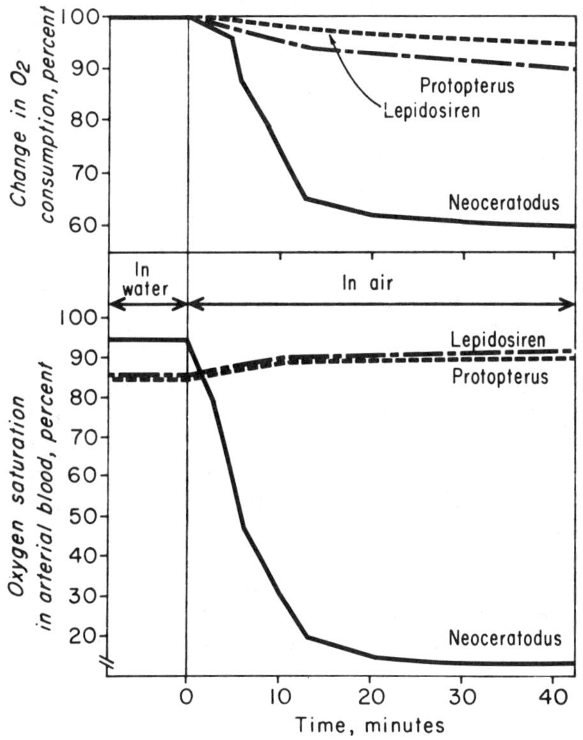

Fig. 11. Arterial O_2 saturation and O_2 uptake during air exposure in the three species of lungfishes. From Johansen *et al.* (1970).

The physiology of estivation in lungfishes has received considerable attention. *Lepidosiren* appears to estivate in wet substrata and does not form a cocoon. *Protopterus* estivates in hardened dry soil at temperatures that can exceed 35-40 °C. This genus becomes encapsulated in a cocoon formed by skin secretions. The cocoon is essential in minimizing desiccation and also offers additional protection against microbial infection from the soil. *Protopterus* in their natural habitat have been reported to estivate for as long as 3.5 years, although an annual estivation cycle is the most common (Johnels and Svensson, 1954). The respiratory physiology of estivation in *Protopterus* was first studied by Dubois (1892), followed by the famous works of Smith (1930, 1931, 1935) on metabolism and excretion. Smith (1930) showed that both chronic fasting of active lungfish in water and estivation induced artificially in the laboratory caused a marked decline in O_2 uptake. In recent years Delaney *et al.* (1974, 1977) and Delaney and Fishman (1977) have quantified various aspects of respiratory physiology in *Protopterus aethiopicus* induced to estivate in the laboratory for periods of 0.5-9.5 months. Oxygen consumption declines sharply at the onset of air exposure. Extensive cardiopulmonary changes, including bradycardia, decreased blood pressure, hyperventilation and respiratory acidosis, were also reported, but their onset was much more gradual than the decline in O_2 uptake.

Remarkably, lungfish entering into estivation in their natural habitat and transferred intact in their cocoon to the laboratory have lived for as long as 7 years (Johansen and Lomholt, unpublished). Respiratory parameters in *Protopterus amphibius* measured both in water and during extremely long periods of estivation are compared in Table II. O_2 uptake falls dramatically in the estivating state, and consequently O_2 extraction from the lung is lower and PO_2 of end expired gas higher than in quiescent fish in water. The end expired PCO_2 in the aquatic *Protopterus* is similar to that of other obligate air breathing fish in water, while in the estivating lungfish it reflects a value typical of vertebrates supporting gas exchange on air breathing alone. The gas exchange ratios for the lung parallel this and emphasize the importance of aquatic gas exchange for CO_2 elimination when the lungfish is in water, compared to sole use of the lung as a gas exchanger during estivation.

After 6 years of estivation there is a 10-fold increase in mass-specific lung volume (Table II), probably related to the inevitable loss of body mass that must occur in the metabolising but non-feeding lungfish undergoing estivation. Unless the lungfish replaced its progressive loss of body mass with an increase in lung volume, the relatively fragile cocoon material surrounding the fish body might fracture and collapse, leading to dehydration and death.

The breathing pattern of estivating lungfish changed from the aquatic pattern, a low frequency of single air breaths with large tidal volume (equal to lung volume), to an estivation pattern of sequences of very small air breaths interrupted by long

Table II. Comparison of respiratory parameters in active and estivating *Protopterus amphibius*.

	Active	Estivating
Temperature (^{o}C)	25-30	22-25
VO_2 ($\mu l\ g^{-1}\ h^{-1}$)	35-40	2-4
V_L (ml kg^{-1})	50-60	500
V_T (ml $kg^{-1}\ h^{-1}$)	100-250	20-70
F (breaths h^{-1})	2-5	10-35
PEO_2 (mm Hg)	40	100
$PECO_2$ (mm Hg)	15	45
R_E (for lung)	0.15	0.19
V_L/VO_2	3-6	10-17
% O_2 Extraction from lung	73	33

breath-hold intervals. This pattern results in an overall reduction in pulmonary ventilation volume during estivation (Table II). The very small tidal volumes may be related to the fact that large and rapid changes in volume of the fish related to breathing could also endanger the physical continuity of the cocoon. The reduced lung ventilation occurring during estivation is a clear consequence of the reduced metabolic rate. Additionally, this reduced ventilation may be very important in minimizing respiratory water loss. Delaney and Fishman (1977), working on *Protopterus aethiopicus* induced to estivate in burlap bags, reported that minute ventilation increased by more than 15 times after 7 months of estivation. Yet, in an earlier study these authors had reported a clear respiratory acidosis during estivation in this species, which seems incompatible with increased lung ventilation. In our judgement such an increase in pulmonary ventilation under natural estivation conditions would lead to a serious respiratory loss of water.

Blood respiratory properties

O_2 binding properties of blood (*e.g.* hemoglobin concentration, O_2-Hb affinity, Bohr factor, heme cooperativity) are major factors influencing both the movement of gases across the respiratory membrane and their transport in the blood. The respiratory properties of the blood of phyletically ancient fishes reflect both phylogenetic and environmental influences.

The hemoglobin of hagfishes and lampreys occurs in a single unit, monomeric configuration, particularly when oxygenated in dilute solutions of neutral pH (see

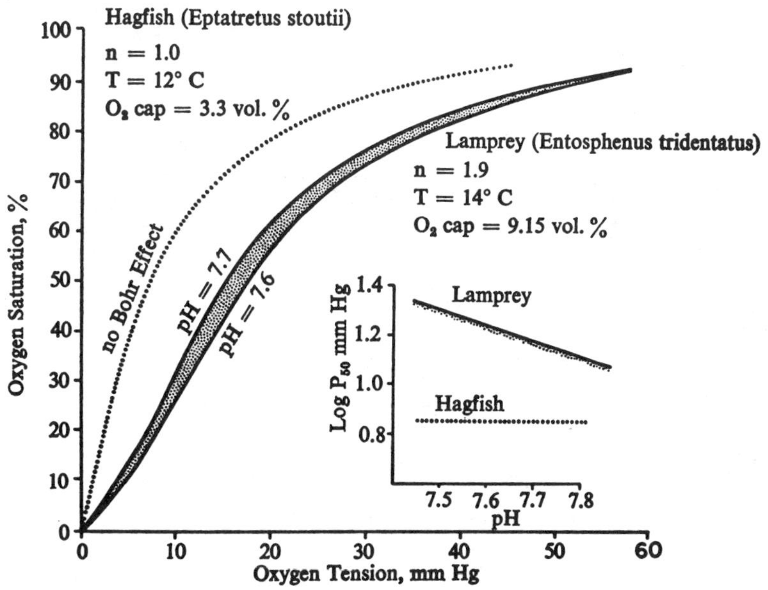

Fig. 12. O_2 dissociation curves and Bohr shifts (inset) of a lamprey and hagfish. From Johansen and Lenfant (1972).

Bannai *et al.*, 1972; Bauer *et al.*, 1975; Macey and Potter, 1982). This contrasts with the tetrameric configuration of all other vertebrate hemoglobins (Perutz, 1969). In the absence of any interaction between heme monomers, the curve describing blood oxygenation as a function of blood PO_2 (the oxygen equilibrium curve) should be hyperbolic and there should be no Bohr factor (effect of hydrogen ion on O_2-Hb binding). Indeed, this is the case for the hagfish *Myxine glutinosa* (Fig. 12). A high O_2-Hb affinity is imparted by the hyperbolic rather than sigmoid equilibrium curve and this will facilitate the uptake of environmental oxygen. This may be particularly appropriate for an animal like the hagfish that may encounter hypoxic conditions, either in its burrows in stagnant muddy bottoms or when gill ventilation is compromised during feeding (Johansen and Lenfant, 1972). Interestingly, the oxygen equilibrium curve of lamprey blood is sigmoidal rather than hyperbolic as predicted for a strictly monomeric hemoglobin (Fig. 12). Although monomeric when oxygenated, the hemoglobin of lampreys tends to aggregate into dimers or tetramers when deoxygenated (Briehl, 1963; Riggs, 1972), imparting a significant Bohr effect and a lower O_2-Hb affinity. These particular characteristics of O_2-Hb interaction, typically absent in monomeric hemoglobins, can enhance oxygen unloading at the tissues compared with monomeric hemoglobins *if* environmental oxygen levels remain comparatively high. The lamprey tends to inhabit more highly-oxygenated waters than does the hagfish, and feeding probably does not introduce a functional reduction in gill ventilation as it does in hagfishes (Johansen *et al.*, 1973).

The natural occurrence of functionally monomeric hemoglobins in the hagfish and lampreys represents the most obvious *functional* hematological difference related to phylogeny in phyletically ancient fishes. All other fishes (indeed, all other vertebrates) have sigmoidal O_2 equilibrium curves as a consequence of typically tetrameric heme-heme interactions. Blood respiratory properties have been quantified for the sturgeon (Burggren and Randall, 1978), the coelacanth (Hughes and Itazawa, 1972; Wood *et al.*, 1972; Weber *et al.*, 1973), the bowfin (Weber *et al.*, 1976; Randall *et al.*, 1981b), the garfish (Smatresk and Cameron, 1982), lungfishes (Johansen *et al.*, 1976; Lenfant *et al.*, 1967), numerous sharks and rays (Hughes and Wood, 1974; Weber *et al.*, 1983), and primitive teleosts such as the osteoglossids (Johansen *et al.*, 1978). The considerable variability in the O_2 binding properties of blood of this diverse range of fishes cannot be fully explained by phylogenetic specialization. Instead, this variability results from the malleability of hemoglobin-O_2 affinity in accordance with the physio-chemical characteristics of the environment in which animals grow, live and evolve (Johansen and Weber, 1976; Wood, 1980).

Amongst phyletically ancient fishes we find several excellent examples of this interdependence of hemoglobin function with environment. For instance, the ammocoete larvae of lampreys occupy benthic habitats more prone to oxygen depletion than those of the adults (see Hardisty, 1979; Macey and Potter, 1982). It has long been recognized that, at constant temperature and pH, the blood of the ammocoete larvae of lampreys has a much higher O_2-Hb affinity than in the adults (Adinolfi *et al.*, 1959; Manwell, 1963; Potter and Nicol, 1968; Bird *et al.*, 1976; Potter and Beamish, 1978; Macey and Potter, 1982) (Fig. 13). The larval hemoglobins are progressively replaced by hemoglobins with intrinsically lower oxygen affinity as development occurs, analogous to the similar fetal-adult shifts that occur in higher vertebrates.

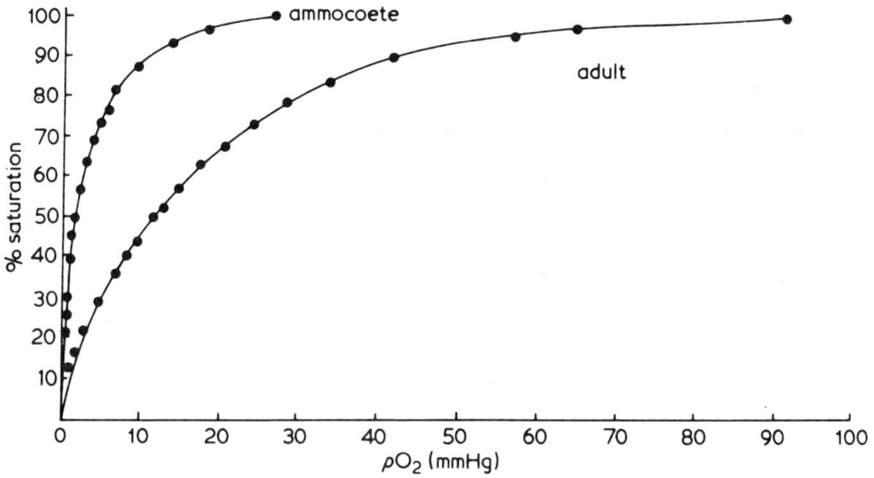

Fig. 13. O_2 dissociation curves for the hemoglobins of ammocoetes and adults of the non-parasitic lamprey, *Lampetra planeri*. From Bird *et al.* (1976).

Changes in the respiratory properties of the blood of phyletically ancient fishes are also associated with the evolution of air breathing which, as stated above, is surprisingly prominent in these fishes. Detailed studies have been made of the family Osteoglossidae, which includes only five living species of limited phyletic diversity. Two Amazonian species, *Osteoglossum bicirrhosum*, exclusively a water breather, and the large *Arapaima gigas*, an obligatory air breathing fish, coinhabit habitats characteristically low in oxygen. In both, the blood has very similar values for hematocrit, O_2 capacity, and erythrocytic concentrations of the nucleotide triphosphates ATP and GTP (potent modulators of O_2-Hb affinity in all fishes) (Johansen *et al.*, 1978). Yet O_2 affinity is strikingly different in the two species (Fig. 14). At a pH of 7.4 at 28-30°C the P_{50} for the blood of the solely water breathing *Osteoglossum* and the air breathing *Arapaima* is 6 and 21 mm Hg, respectively. The Bohr factor is also greater for *Osteoglossum*.

The physiological consequences of these differences are very clear. The O_2 partial pressure of the water in which both osteoglossids live can fall to as low as 15 mm Hg. The exclusively water breathing *Osteoglossum* can maintain its arterial blood near 80% oxygen saturation even at this level of water PO_2, since its O_2-Hb affinity is comparatively high. A high blood-O_2 affinity can be less effective in terms of oxygen unloading at the tissues, but *Osteoglossum* has a comparatively low metabolic rate (Johansen *et al.*, 1978). Contrast this with the obligate air breather, *Arapaima*, whose arterial blood could maximally be about 20% O_2 saturated if forced to breathe water exclusively, since its O_2-Hb affinity is comparatively low. Because *Arapaima* can breathe air, however, it achieves full O_2 saturation of blood leaving the gas bladder. The lower O_2 affinity associated with the obligatory air breathing habit of *Arapaima* offers more efficient O_2 unloading from hemoglobin. This is appropriate for *Arapaima*, which has a resting O_2 uptake twice that of *Osteoglossum*.

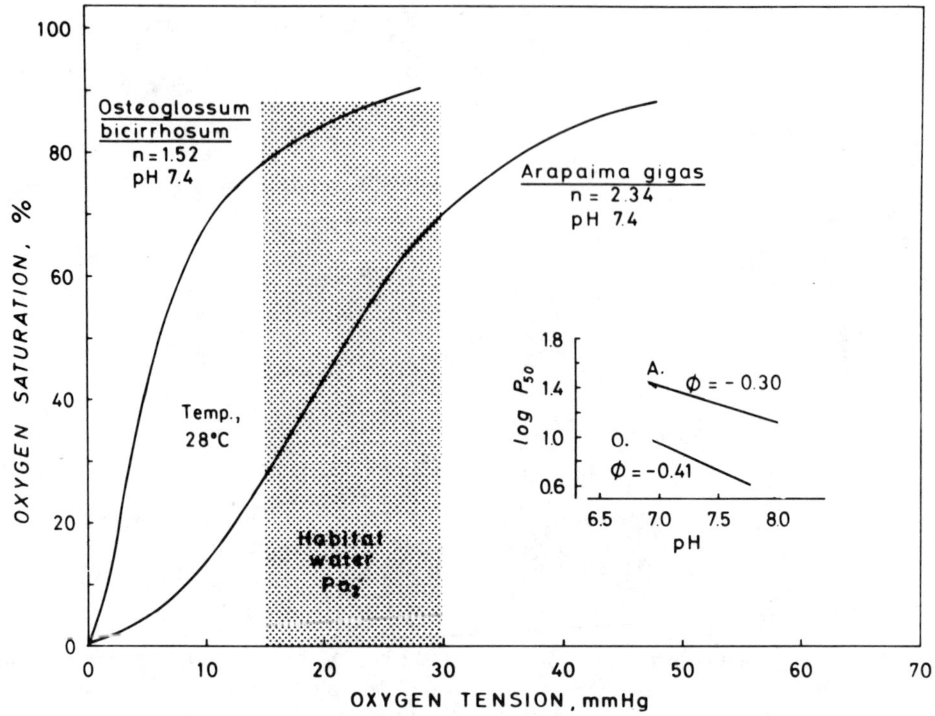

Fig. 14. O_2 dissociation curves and Bohr shifts (inset) of red cell suspensions for *Osteoglossum*, a strictly aquatic fish, and *Arapaima*, an obligative air breather. The rectangular hatched area shows the diurnal range of water PO_2 for these fishes. From Johansen *et al.* (1978).

Three possible explanations could account for these large differences in blood O_2 affinity. First, the hemoglobin molecules themselves could have intrinsically different O_2 binding qualities. Secondly, the intra-erythrocytic cofactors affecting O_2 binding *in vivo* could differ in type or concentration. Finally, the hemoglobins could differ in their binding (and physiological response) to identical concentrations and types of cofactors. The presence of the last two mechanisms has been demonstrated repeatedly in fishes, both phyletically ancient and advanced (Wood and Johansen, 1972; Weber *et al.*, 1975; Johansen and Weber, 1976). However, the very marked differences in blood-O_2 affinity of *Osteoglossum* and *Arapaima* persisted when the hemoglobins were purified and stripped of all intra-erythrocytic co-factors to O_2 binding (Johansen *et al.*, 1978). Hence, the conspicuous differences in the O_2-Hb affinities must reside in different molecular properties of the two hemoglobins, rather than in differing intra-erythrocytic chemical environments. That such profound differences occur in such closely related species of limited phyletic diversity supports the hypothesis of Goodman *et al.* (1975) that changes in a small number of amino acids may result in profound changes in the O_2 binding properties of a respiratory protein.

Interestingly, a low O_2-Hb affinity blood, correlated with the air breathing habit, also appears within the three genera of extant lungfishes. The O_2-Hb affinity of the blood of the more aquatic lungfishes, *Neoceratodus* and *Lepidosiren*, is considerably higher than that of *Protopterus*, the lungfish showing the greatest reliance on air breathing (Lenfant *et al.*, 1967; Swan and Hall, 1966; Johansen and Lenfant, 1967).

Marked changes in hemoglobin-O_2 binding are associated with estivation in lungfishes. Hematocrit, O_2 capacity and blood hemoglobin concentration all increase by about 50%, while P_{50} at pH 7.5 decreases from 33 mm Hg in fish in water to only 9 mm Hg during estivation (Johansen *et al.*, 1976). These changes with estivation were brought about largely by a decrease in intra-erythrocytic concentration of guanosine triphosphate, rather than any change in the hemoglobins themselves. The reasons why such changes accompany estivation are not clear. The lungfish is not necessarily hypoxic during estivation, since the PO_2 of blood and lung gas does not fall during estivation (Table II; Delaney *et al.*, 1974). More physiological information on this most fascinating condition is required.

Circulation in phyletically ancient fishes

Effective gas exchange in either gills, skin or air breathing organ requires equally effective cardiovascular function if gas exchange at the level of the tissues is to be maximized.

The cardiovascular gross morphology of most phyletically ancient fishes - Chondrostei, Chondrichthyes, Holostei, Coelacanthini - is qualitatively similar to the general pattern of more advanced bony fishes. Generally, the single heart, consisting of sinus venosus, atrium and ventricle, ejects blood into a single ventral aorta. This vessel conveys blood in a closed circulation to the capillary bed of the gills, where gas exchange occurs. The dorsal aorta forms from the confluence of the branchial efferent vessels, and carries blood directly on to the systemic vascular bed. Deoxygenated blood draining the tissues returns *via* veins directly to the sinus venosus.

This basic arrangement of the systemic tissues in series with, and downstream from, the gills imposes specific hemodynamic constraints and demands on the circulation, regardless of phylogeny (Randall, 1970, 1984). The gills, for example, represent a variable but large proportion of the total vascular resistance of fishes, and consequently impose a 25-50% reduction in mean pressure of the dorsal aorta compared with the ventral aorta in every gnathostome fish that has been examined. Both branchial and systemic vascular resistances can be neurally and hormonally regulated, and in concert with adjustments in heart rate and stroke volume, fishes exhibit a wide range of cardiovascular performance suitable for rest, exercise or hypoxia.

Though data are rather incomplete (except for elasmobranchs), the cardiovascular physiology of most phyletically ancient fishes thus far appears unremarkable compared with more advanced fishes. However, the hagfishes, lampreys, and the lungfishes (and to a lesser extent, other phyletically ancient fishes that breathe air) represent striking exceptions to this general piscine circulatory pattern.

Hagfishes and Lampreys

The circulation of the hagfish has several apparently primitive features.

The hagfish's branchial heart is considered to be homologous to all other vertebrate hearts, but has the most primitive features. The sinus venosus, atrium and ventricle are all very distinctively set off from one another, somewhat reminiscent of separate chambers along the length of a pulsatile vessel (see Johansen, 1963; Fänge, 1972). The heart of the hagfish has no coronary circulation nor any innervation, unlike the hearts of all gnathostome fishes (Chapman *et al.*, 1963; Jensen, 1965). Arterial blood pressure in hagfishes is generally very low, ranging from 1-5 mm Hg in the resting animal, rising to a maximum of 25 mm Hg during exercise (Johansen, 1960; Chapman *et al.*, 1963; Jensen, 1965).

The vascular anatomy similarly shows many primitive characters (Fig. 15). Whereas the gills, gut and much of the skeletal musculature are drained via a discrete set of venules and veins as in more advanced fishes, some of the head and sub-cutaneous caudal drainage occurs *via* large, open sinuses reminiscent of 'open' invertebrate circulations (Johansen, 1963; Hardisty, 1979). As probable consequences of these large sinus spaces, blood volume in the cyclostomes (lampreys in particular) is larger than most gnathostome fishes (Robertson, 1974), and venous blood pressure is very low.

Return of venous blood to the branchial heart of the hagfish is assisted by two unusual features - accessory hearts and extensive valving to prevent backflow. The hagfish has three sets of accessory hearts; a pair of cardinal hearts pumping venous blood from the head sinus into the anterior cardinal veins, an aneural portal heart pumping blood from the gut and gonads (as well as from the left anterior cardinal vein) into the hepatic veins, and a caudal heart innervated by spinal nerves that pumps blood from the sub-cutaneous sinus into the caudal vein (Fig. 15). The

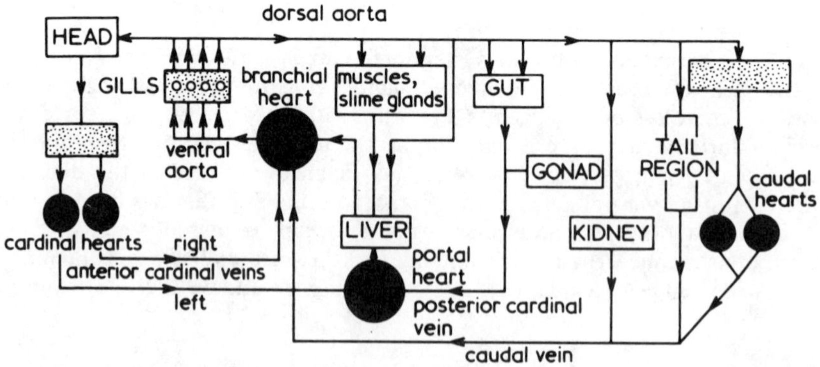

Fig. 15. Diagrammatic representation of the cardiovascular system of a hagfish. Black circles represent contractile structures ("hearts") while sinuses are represented by shaded areas. From Hardisty (1979) based on Jensen (1966).

relative contributions of these accessory hearts to maintenance of blood flow remains enigmatic, particularly since contractions are not synchronized, and all of the hearts, including the branchial heart, show sporadic periods of inactivity (Jensen, 1965). Although the unique structure and pumping action of the caudal heart of the hagfish has long been appreciated (Retzius, 1890) and is frequently described, it is quite small relative to the other accessory hearts or the branchial heart (Jensen, 1965). The caudal heart's contribution to venous return is equivocal in the animal at rest, and may be insignificant during exercise when compared with the combined effects of body movements and extensive valving in the venous circulation (Hardisty, 1979).

The cardiovascular morphology of the lamprey appears intermediate between that of the hagfish and more advanced fishes. The extensive series of accessory hearts typical of *Myxine* are not present in the lampreys, and the single branchial heart is vagally innervated as in gnathostome fishes. Like the hagfish, however, the vascular system is not entirely confined within closed capillary networks. Extensive sinuses are retained primarily in the branchial regions, where respiratory movements also play a significant role in moving blood (Hardisty, 1979).

The Dipnoi (and other air breathers)

The specializations of the lungfish circulation relate primarily to the air breathing habit of these fish. All three extant genera have a highly vascularized lung (homologous to the ammniote lung) supplied with efferent branchial blood derived from the sixth branchial arch (Fig. 16). Importantly, the lungfish has evolved a separate pulmonary vein drain directly into the heart. A peculiar cardiac structure termed the atrioventricular plug (Bugge, 1960) functionally divides the atrium into discrete left and right compartments, which receive pulmonary and systemic venous return, respectively. These features distinguish the lungfish from all other air breathing fish, in which the blood from the air breathing organ drains back into the general systemic venous circulation (see below). Lungfish also possess

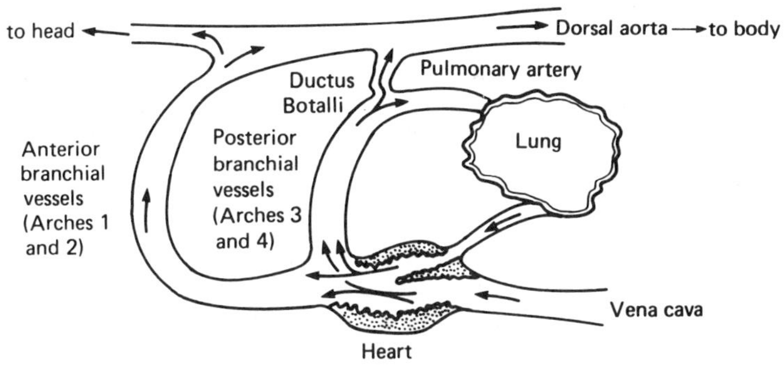

Fig. 16. Highly schematic diagram of the anterior circulation of the lungfish. From Randall *et al.* (1981a) after Johansen *et al.* (1968).

a pair of prominent spiral valves running much of the length of the ventral aorta. These valves functionally divide the proximal region of the ventral aorta into two discrete channels. One channel carries blood to the two anterior-most arches, which are largely devoid of gill filaments and function primarily as shunt vessels to the dorsal aorta. The other channel conveys blood primarily to the two posterior-most gills and to the lung. In part because of the separate entrance into the ventricle of oxygenated and deoxygenated blood, comparatively little admixture occurs in the ventricle and two relatively discrete, parallel blood streams can be ejected simultaneously into the two channels of the ventral aorta. Immediately following an air breath, for example, approximately 90% of the blood entering the dorsal aorta from the two anterior branchial arches is derived from oxygenated blood draining the lung (Johansen *et al.*, 1968). The distribution of cardiac output between the anterior shunt arches, the filament-bearing posterior arches and the lung itself is finely regulated, with pulmonary flow being highest following an air breath and lowest after a period of apnea (see Johansen, 1985 and Fishman *et al.*, 1985 for reviews).

The pulmonary vein and separate right and left atrial compartments of the Dipnoi are highly derived structures, qualitatively distinguishing the lungfish from all other air breathing fish, both 'primitive' and advanced. In all other phyletically ancient air breathing fishes, as well as in almost all teleosts, blood draining the air breathing organ enters into the general systemic venous drainage well before the heart. There is thus no selective pressure for the evolution of mechanisms or structures for the separation of blood flow within the heart or ventral aorta.

In spite of their relative simplicity, the circulations of *Amia*, *Lepisosteus*, *Calamoichthys*, and *Polypterus* are not without interest to the physiologist. These phyletically ancient fishes show many specializations to improve the efficiency of the circulation that, while perhaps not as 'spectacular' as in the Dipnoi, are clearly related to air breathing. Of particular interest is the derivation of the afferent blood supply to the air breathing organ, as well as the potential for redistribution of cardiac output between gills and air breathing organ. In *Amia*, for example, which is probably the best understood of the four above-mentioned genera, both the systemic circulation and swimbladder are in series and downstream from the gills. Unlike many air breathing fishes, the gills of *Amia* show neither a marked reduction in surface area nor differences between anterior and posterior branchial arches (Daxboeck *et al.*, 1981). The afferent blood supply of the air bladder is derived from the efferent artery of the sixth gill arch, placing the air bladder in parallel with the rest of the systemic tissues. Such a vascular arrangement in any vertebrate potentially allows variable distribution of cardiac output between two vascular beds in parallel, provided mechanisms exist to vary their relative impedances (see Johansen and Burggren, 1980).

Studies by Johansen *et al.* (1970) and Randall *et al.* (1981b) suggest that in *Amia* the distribution of cardiac output between air bladder and systemic tissues can, in fact, be regulated. Randall *et al.* (1981b) calculated a cardiac output of 69.1 ml min^{-1} kg^{-1} at 30°C in normoxic water. This is higher than typical for teleosts of similar size and activity level to *Amia*, and they speculate that this results from having the gas exchanger and systemic tissues in parallel and thus 'competing' for cardiac output. They calculated that in normoxia at rest about 35-40% of the cardiac output was distributed to the swimbladder, with the remainder perfusing the systemic tissues. In hypoxic water, cardiac output increased by about 50%, while its distribution changed in favour of the air breathing organ, which received nearly 60% of cardiac output. Hypoxia induces a similar redistribution of cardiac output between systemic tissues and swimbladder in *Lepisosteus* (Smatresk and Cameron, 1982).

Finally, it should be emphasized that several of the cardiovascular specializations mentioned above for *Amia* (*e.g.* specialized blood supply to air breathing organ, control of cardiac output distribution) have evolved independently in a number of advanced air-breathing teleosts, and apparently are associated with air breathing *per se* rather than with ancient ancestry.

Conclusion

Consideration of the morphological features of the phyletically ancient fishes, and the systematic relationships that these features suggest, often gives an impression of "simple", "primitive" or "non-specialized". Yet, our overwhelming impression from reviewing respiration in phyletically ancient fishes is that, physiologically speaking, they are actually complex and sophisticated. Presented with unique physiological problems, the extant phyletically ancient fishes have survived through the evolution of unique physiological solutions. The living phylogenetically ancient fishes hold an evolutionarily venerated position; the apparent extraordinary success of the teleosts has yet to be measured against geologic time.

Literature cited

ADINOLFI, M., G. CHIEFFI, and M. SINISCALCO. 1959. Haemoglobin pattern of the cyclostome, *Petromyzon planeri*, during the course of development. Nature **184**: 1325-1326

BANNAI, S., Y. SUGITA, and Y. YONEYAMA. 1972. Studies on haemoglobin from the hagfish, *Eptatretus burgeri*. J. biol. Chem. **247**: 505-510.

BAUER, C., U. ENGELS, and S. PALEUS. 1975. Oxygen binding to haemoglobins of the primitive vertebrate *Myxine glutinosa*. L. Nature **256**: 66-68.

BEAMISH, F.W.H. 1973. Oxygen consumption of adult *Petromyzon marinus* in relation to body weight and temperature. J. Fish. Res. Bd. Can. **30**: 1367-1370.

BIRD, D., P. LUTZ, and I. POTTER. 1976. Oxygen dissociation curves of the blood of larval and adult lampreys (*Lampetra fluviatilis*). J. exp. Biol. **65**: 449-458.

BISHOP, I.R., and G.E.H. FOXON. 1968. The mechanism of breathing in the South American lungfish *Lepidosiren paradoxa*: radiological study. J. Zool. (Lond.) **154**: 263-272.

BRIEHL, R.W. 1963. The relation between the oxygen equilibrium and aggregation of subunits in lamprey haemoglobin. J. biol. Chem. **238**: 2361-2366.

BUGGE, J. 1960. The heart of the African lungfish, *Protopterus*. Vidensk. Meddr dansk naturh. Foren. **123**: 193-210.

BURGGREN, W.W. 1978. Gill ventilation in the sturgeon, *Acipenser transmontanus*: unusual adaptations for bottom dwelling. Respir. Physiol. **34**: 153-170.

BURGGREN, W.W. 1982. "Air gulping" improves blood oxygen transport during aquatic hypoxia in the goldfish *Carassius auratus*. Physiol. Zool. **55**: 327-334.

BURGGREN, W., J. DUNN, and K. BARNARD. 1979. Branchial circulation and gill morphometrics in the sturgeon *Acipenser transmontanus*, an ancient chondrostean fish. Can. J. Zool. **59**: 2160-2170.

BURGGREN, W.W., and M.S. HASWELL. 1979. Aerial CO_2 excretion in the obligate air breathing fish, *Trichogaster trichopterus*: a role for carbonic anhydrase. J. exp. Biol. **82**: 215-225.

BURGGREN, W.W., and D.J. RANDALL. 1978. Oxygen uptake and transport during hypoxic exposure in the sturgeon, *Acipenser transmontanus*. Resp. Physiol. **34**: 171-183.

BYCZKOWSKA-SMYK, W. 1962. Vascularization and size of the respiratory surface in *Acipenser stellatus*. Respir. Physiol. **34**: 171-183.

CARTER, G.S., and L.C. BEADLE. 1931. The fauna of the swamps of the Paraguayan Chaco in relation to its environment. II. Respiratory adaptations in the fishes. J. Linn. Soc. (Lond.) **37**: 327-366.

CHAPMAN, C.B., D. JENSEN, and K. WILDENTHAL. 1963. On circulatory control mechanisms in the Pacific hagfish. Circ. Res. **12**: 427-440.

CLARIDGE, P.N., and I.C. POTTER. 1975. Oxygen consumption, ventilatory frequency and heart rate of lampreys, *Lampetra fluviatilis*, during their spawning run. J. exp. Biol. **63**: 193-206.

DAXBOECK, C., D.K. BARNARD, and D.J. RANDALL. 1981. Functional morphology of the gills of the bowfin, *Amia calva*, with special reference to their significance during air exposure. Respir. Physiol. **43**: 349-364.

DELANEY, R.G, S. LAHIRI, and A.P. FISHMAN. 1974. Aestivation of the African lungfish, *Protopterus aethiopicus*: cardiovascular and respiratory functions. J. exp. Biol. **61**: 111-128.

DELANEY, R.G., and A.P. FISHMAN. 1977. Analysis of lung ventilation in the aestivating lungfish *Protopterus aethiopicus*. Amer. J. Physiol. **233**: R181-R187.

DELANEY, R.G., S. LAHIRI, R. HAMILTON, and A.P. FISHMAN. 1974. Acid-base balance and plasma composition in the aestivating lungfish, *Protopterus*. Amer. J. Physiol. **232**: R10-R17.

DUBOIS, R. 1892. Du mechanisme respiratoire du Dipnoiques. Annls. Soc. Linn. (Lyon) **36**: 65.

FÄNGE, R. 1972. The circulatory system. pp. 241-259 *In* Hardisty, M.W., and I.C. Potter [eds.] The biology of lampreys, vol. 2. Academic Press, London.

FARRELL, A. and D. RANDALL. 1978. Air-breathing mechanics in two Amazonian teleosts, *Arapaima gigas* and *Hoplerythrinus unitaeniatus*. Can. J. Zool. **56**: 939-945.

FEDER, M.E., and W. BURGGREN. 1985. Cutaneous gas exchange in vertebrates: design, patterns, control and implications. Biol. Rev. (in press).

FISHMAN, A.F., R.G. DELANEY, P. LAURENT, and J.P. SZIDON. 1985. Blood shunting in the lungfish and humans. *In* Johansen, K., and W. Burggren [eds.] Cardiovascular shunts: phylogenetic, ontogenetic and clinical aspects. Munksgaard, Copenhagen (in press).

GOODMAN, M., G.W. MOORE, and G. MATSUDA. 1975. Darwinian evolution in the geneology of haemoglobin. Nature **253**: 603-608.

GREENWOOD, P.H. 1958. Reproduction in the East African lungfish *Protopterus aethiopicus*. Proc. Zool. Soc. (Lond.) **130**: 547-567.

GREENWOOD, P.H., and K.F. LIEM. 1984. Aspiratory respiration in *Arapaima gigas* (Teleostei, Osteoglossomorpha): a reappraisal. J. Zool. (Lond.) **203**: 411-425.

GRIGG, C. 1965. Studies of the Queensland lungfish *Neoceratodus forsteri* (Krefft). I. Anatomy, histology and functioning of the lung. Aust. J. Zool. **13**: 243-253.

HANS, M., and Z. TABENCKA. 1938. Über die Blutgefässe der Haut von *Myxine glutinosa* L. Bull. Acad. Pol. Sci. **11**: 69-77.

HARDISTY, M.W. 1979. The biology of the cyclostomes. Chapman and Hall, London. 428 p.

HEISLER, N. 1984. Acid-base regulation in fishes. pp. 315-400 *In* Hoar, W.S., and D.J. Randall [eds.] Fish physiology, vol. X, part A. Academic Press, London.

HUGHES, G.M. 1984. General anatomy of the gills. pp. 1-72 *In* Hoar, W.S., and D.J. Randall [eds.] Fish physiology, vol. X, part A. Academic Press, London.

HUGHES, G.M., and C. BALLINTIJN. 1965. The muscular basis of the respiratory pumps in the dogfish (*Scyliorhinus canicula*). J. Exp. Biol. **43**: 363-383.

HUGHES, G., and Y. ITAZAWA. 1972. The effect of temperature on the respiratory function of coelacanth blood. Experientia **28**: 1247.

HUGHES, G.M., and M. MORGAN. 1973. The structure of fish gills in relation to their respiratory function. Biol. Rev. **48**: 419-475.

HUGHES, G.M., and S. WOOD. 1974. Respiratory properties of the blood of the thornback ray. Experientia **30**: 167-168.

JARVIK, E. 1980. Basic structure and evolution of vertebrates, vol. 1. Academic Press, London.

JENSEN, D. 1965. The aneural heart of the hagfish. Ann. N.Y. Acad. Sci. **127**: 443-458.

JENSEN, D. 1966. The hagfish. Sci. Amer. **214**: 82-90.

JOHANSEN, K. 1960. Circulation in the hagfish, *Myxine glutinosa* L. Biol. Bull. **118**: 289-295.

JOHANSEN, K. 1963. The cardiovascular system of *Myxine glutinosa* L. *In* Brodal, A., and R. Fänge [eds.] The biology of *Myxine*. Universitetsforlaget, Oslo.

JOHANSEN, K. 1970. Air breathing in fishes. pp. 361-408 *In* Hoar, W.S. and D.J. Randall [eds.] Fish physiology. vol. IV. Academic Press, London.

JOHANSEN, K. 1985. A phylogenetic overview of cardiovascular shunts. *In* Johansen, K., and W. Burggren [eds.] Cardiovascular shunts: phylogenetic, ontogenetic and clinical aspects. Munksgaard, Copenhagen (in press).

JOHANSEN, K., and W. BURGGREN. 1980. Cardiovascular function in lower vertebrates. pp. 61-118 *In* Bourne, G.H. [ed.] Hearts and heart-like organs, vol. 1. Academic Press, London.

JOHANSEN, K., HANSON, D., and C. LENFANT. 1970. Respiration in a primitive air breather, *Amia calva*. Respir. Physiol. **9**: 162-174.

JOHANSEN, K., and C. LENFANT. 1967. Respiratory function in the South American lungfish, *Lepidosiren paradoxa* (Fitz.). J. exp. Biol. **46**: 205-218.

JOHANSEN, K., and C. LENFANT. 1972. A comparative approach to the adaptability of O_2-Hb affinity. Proc. A. Benzon Symp. **4**: 750-780.

JOHANSEN, K., C. LENFANT, and D. HANSON. 1968. Cardiovascular dynamics in the lungfish. Z. vergl. Physiol. **59**: 157-186.

JOHANSEN, K., C. LENFANT, and D. HANSON. 1973. Gas exchange in the lamprey, *Entosphenus tridentata*. Comp. Biochem. Physiol. **44A**: 107-119.

JOHANSEN, K., J.P. LOMHOLT, and G.M.O. MALOIY. 1976. Importance of air and water breathing in relation to size of the African lungfish *Protopterus amphibius* Peters. J. exp. Biol. **65**: 395-399.

JOHANSEN, K., G. LYKKEBOE, R. WEBER, ands G. MALOIY. 1976. Respiratory properties of blood in awake and estivating lungfish, *Protopterus amphibius*. Respir. Physiol. **27**: 335-345.

JOHANSEN, K., C. MANGUM, and R. WEBER. 1978. Reduced blood O_2 affinity associated with air breathing in osteoglossid fishes. Can. J. Zool. **56**: 891-897.

JOHANSEN, K., and R. STRAHAN. 1963. The respiratory system of *Myxine glutinosa*. pp. 352-371 *In* Brodal, A. and R. Fänge [eds.] The biology of *Myxine*. Universitetsforlaget, Oslo.

JOHANSEN, K., and R. WEBER. 1976. On the adaptability of haemoglobin function to environmental conditions. Zool. Persp. exp. Biol. 1.

JOHNELS, A.G., and G.S.O. SVENSSON. 1954. On the biology of *Protopterus annectens*. Arkiv f. Zool. **7**: 131-158.

KOROLEWA, N.W. 1964. Water respiration of lamprey and survival in a moist atmosphere. Isv. vses. nauchno-issled. Inst. ozern. rechn. ryb. Khoz. **58**: 186-190 (in Russian).

LAURENT, P. 1984. Gill internal morphology. pp. 73-184 *In* Hoar, W.S., and D.J. Randall [eds.] Fish physiology, vol. X, part A. Academic Press, London.

LENFANT, C., and K. JOHANSEN. 1968. Respiration in the African lungfish *Protopterus aethiopicus* I. Respiratory properties of blood and normal patterns of breathing and gas exchange. J. exp. Biol. **49**: 437-452.

LENFANT, C., K. JOHANSEN, and G.C. GRIGG. 1967. Respiratory properties of blood and pattern of gas exchange in the lungfish *Neoceratodus forsteri* (Krefft). Respir. Physiol. **2**: 1-12.

LENFANT, C., K. JOHANSEN, and D. HANSON. 1970. Bimodal gas exchange and ventilation-perfusion relationships in lower vertebrates. Fed. Proc. **29**: 1124-1129.

LEWIS, S.V. 1976. Respiration and gill morphology of the paired species of lampreys, *Lampetra fluviatilis* (L.) and *Lampetra planeri* (Bloch). Ph.D. thesis, University of Bath, U.K.

LEWIS, S.V., and I.C. POTTER. 1976. Gill morphometrics of the lampreys, *Lampetra fluviatilis* (L.) and *Lampetra planeri* (Bloch). Acta Zool. (Stockh.) **57**: 103-112.

LIEM, K. 1982. Larvae of air-breathing fishes as countercurrent flow devices in hypoxic environments. Science **211**: 1177-1179.

MACEY, D., and I.C. POTTER. 1982. The effect of temperature on the oxygen dissociation curves of whole blood of larval and adult lampreys (*Geotria australis*). J. exp. Biol. **97**: 253-262.

MAGID, A. 1966. Breathing and function of the spiracles in *Polypterus senegalus*. Anim. Behav. **14**: 530-533.

MANWELL, C. 1963. The blood proteins of cyclostomes. A study in phylogenetic and ontogenetic biochemistry. pp. 372-455 *In* Hardisty, M.W., and I.C. Potter [eds.] The biology of lampreys, vol. 2. Academic Press, London.

McMAHON, B. 1969. A functional analysis of the aquatic and aerial respiratory movements of an African lungfish, *Protopterus aethiopicus*, with references to the evolution of the lung-ventilation mechanism in vertebrates. J. exp. Biol. **51**: 407-430.

McMAHON, B. 1970. The relative efficiency of gaseous exchange across the lungs

and gills of an African lungfish *Protopterus aethiopicus*. J. exp. Biol. **52**: 1-15.
MUNZ, F.W., and R.W. MORRIS. 1965. Metabolic rate of the hagfish *Eptatretus stouti* (Lockington) 1878. Comp. Biochem. Physiol. **16**: 1-5.
NAKAO, T., and K. UCHINOMIYA. 1978. A study on the blood vascular system of the lamprey gill filament. Amer. J. Anat. **151**: 239-264.
NEILL, W.T. 1950. An estivating bowfin. Copeia **1950**: 240.
PERUTZ, M.F. 1969. The haemoglobin molecule. Proc. R. Soc. (Lond.) **173B**: 113-140.
PIIPER, J., and P. SCHEID. 1984. Model analysis of gas transfer in fish gills. pp. 230-262 *In* Hoar, W.S. and D.J. Randall [eds.] Fish physiology, vol. X, part A. Academic Press, London.
POLL, N. 1962. XI. Etude sur la structure adulte et la formation des sacs pulmonaires des Protoptères. Annls Mus. r. Afr. cent. Sér. 8vo. **103**: 131-171.
POTTER, I.C., and F.W.H. BEAMISH. 1978. Changes in haematocrit and haemoglobin concentrations during the life cycle of the anadromous sea lamprey, *Petromyzon marinus* L. Comp. Biochem. Physiol. **60A**: 431-434.
POTTER, I.C., and P.I. NICOL. 1968. Electrophoretic studies on the haemoglobin of Australian lampreys. Aust. J. exp. Biol. Med. Sci. **46**: 639-641.
PURSER, L.G. 1926. *Calamoichthys calabaricus* J.A. Smith. Part I. The alimentary and respiratory system. Trans. R. Soc. (Edinb.) **54**: 767- 784.
RAHN, H., K. RAHN, B.J. HOWELL, C. GANS, and S.M. TENNEY. 1971. Air breathing of the garfish, *Lepisosteus osseus*. Respir. Physiol. **11**: 285-307.
RANDALL, D.J. 1970. The circulatory system. pp. 133-172 *In* Hoar, W.S., and D.J. Randall [eds.] Fish physiology, vol. IV. Academic Press, London.
RANDALL, D.J. 1972. Respiration. pp. 287-306 *In* Hardisty, M.W., and I.C. Potter [eds.] The biology of lampreys, vol. 2. Academic Press, London.
RANDALL, D.J. 1984. Oxygen and carbon dioxide transfer across fish gills. pp. 263-314 *In* Hoar, W.S., and D.J. Randall [eds.] Fish physiology, vol. X, part A. Academic Press, London.
RANDALL, D.J., W.W. BURGGREN, A.P. FARRELL, and M.S. HASWELL. 1981a. The evolution of air breathing in vertebrates. Cambridge University Press, Cambridge, U.K.
RANDALL, D.J., J.N. CAMERON, C. DAXBOECK, and N. SMATRESK. 1981b. Aspects of bimodal gas exchange in the bowfin, *Amia calva* L. (Actinopterygii: Amigormes). Respir. Physiol. **43**: 339-348.
RETZIUS, G. 1890. Ueber Zellenteilung bei *Myxine glutinosa*. Biol. Foren. Stockh. Forhandl. **11**: 50-90.
RIGGS, A. 1972. The haemoglobins. pp. 261-286 *In* Hardisty, M.W., and I.C. Potter [eds.] The biology of lampreys, vol. 2. Academic Press, London.
ROBERTSON, J.D. 1974. Osmotic and ionic regulation in cyclostomes. pp. 149-193 *In* Florkin, M, and B.T. Scheer [eds.] Chemical zoology, vol. 8. Academic Press, London.
ROVAINEN, C.M., and M.H. SCHIEBER. 1975. Ventilation of larval lampreys. J. comp. Physiol. **104**: 185-203.
SACCA, R., and W.W. BURGGREN. 1982. Oxygen uptake in air and water in the air-breathing reedfish, *Calamoichthys calabaricus*: role of skin, gills and lungs. J. exp. Biol. **97**: 179-186.
SCHEID, P., and J. PIIPER. 1976. Quantitative functional analysis of branchial gas transfer: theory and application to *Scyliorhinus stellaris* (Elasmobranchii). pp. 17-38 *In* Hughes, G.M. [ed.] Respiration of amphibious vertebrates. Academic Press, London.

SHELTON, G. 1970. The regulation of breathing. pp. 293-359 *In* Hoar, W.S. and D.J. Randall [eds.] Fish Physiology. vol. 4. Academic Press, N.Y.

SMATRESK, N., and J. CAMERON. 1982. Respiration and acid-base physiology of the spotted gar, a bimodal breather. I. Normal values and the response to severe hypoxia. J. exp. Biol. **96**: 263-280.

SMITH, H.W. 1930. Metabolism of the lungfish. J. biol. Chem. **88**: 97-130.

SMITH, H.W. 1931. Observations on the African lungfish *Protopterus aethiopicus*, and on evolution from water to land environments. Ecology **12**: 164-181.

SMITH, H.W. 1935. The metabolism of the lungfish. J. cell. comp. Physiol. **6**: 43-67.

STEFFENSEN, J.F., JOHANSEN, K., C.D. SINDBERG, J.H. SORENSEN, and J.L. MOOLER. 1984. Ventilation and oxygen comsumption in the hagfish, *Myxine glutinosa* L. J. exp. mar. Biol. Ecol. **84**: 173-178.

STRAHAN, R. 1958. The velum and respiratory current of *Myxine*. Acta Zool. (Stockh.) **16**: 227-240.

SWAN, H., and F.G. HALL. 1966. Oxygen-hemoglobin dissociation in *Protopterus aethiopicus*. Amer. J. Physiol. **210**: 487-489.

TAPPAN, H. 1974. Molecular oxygen and evolution. pp. 81-135 *In* Hayaishi, O. [ed.] Molecular oxygen in biology. North Holland/Elsevier, Amsterdam.

WEBER, R., J. BOL, K. JOHANSEN, and S. WOOD. 1973. Physiochemical properties of coelacanth hemoglobin. Arch. Biochem. Biophys. **154**: 96-105.

WEBER, R., G. LYKKEBOE, and K. JOHANSEN. 1975. Biochemical aspects of the adaptation of hemoglobin-oxygen affinity of eels to hypoxia. Life Sci. **17**: 1345-1350.

WEBER, R., R. WELLS, and J. ROSSETTI. 1983. Allosteric interactions governing oxygen equilibria in the haemoglobin system of the spiny dogfish, *Squalus acanthias*. J. exp. Biol. **103**: 109-120.

WEBER, R., B. SULLIVAN, J. BONAVENTURA, and C. BONAVENTURA. 1976. The hemoglobin system of the primitive fish, *Amia calva*: isolation and functional characterization of the individual hemoglobin components. Biochim. Biophys. Acta **434**: 18-30.

WHITING, H.P., and Q. BONE. 1980. Ciliary cells in the epidermis of the larval Australian dipnoan, *Neoceratodus*. J. Linn. Soc. Lond. Zool. **68**: 125-137.

WOOD, S. 1980. Adaptation of red cell function to hypoxia and temperature in ectothermic vertebrates. Amer. Zool. **20**: 163-172.

WOOD, S., and K. JOHANSEN. 1972. Adaptation to hypoxia by increased HbO_2 affinity and decreased red cell ATP concentration. Nature **237**: 278-279.

WOOD, S., K. JOHANSEN, and R. WEBER. 1972. Haemoglobin of the coelacanth. Nature **239**: 283-285.

YOUSON, J.H., and P.A. FREEMAN. 1976. Morphology of the gills of larval and parasitic adult sea lampreys, *Petromyzon marinus*. J. Morphol. **149**: 73-104.

REGULATION OF BLOOD AND BODY FLUIDS IN PRIMITIVE FISH GROUPS

Ragnar Fänge

Department of Zoophysiology
PB 25059
S-40031 Göteborg, Sweden

Introduction

Primitive is a controversial concept in ichthyology as in other branches of zoology. What is 'advanced' as opposed to 'primitive' is not always clear. Teleosts are considered more advanced than non-teleostean fishes. But among the latter, the dipnoans (lungfishes), the coelacanth (*Latimeria*) and the brachiopterygians (bichirs: *Polypterus, Erpetoichthys*) show relationships to the tetrapods, *i.e.* the higher vertebrates, and certain sharks have a remarkably large brain volume, a feature usually regarded as 'advanced' (Bauchot *et al.*, 1976).

The myxinoids (hagfishes) and petromyzonids (lampreys) undoubtedly are primitive, but some biologists put these agnathan groups at the side of, not within, the systematic category of fishes. The non-teleostean fishes, if, for practical reasons, they are considered as primitive, comprise an extremely heterogenous group. This survey will discuss aspects of body fluids in non-teleostean fishes, but it is necessary to include the teleosts, which have been investigated more than the non-teleosts.

The regulation of blood and body fluids in fishes has been treated in excellent ways by several authors (Robertson, 1957; Holmes and Donaldson, 1969; Love, 1980).

Body fluid compartments

The body fluids are blood, lymph, interstitial fluid and transepithelial fluids (cerebrospinal, peritoneal and pericardial fluids, endolymph of the inner ear *etc.*; bile and other secreted fluids may be included). The transepithelial fluids are formed by filtration or by transport (secretion) through epithelial layers.

Cerebrospinal fluid and endolymph resemble filtrates of the blood in composition, but endolymph often has a high potassium concentration (Fänge *et al.*, 1972).

The total body water makes up roughly 70% of the body weight (or volume) of fishes and other vertebrates. Rather higher values are found for cyclostomes than for fishes generally. Thorson (1961) reported 75.6% for a lamprey (*Petromyzon*), and 70.8% for a marine teleost.

The extracellular volume may be defined as the sucrose space, and the plasma volume as the T 1824 (Evans blue) space. The interstitial fluid volume is the sucrose space minus the plasma volume, and blood volume is plasma volume plus the blood cell volume (determined by hematocrit). The values obtained for these volumes depend much on the methods used (Holmes and Donaldson, 1969).

Cyclostomes have high blood volumes (8.5-16.9%), which can be correlated with the presence of large blood sinuses. High blood volumes also characterize chondrichthyans (sharks, rays, chimaeroids), which also possess blood sinuses. Relatively small blood volumes are recorded for chondrosteans (sturgeons), a holostean (*Lepisosteus*) and many teleosts. However, Laurs *et al.* (1978) determined blood volumes of between 8.2 and 19.7% in the albacore (*Thunnus thunnus*), a fast-swimming teleost fish. Obviously all teleosts do not have a small blood volume. The blood volume may depend more on eco-physiological factors than on the evolutionary position (Table 1).

Mechanisms for keeping blood volume constant in the living fish are not well understood. Hormones may be important. In mammals, mechanical stretch of granulated cardiac cells cause release of a peptidic blood volume regulatory hormone

Table I. Volumes of extracellular fluid compartments in fish groups in percent of body weight/volume (from Thorson, 1961; Holmes and Donaldson, 1969; Laurs *et al.*, 1978).

Fish Group	Extracellular fluid	Plasma volume	Blood volume
Cyclostomes			
Lamprey	23.9	5.5	8.5
Hagfish	25.9	13.8	18.7
Elasmobranch	21.2	5.4	6.6
Holocephalan	---	5.2	5.2
Chondrostean	18.4	2.5	3.4
Holostean	16.0	2.1	3.6
Teleosts			
Several	15.4	1.9	2.9
Albacore	---	---	8.2-19.7

(Lang *et al.*, 1985). Jensen (1963) reported the presence of a cardioactive substance, eptatretin, in the heart of the hagfish, *Eptatretus*.

Lymph

Vessels and spaces containing lymph are found in fishes of different groups (Kampmeier, 1969). Tiny lymph-filled vessels occur at the surface of the heart and the intestine of myxinoids (Fänge, 1973), but the caudal heart and the caudal sinus of the same animals contain blood, not lymph (Johansen *et al.*, 1962). Elasmobranchs have very thin veins which may function in part like lymph vessels.

Teleosts have a highly developed lymph vascular system, but according to Vogel and Claviez (1981) this system consists of secondary blood vessels instead of lymph vessels comparable to those of mammals, and their content is formed by a plasma skimming process rather than filtration. Many teleosts possess a lymph-filled spinal or supraneural duct which collects lymph from the skeletal muscles. Opercular movements are supposed to act in pumping fluid from the rigid spinal duct into the venous system. Extensive lymph-filled spaces occur in the connective tissue of the orbit, for example in the pike (*Esox*) and the cod (*Gadus*). These structures may facilitate movements of the eye ball. The eel (*Anguilla*) and a few other teleosts possess lymph hearts in the tail. The skeletal muscles are richly supplied with lymph. In the plaice (*Pleuronectes platessa*) the muscles contain about 70 times more lymph than blood (Wardle, 1971). The blood capillaries of fishes have a high permeability, and the protein concentration of the lymph is only slightly lower than in the blood (Hargens *et al.*, 1974).

Inorganic composition of body fluids

Vertebrate blood plasma, irrespective of the habitat, contains sodium, potassium and chloride in about the same proportions as in seawater, and similar proportions are used in Ringer solutions. However, the total ionic concentration in the plasma is only 1/4-1/3 of that in seawater except in the myxinoids (hagfishes), which are iso-osmotic with seawater. It is not necessary to go into details about osmoregulation in fishes, because several surveys have been published on this matter, but it may be of interest to discuss certain relationships of ion and water balance.

Calcium

The calcium concentration in fish blood plasma varies around 2-7 mM, but may be much higher in females during reproduction. Myxinoids, holocephalans and elasmobranchs have slightly higher values than the rest of the fishes, and the lowest values are found in dipnoans and chondrosteans (Urist *et al.*, 1972). The skeleton serves as a calcium reserve in terrestrial vertebrates, and calcium exchange between the blood and the skeleton is controlled by hormones. No marked differences seem to be found in the blood calcium between fish groups with and those without a calcified skeleton. Fishes lack parathyroid glands and hormone but have calcitonin and vitamin D_3. Calcium-regulating hormones may have other functions in fishes than in higher vertebrates (Björnsson, 1985).

Renal regulation of sodium, chloride and water

Several organs influence the salt and water balance in fishes. The skin, the digestive system, the rectal gland of elasmobranchs, holocephalans and *Latimeria*, and the kidney, contain ion-transporting epithelial cells. The great importance of the kidney for maintenance of constant composition of the body fluids was described in masterly detail by Homer W. Smith in "From Fish to Philosopher" (1953).

Glomerulus. The glomerulus is a device, unique to vertebrates, which is particularly efficient in the elimination of water. The sizes and the total filtering area of the glomeruli in an animal are correlated with the habitat of that animal. Freshwater fishes and freshwater-inhabiting amphibians such as urodeles (salamanders), almost without exception, possess prominent glomeruli with a large total filtering area. On the other hand, certain marine teleosts lack functioning glomeruli or have small or degenerate ones (*Lophius, Opsanus*, syngnathids, Antarctic icefish), and some desert frogs possess degenerate glomeruli (Dawson, 1951).

However, myxinoids (hagfishes) and marine elasmobranchs (sharks, rays), although living in the ocean, possess remarkably large glomeruli. *Myxine* has a total filtration area of its glomeruli larger than that of most marine teleosts, and approaching that of freshwater teleosts (Nash, 1931). Myxinoids and elasmobranchs, although by different mechanisms, are both iso-osmotic or slightly hyperosmotic to seawater and thus have few problems in obtaining water from the environment. Like freshwater vertebrates they might need a well functioning water excretory system.

Tubular reabsorption of salt. Production of hypotonic urine is a common feature in fishes. It depends upon tubular reabsorption of sodium and chloride. This capacity of the renal tubules to reabsorb inorganic ions from the urine is immensely important in fishes living in freshwater and amphibians, and in terrestrial vertebrates obtaining inorganic ions from food and water poor in salt.

It is a paradox that marine teleosts, surrounded by water rich in salt, absorb ions from the urine resulting in urine low in salt. Tubular resorption of sodium and chloride also has been observed in chondrosteans (sturgeons) in the Caspian sea (Natochin *et al.*, 1985), and in marine elasmobranchs (Hickman and Trump, 1969). The coelacanth, *Latimeria*, resorbs more chloride than sodium from the urine (Griffith *et al.*, 1976; Griffith and Pang, 1979), and myxinoids (hagfishes) show a weak but measurable resorption of sodium from the urine (McInerney, 1974).

The tubular resorption of sodium and chloride in the kidneys of marine fishes may be a legacy from ion-saving mechanisms of early freshwater vertebrates. When, during phylogenesis, they invaded salt water, the tubular salt resorption became unnecessary or even unfavourable. The hagfishes, during their long adaptation to marine life, seem to have diminished salt reabsorption to a minimum by anatomical reduction of the renal tubular system. The kidney of *Myxine* lacks tubules almost completely (Fänge and Krog, 1963). However, hagfishes are not completely restricted to high salinity environments. The Pacific hagfish, *Eptatretus stouti*, is able to adapt to salinities down to 24-25 ^{o}/oo in laboratory experiments, and seems to tolerate slightly diluted seawater in its natural environment (McFarland and Munz, 1958; McInerney and Evans, 1970). Their capacity for cellular volume regulation (Cholette *et al.*, 1970) indicates that they possess some, although strictly limited, ability to survive changes of osmolarity.

Nephrostomes and peritoneal funnels - vestigial water excretory system? Ciliated canals which drain the coelom are important in water balance of invertebrates such as annelids. Somewhat similar structures occur in the renal excretory system of certain water-inhabiting vertebrates, especially in the larvae.

During embryogenesis, three generations of vertebrate kidneys develop: pro-, meso- and metanephros, all considered as parts of a more or less segmentally-arranged holonephros. The pronephros is often absent or vestigial, but it functions as a well-developed organ during a short period of the embryonic development in petromyzonids (lampreys), dipnoans (lungfishes) and many teleosts. The pronephros reaches its highest development in the tadpole larvae of amphibians, notably urodeles (salamanders). If the pronephros is damaged, salamander larvae become edematous. Apparently the pronephros functions as a water-eliminating structure (Swingle, 1919; Fox, 1963; Christensen, 1964).

In adult salamanders the pronephros has disappeared, but ciliated funnels of the mesonephros carry peritoneal fluid into the nephrons. In adult anurans (frogs) the ciliated funnels lose the connection with the nephrons and join the renal venous system early in embryonic development. Especially in desert frogs, this seems to have a water-conserving effect. Fluid is transported back into the circulatory system (Dawson, 1951). Morris (1981), using scanning electron microscopy, counted 600-800 ciliated openings at the surface of each kidney of the toad, *Bufo marinus*.

In myxinoids (hagfishes), probably also in ammocoete larvae of lampreys, pronephric ciliated tubules or nephrostomes transport material from the peritoneal cavity into lymphoid cell masses associated with the venous system (Fänge, 1973), and in certain adult elasmobranchs (*Squalus, Squatina*), ciliated funnels transport fluid and particles from the peritoneal cavity into lymphoid cell masses at the surface of the kidney (Schneider, 1897). Transport of antigenic material from the peritoneal cavity into the lymphoid structures may be of immunologic importance.

Whatever functions ciliated kidney-associated canals have in adult animals, it seems plausible that the original function might have been that of a water excretory system. In the water excretory system of early vertebrates the whole body cavity, with vascular tufts (glomus) in its wall, might have functionally resembled the renal malpighian corpuscles with their glomeruli. According to Stensiö (1927), extinct cephalaspidomorph paleozic agnathans probably had a pronephros of considerable size. One can speculate whether this hypothetical adult pronephros of primitive jawless vertebrates functioned in water balance, or if it had transformed into lymphohemopoietic structures like the anterior part of the kidney of many fishes living now.

Urea retention

Chondrichthyans (elasmobranchs: sharks, rays; holocephalans: chimaeroids), the coelacanth (*Latimeria*), the aestivating African lungfish (*Protopterus*) and the crab-eating frog (*Rana cancrivora*) protect themselves against osmotic loss of water by retention of urea and other nitrogenous compounds (trimethylamine oxide). Water regulation by urea was necessary for the evolution of viviparity and ovoviviparity in elasmobranchs. The early larvae of sharks and rays lack the capacity of osmoregulation and must spend their early embryonic development in a urea-containing medium inside the female body, or enclosed within an egg capsule (Price and Daiber, 1967).

The use of urea in osmoregulation probably evolved independently in different vertebrate groups (Griffith and Pang, 1979).

Water balance and early vertebrate habitats

Smith (1953) proposed the hypothesis that ancestral vertebrates, early in their evolution, lived in freshwater and developed renal glomeruli because efficient water excretion was needed. Romer (1955) concluded from paleontological evidence that paleozoic vertebrates lived mainly in freshwater and he supported the ideas of a freshwater origin. Robertson (1957) suggested as an alternative hypothesis that glomeruli evolved during marine life, and this may have preadapted early vertebrates for later invasion of freshwater. Paleontological data provide few clear answers to these problems. Lancelet-like chordates have been found in the Middle Cambrian (*Pikaya* in Burgess shale; Morris and Whittington, 1979), and fragments of the calcified armor of heterostracan agnathans occur together with remains of marine invertebrates in late Cambrian and Ordovician layers (Repetsky, 1978). This indicates that vertebrates lived in the sea very early during their phylogenesis, but fossils from later paleozoic periods (Silurian, Devonian) indicate that ancestors of fishes lived in both marine, brackish and freshwater environments.

Lutz (1975) concluded from the composition of the body fluids of different groups that, while the myxinoids (hagfishes) probably never left the sea, other groups of fishes may have invaded freshwater very early. The ancestors of brachiopterygians (bichirs) and dipnoans (lungfishes) never left freshwater, but other groups moved to the sea, and some returned to freshwater. Lutz presented a logical diagram of the habitat changes during evolution of the fishes.

It might be assumed that, at their very first beginning, vertebrates evolved from marine chordates related to the lancelet (amphioxus) and the ascidians, but further evolution occurred in fresh or brackish water. The highly variable physical and chemical conditions in river mouths and shallow lagoons stimulated differentiation into new forms (mutants) more than the relatively constant oceanic environment. Several features in the structure and function of the kidney and in the mode of osmoregulation of marine fishes are best understood as results of previous adaptation to freshwater. If this hypothesis is correct, which of course is impossible to prove, the ancestors of myxinoids developed large glomeruli, a functioning pronephros, and perhaps an ion- reabsorbing system of renal tubules during life in freshwater. When the animals moved to the sea the now unnecessary tubular ion resorption was diminished by reduction of the tubules, and the pronephric duct degenerated and was replaced by a lymphoid structure. The "proto-myxinoids" neither developed hypo-osmotic, nor ureo-osmotic regulatory mechanisms, but adapted to seawater in a lazy way by being ionic conformers, as are all marine invertebrates. Only the bivalent ions, *i.e.* magnesium, calcium and sulfate, are controlled by the hagfish kidney and liver cells.

Proteins of body fluids

Mammalian plasma has a colloid osmotic pressure of about 25 mm Hg. Albumin contributes to more than half of the osmotic pressure of the proteins.

In many fishes albumins are lacking in the plasma and colloid osmotic pressure is low (5-10 mm Hg; Yoffey and Courtice, 1970; Hargens *et al.*, 1974). The plasma albumin fraction is missing in elasmobranchs and some teleosts (Sulya *et al.*, 1961), but fractions of globulins are always present.

Iron-transporting proteins, transferrins, occur in all fishes. Transferrins from holocephalans and elasmobranchs are immunologically alike indicating that these fish groups are phylogenetically related to each other (Burch *et al.*, 1984). Few comparative studies of plasma proteins of fishes have been published. With modern techniques of protein separation such studies may be fruitful.

Blood Cells

Erythrocytes

Fish erythrocytes typically are oval and nucleated. In petromyzonids (lampreys) they are biconcave with a circular outline, rather small and remarkably similar to mammalian red cells (Potter *et al.*, 1982).

Myxinoids (hagfishes), chondrichthyans (sharks, rays, chimaeroids) and dipnoans (lungfishes) possess large or very large erythrocytes, while teleosts have relatively small ones. A few deep sea teleosts have small anucleate erythrocytes (*Maurolicus*: Wingstrand, 1956). The hemoglobin of teleost erythrocytes is often in a semicrystalline state (Thomas, 1971).

Cell size and nuclear DNA. The size of the erythrocytes and other cells is correlated to the genome size, *i.e.* the amount of nuclear DNA (Olmo and Morescalchi, 1978). The amount of nuclear DNA increases with the complexity of the organism (Schmidke *et al.*, 1979) and by multiplication of chromosomes or gene sequences. Mutations during early phases of vertebrate evolution seem to have caused extensive gene multiplications (Ohno, 1970). Multiplication of gene material in elasmobranchs, dipnoans, and urodeles (salamanders) among the amphibians have resulted in the formation of remarkably large cells (Table II; Fig. 1).

In the teleosts, regarded as 'advanced' or specialized, phylogenesis was accompanied by economizing with the genetic material, in that repetitive DNA-

Table II. Sizes of blood cells (length or diameter in μm) and amounts of nuclear DNA (pg/N) in fishes of various groups. From Fange and Lundblad, 1985; Hinegardner, 1976; Ohno, 1970; Millot *et al.*, 1978).

Fish	Erythrocytes	Granulocytes	DNA
Cyclostomes			
Petromyzon	11	--	2.8
Eptaretus	18	14-15	5.6
Elasmobranchs			
Torpedo	30-33	19-25	--
and others			
Squalus	21	15	14.6
Holocephalans			
Hydrolagus	--	--	*3.1*
Chimaera	18	17	--
Coelacanth			
Latimeria	15	--	7.2
Dipnoans			
Protopterus	40	44	160-284
Chondrosteans			
Acipenser	18	14	--
Holostean			
Amia	--	--	2.4
Teleosts			
several	10-15	--	0.8-6.6

sequences were eliminated. As a consequence teleost cells are relatively small, with amounts of DNA down to about 1 pg per nucleus (Hinegardner and Rosen, 1972). Erythrocytes of dipnoans (lungfishes), and urodeles (salamanders) among the amphibians, due to duplications of the genetic material, may contain up to 200 pg DNA per nucleus.

The erythrocyte dimensions have physiological significance. Due to a large surface area to volume ratio, small erythrocytes allow faster oxygenation and ion exchange than large ones (Holland and Forster, 1966). The smallest nuclear DNA values of teleosts are comparable with those of the amphioxus (*Branchiostoma*), 1.2 pg/N (Ohno, 1970).

Immature red cells with persisting cytoplasmic organelles such as mitochondria are common in the peripheral blood of fishes, especially myxinoids and elasmobranchs (Zapata and Carrato, 1981).

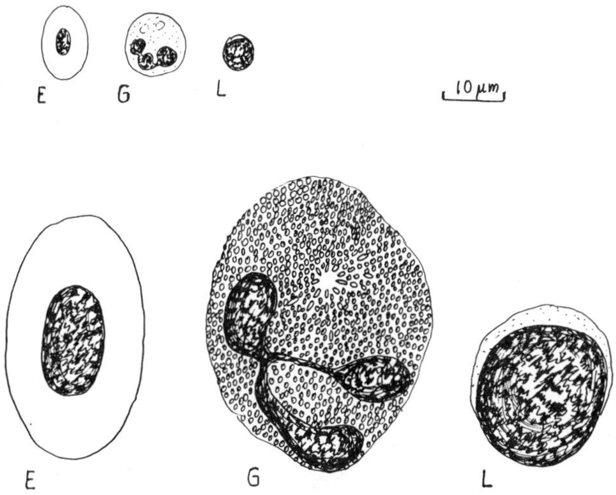

Fig. 1. Erythrocyte (*E*), granulocyte (*G*) and lymphocyte (*L*) from a teleost, *Gadus* (upper row), and a dipnoan, *Protopterus* (lower row). The granulocyte of the cod (*Gadus*) has indistinct granules, that of the lungfish (*Protopterus*) has large, eosinophilic granules. Camera lucida drawings at same scale of May-Grünwald-Giemsa stained blood smears (From Fänge and Lundblad, 1985).

Leucocytes

The leucocyte/erythrocyte ratio in the blood is larger for fish than for higher vertebrates (Table III). However, leucocytes probably exert their functions in the tissues rather than in the blood. In mammals, 60 times more granulocytes and up to 400 times more lymphocytes are found in the tissues than in the blood (Antonioli, 1961). The lymphocytes form the basis of the immune system. B and T lymphocytes probably occur in fishes as in higher vertebrates (McCumber *et al.*, 1982).

The classification of fish granulocytes is in a confused state, as the routine differential staining methods used on mammalian blood do not work well on fish material (Ellis, 1977). Myxinoids (hagfishes) have only one category of granulocytes which show some similarities to mammalian nutrophils (Mattisson and Fänge, 1977). Granulocytes with large eosinophilic cytoplasmic granules are found in elasmobranchs, holocephalans and dipnoans (Fänge, 1984; Fänge and Lundblad, 1985), and in the coelacanth, *Latimeria* (Millot *et al.*, 1978; Fig. 1, lower part).

The teleost granulated white cells are small and insignificant looking, with indistinct granules (Fig. 1, upper part). Eosinophils are found in some species, not in others.

Table III. Leucocytes/erythrocytes ratio in fishes compared with that of man (based on values from Grodzinski, 1938).

Group	Ratio
Cyclostomes (hagfish)	0.06
Elasmobranchs (sharks)	0.02-0.25
Teleosts (bony fishes)	0.01-0.1
Chondrostean (sturgeon)	0.1
Man	0.001

Hemoglobin, organic phosphates and carbonic anhydrase of erythrocytes.

The properties and the concentration of erythrocytic hemoglobin in fish blood vary with ecological conditions and phylogenetic positions. Grigg (1974) concluded that it is difficult to draw phylogenetic relationships, other than that the blood of cyclostomes and elasmobranchs have lower oxygen capacities than the blood of teleosts.

In contrast to other vertebrate hemoglobins, which are tetrameric, that of cyclostomes is monomeric and the molecule has an extra tail of nine amino acids. The hemoglobin molecules of myxinoids and petromyzonids differ from each other by 88 amino acids, and both differ from hemoglobin of shark, carp or man by more than 100 amino acids. This indicates that the hagfish and the lamprey are a little more related to each other than they are to other vertebrates (Hardisty, 1979; Liljeqvist, 1985). Hagfishes and lampreys probably have evolved along separate pathways for hundreds of millions of years.

The oxygen binding capacity depends both on the structure of the respiratory pigment molecule itself and on the modulatory action of organic phosphates present within the erythrocytes. Lamprey erythrocytes, like mammalian erythrocytes, contain 2,3-diphosphoglycerate, while hagfish erythrocytes contain high concentrations of ATP. The red cells of the elasmobranch, *Squalus*, the chondrostean, *Acipenser*, and the holostean, *Amia*, contain 2,3-diphosphoglycerate and ATP. In teleosts, the oxygen transporting properties of erythrocytic hemoglobin are modulated by ATP, guanosine triphosphate and inositol hexaphosphate (Bartlett, 1982a,b).

The enzyme carbonic anhydrase occurs together with hemoglobin inside erythrocytes. Red cell carbonic anhydrase from hagfishes and lampreys, like the same enzyme in most vertebrates, has a molecular weight of about 20,000 (Carlsson *et al.*, 1980; Berglund *et al.*, 1980). *Myxine* carbonic anhydrase binds Zn less firmly than that of other vertebrates. Perhaps as a consequence of this, the Zn content of the plasma of the hagfish is much higher (40 µmol/ml) than in other vertebrates (Maren and Friedland, 1978).

Osmotic properties of the blood cells.

Erythrocytes hemolyse in diluted salt solutions. Ezell *et al.* (1969) reported that the erythrocytes of the holostean, *Lepisosteus*, were markedly resistant to hypotonic media. Personal observations (Fänge, 1983 unpublished) show that the erythrocytes of two marine teleosts (*Labrus beggylta*; *Gadus morhua*) hemolyse in 0.05-0.08 M NaCl solutions, those of the hagfish (*Myxine glutinosa*) in 0.07-0.1 M NaCl solutions, and the red cells from an elasmobranch (*Somniosus microcephalus*) in 0.13-0.21 M NaCl solutions. The cells were incubated at 18° C for 6 hours in the test solutions.

Green and Hoffman (1953) determined concentrations of NaCl solutions which were isotonic for teleost red cells (0.1-0.26 M) and elasmobranch red cells (0.33-0.35 M NaCl).

Fugelli (1967) showed that taurine and other amino acids play a volume regulatory role in osmotically stressed fish red cells (teleost: *Platichthys flesus*). Intracellular amino acids are important in osmotic volume regulation in red cells of elasmobranchs (*Squalus*: Bedford, 1983; *Raja*: Goldstein and Boyd, 1978).

The data are still too few to reveal whether there are any correlations between osmotic properties of fish red blood cells and phylogenetic position.

Lymphohemopoietic tissues

Instead of bone marrow and lymph nodes, fishes possess other types of lymphohemopoietic tissues (Fänge, 1984). New blood cells originate within these tissues and to some extent in the circulating blood.

Hemopoiesis relies on multipotent stem cells, supposedly lymphocyte-like, which are transported by the blood. Stem cells from the blood settle at different sites in the organism and start to proliferate, forming lymphohemopoietic tissues or organs. Probably under the influence of microenvironmental factors (carbon dioxide, oxygen, pH, hormones), they transform into blast cells which divide and differentiate into mature blood cells: erythrocytes, lymphocytes, granulocytes and so on.

Lymphohemopoietic tissues, such as the epigonal and Leydig organs of elasmobranch fishes, are characterized by a continuous flux of cells. They may be considered as aggregations of dividing blood cells, cell cultures, rather than well defined organs. However, because the dividing blood cells have a predilection for certain sites in the organism, the lymphohemopoietic tissues may appear as structurally rather well defined organs. The localization of the sites for lymphohemopoietic activity probably is phylogenetically anchored.

Table IV. Distribution of lymphohemopoietic tissues in various groups of fishes (based on Fänge, 1982,1984; Millot *et al.*, 1978; and other sources). See text re: renal tissue.

Fish group	Thymus	Spleen	Intestine	Oesophagus	Meninges/ neural arch	Skeleton
Cyclostomes						
Lamprey[a]	0	0	(+)	0	+	0
Hagfish	0	0	+	0	0	0
Holocephalans	+	+	(+)	0	0	+
Elasmobranchs	+	+	(+)	+/0	(+)	0
Coelacanth	+	+	(+)	0	0	0
Dipnoans	+	+	+	0	0	0
Brachiopterygians	+	+	(+)	0	+	0
Chondrosteans	+	+	(+)	0	+	0
Holosteans	+	+	(+)	0	+	0
Teleosts	+	+	(+)	(+)/0	0	0

+ = present; (+) = present in small amounts, or diffusely distributed; 0 = not present. Details of the table may need future revision. The distribution of lymphohemopoietic tissues is insufficiently known in non-teleostean fishes.

[a] During metamorphosis of the lamprey larvae the major sites of hemopoiesis change from the kidney and the intestinal typhlosole to the supraneural organ (fat column).

The intestinal submucosa, the pronephros and the peripheral blood are the main sites for production of new blood cells in myxinoids (hagfishes). In petromyzonids (lampreys) the main locus for hemopoiesis moves from the intestine (typhlosole, spiral valve) to the supraneural organ. Neither myxinoids nor petromyzonids have a thymus, but this probably exists in all other fishes (Table IV).

In the elasmobranchs (sharks, rays) erythropoiesis takes place in the spleen and in the peripheral blood, while leucocytes differentiate mainly in the submucosa of the oesophagus (Leydig organ) or in the gonadal mesenteries (epigonal organ). The meninges of the brain and the anterior spinal cord are an important site of leucocytopoiesis in chondrosteans (sturgeons) and holosteans (bowfin, gars), and probably to some extent also in brachiopterygians (bichirs) and certain elasmobranchs. In chondrosteans and holosteans the heavily leucocyte-infiltrated meninges form a distinct 'meningeal' or 'epimyelencephalic organ' (Grodzinski, 1938; Waldschmidt, 1887; Fänge, 1984). According to Bjerring (1984) certain depressions or canals in the cranium of extinct Devonian fishes indicate that those had a well-developed 'epimyelencephalic organ'. The microscopic structure of the meningeal lymphohemopoietic tissues is strikingly similar to that of tetrapod hemopoietic bone marrow (Fig. 2).

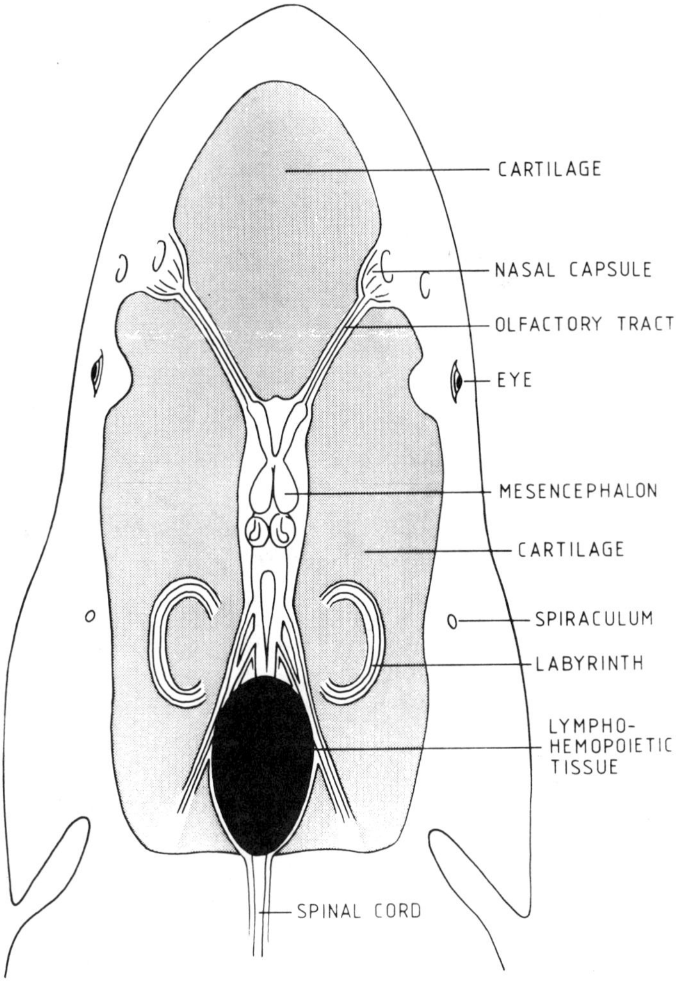

Fig. 2. Meningeal lymphohemopoietic tissue in the head of a sturgeon (*Acipenser*). (From Fänge and Lundblad, 1985).

In holocephalans (chimaeroids) bone marrow-like tissue is situated in cavities of the cartilage skeleton in a way somewhat resembling that of the bone marrow of tetrapods (Fänge, 1984; Fig. 3). In many fishes such as chondrosteans (sturgeons), holosteans (bowfin, gars), brachiopterygians (bichirs), dipnoans (lungfishes) and teleosts the anterior part of the kidney is important in hemopoiesis, especially erythropoiesis. The central mass of the pronephros in myxinoids is a lymph node-like structure. Table IV shows the main sites of lymphohemopoietic tissues (or activities) in different fish groups.

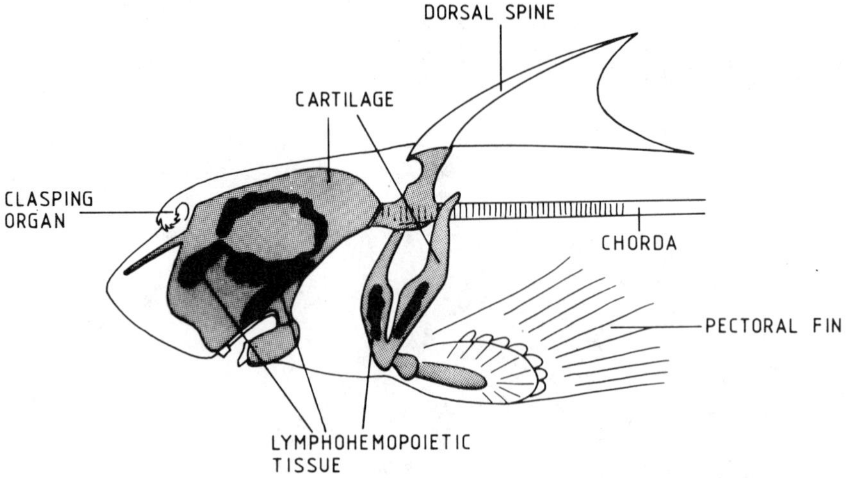

Fig. 3. Bone marrow-like lymphohemopoietic tissue in the cartilage skeleton of chimaeroid fish (*Hydrolagus, Chimaera*; diagram). (From Fänge and Lundblad, 1985).

The lymphohemopoietic tissues usually contain large numbers of lymphocytes and may serve functions similar to those of mammalian lymph nodes. Plasma cells, regarded as the main source of immunoglobulins, occur in lymphomyeloid tissues of most groups of fishes (Zapata *et al.*, 1984).

Defence systems

Cyclostomes have a weak antibody production, but elasmobranchs and teleosts are good producers of immunoglobulins.

Information is largely lacking on immune responses in non-teleost fish groups except elasmobranchs and cyclostomes. Probably chondrosteans and dipnoans *etc.* have well functioning immune systems.

The habitat may influence the degree of development of the immune apparatus. Among chondrosteans (sturgeons), the paddlefish (*Polyodon*) possesses extensive lymphoid tissues in its digestive tract, while another chondrostean, *Scaphirhynchus*, has weakly developed lymphoid tissue. It was noted that the paddlefish suffers from numerous parasites, which apparently activate the lymphoid system (Weisel, 1979).

Certain sturgeons and sharks, which grow to large size, during their long life may be exposed to repeated infections by disease-producing agents. As a consequence these fishes might develop especially efficient immune systems. Sturgeons and sharks possess voluminous highly-differentiated lymphohemopoietic tissues (Fänge, 1984).

Fish immunoglobulins are analogous to mammalian IgM. Elasmobranch immunoglobulins are pentameric or dimeric, those of teleosts tetrameric (Warr and Marchalonis, 1982; Warr, 1983).

Holocephalans (chimaeroids) possess immunoglobulin-like components in their plasma (*Chimaera*: Fänge and Sundell, 1969). The plasma of another chimaeroid fish, *Callorhynchus*, contains a pentameric natural immunoglobulin. This has hemagglutinating activity and shows a mannose/galactose ratio similar to that of elasmobranch immunoglobulins (Sánchez *et al.*, 1980). This emphasizes that holocephalans are phylogenetically related to elasmobranchs.

The nurse shark, *Ginglymostoma cirratum*, has a remarkably well developed epigonal organ (Fänge and Mattisson, 1981). In the adults, about 50% of the plasma proteins are stated to be immunoglobulins. The nurse shark has a complement system in its plasma. The elasmobranch complement system functions in a similar way to that of higher vertebrates, but the complement of cyclostomes participates in reactions or pathways which are more primitive than the 'classical' pathway (Day *et al.*, 1970; Fujii and Murakawa, 1981).

Phagocytosis

Phagocytic systems exist in all vertebrates. In myxinoids (hagfish) remarkably active macrophages patrol the peritoneal cavity, especially the surface of the gonad. The peritoneal macrophages of *Myxine* show both monocytic and granulocytic features. They ingest yeast cells and other foreign material which is injected into the peritoneal cavity (Fänge and Gidholm, 1968). Peritoneal macrophages also occur in elasmobranchs, teleosts and other fishes. In the holostean gar, *Lepisosteus*, macrophages and monocytes are capable of phagocytosis but blood granulocytes seem incapable of this (McKinney *et al.*, 1977; McCumber *et al.*, 1982).

In hagfish (*Myxine*), granulocytes of the blood are less efficient phagocytes than monocytes and macrophages (Mattisson and Fänge, 1977).

Various protective substances

As a part of the defense against parasites and microbes, body fluids and cells contain various compounds with non-specific defense activities. The leucocytes contain hydrolytic enzymes, among them lysozyme, chitinase and several others (Fänge and Lundblad, 1985).

Iron-transporting proteins, transferrins, may protect against infections by depriving the body fluids of iron ions necessary for the growth of microbes.

Leucocytic peroxidase is known to act in a halide-H_2O_2-dependent bacteria-killing system. Peroxidase occurs at high activity in the granulocytes of teleosts and in part of the neutrophils (heterophils) of elasmobranch blood (Fey, 1966; Grimaldi *et al.*, 1983). Mammalian eosinophils are supposed to form a defense system against parasites. It is not known whether eosinophils of fishes contain substances active against parasites.

Some conclusions

The blood volume and the concentration of erythrocytic hemoglobin depend more upon eco-physiological conditions than upon phylogenetic relationships.

Certain structural and functional features of the kidney of marine fishes, including myxinoids (hagfishes), indicate that ancestors of these fishes lived in freshwater. Different groups of marine fishes have adapted in different ways to salt water surroundings.

Variations in size of fish blood cells are correlated with the size of the genome.

The localization of hemopoietic tissues probably has some phylogenetic significance.

All fishes show immune responses, but the production of immunoglobulins is weak in petromyzonids and myxinoids. Fishes belonging to different groups may have evolved different non-specific defense systems, such as the production of compounds which protect against microbes and parasites.

Acknowledgements

I want to thank Professor Sergej Doroshov (University of California, Davis) and Dr. Ron Foreman (Bamfield Marine Station, British Columbia) for material of *Acipenser transmontanus* and *Hydrolagus colliei* used in comparative studies of hemopoietic structures. Permission to publish figures 1,2 and 3 was kindly provided by Bioscience Ediprint Inc., Geneva (Mrs. R.C. Sudan).

Literature cited

ANTONIOLI, J.A. 1961. Metabolism of the white blood cell inside and outside the blood stream. pp. 92-102 *In* Biological activity of the leucocyte. Ciba Foundation study group 10, Churchill, London.

BARTLETT, G.R. 1982a. Phosphate compounds in red cells of two dogfish sharks: *Squalus acanthias* and *Mustelus canis*. Comp. Biochem. Physiol. **73A**: 135-140.

BARTLETT, G.R. 1982b. Phosphates in red cells of a hagfish and a lamprey. Comp. Biochem. Physiol. **73A**: 141-145.

BAUCHOT, R., R. PLATEL, and J.-M. RIDET. 1976. Brain-body weight relationships in Selachii. Copeia **1976**: 305-310.

BEDFORD, J.J. 1983. The effect of reduced salinity on tissue and plasma composition of the dogfish, *Squalus acanthias*. Comp. Biochem. Physiol. **76A**: 81-84.

BERGLUND, L., U. CARLSSON, and B. KJELLSTRÖM. 1980. Cyclostome carbonic anhydrase: purification and some properties of the enzyme from erythrocytes of lamprey. Acta Chem. Scand. Short Comm. B 1517.

BJERRING, H.C. 1984. The term 'fossa bridgei' and five endocranial fossae in teleostome fishes. Zool. Scripta **13**: 231-238.

BJÖRNSSON, B.T. 1985. Calcium balance in teleost fish: views on endocrine control. Ph.D. thesis, University of Göteborg, Sweden.

BURCH, S.J., R. LAWSON, and D.H. DAVIES. 1984. The relationship of cartilaginous fishes: an immunological study of serum transferrins of holocephalans and elasmobranchs. J. Zool. (Lond.) **203**: 303-317.

CARLSSON, U., B. KJELLSTRÖM, and B. ANTONSSON. 1980. Purification and properties of cyclostome carbonic anhydrase from erythrocytes of hagfish. Biochem. Biophys. Acta **612**: 160-170.

CHOLETTE, C., A. GAGNON, and P. GERMAIN. 1970. Isosmotic adaptation in *Myxine glutinosa* L. - I. Variations of some parameters and role of the amino acid pool of the muscle cells. Comp. Biochem. Physiol. **33**: 333-346.

CHRISTENSEN, A.K. 1964. The structure of the functional pronephros in larvae of *Ambystoma opacum* as studied by light and electron microscopy. Amer. J. Anat. **115**: 257-258.

DAWSON, A.B. 1951. Functional and degenerate or rudimentary glomeruli in the kidney of the Australian frog *Cyclorana* (*Chiroleptes*) *platycephalus* and *alboguttatus*. Anat. Rec. **109**: 417-424.

DAY, N.K.B., H. GEWURZ, R. JOHANNSEN, J. FINSTAD, and R.A. GOOD. 1970. Complement and complement-like activity in lower vertebrates and invertebrates. J. exp. Med. **132**: 941.

ELLIS, A.E. 1977. The leucocytes of fish: a review. J. Fish Biol. **11**: 453-491.

EZELL, G.H., L.L. SULYA, and C.L. DODGEN. 1969. The osmotic fragility of some fish erythrocytes in hypotonic saline. Comp. Biochem. Physiol. **28**: 409-415.

FÄNGE, R. 1973. The lymphatic system of *Myxine*. Acta Reg. Soc. Sci. Litt. Gothoburg. Zool. **8**: 57.

FÄNGE, R. 1982. A comparative study of lymphomyeloid tissue in fish. Developm. comp. Immunol. Suppl. **2**: 23.

FÄNGE, R. 1984. Lymphomyeloid tissues in fish. Vidensk. Meddr dansk naturh. Foren. **145**: 143-162.

FÄNGE, R., and L. GIDHOLM. 1968. A macrophage system in *Myxine glutinosa* L. Naturwiss. **55**: 44.

FÄNGE, R., and J. KROG. 1963. Inability of the kidney of the hagfish to secrete phenol red. Nature **199**: 713.

FÄNGE, R., and G. LUNDBLAD. 1985. Leucocytes, lymphohemopoietic tissues and lysosomal enzymes in fishes. *In* Comparative aspects on Inflammation. Bioscience Ediprint Inc., Geneva (in press).

FÄNGE, R., Å. LARSSON, and U. LIDMAN. 1972. Fluids and jellies of the acusticolateralis system in relation to body fluids in *Coryphaenoides rupestris* and other fishes. Mar. Biol. **17**: 180-185.

FÄNGE, R., and A. MATTISSON. 1981. The lymphomyeloid (hemopoietic) system of the Atlantic nurse shark, *Ginglymostoma cirratum*. Biol. Bull. **160**: 240-249.

FÄNGE, R., and G. SUNDELL. 1969. Lymphomyeloid tissues, blood cells and plasma proteins in *Chimaera monstrosa* (Pisces, Holocephali). Acta Zool. (Stockh.) **50**: 155-168.

FEY, F. 1966. Vergleichende Hämozytologie niederer Vertebraten. III. Granulozyten. Folia Haematologica **86**: 1.

FOX, H. 1963. The amphibian pronephros. Quart. Rev. Biol. **38**: 1-25.

FUGELLI, K. 1967. Regulation of cell volume in flounder (*Pleuronectes flesus*) erythrocytes accompanying a decrease in plasma osmolarity. Comp. Biochem. Physiol. **22**: 253-260.

FUGELLI, K. 1976. Regulation of taurine, gamma-aminobutyric acid, and inorganic ions between cell volume, plasma and erythrocytes in flounder (*Platichthys flesus*) at different plasma osmolarities. Comp. Biochem. Physiol. **55A**: 173-177.

FUJII, T., and S. MURAKAWA. 1981. Immunity in lamprey. III. Occurrence of the complement-like activity. Developm. comp. Immunol. **5**: 251.

GOLDSTEIN, L., and T.A. BOYD. 1978. Regulation of ß-alanine transport in skate (*Raja erinacea*) erythrocytes. Comp. Biochem. Physiol. **60**: 319.

GREEN, J.W., and J.F. HOFFMAN. 1953. A study of isotonic solutions for the erythrocytes of some marine teleosts and elasmobranchs. Biol. Bull. **105**: 289-295.

GRIFFITH, R.W., and P.K.T. PANG. 1979. Mechanisms of osmoregulation in the coelacanth: evolutionary implications. Occ. Papers Calif. Acad. Sci. (San Francisco) **134**: 79-93.

GRIFFITH, R.W., B.L. UMMINGER, B.F. GRANT, P.K.T. PANG, L. GOLDSTEIN, and G.E. PICKFORD. 1976. Composition of bladder urine of the coelacanth, *Latimeria chalumnae* Smith. J. exp. Zool. **196**: 371.

GRIGG, G.C. 1974. Respiratory function of blood in fishes. *In* Hardisty, M.W., and I.C. Potter [eds.] The biology of lampreys, vol. 2. Academic Press, New York.

GRIMALDI, M.C., S. D'IPPOLITO, A. PICA, and F. DELLA CORTE. 1983. Cytochemical identification of the leukocytes of torpedoes (*Torpedo marmorata* and *Torpedo ocellata* Rafinesque). Bas. Appl. Histochem. **27**: 311-317.

GRODZINSKI, Z. 1938. Echte Fische, Blut und blutbildende Organe. *In* Bronns H.G. [ed.] Klassen und Ordnungen des Tierreichs, Bd. 6, Abt. 1, 2. Buch, Teil 2, Lief. 1.

HARGENS, A.R., R.W. MILLARD, and K. JOHANSEN. 1974. High capillary permeability in fishes. Comp. Biochem. Physiol. **48A**: 675-680.

HARDISTY, M.W. 1979. Biology of cyclostomes. Chapman and Hall, London.

HICKMAN, C.P. Jr. and B.F. TRUMP. 1969. The kidney. pp. 91-239 *In* Hoar, W.S., and D.J. Randall [eds.] Fish physiology, vol. 1. Academic Press, New York.

HINEGARDNER, R. 1976. The cellular DNA content of sharks, rays and some other fishes. Comp. Biochem. Physiol. **55B**: 367.

HINEGARDNER, R. and D.E. ROSEN. 1972. Cellular DNA content and the evolution of teleostean fishes. Amer. Nat. **106**: 621-644.

HOLLAND, R.A.B. and R.E. FORSTER. 1966. The effect of size of red cells on the kinetics of their oxygen uptake. J. gen. Physiol. **49**: 727-742.

HOLMES, W.N. and E.M. DONALDSON. 1969. The body compartments and the distribution of electrolytes. pp. 1-89 *In* Hoar, W.S., and D.J. Randall [eds.] Fish physiology, vol. 1. Academic Press, New York.

JENSEN, D. 1963. Eptatretin: a potent cardioactive agent from the branchial heart of the Pacific hagfish, *Eptatretus stouti*. Comp. Biochem. Physiol. **10**: 129-152.

JOHANSEN, K., R. FÄNGE, and M.W. JOHANNESSEN. 1962. Relations between blood, sinus fluid and lymph in *Myxine glutinosa* L. Comp. Biochem. Physiol. **7**: 23-28.

KAMPMEIER, O.F. 1969. Evolution and comparative morphology of the lymphatic system. C.C. Thomas, Springfield, Ill.

LANG, R.E., H. THÖLKEN, D. GANTEN, F.C. LUFT, H. FUSKOAHO, and T. UNGER. 1985. Atrial natriuretic factor - a circulating hormone stimulated by volume loading. Nature **314**: 264-266.

LAURS, R.M., R. ULEVITCH, and D.C. MORRISON. 1978. Estimates of blood volume in the albacore tuna. pp. 135-139 *In* Sharp, G.D., and A.E. Dizon [eds.] The physiological ecology of tunas. Academic Press, New York.

LILJEQVIST, G. 1985. Die Hämoglobine von *Myxine glutinosa* L. (Cyclostomata). Primärstruktur des monomeren Hämoglobins III und Untersuchung von Funktion und Evolution. Ph.D. thesis, Stockholm University, Sweden.

LOVE, R.M. 1980. The chemical biology of fishes, vol. 2. Academic Press, New York. 943 p.

LUTZ, P.L. 1975. Adaptive and evolutionary aspects of the ionic content of fishes. Copeia **1975**: 369.

MAREN, T.H., and B.R. FRIEDLAND. 1978. Further studies on the phylogeny of vertebrate carbonic anhydrase in red cells and secretory organs. Bull. Mount Desert Island Biol. Lab. **18**: 79.

MATTISSON, A.G.M., and R. FÄNGE. 1977. Light- and electronmicroscopic observations on the blood cells of the Atlantic hagfish, *Myxine glutinosa* (L.). Acta Zool. (Stockh.) **58**: 205.

McCUMBER, L.J., M.M. SIGEL, R.J. TRAUGER, and M.A. CUCHENS. 1982. Reticuloendothelial system structure and function of the fishes. *In* Cohen, N- and M.M. Sigel [eds.] The reticuloendothelial system, vol. 3: Phylogeny and ontogeny. Plenum Press, New York.

McFARLAND, W.N. and F.W. MUNZ. 1958. A re-examination of the osmotic properties of the Pacific hagfish, *Polistotrema stouti*. Biol. Bull. **114**: 348.

McINERNEY, J.E. 1974. Renal reabsorption in the hagfish, *Eptatretus stouti*. Comp. Biochem. Physiol. **49A**: 273.

McINERNEY, J.E. and D.O. EVANS. 1970. Habitat characteristics of the Pacific hagfish, *Polistotrema stouti*. J. Fish. Res. Bd. Can. **27**: 966.

McKINNEY, E.C., S.B. SMITH, H.B. GAINES, and M.M. SIGEL. 1977. Phagocytosis by fish cells. J. Reticuloendothel. Soc. **21**: 89.

MILLOT, J., J. ANTHONY, and D. ROBINEAU. 1978. Anatomie de *Latimeria chalumnae*. III. Éditions de Centre National de Rech. Scient., Paris.

MORRIS, J.L. 1981. Structure and function of ciliated peritoneal funnels in the toad kidney (*Bufo marinus*). Cell Tissue Res. **217**: 599.

MORRIS, S.C., and H.B. WHITTINGTON. 1979. The animals of the Burgess shale. Scient. Amer. **241**: 110.

NASH, J. 1931. The number and size of glomeruli in the kidneys of fishes, with observations on the morphology of the renal tubules of fishes. Amer. J. Anat. **47**: 445.

NATOCHIN, Y.V., V.I. LUKIANENKO, V.I. KIRSANOV, E.A., E.A. LAVROVA, G.F. MATELLOV, and E.I. SHAKMATOVA. 1985. Features of osmotic and ionic regulations in Russian sturgeon (*Acipenser guldenstadti* Brandt). Comp. Biochem. Physiol. **80A**: 297.

OHNO, S. 1970. Evolution by gene duplication. Springer Verlag, Berlin.

OLMO, E., and A. MORESCALCHI. 1978. Genome and cell sizes in frogs: a comparison with salamanders. Experientia **34**: 44.

POTTER, I.C., L.R. PERCY, D.L. BARBER, and D.J. MACEY. 1982. The morphology, development and physiology of blood cells. pp. 233-292 *In* Hardisty, M.W., and I.C. Potter [eds.] The biology of lampreys, vol. 4A. Academic press, New York.

PRICE, K.S., and F.C. DAIBER. 1967. Osmotic environments during development of dogfish *Mustelus canis* (Mitchell) and *Squalus acanthias*, and some comparisons with skates and rays. Physiol. Zool. **40**: 248.

REPETSKY, J.E. 1978. A fish from the Upper Cambrian of North America. Science **200**: 529.

ROBERTSON, J.D. 1957. The habitat of early vertebrates. Biol. Rev. **32**: 156.

ROBERTSON, J.D. 1974. Osmotic and ionic regulation in cyclostomes. *In* Florkin, M. and B.T. Scheer [eds.] Chemical zoology, vol. VIII. Academic press, New York.

ROMER, A.S. 1955. Fish origins - fresh or salt water? Papers in Mar. Biol. and Oceanogr. 261. Pergamon Press, London.

SÁNCHEZ, G.A., M.K. GAJARDO, and A.E. DE IOANNES. 1980. IgM-like natural hemagglutinin from ratfish serum: isolation and physico-chemical characterization. (*Callorhynchus callorhynchus*) 1. Developm. comp. Immunol. **4**: 667.

SCHMIDKE, J., E. SCHMITT, M. LEIPOLDT, and W. ENGEL. 1979. Amount of repeated and non-repeated DNA in the genomes of closely related fish with varying genome sizes. Comp. Biochem. Physiol. **64B**: 117.

SCHNEIDER, G. 1897. Ueber die Niere und ihre Abdominalporen von *Squatina angelus*. Anat. Anz. **13**: 393.

SMITH, H.W. 1953. From fish to philosopher. Little, Brown and Co., Boston.

STENSIÖ, E.A. 1927. The Downtonian and Devonian vertebrates in Spitsbergen. No. 12, Part 1. Family Cephalaspidae. A. Det Norske Videnskaps-Akademi i Oslo. Skrifter om Svalbard of Dordishavet. pp. 1-391.

SULYA, L.L., B.E. BOX and G. GUNTER. 1961. Plasma proteins in the blood of fishes from the Gulf of Mexico. Amer. J. Physiol. **200**: 152-154.

SWINGLE, W.W. 1919. On the experimental production of edema by nephrectomy. J. gen. Physiol. **1**: 508-514.

THOMAS, N.W. 1971. The form of haemoglobin in the erythrocytes of the cod, *Gadus callarias*. J. Cell Sci. **8**: 407-412.

THORSON, T.B. 1961. The partitioning of body water in Osteichthyes; phylogenetic and ecological implications in aquatic vertebrates. Biol. Bull. **20**: 238-254.

URIST, M.R., S. UYENO, E. KING, M. OKADA, and S. APPLEGATE. 1972. Calcium and phosphorus in the skeleton and blood of the lungfish *Lepidosiren paradoxa*, with comment on humoral factors in calcium homeostasis in the Osteichthyes. Comp. Biochem. Physiol. **42A**: 393-408.

VOGEL, W.O.P. 1981. Struktur und Organisationprinzip im Gefässsystem der Knochenfische. Gegenbaurs morph. Jb. **127**: 772-784.

VOGEL, W.O.P. and M. CLAVIEZ. 1981. Vascular specialization in fish, but no evidence for lymphatics. Z. Naturforsch. **36C**: 490.

WALDSCHMIDT, J. 1887. Beitrag zur Anatomie des Zentralnervensystems und des Geruchsorgan von *Polypterus bichir*. Anat. Anz. **2**: 308-322.

WARDLE, C.S. 1971. New observations on the lymph system of the plaice *Pleuronectes platessa* and other teleosts. J. mar. biol. Assoc. U.K. **52**: 977-990.

WARR, G.W. 1983. Immunoglobulin of the toadfish, *Spheroides glaber*. Comp. Biochem. Physiol. **76B**: 507-514.

WARR, G.W. and J.J. MARCHALONIS. 1982. Molecular basis of self/nonself discrimination in the ectothermic vertebrates. pp. 541-567. *In* Cohen, N., and M.M. Sigel [eds.] The reticuloendothelial system: a comprehensive treatise, vol. 3. Phylogeny and ontogeny. Plenum Press, New York.

WEISEL, G.F. 1979. Histology of the feeding and digestive organs of the shovelnose sturgeon, *Scaphirhynchus platorhynchus*. Copeia **1979**: 518-525.

WINGSTRAND, K.G. 1956. Non-nucleated erythrocytes in a teleostean fish, *Maurolicus mulleri* (Gmelin). Z. Zellforsch. **45**: 195-200.

YOFFEY, J.M. and F.C. COURTICE. 1970. Lymphatics, lymph and lymphomyeloid complex. Academic Press, New York.

ZAPATA, A. and A. CARRATO. 1981. Ultrastructure of elasmobranch and teleost erythrocytes. Acta Zool. (Stockh.) **62**: 129-135.

ZAPATA, A., R. FÄNGE, A. MATTISSON, and A. VILLENA. 1984. Plasma cells in adult Atlantic hagfish, *Myxine glutinosa*. Cell Tissue Res. **235**: 695.

EVOLUTION OF THE RENIN-ANGIOTENSIN SYSTEM AND ITS ROLE IN CONTROL OF CARDIOVASCULAR FUNCTION IN FISHES

Hiroko Nishimura

Department of Physiology and Biophysics
University of Tennessee Center for the Health Sciences
Memphis, Tennessee 38163

Introduction

Renin, a protein enzyme synthesized by the juxtaglomerular cells in the kidney, is released into the circulation and possibly into the renal lymph (Morgan *et al.*, 1982). In mammals, renin acts on angiotensinogen (renin substrate), an α_2-globulin in plasma, to form angiotensin I, a decapeptide, which is subsequently converted by converting enzymes to active octapeptide angiotensin II (ANG II), which plays an important role in maintaining cardiovascular and hydromineral homeostasis (Fig. 1) (for review, see Peach, 1977; Skeggs *et al.*, 1974; Vane, 1974). A similar renin-angiotensin system has been shown in teleost and nonmammalian tetrapods (for review, see Sokabe *et al.*, 1969; Nishimura *et al.*, 1973), but evolution and function of this enzyme cascade among more primitive fishes is uncertain (Nishimura *et al.*, 1970).

In mammals, the juxtaglomerular (JG) apparatus consists of granulated cells in the wall of afferent arterioles (JG cells), specialized macula densa cells in the early distal tubules that are in close contact with the glomerular vascular poles, extraglomerular mesangium, and sympathetic nerves densely innervating the afferent arterioles (Davis and Freeman, 1976). Renin secretion is principally controlled by 1) an intrarenal baroreceptor, presumably located on or near JG cells, that is believed to sense changes in intraluminal pressure or a transluminal pressure gradient at the afferent arteriole, 2) the rate of NaCl transport across the macula densa cells, 3) the sympathetic nervous system and humorally released catecholamines, and 4) various other humoral factors including prostaglandins, vasopressin, steroid hormones and plasma electrolytes (for review, see Keeton and Campbell, 1980; Davis and Freeman, 1976). From a phylogenetic point of view, however, each component of the JG apparatus and, accordingly, the factors that control renin release, appear to have evolved at different stages of vertebrate evolution (Sokabe and Ogawa, 1974; Nishimura, 1980).

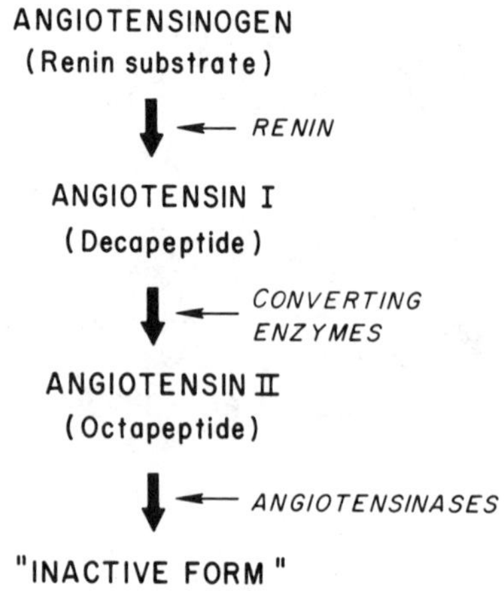

Fig. 1. Cascade of the renin-angiotensin system.

Angiotensins I and II appear to be stable molecules throughout the vertebrate scale, and the amino acid sequence of decapeptide ANG I identified in various species of nonmammalian and mammalian vertebrates (Nakajima *et al.*, 1978; Khosla *et al.*, 1983) varies in positions 1, 5, and 9. In mammals, octapeptide ANG II evokes contraction of vascular smooth muscles, stimulates drinking and a release of antidiuretic hormone in the central nervous system, releases catecholamines from both the adrenergic nerve terminals and the adrenal medulla, exerts glomerular and tubular actions in the kidney, and promotes glycogenolysis in the liver (Peach, 1977; Campanile *et al.*, 1982). Renin and/or angiotensin activities have been found, more recently, in a variety of organs and tissues other than the kidney, including various areas of the central nervous system, blood vessels, uterus, and adrenal glands (Peach, 1977), and their function as locally produced hormones has been suggested. In nonmammalian vertebrates, however, such extrarenal localization of renin has not been demonstrated except in the corpuscles of Stannius of teleosts.

In this chapter, I will review morphological and biochemical evidence that suggests the presence or absence of the renin-angiotensin system in primitive fishes including cyclostomes, elasmobranchs, holocephalans and primitive bony fishes. For comparison, a few biochemical and functional aspects of teleosts are included. Details of comparative morphology and physiology of the renin-angiotensin system have been reviewed previously (Nishimura and Ogawa, 1973; Sokabe and Ogawa, 1974; Nishimura, 1980; Wilson, 1984). Presence or absence of the renin angiotensin system in primitive vertebrates has been determined according to the following criteria (Sokabe *et al.*, 1969; Nishimura *et al.*, 1973): 1) granulated cells morphologically and histochemically resembling JG cells are present in the kidney; 2) incubation of homologous plasma (substrate) and kidney extract (renin source) under sufficient inhibition of angiotensinases (degrading enzymes) forms an angiotensin (or angiotensin-like) pressor substance which increases with prolongation of incubation time; heating either plasma or kidney extract prevents formation of this product; 3) formed product resembles angiotensin in its pressor responses in the rat, being resistant to alpha adrenergic blockade, dialyzable and heat stable, susceptible to digestion by α-chymotrypsin, and adsorbed onto Dowex 50W-X2 resin.

Cyclostomes

Juxtaglomerular cells and renal renin activity

Studies of the renin-angiotensin system in cyclostomes are few. The nephron structure of hagfish and lampreys is rather primitive, and granulated cells stainable by Bowie's method have not been seen in renal arteries and arterioles of *Paramyxine atami* and *Lampetra japonica* (Nishimura *et al.*, 1970; Oguri *et al.*, 1970). The renal tubular component of the JG apparatus is absent as well. Capréol and Sutherland (1968) also reported the absence of JG cells in larval and adult lampreys as well as in the hagfish. Incubation of kidney extracts from *Paramyxine* or *Lampetra* with homologous plasma, or the plasma from the rat or carp, did not time-dependently produce pressor substance, despite adequate inhibition of angiotensinases (Table I). Similarly, kidney extracts from the rat or carp did not form angiotensin upon incubation with cyclostome plasma. Henderson *et al.* (1980, data are not shown) found, however, that renal extracts of *Lampetra fluviatilis* incubated with dog renin substrate generated a pressor substance similar to angiotensin when assayed in the rat. Proteolytic enzymes, such as pepsin, trypsin, chymotrypsin (Croxatto, 1974; Ikeda *et al.*, 1977) and cathepsin D (Reid, 1977; Figueiredo *et al.*, 1983), however, are known to hydrolyze renin substrate, and it is thus necessary to determine whether the above pressor activity is indeed formed by renal renin or by other endogenous peptidases.

Table I. Renal renin activity[a] in Cyclostomes.

Kidney extract	Plasma			Dog substrate
	Paramyxine	*Lampetra*	Rat or Carp	
Paramyxine atami	-		-	
Lampetra japonica		-		
Lampetra fluviatilis				+[b]
Rat or carp	-	-		

From: Nishimura *et al.* (1970)

[a] See "Introduction" for criteria for renal renin activity.
[b] Pressor activity in rats, Henderson *et al.* (1980).

Effect of exogenously administered angiotensin

Although the presence of the renin-angiotensin system is obscure in cyclostomes, intra-arterial injection of synthetic [Asn^1,Val^5]ANG II (native ANG II from Japanese goosefish, *Lophius litulon*) at the dose of 2 μg kg^{-1} increased dorsal aortic pressure (mm Hg) of the conscious hagfish, *Myxine glutinosa*, from 6.6 ± 0.9 to 10.0 ± 0.6 (n=3, $P<0.05$) (Carroll and Opdyke, 1982). Moreover, phentolamine, an α-adrenergic blocking drug, decreased the resting blood pressure level (BP) to 4.0 mm Hg, and totally inhibited the pressor response to ANG II, suggesting that the vasopressor action of ANG II in the hagfish may be ascribed to the release of catecholamines (Carroll and Opdyke, 1982). It is not known whether this angiotensin effect is mediated through specific angiotensin receptors. Kobayashi *et al.* (1983) have examined stimulation of water intake by ANG II in a variety of cartilaginous and bony fishes. [Asn^1,Val^5]ANG II at as large a dose as 500 μg kg^{-1} (i.p.) neither induced drinking in the Arctic lamprey, *Lampetra japonica* nor increased significantly the rate of water intake (2.6 ± 0.6 μL 10 g body wt^{-1}) in the hagfish *Myxine glutinosa*. Therefore, at present, there is no clear evidence that the renin-angiotensin system exists in cyclostomes, although it is interesting and possibly pertinent that exogenous ANG II increases BP in the hagfish.

Elasmobranchs

Juxtaglomerular cells and renal renin activity

No granulated epithelioid cells were observed in the walls of renal arteries and arterioles of four species of marine sharks, *Triakis scyllia*, *Heterodontus japonicus*, *Orectolobus japonicus*, and *Acanthias vulgaris*, two species of marine rays, *Dasyatis akaei* and *Raja laevis*, and a freshwater stingray, *Potamotrygon circularis* (Bohle and Walvig, 1964; Capréol and Sutherland, 1968; Nishimura *et al.*, 1970; Oguri *et al.*, 1970). Crockett *et al.* (1973) examined juxtaglomerular cells in six elasmobranch species from different environmental salinities. Histologic examination of the afferent and efferent arterioles, and the renal tubules failed to reveal the presence of juxtaglomerular cells in any of the elasmobranch species examined. In elasmobranchs, the early segment of the distal tubule is in close contact with the afferent arteriole at the vascular pole of the glomerulus, but no specialized macula densa cells are present (Nishimura *et al.*, 1970). Similarly, no time-dependent angiotensin formation was noted during incubation of homologous plasma with kidney extract from *Triakis, Heterodontus, Orectolobus, Dasyatis* (Nishimura *et al.*, 1970) and *Squalus acanthias* (unpublished) (Table II), despite sufficient suppression of angiotensinase activities and protection of formed angiotensin, if any, by absorbing to Dowex resin. Incubation of shark or ray kidneys with rat or carp plasma or, conversely, rat or carp kidney extracts with shark or ray plasmas did not form angiotensin-like pressor substance (Nishimura *et al.*, 1970). Henderson *et al.* (1980) reported, however, that renal extracts from dogfish, *Scyliorhinus canicula*, incubated with rat substrate, or injection of renal extract itself, produced a pressor response similar to that of angiotensin in the anesthetized rat (Fig. 2). Thus it is possible that the renin substrate level in elasmobranch plasma is too low to produce sufficient angiotensin to be detected by bioassay without the use of added, more concentrated substrate. However, biochemical identification of renin activity is

Table II. Renal renin activity[a] in Chondrichthyes

Kidney Extract	Plasma							Rat substrate
	Triakis	*Heterodontus*	*Orectolobus*	*Squalus*	*Dasyatis*	*Hydrolagus*	Rat or carp	
Triakis scyllia	-						-	
Heterodontus japonicus		-					-	
Orectolobus japonicus			-				-	
Squalus acanthias				-				
Dasyatis akaei					-		-	
Scyliorhinus canicula								+[b]
Hydrolagus colliei						+		
Rat or carp	-		-		-			

From: Nishimura *et al.*, 1970.

[a]See Introduction: for criteria for renal renin activity
[b]Pressor activity in rats, Henderson *et al.*, 1980

necessary before a conclusion is made as to the presence of renal renin in elasmobranchs. Furthermore, since unidentified pressor substances are present in plasmas from primitive fishes (Nishimura *et al.*, 1973), it is important to determine that production of pressor activity increases as a function of incubation duration.

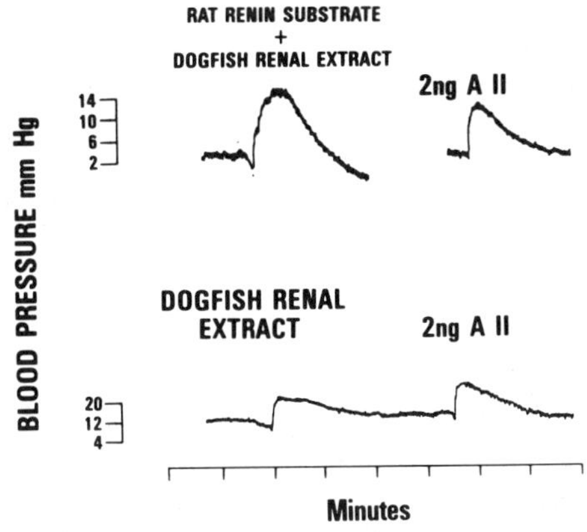

Fig. 2. Renin-like material in dogfish (*Scyliorhinus canicula*) kidney extracts assayed in Inactin-anesthetized, nephrectomized, pentolinium-treated rat. *Upper panel*: Carotid arterial pressure (*BP*) response to the product generated from incubation of rat angiotensinogen with dogfish renal extract (pH 6.0, 6°C, 24 h). *Lower panel*: BP response to dogfish kidney extract. AII: responses to standard (Hypertension, CIBA) angiotensin II. (Reproduced with permission from Henderson *et al.*, 1980).

Effects of exogenously administered angiotensins

Cardiovascular effects of exogenous angiotensins in the dogfish, *Squalus acanthias*, were extensively studied by Opdyke, Carroll and coworkers (Table III). They demonstrated: 1) intra-arterial injection of [Asp^1,Ile^5,His^9]ANG I (mammalian ANG I, 20 μg $fish^{-1}$) increased BP in conscious dogfish, which was blocked by pretreatment of fish with an angiotensin-converting enzyme inhibitor, SQ 20, 881 (Squibb), suggesting that conversion of ANG I to biologically active ANG II takes place in the shark (Opdyke and Holcombe, 1976). 2) [Asn^1,Val^5]ANG II increased BP in a dose-related fashion (Carroll, 1981), and this pressor response was entirely abolished by an alpha adrenergic blocking agent, phentolamine (Opdyke and Holcombe, 1976). 3) Moreover, ANGs I and II perfused into the blood vessels of an isolated gut preparation or into whole body vascular bed failed to alter the resistance to flow, while epinephrine caused a marked increase in flow resistance (Opdyke and Holcombe, 1978). 4) Similarly, [Asn^1,Val^5]ANG II did not evoke contraction of helical strips from dogfish celiac artery or anterior intestinal vein (Fig. 3; Carroll, 1981). 5) After addition of chromaffin tissue in the bath, however, ANG II produced contraction of isolated arterial strips (Carroll, 1981). 6) Intra-arterial injection of [Asn^1,Val^5]ANG II (5 μg kg^{-1}) indeed increased plasma levels of norepinephrine and epinephrine by 4 - 8 fold (Opdyke *et al.*, 1981). These results indicate that the vasopressor action of angiotensin in the dogfish is indirect, being mediated by catecholamines. It would be interesting to see whether a binding site (or sites) specific to angiotensin exist(s) on the chromaffin tissues and sympathetic ganglions.

In mammals, ANG II analogs with the 8th amino acid replaced competitively antagonize the receptor binding of ANG II and, thus, block its biological action (Türker *et al.*, 1974). In the dogfish, however, [Sar^1,Ile^8]ANG II produces a considerable agonist pressor effect and does not inhibit ANG II action (Opdyke, personal communication). [Sar^1,Thr^8]ANG II, another mammalian ANG II antagonist that has no agonist action itself in the dogfish, did not antagonize the pressor response to ANG II either, suggesting that ANG II receptor, if it exists, in the dogfish may have different properties from the mammalian vascular angiotensin receptor.

Since the renin-angiotensin system is a potent regulator of aldosterone secretion in mammals, Hazon and Henderson (1985) sought a homologous action in conscious chronically cannulated dogfish, *Scyliorhinus canicula.* They found that [Asn^1,Val^5]ANG II (0.6 μg $kg^{-1} \cdot min^{-1}$, i.a.) as well as homologous renal extract of *Squalus* kidneys increased plasma concentrations of 1 α-hydroxycorticosterone, a naturally occurring interrenal steroid hormone in elasmobranchs, while the metabolic clearance rate of this steroid remained unchanged, suggesting that the rise in plasma level is due to an increase in the rate of production. Intraperitoneal injection of [Asn^1,Val^5]ANG II (10 - 1000 ng kg^{-1}), however, failed to stimulate water intake in conscious dogfish, *Triakis scyllia* and *Heterodontus japonicus* (Kobayashi *et al.*, 1983).

Table III. Effects of exogenously administered angiotensin II in fishes

Class & species	*Blood Pressure* ANG II	α-Adrenergic blocker + ANG II (% decrease)	Arterial strip Contraction	Plasma Catecholamines	Drinking Stimulation	Steroid Secretion	JG Cells
CYCLOSTOMES							
Myxine glutinosa[b]	↑	100					
Eptatretus burgeri[c]					(-)		
Lampetra japonica[c,d]					(-)		(-)
ELASMOBRANCHS							
Squalus acanthias[e,f,g]	↑	100	(-)	EP↑NE↑			
Triakis scyllia[c,d]					(-)		(-)
Heterodontus japonicus[c,d]					(-)		(-)
Scyliorhinus canicula[h]						(+)	
TELEOSTS							
Anguilla rostrata[i,k]	↑	30-70	(+)[a]				
Anguilla anguilla[j,l,m]	↑				(+)	(+)	(+)
Cyclopterus lumpus[b]	↑			EP↑NE↑			
Myoxocephalus octodecimspinosus[e]			(+)				

EP = epinephrine NE = norepinephrine

[a]Khairrallah and Nishimura (unpublished)
[b]Carroll and Opdyke (1982)
[c]Kobayashi *et al.* (1983)
[d]Nishimura *et al.* (1970)
[e]Carroll (1981)
[f]Opdyke and Holcombe (1976)
[g]Opdyke *et al.* (1981)
[h]Hazon and Henderson (1985)
[i]Capreol and Sutherland (1968)
[j]Takei *et al.* (1979)
[k]Nishimura *et al.* (1978)
[l]Henderson *et al.* (1976)
[m]Sokabe and Ogawa (1974)

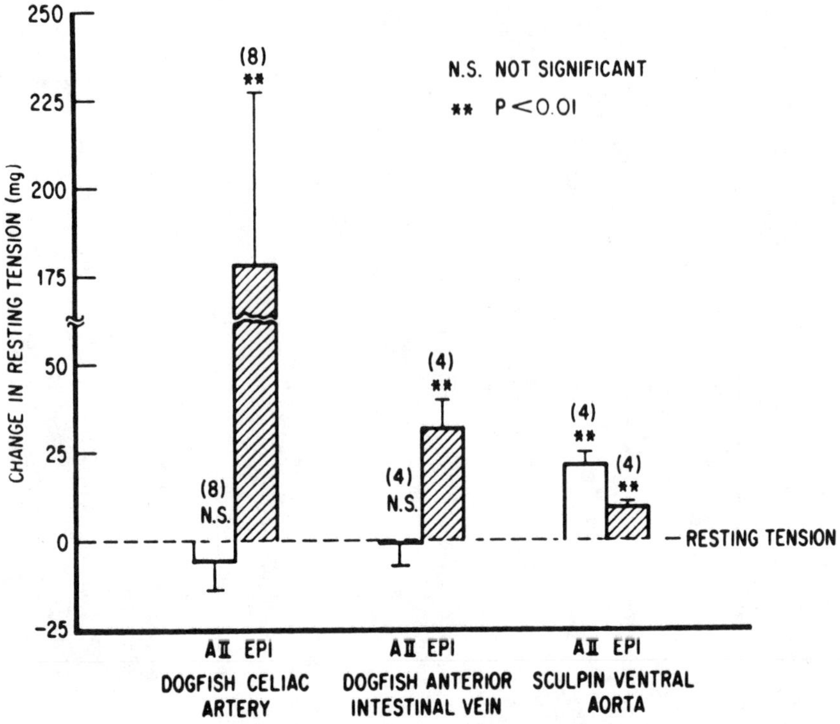

Fig. 3. Reactivity of helically cut blood vessels from the dogfish, *Squalus acanthias*, and from a teleost, the sculpin, *Myoxocephalus octodecimspinosus*, to epinephrine (EPI) and [Asn^1, Val^5] ANG II (AII). Isometric contraction was determined by measuring the changes in tension at 16°C using elasmobranch saline bubbled with 95% O_2 + 5% CO_2. Values shown are means ± SE. Number of trials are shown above each bar. Resting tension at a preload of >2g taken as 0 point. (Reproduced with permission from Carroll, 1981).

Holocephalans

In contrast to the lack in elasmobranchs of granulated cells resembling JG cells, granulated epithelioid cells stainable with Bowie's method are present in tunica media of the arterioles adjacent to glomeruli in two species of holocephalans, the ratfish, *Hydrolagus colliei* (Nishimura *et al.*, 1973; Oguri, 1978) and the rabbitfish, *Chimaera monstrosa* (Oguri, 1978). Differing from the JG granules in teleostean kidneys, which are minute in size and stained homogenously, holocephalan JG granules are more coarse and are not stained with periodic acid-Schiff (PAS) reagent (Oguri, 1978). As in elasmobranchs, the early distal tubule of holocephalans is in close contact with the vascular pole of the glomerulus (Fig. 4), but no specialized

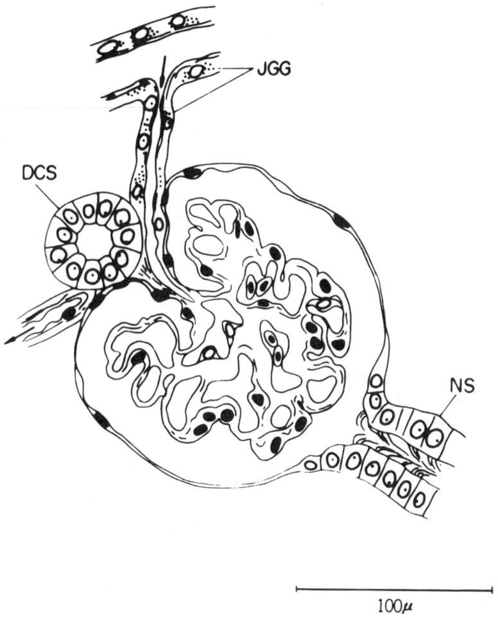

Fig. 4. Schematic illustration of the juxtaglomerular area of the ratfish (*Hydrolagus colliei*). Renal distal tubule shows a close apposition to the afferent arteriole near the vascular pole, but no macula densa cells were recognized. The cells containing granules are distributed along the afferent arteriole, but they are not as thick as juxtaglomerular cells of teleosts or tetrapods. Glomerulus : spherical, 150 x 150μ . (Reproduced from Nishimura *et al.*, 1973).

tubular cells resembling macula densa cells are present (Nishimura *et al.*, 1973; Oguri, 1978).

A pressor substance biologically similar to angiotensin is produced when *Hydrolagus* kidney extract is incubated with homologous plasma, although the plasma angiotensinogen level appears to be low (Table IV; Nishimura *et al.*, 1973). Teleostean kidney (toadfish, *Opsanus tau*) did not form angiotensin-like pressor substance from *Hydrolagus* plasma (Nishimura, unpublished). No study has reported the effect of exogenous or endogenous angiotensin in holocephalans. It is interesting that presence of a renin-angiotensin system is clearer in holocephalans than in elasmobranchs, although both belong to the Chondrichthyes. Although holocephalans resemble elasmobranchs in sharing certain morphological characteristics and osmoregulatory properties, they represent a line of evolution which has long been distinct from that leading to the elasmobranchs. It has been reported that holocephalans differ from elasmobranchs in certain endocrinological aspects (Sawyer, 1968; Idler, 1970).

Table IV. Renin activity and plasma angiotensinogen level in primitive bony fishes and in a holocephalan (from Nishimura *et al.*, 1973)

Species	No.	Kidney renin ($K \times 10^2$)	Angiotensinogen ($\mu g\ mL^{-1}$)
Coelacanth	1	11.4	0.12
African lungfish	2	3.1	1.05
		1.8	0.49
South American lungfish	4	5.5	0.53
		5.0	0.14
Bowfin	4	9.8	0.21
		41.3	0.19
		12.4	0.29
Gar-pike	2	8.2	0.08
Sturgeon	3	+?	
Bichir	2	9.2	0.03
Reedfish	2		
Ratfish	3	4.0	0.01

Primitive bony fishes

Juxtaglomerular cells and renal renin activity

There seems to be a discrepancy between the histological visualization of JG granules and biological demonstration of renal renin activity in primitive bony fishes, suggesting that the histochemical properties of the granules may differ. In three species of chondrosteans, *Polypterus senegalus* (Nile bichir), *Calamoichthys calabaricus* (reedfish) and *Acipenser brevirostris* (shortnose sturgeon), granulated cells resembling JG cells have not been demonstrated, but angiotensin-forming activity is present in *Polypterus* (Nishimura *et al.*, 1973). Pressor substance was formed from *Acipenser* plasma after incubation with homologous renal extract, but it is still unclear from the biological evidence whether or not the formed substance is angiotensin. Both JG cells and renal or plasma renin activities are present in two species of holosteans, *Amia calva* (bowfin) and *Lepisosteus osseus* (longnose gar; Fig. 5; Nishimura *et al.*, 1973 and unpublished), three species of dipnoans, *Neoceratodus forsteri* (Australian lungfish; Blair-West *et al.*, 1977), *Lepidosiren paradoxa* (South American lungfish), *Protopterus aethiopicus* (African lungfish; Nishimura *et al.*, 1973), and in *Latimeria chalumnae* (coelacanth; Nishimura *et al.*, 1973; Lagios, 1974). Thus, the renin-angiotensin system appears to be present among primitive living bony fishes.

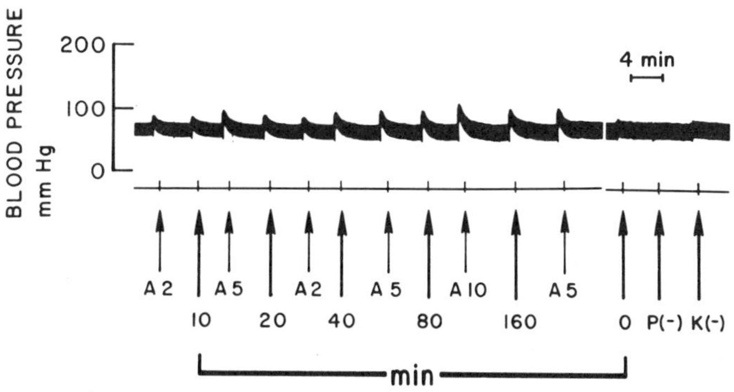

Fig. 5. Bioassay record of pressor activities obtained from the longnose gar, *Lepisosteus osseus*, after incubation of their kidney extract with homologous plasma. A2, A5, and A10 indicate blood pressure rises caused by injecting 0.3 ml of the solution containing 2, 5, or 10 ng of [Asp^1, Val^5] ANG II as standards. 10, 20, --- 160 are responses to 0.3 ml of the product of 10, 20, --- 160 min incubation. 0 min, P (-), and K (-) are controls without incubation, plasma or kidney extract, respectively. (Reproduced from Nishimura, 1971).

Function of the renin-angiotensin system

Physiological studies of the renin-angiotensin system in the fishes mentioned above are limited. [Asn^1,Val^5]ANG II increased BP and caused mild to moderate glomerular diuresis and natriuresis in conscious lungfishes, *Protopterus aethiopicus* (Sawyer, 1970) and *Neoceratodus forsteri* (Sawyer *et al.*, 1976). Moreover, intravenous injection of angiotensin-converting enzyme inhibitor SQ 14,225 (Squibb) decreased the resting BP in *Protopterus* (P.K.T. Pang, personal communication). Iso-osmotic volume expansion in *Neoceratodus*, produced by iso-osmotic saline infusion, reduced plasma renin activity and slightly increased aortic pressure (Blair-West *et al.*, 1977). These findings suggest that the renin-angiotensin system may play a role in control of blood pressure and/or blood volume in lungfish.

Teleosts

The renin-angiotensin system has been studied extensively in teleosts and a detailed review of these findings is beyond the scope of this chapter. Occurrence of JG cells and renal renin, and the comparative physiology of the renin-angiotensin system of teleosts were reviewed previously (Sokabe, 1974; Sokabe and Ogawa, 1974; Taylor, 1977; Nishimura, 1980, 1985; Wilson, 1984). In teleost fishes, ANG II has a cardiovascular action (see below); it stimulates water intake (Takei *et al.*, 1979; Kobayashi *et al.*, 1983; Malvin *et al.*, 1980); it causes catecholamine release (Carroll and Opdyke, 1982), glomerular antidiuresis (Brown *et al.*, 1980), and an increase in circulating cortisol level (Henderson *et al.*, 1976). In this review I will discuss only the cardiovascular action of angiotensin in teleosts in relation to that in primitive fishes.

Juxtaglomerular cells and biochemistry of renin and angiotensin

Granulated cells with the histochemical characteristics of JG cells have been found in the walls of renal arterioles and small arteries from a variety of glomerular and aglomerular teleosts (Capréol and Sutherland, 1968; Oguri and Sokabe, 1974; Sokabe and Ogawa, 1974) and they display several patterns of distribution (Krishnamurthy and Bern, 1969). Apparently, similar granules have been found in the corpuscles of Stannius (Krishnamurthy and Bern, 1969). Renin activities have also been demonstrated in the kidney (for review, see Sokabe and Ogawa, 1974), plasma (Henderson *et al.*, 1976; Nishimura *et al.*, 1976, 1979; Bailey and Randall, 1981), and in the corpuscles of Stannius (Sokabe *et al.*, 1970). The amino acid sequence of decapeptide ANG I has been described in four species of teleost fishes (Fig. 6) in which the amino acids in positions 1 and 9 are different from those of more advanced vertebrates (Nakajima *et al.*, 1978). Valine is in position 5 in all nonmammalian vertebrates examined, while isoleucine is found at that position in most mammalian angiotensins. The chemical structure of renin has not been determined in teleost fishes. No anatomical proximity is found between the JG cells and renal tubules in teleostean kidneys; thus a tubular component of the JG apparatus is absent.

Cardiovascular function of the renin-angiotensin system

Synthetic native [Asn^1,Val^5]ANG II and partially purified homologous angiotensin increased the BP of conscious eels in a dose-related fashion (Nishimura *et al.*, 1978); this is reduced by replacement of Asn^1 with Asp^1 or Sar^1 or by pretreatment with an alpha adrenergic blocker (unpublished; Fig. 7). In contrast to the response in elasmobranchs, however, angiotensin produces a contraction of isolated arterial strips (Carroll, 1981); it increases plasma levels of epinephrine and to a lesser extent norepinephrine (Carroll and Opdyke, 1982). This indicates that

Lophius litulon (Japanese goosefish)	[Asn^1, Val^5, His^9] ANG I	Hayashi *et al.*, 1978
Oncorhynchus keta (chum salmon)	[Asn^1, Val^5, Asn^9] ANG I	Takemoto *et al.*, 1983
Anguilla japonica (Japanese eel)	[Asp^1, Val^5, Gly^9] ANG I (Asn)	Hasegawa *et al.*, 1983
Anguilla rostrata (American eel)	[Asn^1, Val^5, Gly^9] ANG I (Asp)	Khosla *et al.*, 1985

Fig. 6. Amino acid sequence of native angiotensin I in teleosts. In *Anguilla rostrata* major and minor peptides were identified, respectively, as [Asn^1, Val^5, Gly^9] ANG I and [Asp^1, Val^5, Gly^9] ANG I, while in *Anguilla japonica*, aspartyl decapeptide was found to be the major peptide.

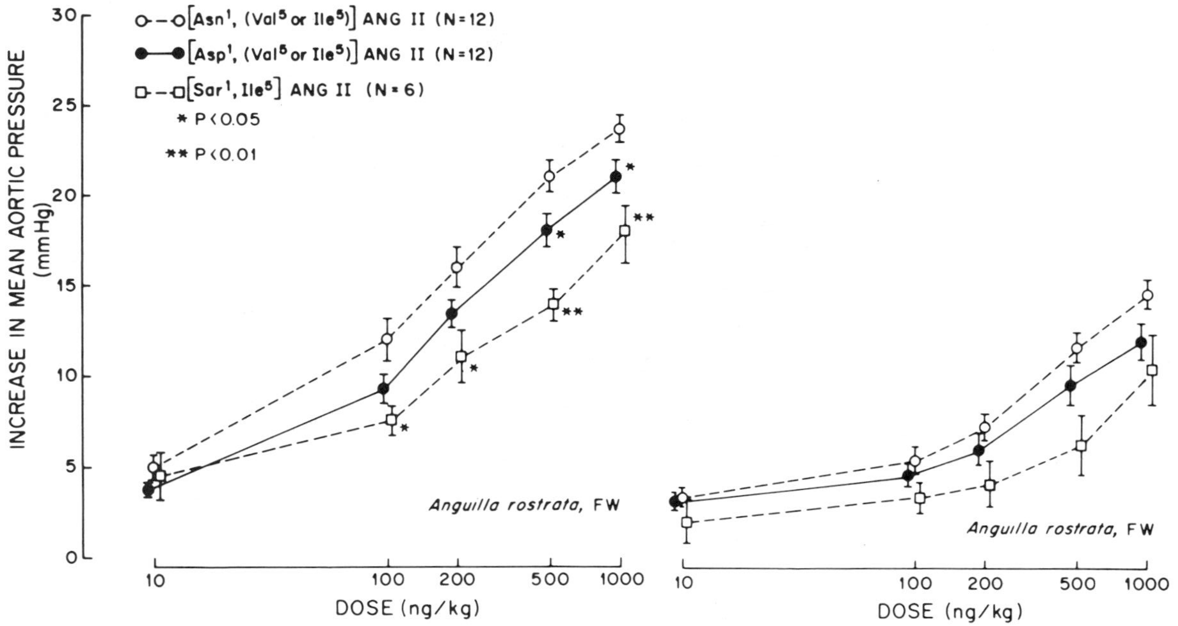

Fig. 7. Vasopressor responses in conscious eels, *Anguilla rostrata*, to angiotension II analogs in which the amino acid of position 1 varies. [Asn^1, Val^5] ANG II is native to *A. rostrata*. There is no difference in the vasopressor action between [Val^5] and [Ile^5] ANG II, and thus the results are pooled. Replacement of [Asn^1] with [Asp^1] or [Sar^1] reduced the vasopressor effect in both control (right panel) and phentolamine-treated (5 mg kg^{-1}) (left panel) eels. Phentolamine reduced vasopressor responses to angiotensin approximately to half.

the vasopressor action of ANG II consists of both a direct vascular contractile action as well as an indirect action through catecholamines. Similar to the situation in elasmobranchs, analogues with the 8th amino acid replaced, [Sar^1,Ile^8]ANG II and [Sar^1,Thr^8]ANG II do not antagonize the vasopressor action of ANG II (Nishimura *et al.*, 1978).

Since the vascular component of the JG apparatus appears to have evolved before the tubular macula densa, a possible baroreceptor function of JG cells has been examined in teleosts. Reduction of blood volume and/or blood pressure by experimental hemorrhage or vasodilatory drugs increased the circulating level of renin by more than ten-fold in toadfish, *Opsanus tau* (Nishimura *et al.*, 1979; Fig. 8). Isoproterenol, a ß-adrenergic drug (1 μg kg^{-1}), and SQ 14,225 (1 mg kg^{-1}) also caused, respectively, a transient and sustained hypotension and increased plasma renin activity by several-fold (Nishimura and Bailey, 1982 and unpublished). Propranolol, a ß-adrenergic blocking drug, inhibited both reduction in BP and the renin response to isoproterenol, while infusion or injection of norepinephrine increased BP with no effect on PRA (Nishimura *et al.*, unpublished). Since these drugs were applied through the systemic circulation, the observed reduction in BP may have stimulated an extrarenal baroreceptor, if it exists, which in turn, caused renin release via a neural pathway. Histochemical examination, however, failed to reveal any monoamine-specific fluorescence in the walls of renal arterioles of the toadfish in close contact with granulated cells, after loading the fish with catecholamines or inhibiting monoamine oxidase activity (Nishimura *et al.*, unpublished). Therefore, it appears likely that there may be a pressure-sensitive mechanism in the kidney that mediates renin release in response to the reduction of renal perfusion pressure. Bailey and Randall (1981) have shown that renin secretion from the kidney of the rainbow trout, *Salmo gairdneri*, perfused *in situ* increased when renal perfusion pressure was lowered. Preliminary studies from our laboratory indicate that acetylcholine (10^{-5} M), but not isoproterenol (10^{-6} M), can stimulate renin secretion from renal slices superfused *in vitro* (unpublished). Since the dose required is high, the physiological significance, and possible participation of cholinergic nerves, in control of renin release remain to be determined.

Evolutionary speculation

There is no clear evidence at present to suggest that a renin-angiotensin system is present in cyclostomes. In elasmobranchs, exogenous administration of synthetic ANG II produces several physiological responses, including a vasopressor action, catecholamine release, and stimulation of 1 α-hydroxycorticosterone production. Although incubation of homologous plasma and kidney extract failed to generate angiotensin, Henderson *et al.* (1980) have suggested that a renin-like enzyme may exist in the dogfish, based on their tests using added renin substrate. However, it is necessary to differentiate biochemical renin activity from that of other naturally-occurring proteolytic enzymes which are known to hydrolyze renin substrate, for example, by examining its pH profile, substrate specificity, and inhibition by specific antagonists. Since plasma renin substrate levels appear to be lower in primitive fishes than in teleosts or higher animals (Table IV), time-dependent formation of angiotensin is difficult to measure by use of the rat vasopressor bioassay. Measurement of renin activity through its action on the rate of ANG I

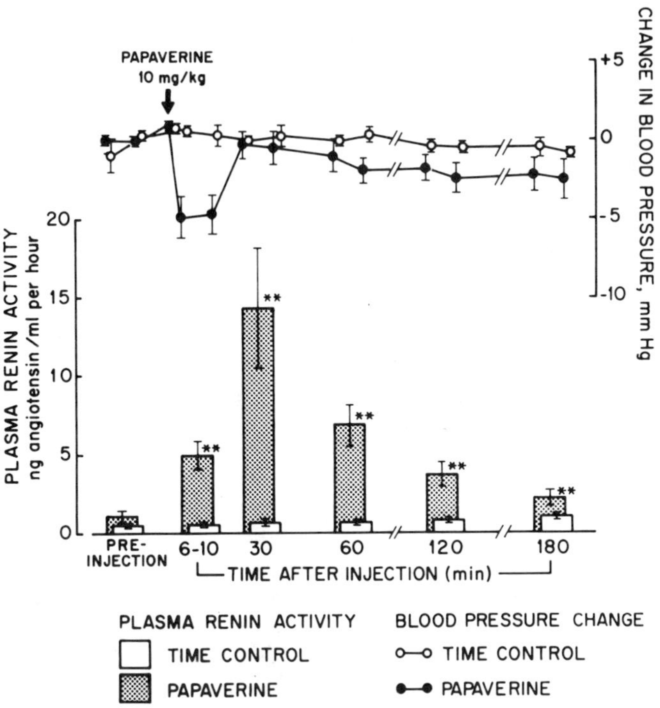

Fig. 8. Effects of papaverine (10 mg kg^{-1}, i.a.) on plasma renin activity (PRA) and blood pressure in conscious toadfish adapted to 50% seawater. Figures are means ± SE. Statistical significance of the differences between resting level PRA and that after papaverine injection was determined by paired *t* test using logs of data (transformed). Time control experiment (injected, solvent) was done in the same fish prior to this experiment. (Reproduced from Nishimura *et al.*, 1979).

generation, with radioimmunoassay, is often not feasible because the variation in the amino acid in position 9 of native ANG I appears to inhibit its binding to the readily available [His^9]ANG I antibody. It may be necessary to increase a concentration of homologous substrate by partial purification or alternatively, to measure ANG II, which is a more stable molecule throughout the vertebrate classes (Nakajima *et al.*, 1978), by radioimmunoassay. Furthermore, the search for genic information for renin and angiotensin with molecular biological techniques may provide a useful approach for elucidating the evolution and physiological significance of this hormonal system in primitive fishes.

The renin-angiotensin system appears to be present in holocephalans and primitive bony fishes, although a more physiological study of the function of angiotensin is needed. The fact that angiotensin stimulates catecholamine release in all vertebrate classes, and that the magnitude of the release is greater in more primitive vertebrates (Carroll and Opdyke, 1982), suggests that one of the important roles of the renin-angiotensin system in primitive fishes may be to modulate the adreno-sympathetic system. The adreno-sympathetic system has a direct role in the control of cardiovascular homeostasis. Evolution of JG cells prior to evolution of a macula densa, and a close relationship between blood pressure and endogenous renin level in teleosts, appear to support this concept. Moreover, specific angiotensin II binding sites in various tissues, such as chromaffin tissues, vascular smooth muscles, adrenocortical cells and glomerulus, should be examined as to whether evolution of angiotensin receptor would agree with evolution of the hormone.

Acknowledgements

Unpublished observations cited in the text were supported by the National Heart, Lung and Blood Institute, grant HL 29364, and the National Science foundation, grant PCM 8302812.

Literature cited

BAILEY, J.R., and D.J. RANDALL. 1981. Renal perfusion pressure and renin secretion in the rainbow trout, *Salmo gairdneri*. Can. J. Zool. **59**: 1220.

BLAIR-WEST, J.R., J.P. COGHLAN, D.A. DENTON, A.P. GIBSON, C.J. ODDIE, W.H. SAWYER, and B.A. SCOGGINS. 1977. Plasma renin activity and blood corticosteroids in the Australian lungfish, *Neoceratodus forsteri*. J. Endocrinol. **74**: 137.

BOHLE, A., and F. WALVIG. 1964. Vergleichende Morphologie der epithelioiden Zellen der Nierenarteriolen. Klin. Wochschr. **42**: 416.

BROWN, J.A., J.A. OLIVER, I.W. HENDERSON, and B.A. JACKSON. 1980. Angiotensin and single nephron glomerular function in the trout *Salmo gairdneri*. Amer. J. Physiol. (Regulatory Integrative Comp. Physiol. 8) **239**: R509.

CAMPANILE, C.P., J.K. CRANE, M.J. PEACH, and J.G. GARRISON. 1982. The hepatic angiotensin II receptor. I. Chracterization of the membrane-binding site and correlation with physiological response in hepatocytes. J. biol. Chem. **257**: 4951.

CAPRÉOL, S.V., and L.E. SUTHERLAND. 1968. Comparative morphology of juxtaglomerular cells. I. Juxtaglomerular cells in fish. Can. J. Zool. **46**: 249.

CARROLL, R.G. 1981. Vascular response of the dogfish and sculpin to angiotensin II. Amer. J. Physiol. (Regulatory Integrative Comp. Physiol. 9) **240**: R139.

CARROLL, R.G., and D.F. OPDYKE. 1982. Evolution of angiotensin II-induced catecholamine release. Amer. J. Physiol. (Regulatory Integrative Comp. Physiol. 12) **243**: R65.

CROCKETT, D.R., J.W. GERST, and S. BLANKENSHIP. 1973. Absence of juxtaglomerular cells in the kidneys of elasmobranch fishes. Comp. Biochem. Physiol. **44A**: 673.

CROXATTO, H.R. 1974. Plasma serum vasopressor peptides other than angiotensins. *In* Page, I.H., and F.M. Bumpus [eds.] Angiotensins. Springer Verlag, New York.

DAVIS, J.O., and R.H. FREEMAN. 1976. Mechanisms regulating renin release. Physiol. Rev. **56**: 1.

FIGUEIREDO, A.F.S., Y. TAKII, H. TSUJI, K. KATO, and T. INAGAMI. 1983. Rat kidney renin and cathepsin D: purification and comparison of properties. Biochemistry **22**: 5476.

HASEGAWA, Y., T. NAKAJIMA, and H. SOKABE. 1983. Chemical structure of angiotensin formed with kidney renin in the Japanese eel, *Anguilla japonica*. Biomed. Res. **4**: 417.

HAYASHI, T., T. NAKAYAMA, T. NAKAJIMA, and H. SOKABE. 1968. Comparative studies on angiotensins. V. Structure of angiotensin formed by the kidney of Japanese goosefish and its identification by dansyl method. Chem. Pharmacol. Bull. **26**: 215.

HAZON, N., and I.W. HENDERSON. 1985. Factors affecting the secretory dynamics of 1 -hydroxycorticosterone in the dogfish, *Scyliorhinus canicula*. Gen. comp. Endocrinol. (in press).

HENDERSON, I.W., V. JOTINSANKASA, W. MOSELY, and M. OGURI. 1976. Endocrine and environmental influences upon plasma cortisol concentrations and plasma renin activity of the eel, *Anguilla anguilla* L. J. Endocrinol. **70**: 81.

HENDERSON, I.W., J.A. OLIVER, A. McKEEVER, and N. HAZON. 1980. Phylogenetic aspects of the renin-angiotensin system. *In* Pethes, G., and V.L. Frenyo [eds.] Advances in physiological sciences: advances in animal and comparative physiology. Pergamon Press, Budapest.

IDLER, D.R. 1970. Some comparative aspects of corticosteroid metabolism. Proc. 3rd Int. Congr. Symp. Hormonal Steroids. Exerpta Med. Int. Cong. Ser. **219**: 14.

IKEDA, M., T. SAKAI, M. YUKI, T. GEJI, and K. ARAKAWA. 1977. Formation of vasoactive substances by trypsin-effect of pH differences on the generation. Jap. Cir. J. **41**: 871.

KEETON, T.K., and W.B. CAMPBELL. 1980. The pharmacologic alteration of renin release. Pharmacol. Rev. **32**: 81.

KHOSLA, M.C., F.M. BUMPUS, H. NISHIMURA, D.F. OPDYKE, and A. COVIELLO. 1983. Synthesis of nonmammalian angiotensins and their comparative pressor properties in dogfish shark, domestic chicken and rat. Hypertension **5** (suppl. V): v-22.

KHOSLA, M.C., H. NISHIMURA, Y. HASEGAWA, and F.M. BUMPUS. 1985. Identification and synthesis of [1-Asparagine, 5-Valine, 9-Glycine] angiotensin I produced from plasma of the American eel *Anguilla rostrata*. Gen. comp. Endocrinol. **57**: 223.

KOBAYASHI, H., H. UEMURA, Y. TAKEI, N. ITATSU, M. OZAWA, and K. ICHINOHE. 1983. Drinking induced by angiotensin II in fishes. Gen. comp. Endocrinol. **49**: 295.

KRISHNAMURTHY, V.G., and H.A. BERN. 1969. Correlative histologic study of the corpuscles of Stannius and the juxtaglomerular cells of teleost fishes. Gen. comp. Endocrinol. **13**: 313.

LAGIOS, M.D. 1974. Granular epithelioid (juxtaglomerular) cell and renovascular morphology of the Coelacanth *Latimeria chalumnae* Smith (Crossopterygii) compared with that of other fishes. Gen. comp. Endocrinol. **22**: 296.

MALVIN, R.L., D. SCHIFF, and S. EIGER. 1980. Angiotensin and drinking rates in the euryhaline killifish. Amer. J. Physiol. (Regulatory Integrative Comp. Physiol. 8) **239**: R31.

MORGAN, T., J. DAVIS, and A. GILLIES. 1982. Release of renin into the

circulation. Kidney Int. **22** (suppl. 12): S-63.
NAKAJIMA, T., M.C. KHOSLA, and S. SAKAKIBARA. 1978. Comparative biochemistry of renins and angiotensin in the vertebrates. Jap. Heart J. **19**: 799.
NISHIMURA, H. 1971. Evolution of the renin-angiotensin system and its possible functions in bony fish. J. Med. Soc. Toho Univ. **18**: 946.
NISHIMURA, H. 1980. Comparative endocrinology of renin and angiotensin I. *In* Johnson, J.A., and R.R. Anderson [eds.] The renin-angiotensin system. Plenum Publishing Corp., New York.
NISHIMURA, H. 1985. Endocrine control of renal handling of solutes and water in vertebrates. *In* Renal physiology. (in press)
NISHIMURA, H., and J.R. BAILEY. 1982. Intrarenal renin-angiotensin system in primitive vertebrates. Kidney Int. **22** (suppl. 12): S-185.
NISHIMURA, H., L.G. LUNDE, and A. ZUCKER. 1979. Renin response to hemorrhage and hypotension in the aglomerular toadfish *Opsanus tau*. Amer. J. Physiol. (Heart Circ. Physiol. 2) **237**: H105.
NISHIMURA, H. V.M. NORTON, and F.M. BUMPUS. 1978. Lack of specific inhibition of angiotensin II in eels by angiotensin antagonists. Amer. J. Physiol. (Heart Circ. Physiol. 1) **235**: H95.
NISHIMURA, H. and M. OGAWA. 1973. The renin-angiotensin system in fishes. Amer. Zool. **13**: 823.
NISHIMURA, H., M. OGAWA, and W.H. SAWYER. 1973. Renin-angiotensin system in primitive bony fishes and a holocephalan. Amer. J. Physiol. **244**: 950.
NISHIMURA, H., M. OGURI, M. OGAWA, H. SOKABE, and M. IMAI. 1970. Absence of renin in kidneys of elasmobranchs and cyclostomes. Amer. J. Physiol. **218**: 911.
NISHIMURA, H., W.H. SAWYER, and R.F. NIGRELLI. 1976. Renin, cortisol and plasma volume in marine teleost fishes adapted to dilute media. J. Endocrinol. **70**: 47.
OGURI, M. 1978. Presence of juxtaglomerular cells in the holocephalan kidney. Gen. comp. Endocrinol. **36**: 170.
OGURI, M., M. OGAWA, and H. SOKABE. 1970. Absence of juxtaglomerular cells in the kidneys of Chondrichthyes and Cyclostomi. Bull. Jap. Soc. scient. Fish. **36**: 881.
OGURI, M., and H. SOKABE. 1974. Comparative histology of the corpuscles of Stannius and the juxtaglomerular cells in the kidneys of teleosts. Bull. Jap. Soc. scient. Fish. **40**: 545.
OPDYKE, D.F., R.G. CARROLL, N.E. KELLER, and A.A. TAYLOR. 1981. Angiotensin II releases catecholamines in dogfish. Comp. Biochem. Physiol. **70C**: 131.
OPDYKE, D.F., and R. HOLCOMBE. 1976. Response to angiotensin I and II and to AI-converting-enzyme inhibitor in a shark. Amer. J. Physiol. **231**: 1750.
OPDYKE, D.F., and R.F. HOLCOMBE. 1978. Effect of angiotensins and epinephrine on vascular resistance of isolated dogfish gut. Amer. J. Physiol. (Regulatory Integrative Comp. Physiol. 3) **234**: R196.
PEACH, M.J. 1977. Renin-angiotensin system: biochemistry and mechanisms of action. Physiol. Rev. **57**: 313.
REID, I.A. 1977. Is there a brain renin-angiotensin system? Circ. Res. **41**: 147.
SAWYER, W.H. 1968. Phylogenetic aspects of the neurohypophysial hormones. *In* Berde, B. [ed.] Handbook of experimental pharmacology. Springer Verlag, Berlin.

SAWYER, W.H. 1970. Vasopressor, diuretic, and natriuretic responses by lungfish to arginine vasotocin. Amer. J. Physiol. **218**: 1789.

SAWYER, W.H., J.R. BLAIR-WEST, P.A. SIMPSON and M.K. SAWYER. 1976. Renal responses of Australian lungfish to vasotocin, angiotensin II, and NaCl infusion. Amer. J. Physiol. **231**: 593.

SKEGGS, L.T., F.E. DORER, J.R. KAHN, K.E. LENTZ, and M. LEVINE. 1974. The biological production of angiotensin. *In* Page, I.H., and F.M. Bumpus [eds.] Angiotensin. Springer-Verlag, New York.

SOKABE, H. 1974. Phylogeny of the renal effects of angiotensin. Kidney Int. **6**: 263.

SOKABE, H., H. NISHIMURA, M. OGAWA, and M. OGURI. 1970. Determination of renin in the corpuscles of Stannius of the teleost. Gen. comp. Endocrinol. **14**: 510.

SOKABE, H., and M. OGAWA. 1974. Comparative studies of the juxtaglomerular apparatus. Int. Rev. Cytol. **37**: 271.

SOKABE, H., M. OGAWA, M. OGURI, and H. NISHIMURA. 1969. Evolution of the juxtaglomerular apparatus in the vertebrate kidneys. Texas Rep. Biol. Med. **27**: 3.

TAKEI, Y., T. HIRANO, and H. KOBAYASHI. 1979. Angiotensin and water intake in the Japanese eel, *Anguilla japonica*. Gen. comp. Endocrinol. **38**: 466.

TAKEMOTO, Y., T. NAKAJIMA, Y. HASEGAWA, T.X. WATANABE, H. SOKABE, S. KUMAGAE, and S. SAKAKIBARA. 1983. Chemical structures of angiotensins formed by incubating plasma with the kidney and the corpuscles of Stannius in the chum salmon, *Oncorynchus keta*. Gen. comp. Endocrinol. **51**: 219.

TAYLOR, A.A. 1977. Comparative physiology of the renin-angiotensin system. Fed. Proc. **36**: 1776.

TURKER, R.K., I.H. PAGE, and F.M. BUMPUS. 1974. Antagonists of angiotensin II. *In* Page, I.H., and F.M. Bumpus [eds.] Angiotensin. Springer-Verlag, New York.

VANE, J.R. 1974. The fate of angiotensin I. *In* Page, I.H., and F.M. Bumpus [eds.] Angiotensin. Springer-Verlag, New York.

WILSON, J.X. 1984. The renin-angiotensin system in nonmammalian vertebrates. Endocrine Rev. **5**: 45.

EVOLUTIONARY ASPECTS OF REPRODUCTION IN CYCLOSTOMES AND CARTILAGINOUS FISHES

J.M. Dodd and M.H.I. Dodd

School of Animal Biology
University College of North Wales
Bangor, Gwynedd, U.K.

Introduction

In this paper we examine what is known of selected morphological and physiological aspects of reproduction in cyclostomes and chondrichthyan fishes and attempt to evaluate the contribution this makes to our knowledge of the ways in which reproduction may have evolved in these animals and in general. The reproductive biology of both groups is of exceptional interest in this context in view of their long phylogenetic history, their long separation from each other, and the diverse range of reproductive specializations they have adopted. Not only are both groups phylogenetically ancient, they both contain two subgroups which are themselves old. The cyclostomes are classified into myxinoids (hagfish) and petromyzonids (lampreys) and, according to Jarvik (1968), their probable respective ancestors, the heterostracans and cephalaspids, diverged during the Pre-Cambrian period, more than 600 million years ago. The chondrichthyans are subdivided into elasmobranchs (sharks and rays) and holocephalans (chimaeras and ratfishes). These are probably sister groups, sharing a common ancestor from which they diverged some 350 million years ago (see Dodd, 1983 for references). As might be expected, the basic difference in ancestry between cyclostomes and chondrichthyans is reflected in the reproductive structures and functions of the two groups.

There are relatively few extant species of cyclostomes (about 40 species of lampreys and 30 of hagfishes) and holocephalans (6 genera and 28 species); the elasmobranchs are much better represented in the contemporary fauna (128 genera and 600 species). For a number of reasons, the two groups that are the subject of the present paper have received much less research attention than the 20,000 species of teleost fish. This is a major constraint in the present exercise; generalisations are vulnerable and findings of major significance in the search for evolutionary trends certainly still await discovery. There are other constraints: neither physiological processes nor soft tissues are recorded in the fossil record, and animals are opportunists in their physiology. Consequently, the evidence with which we are dealing is indirect and therefore conclusions are speculative. Furthermore, as the physiological problems faced by animals have changed, so have the ways in which they are solved, though within the limits set by the biochemical pathways available. Convergent evolution has certainly occurred. It therefore follows that outgroup comparisons between contemporary animals, in an attempt to identify phylogenetic relationships, must be made cautiously; similarities do not necessarily indicate relationships. The similarities that have recently been discovered between elasmobranchs and the coelacanth illustrates the point (see Løvtrup, 1977 for a discussion). Løvtrup enumerates ten characters of the soft anatomy that are shared by the two and writes: "For the reader brought up with the notion that Chondrichthyes and Osteichthyes are two separate and quite distinct taxa this list may not be very impressive." At the same time, he appears to indicate that, in the absence of support for other classificatory alternatives, this evidence may be used to support, for the time being, the idea that Chondrichthyes and Actinistia (coelacanths) are secondary twins. This suggestion that physiological similarities may be used as supporting evidence in phylogenetic studies may be applicable generally.

In the present context, it may be relevant also that the reproductive system is unique in being the only one in the body which is not essential for the individual; indeed, in some cases the individual may be better off without it (F.L. Hisaw Sr., personal reflections). This may have a bearing on the magnitude of mutations that can be tolerated since they would be less likely to be lethal, and, in turn, this might have affected the rate at which the reproductive system evolved. It may account, for example, at least in part, for the apparent ease with which elasmobranchs have achieved viviparity on so many separate occasions in widely separated taxa.

The concept of 'primitiveness' assumes particular importance in connection with the cyclostomes. Extant hagfishes are usually accepted as primitive yet, as we shall see, their ovary is one of the most sophisticated in the vertebrate series. Also, the question arises as to whether some systems may have degenerated during evolutionary time from a more advanced condition because they were no longer necessary. For example, the absence of hypothalamic control of the pituitary in modern hagfish could be either primitive or derived. It is possible to imagine that earlier hagfish, living in shallow seas and having cyclical reproduction, had a hypophyseal portal system and hypothalamic control of pituitary gonadotrophic activity which were lost when they changed to a deep sea habitat in which there was thermal constancy and perpetual darkness.

Contemporary Chondrichthyes also usually are said to be primitive. Certainly their morphological evolution appears to have been conservative and it may be that many characters have been retained with little change. In support of this, Cappetta (1980) has recently, albeit tentatively, placed two Cretaceous elasmobranchs in the genus *Scyliorhinus*. However, the reproductive physiology of extant species is often sophisticated and in them the following reproductive processes either make their appearance for the first time in the vertebrate series or become well established: internal fertilization; the vertebrate pattern of gonadal sex-differentiation; viviparity and placentation. Furthermore, many aspects of reproduction in cartilaginous fishes, including gonadogenesis, sex-determination, origin of the reproductive ducts, low ovarian fecundity and uterine gestation are more closely similar to the situation found in amphibians and amniotes than in other fishes.

With these and other considerations in mind, we shall examine selected aspects of the reproductive biology of these two groups of 'lower' vertebrates, in particular, the ovary, secondary sex characters, brain-pituitary-gonad inter-relations, and viviparity and discuss them in the context of evolution.

Cyclostomata

The ovary of cyclostomes

It is generally accepted, though on the basis of indirect evidence (Gorbman, 1983), that hagfish breed over several years, whereas lampreys spawn only once in their lifetime and then die. These different patterns of reproduction undoubtedly account for some of the differences that are found between the ovaries of the two groups of cyclostomes.

The hagfish ovary. The level of sophistication achieved by the hagfish ovary (Fig. 1b,c) is truly remarkable for an animal that is said to be primitive; Gorbman (1983) has described the morphology of the ovary of *Eptatretus stouti*. The stroma is sparse and consists of a thin membranous curtain of tissue attached to the dorsal body wall on one side of the gut. The presumptive oogonia occupy the ventral margin of the ovary and from these oocytes proliferate, which are believed to give rise to successive clutches of eggs. As these mature, they appear to move dorsalwards and when they reach a diameter of 2-3 mm folliculogenesis starts. At first the follicles are spherical, but soon they assume the elongated ovoid shape characteristic of the mature oocyte and begin to protrude from the surface of the ovary, becoming 'stalked'. By the end of the growth phase, they reach a length of 25 mm. Tsuneki and Gorbman (1977) have described the ultrastructure of the ovary of *Eptatretus stouti* and reviewed earlier relevant literature. They found that the follicular wall, as in other vertebrates, consists of a granulosa and a double-layered theca; they also described the structure of post-ovulatory follicles (Fig. 1c) and pre-ovulatory atretic follicles. However, no cells having the ultrastructure of steroid-secreting cells were identified in any of the ovarian constituents examined. This is a point of considerable significance since steroid secretion is an important function of all other vertebrate ovaries, including lampreys. As Tsuneki and Gorbman point out, their observations do not conclusively exclude the possibility that the hagfish ovary has a steroidogenic function. Moreover, sex steroids have been demonstrated in hagfish plasma, though in exceedingly small amounts and not in all the animals examined.

A unique feature of the hagfish follicle is its ability to secrete a 'shell' around the oocyte; not merely a simple investment, but one with a micropyle for sperm entry and, at each pole, a fan-like array of hooks. Another feature of the hagfish ovary, attesting to its sophistication, is its ability to restrict, by controlled atresia, each clutch of developing oocytes to approximately 20, from the considerable number that enter the growth phase. Gorbman and Dickhoff (1978) have examined the nature of this selection process. The point of interest in the present context is that, as in the mammals and most other vertebrates, atresia is the mechanism by

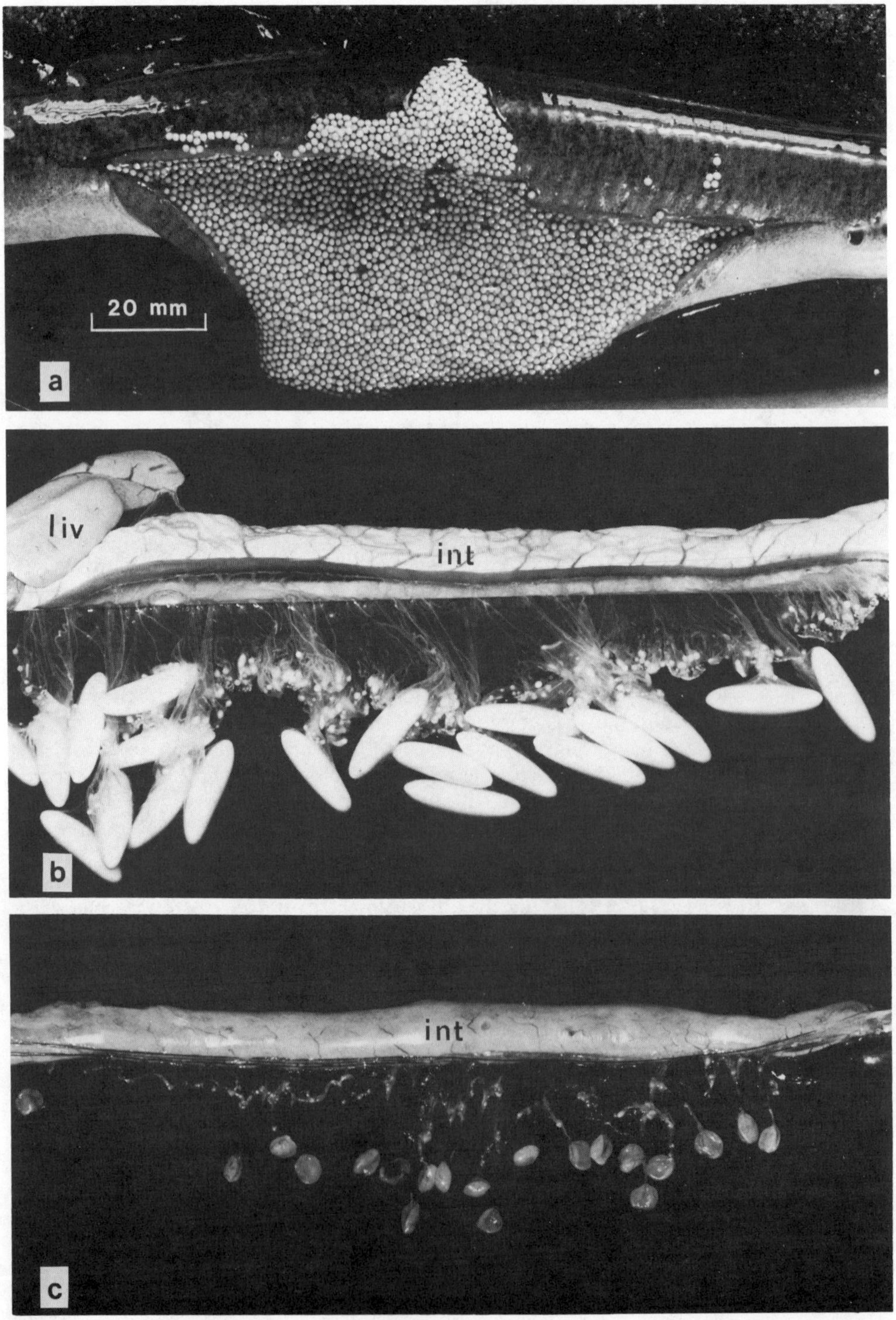
20 mm
a
liv
int
b
int
c

which the appropriate number of oocytes are selected for further development from the many contenders.

Patzner (1978) reports that the post-ovulatory follicles in hagfish show no signs of secretory activity; they merely shrink and are ultimately removed, presumably by phagocytes. The process is slow and Patzner records that some animals may have three generations of resorbing post-ovulatory follicles in their ovaries.

Vitellogenesis is an important function of the hagfish ovary and it has recently been shown that, as in all other vertebrates, oestrogens stimulate hepatic vitellogenesis in hagfish of both sexes (Yu *et al.*, 1981). Furthermore, Turner *et al.* (1982) have demonstrated that liver cells of mature *Eptatretus stouti* have a single class of high affinity nuclear receptors for oestrogens. As Gorbman (1983) has pointed out, a shared property like this between lampreys and hagfishes, which themselves diverged some 400 million years ago, must indicate that oestrogenic stimulation of vitelloprotein synthesis by the liver is a phylogenetically ancient function.

The lamprey ovary. Ovarian morphology in lampreys (Fig. 1a) has been described in detail by a number of authors (Lewis and McMillan, 1965; Busson-Mabillot, 1967a,b; Hardisty, 1979; Dodd and Sumpter, 1984). In *Lampetra planeri*, the brook lamprey, the ovary is unpaired and lobulated and it virtually fills the body cavity at maturity. Stroma is sparse and the follicles develop synchronously. The follicle wall, as in other vertebrates, consists of a granulosa in contact with the oocyte, a two-layered theca and an outer investment of squamous cells. The granulosa is exceptional among vertebrates in being restricted to one pole of the follicle, the oocyte sitting in it like an egg in an egg cup. Ovarian fecundity varies widely; Hardisty (1971) recognizes four distinct levels in lampreys, ranging between 170,000 eggs in *Petromyzon marinus* to as few as 500-2,500 in the non-parasitic freshwater *Lampetra planeri*. Even the latter is appreciably more fecund than the hagfishes, which produce clutches of 20-30 eggs.

Atresia is a feature of the lamprey ovary, as of all other vertebrate ovaries, but in most species, other than *Petromyzon marinus*, it is restricted to oocytes in early meiotic prophase. Hardisty (1971) has estimated that in *Lampetra planeri* as many as 80% of the oocytes that enter meiotic prophase undergo atresia, recalling the situation in mammals. The spent ovary of lampreys consists merely of stroma and post-ovulatory follicles. Since the animals die immediately after spawning, there is no possibility that the latter have any function.

Fig. 1. Cyclostome ovaries. *a*. Ovary of *Petromyzon fluviatilis* at the time of ovulation (From Dodd, 1972). *b*. Mature ovary of *Eptatretus stouti*, adult female, 58 cm long, eggs 22-24 mm in length. Note small eggs developing along the free ventral edge of the ovary and more dorsal atretic follicles (From Gorbman, 1983). *int*, intestine; *liv*, liver. *c*., Ovary of *Myxine glutinosa* after ovulation showing corpora lutea and corpora atretica (photograph by Dr. Finn Walvig, from Dodd, 1972).

Secondary sexual characters

Myxinoids have no recognisable external secondary sexual characters; this is not unique among vertebrates, though it is unusual. The absence of oviducts, however, is shared only with lampreys. In both groups the genital products are shed through openings in the posterior regions of the urinary ducts which become patent at the time of spawning.

In lampreys, both sexes develop secondary sexual characters, though these involve mainly modifications of existing structures (Dodd *et al.*, 1960). In both sexes, the fins enlarge at the time of sexual maturity, the two dorsal fins becoming contiguous; a post-anal fin appears ventrally in the female. Cloacal labia develop in both males and females, and a penis-like structure, erectile by vasodilation, develops in the cloacal region. The tail of the female curves sharply upwards at sexual maturity and in the male there is a slight downward curvature. These sexual characters have been shown to be under the influence of sex hormones as in other vertebrates. Hypophysectomy prevents their appearance though, presumably, this is a secondary effect since treatment with sex hormones causes them to reappear.

Regulation of reproduction by pituitary gland hypothalamus

In all vertebrates other than hagfishes, and to some extent lampreys, hypothalamus and pituitary glands have well-defined roles in the control of reproduction. The hypothalamus receives cues from both the internal and the external environment, transduces them and translates them into surges of gonadotrophin - releasing hormone (GnRH) which are carried to the pituitary by a short loop vascular link, the hypophysial portal system, here to release gonadotrophin. It seems unlikely that a system as complicated as this was present in the early vertebrates, and it is of interest to ask to what extent contemporary cyclostomes have the cellular and anatomical bases through which such functions could be mediated.

In hagfishes, Matty *et al.* (1976) found no evidence for the existence of a gonadotrophic hormone in the pituitary gland of *Eptatretus stouti*. Animals from which the pituitary had been removed completed vitellogenesis, ovulated and laid apparently normal eggs. Furthermore, studies on the vasculature and innervation of the hypothalamo-hypophysial region of *E. stouti* have failed to demonstrate either a hypophysial portal system, or nervous connections to the pituitary (Gorbman, 1965). Also, an immunocytochemical search for immunoreactive GnRH in *E. stouti* (Crim *et al.*, 1979a) and *E. burgeri* (Nozaki and Kobayashi, 1979) failed to yield any evidence that the releaser was present. However, there have been some studies in which minor effects of hypophysectomy on the gonads have been noted (Patzner and Ichikawa, 1977) and it has been tentatively suggested that a median eminence-like structure may be present in the hypothalamus of *E. burgeri* (Kobayashi, 1972). However, in view of the absence of demonstrable gonadotrophin in the hagfish pituitary and the similar absence of immunoreactive GnRH in the brain, it must be concluded, on present evidence, that the hypothalamus and pituitary play little or no part in reproductive control in hagfish (see Gorbman, 1983). This is perhaps surprising in the case of *E. burgeri* which is a cyclical breeder and might therefore be expected to have some degree of hypothalamic control.

In lampreys, the situation is different and there are some signs of advances towards the situation found in other vertebrates. The adenohypophysis of the lamprey pituitary is clearly subdivided into rostral and proximal pars distalis and pars intermedia, though there is no segregated lobe such as is found in the chondrichthyan fishes. Histochemical studies and partial hypophysectomy have shown that the main gonadotrophic lobe of the pituitary is the proximal pars distalis (Evennett and Dodd, 1963; Larsen, 1969). However, removal of the lobe, unlike hypophysectomy in other vertebrates, does not halt gametogenesis, it has merely a rate-limiting effect; in both sexes the process goes to completion though at a slower pace. It appears that the pituitary has not fully 'captured' the gonads at this stage of evolution, though hypophysectomy prevents the appearance of the secondary sexual characters, which are steroid-dependent (Dodd *et al.*, 1960; Evennett and Dodd, 1963; Larsen, 1969).

As in hagfish, there is no hypophysial portal system in lampreys nor are there any nervous connections between pituitary and hypothalamus (Gorbman, 1965; Tsuneki and Gorbman, 1975a,b). However, Crim *et al.* (1979a,b) have shown that immunoreactive GnRH is present in the lamprey hypothalamus (*Entosphenus tridentata* and *Lampetra richardsoni*) and that it varies in amount with the state of sexual maturity. In the absence of hypothalamo-hypophysial links, it must be assumed that the GnRH reaches the pituitary either by a systemic route or by simple diffusion. The absence of a feed-back mechanism between gonads and hypothalamus (Larsen, 1974), and the fact that lampreys kept in darkness at a constant temperature showed normal sexual development and cyclicity (Larsen, 1978) throws further doubt on the existence of a hypothalamo-hypophysial axis, though the situation must be regarded as unresolved.

Evolutionary considerations

The extant cyclostomes, as we have already indicated, are probably not good animals from which to draw evolutionary conclusions. The contemporary myxinoids may well be secondarily degenerate and give no clue to the earlier reproductive adaptations, and lamprey reproduction is unique in that they breed only once and then die. The suggestions made here must be evaluated in the light of these reservations.

The marked differences in reproductive patterns, structures and physiology between hagfishes and lampreys support the view, based on other lines of evidence (Jarvik, 1968; Stensiö, 1968), that the two groups are diphyletic in origin. Yet, they also have a good deal in common. Features that may testify to an ancient link between them, or to the fact that the structures and functions they share are themselves ancient, are: ovarian structure is basically similar, though superficially different; sex steroids appear to be present in both, at low titre in myxinoids, though this does not necessarily indicate a low functional level (Gorbman, 1983); oestrogen-stimulated, liver-based, vitellogenesis is found in both, as in all non-mammalian vertebrates; atresia of oocytes, a universal phenomenon in vertebrates, is encountered in both groups and, at least in myxinoids, appears to have an important function; post-ovulatory follicles, a concomitant of ovulation, may be destined only for resorption. They are clearly functionless in lampreys, and in myxinoids there is no information as to whether they subserve any function.

In myxinoids, a structure is present at the base of hypothalamus which has been called a pituitary. However, in view of the recent embryological studies of Gorbman (this volume), in which it is shown to be endodermal in origin, and earlier work in which no adenohypophysial functions could be ascribed to it, it is probably neither the structural nor the functional homologue of the vertebrate adenohypophysis. This structure and its functions, if any, and the absence of GnRH from the hagfish hypothalamus, must clearly be given full consideration in future studies on the evolution of the pituitary and its relationships with the brain.

The absence of oviducts of paramesonephric origin in the two groups is not unique; they are absent also in the teleosts, though here they are replaced by posterior extensions of the ovarian wall. It may be suggested that the early vertebrates, like present day cyclostomes, made use of existing renal ducts which, at the appropriate time, acquired perforations between coelom and urinary sinus through which the genital products were shed.

Finally, we may note that, although provisions for internal fertilisation are absent in contemporary hagfish, a penis-like structure, erectile by vasodilation, is present in lampreys, though not used for intromission of sperm.

Chondrichthyes

The ovary in Chondrichthyes

The vertebrate ovary shows extreme morphological variation both between, and within, species at different times of the year but is virtually invariable in basic structure. Indeed, it could have been the ovary that Milne Edwards had in mind when he wrote: "Nature is profligate in variety but niggard in invention"!

The elasmobranch ovary. The elasmobranch ovary (Fig. 2a,b) resembles closely that of all vertebrates with yolky eggs. Even in viviparous species and, as we have said, these constitute a considerable majority, the oocytes are usually heavily yolked, though they vary considerably in size at the time of ovulation. In *Scoliodon sorrakowah*, they are about 1 mm in diameter, whereas in *Chlamydoselachus anguineus* they may reach 120 mm and each female contains 12 of these (Gudger, 1940, quoted by Wourms, 1977). Unlike many teleosts, ovarian fecundity is low. In *Squalus acanthias*, which is ovoviviparous, of 50 eggs which initially become vitellogenic, only seven or so are ovulated; the rest becoming atretic. In *Scyliorhinus canicula*, an oviparous species, about 30 are ovulated during the extended breeding season, and in the placental *Carcharhinus dussumieri* only two are ovulated.

→

Fig. 2. *a. Scyliorhinus canicula*, ventral view of a partly dissected mature ovary (From Dodd, 1983). *b. S. canicula*, mature ovary from which vitellogenic eggs have been removed and placed peripherally to show the paired hierarchy (From Dodd, 1983). *c. Hydrolagus colliei*, paired ovaries; note size hierarchy. *E*, epigonal organ; *O*, follicular oocyte; *pof.*, post-ovulatory follicle.

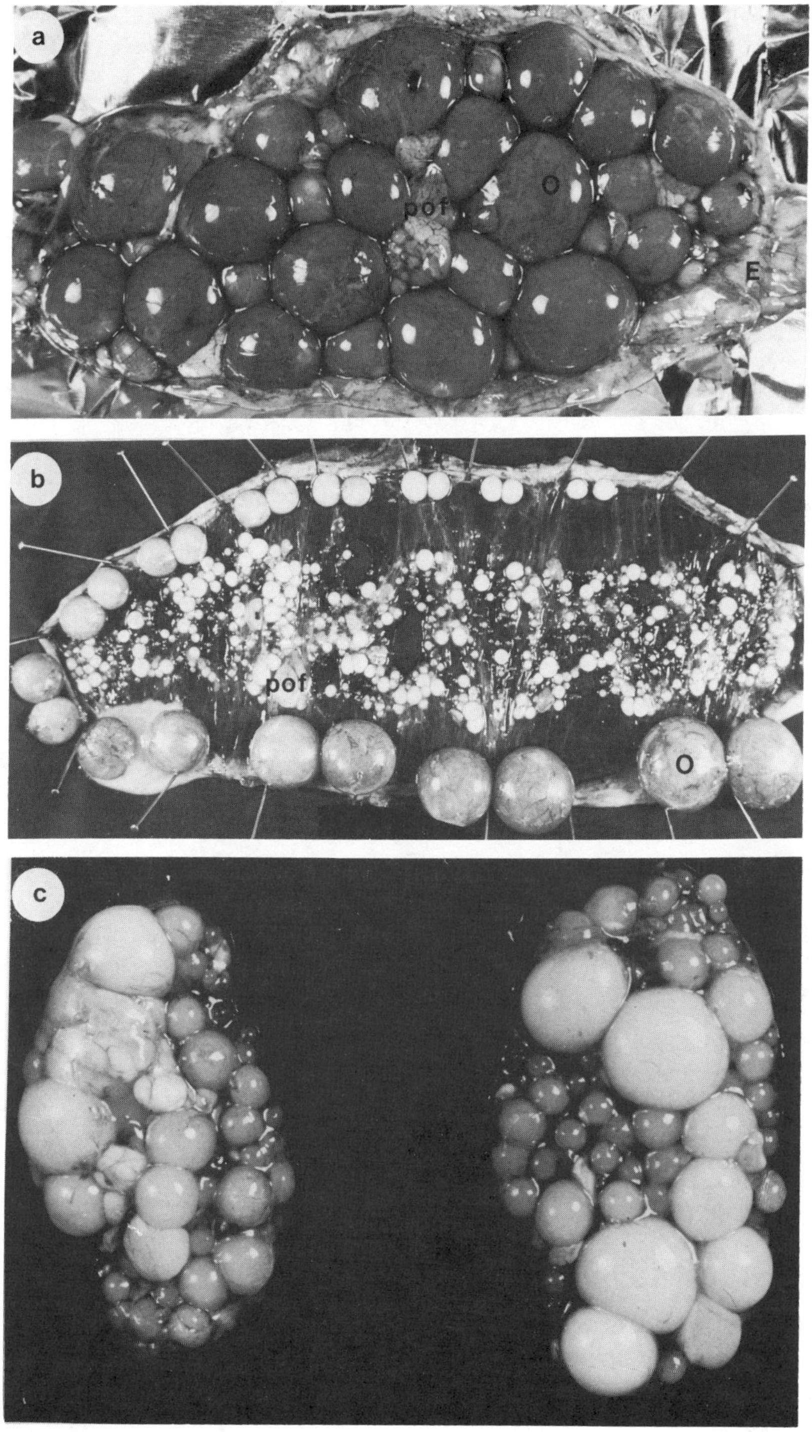
a
pof
O
E
b
pof
O
c

The single ovary of *Scyliorhinus canicula* (Dodd, 1972, 1977; Fig. 2a,b) is typical of most elasmobranchs, even those that are viviparous. It develops from the right primordium and is suspended from the dorsal body wall by the mesovarium. An unusual feature of the elasmobranch gonad, though not of the holocephalan, is its close association with an investment of haemopoietic tissue, the epigonal organ; the stromal and germinal elements of the ovary seem to be embedded in the latter. The stroma is sparse and the germinal elements in the fully developed ovary consist of yolky oocytes, ranging in weight from 2.5 g to a few mg arranged in a paired-size hierarchy, pre-vitellogenic oocytes, corpora atretica and post ovulatory follicles. As in all other vertebrates, except bony fishes and reptiles, there are no oogonia. The follicular investments consist of a single layered granulosa, a two layered theca and an outer squamous investment. The theca interna is separated from the follicle by a basement membrane which supports a rich vasculature. These are constituents of the vitellogenic follicles of all vertebrates. Some of the vessels are perforated, and yolk precursors are believed to pass through the perforations and across the basement membrane to reach the oocyte *via* spaces between follicle cells and to be incorporated into the oocyte by micropinocytosis. The oocyte communicates with the granulosa by means of interdigitating villi which form a zona radiata (see Dodd, 1983).

As in all other vertebrates, the ovary may contain atretic follicles (corpora atretica) in which the oocyte has died and is being removed by phagocytic invasion by the granulosa cells. Atresia affects previtellogenic as well as vitellogenic follicles. In the former case it may serve to limit the size of the annual 'clutch'; in the latter it removes yolky eggs which for some reason have lost their integrity or failed to be ovulated. Various authors have, on the basis of indirect evidence, ascribed an endocrine function to these bodies and others believe that they are merely engaged in removing moribund oocytes. Dodd (1983) has reviewed the evidence for a hormonal function and shown it to be inconclusive.

The mature ovulating elasmobranch ovary also contains post-ovulatory follicles, sometimes called 'corpora lutea', an unfortunate term since it suggests homology with mammalian corpora lutea which are functional endocrine structures. In the majority of elasmobranchs these structures are merely resorbed or removed by phagocytes. Shrinkage of the follicle after ovulation gives the impression of an increase in granulosa cell activity, though mitoses are not seen, and the presence of steroidogenic enzymes probably represents merely previous activity which persists for a day or two after ovulation before the granulosa cells die and are resorbed. However, Chieffi (1967) believes that 'true' corpora lutea (that is, in the mammalian functional sense) are found in some elasmobranchs, both oviparous and viviparous, and that these may develop from either corpora atretica or post-ovulatory follicles. This is an important point, bearing on the evolution of corpora lutea, but the evidence for a functional role is both indirect and contradictory.

The holocephalan ovary. The holocephalan ovary (Fig. 2c), unlike that of most elasmobranchs, is paired. General accounts of the development and histological structure of the ovaries of *Chimaera monstrosa* and *Hydrolagus colliei* have been provided by Vu Tan Tue (1972) and Stanley (1963) respectively. The fine structure of the holocephalan ovary is unknown, though histological studies have established that, at the light microscope level, ovarian structure is virtually identical in the two chondrichthyan groups. In gross morphology also they are closely similar, and both show a paired size hierarchy. The two largest follicles, next in line for ovulation, may be both in the same ovary or there may be one in each ovary.

As in elasmobranchs, corpora atretica are usually present in mature, egg-laying females; post-ovulatory follicles are also found. Hisaw and Hisaw (1959) have described the histology of these structures in *Hydrolagus colliei*, but their function, if other than removal of moribund follicles, is unknown. We have seen that in most elasmobranchs the ovary is closely associated with and, indeed, embedded in a mass of lymphomyeloid tissue, the epigonal organ (Fänge and Mattison, 1981; Dodd, 1983); such an association is absent in holocephalans.

Secondary sexual characters

In chondrichthyan fishes, as in other vertebrates, secondary sexual characters, morphological, physiological and behavioural, are present. In the female, the external morphological characters are restricted to body shape and a more spacious glandular cloaca. The internal characters comprise the oviducts and extensive ciliation of the peritoneal epithelium. The specialised oviducts are a marked advance on the situation found in cyclostomes. They are said by Chieffi (1967) to be derived from kidney ducts by longitudinal division of the mesonephric (Wolffian) ducts; this nephric origin is more in line with the derivation of the oviduct in the rest of the vertebrates, other than teleosts, though in these, it develops from the paramesonephric (Mullerian) ducts which arise *de novo* alongside the mesonephric ducts. The oviducts open anteriorly into the body cavity *via* the ostium, a surviving nephrostome of a pronephric tubule (Balinsky, 1981), and posteriorly into the cloaca in the mature female. The oviducts are simple tubes in immature females, but they subsequently undergo a degree of regional differentiation which varies with the mode of reproduction (Figs. 3,4,5), additional modifications occurring to accomodate pregnancy (Figs. 4,5).

In the male, the most striking external secondary sexual characters are the claspers. These are derived from the margins of the pelvic fins and used, in conjunction with muscular sacs or siphons, for intromission of sperm (see Wourms, 1977 and Dodd and Sumpter, 1984). They have a skeleton of articulated cartilaginous rods which, with fin tissue, form a pair of scroll-like tubes. Claspers have a long evolutionary history though they are not universally found in early chondrichthyans (Løvtrup, 1977). However, they appear to have been present in cladodonts, hybodonts (*Xenacanthus*) and all the Jurassic sharks except *Chladoselache* (Breder and Rosen, 1966; Schaeffer, 1967). The reproductive ducts in male chondrichthyans, as in most vertebrates, consist of modified pro- and mesonephric (Wolffian) ducts.

The situation in female holocephalans *vis à vis* secondary sexual characters is identical to that found in female elasmobranchs. In the male, in addition to well-developed claspers, there is an erectile frontal tentacle, the swollen extremity of which is covered with recurved hooks and which is, presumably, used in copulation. The oviducts of holocephalans are closely similar to those of elasmobranchs though, unlike the latter, they open separately on the body surface, not into the cloaca; this is considered to be more primitive.

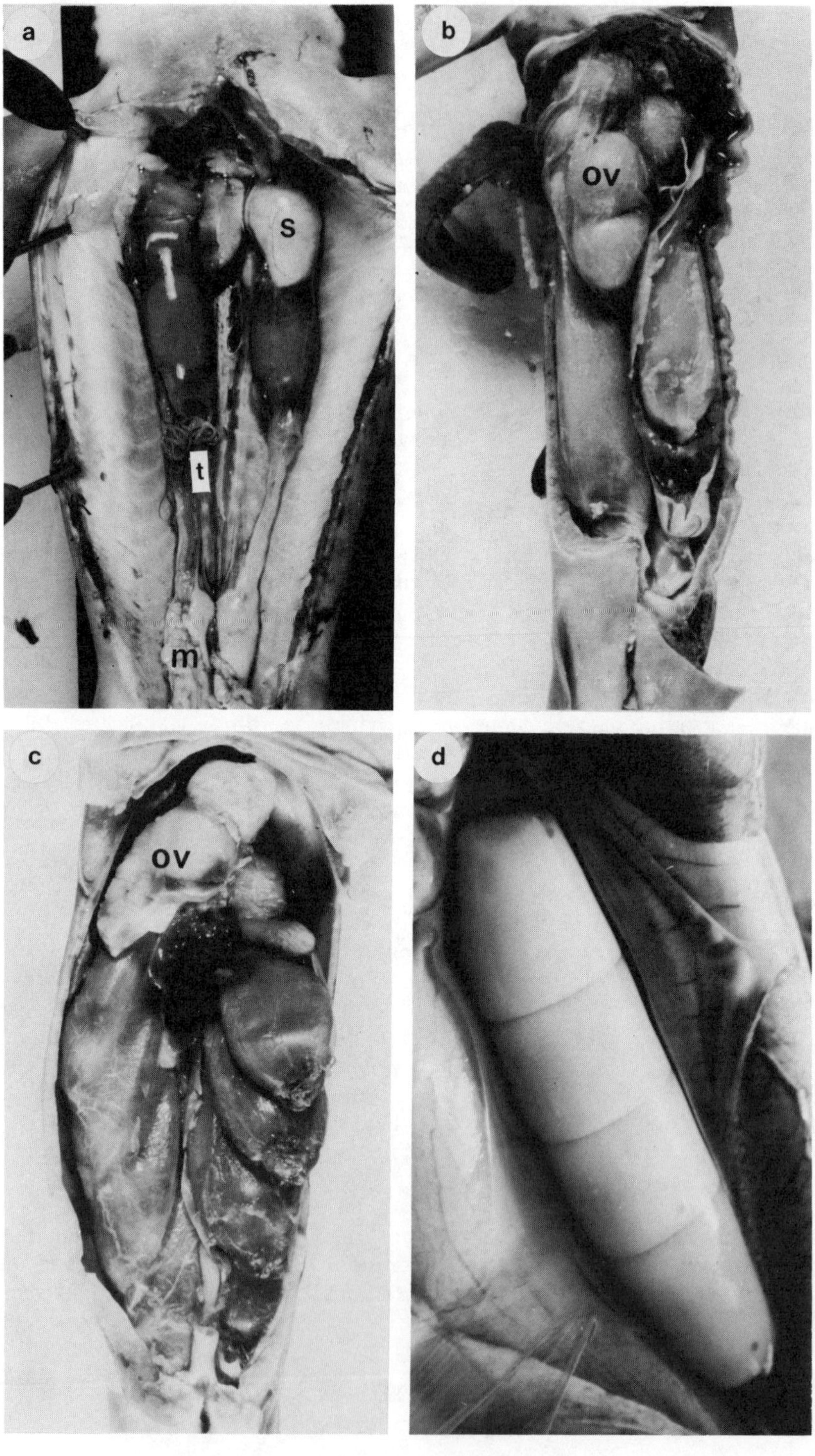
a
S
t
m
b
ov
c
ov
d

Fig. 3. *a. S. canicula*, mature female dissected to show the two oviducts, each containing a shelled egg; right oviduct opened. Note shell ('purse') with prominent tendrils for attachment to substratum during lengthy incubation. *b. Proscyllium haberari*. As in *S. canicula*, each oviduct contains only a single shelled egg at any one time but they are retained during incubation. Note absence of tendrils. (Left oviduct opened). *c. Halaelurus burgeri*. Here, each oviduct contains four shelled eggs; all are retained during incubation. Note very reduced tendrils. (Left oviduct opened). *d. Squalus acanthias*. Oviduct opened to show 'candle' consisting of four heavily yoked eggs enclosed in a membranous sheath. These are retained throughout the 22 month gestation period. *m*, muscular segment of oviduct; *ov*, ovary; *s*, shell gland; *t*, posterior tendrils of egg case.

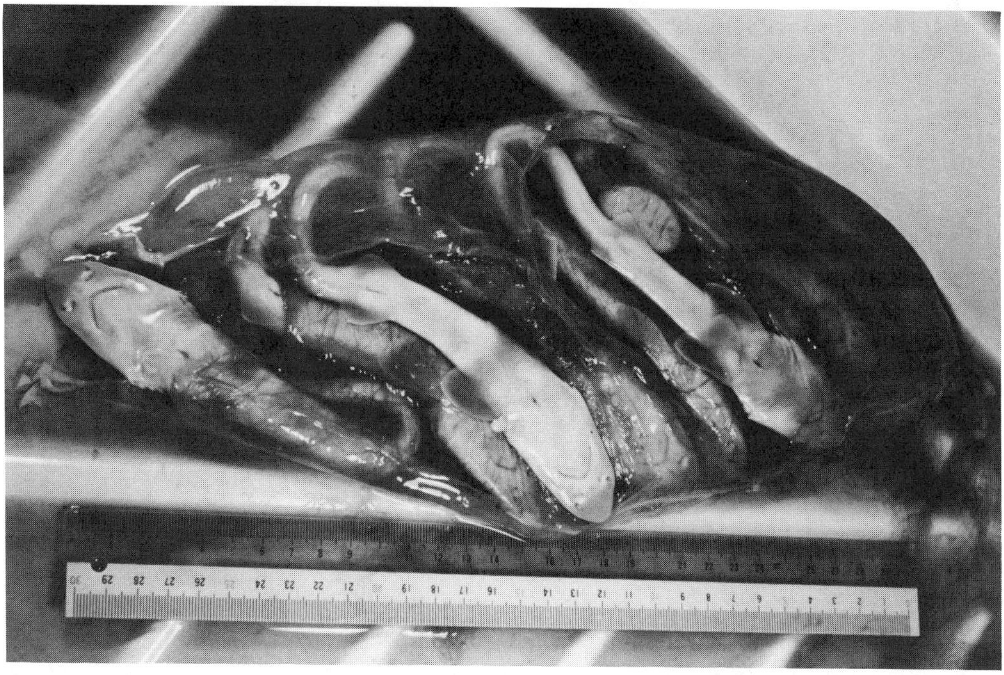

Fig. 4. Late embryos of the aplacental shark *Mustelus manazo* lying in uterine compartments (photograph by courtesy of Dr. K. Teshima).

Thus, in Chondrichthyes, especially in the male, well developed secondary sex characters are present. These appear to be somatic structures, only partly under the control of sex hormones (Dodd and Goddard, 1960). In support of this view, we have recently encountered a male *Hydrolagus* with a large tumour in the region of

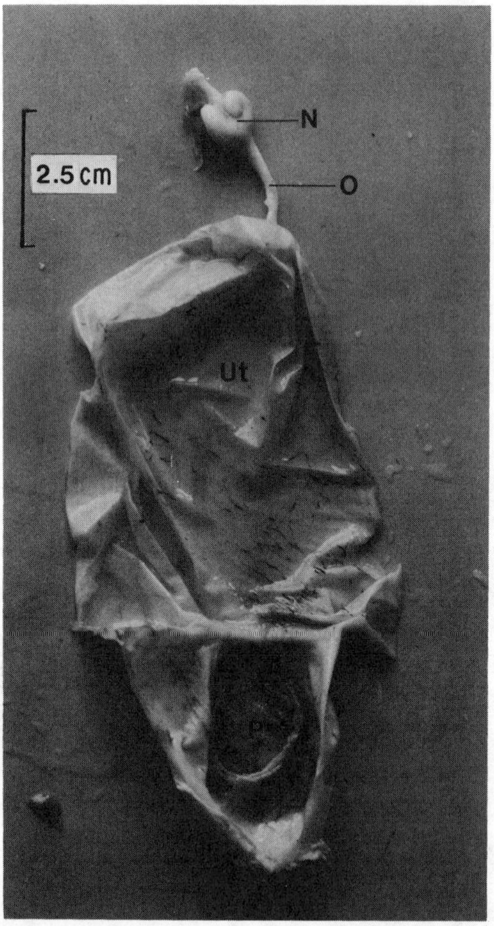

Fig. 5. *Carcharhinus dussumieri*, a placental shark. Oviduct ('uterus') dissected to show maternal region of the placenta (*P*). *N*, nidamentary gland; *O*, upper oviduct; *Ut*, uterus. (From Teshima and Mizue, 1972).

the gonadotrophic lobe of the pituitary (see below) which had apparently destroyed the latter. Although this fish was fully grown, indeed, larger than is usual for males, its gonads and reproductive ducts were completely undifferentiated, yet the claspers were developed. This 'natural' experiment argues in favour of the view that the claspers are somatic characters which came under the influence of sex hormones at some stage of evolution.

Regulation of reproduction by pituitary gland and hypothalamus

The pituitary gland of elasmobranchs and holocephalans (Fig. 6a,b) is subdivided into separate lobes to a degree that is not found in other vertebrates

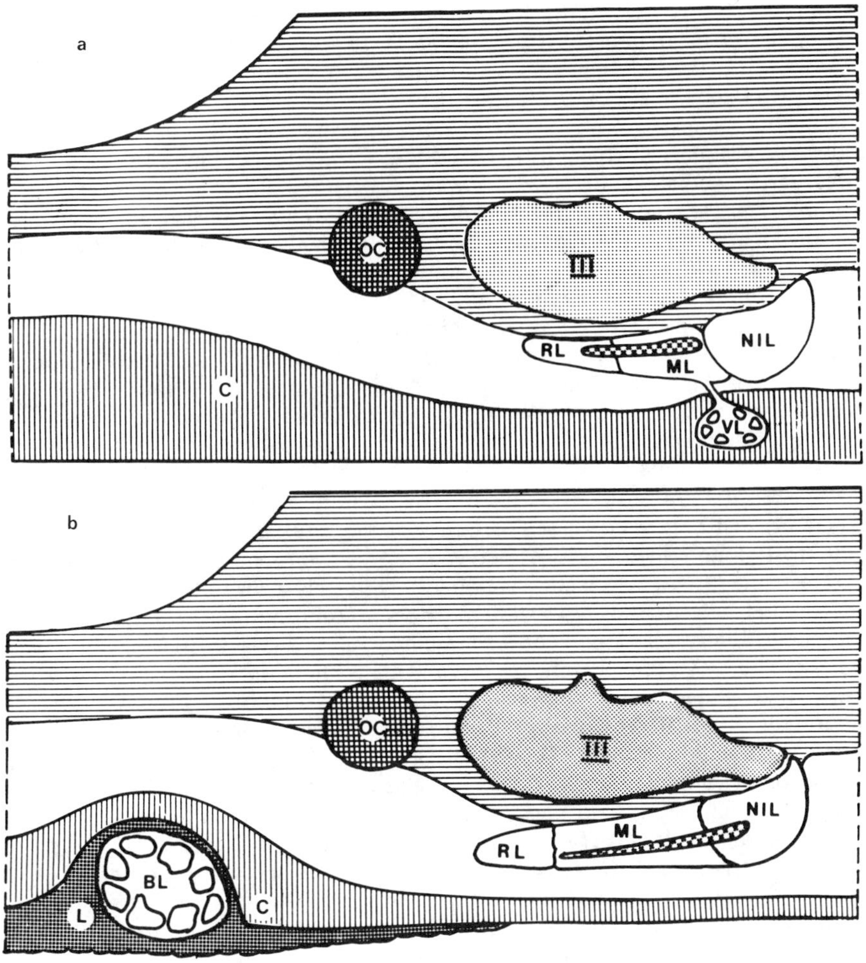

Fig. 6. Diagrammatic sagittal sections of an elasmobranch (*a*) and a holocephalan (*b*) pituitary gland and associated structures to show positions and relationships of the individual lobes. *BL*, buccal lobe; *RL*, rostral lobe; *ML*, median lobe; *NIL*, neurointermediate lobe; *VL*, ventral lobe; *C*, cartilage of the roof of the mouth; *L*, lymphoid tissue; *OC*, optic chiasma; *III*, third ventricle.

(Norris, 1941; Dodd, 1975, 1983; Holmes and Ball, 1974; Knowles *et al.*, 1975). The intracranial lobes, rostral, median and neuro-intermediate, are separated from the ventral lobe (in elasmobranchs) and buccal lobe (in holocephalans), though in the former, a slender stalk of tissue connects the ventral lobe with the posterior region of the median lobe. The ventral lobe in Squaliformes (sharks and dogfishes) lies embedded in the cartilage of the floor of the skull, whereas in Rajiformes (skates and rays), it lies in a superficial groove, is largely intracranial and has a broader connection with the median lobe. In mature Holocephali, the buccal lobe is completely isolated in a ventral-facing cavity in the roof of the mouth. In the context of this paper it is important to note that the isolated lobes are the main gonadotrophic regions of the pituitary (Dodd *et al.*, 1960; Sumpter *et al.*, 1978; Knowles *et al.*, 1975; Dodd *et al.*, 1982). Bioassay studies have shown that in *Scyliorhinus canicula* 98.8% of the gonadotrophic activity of the pituitary resides in the ventral lobe, 0.3% in the median lobe and 0.9% in the neuro-intermediate lobe. In *Hydrolagus colliei* the buccal lobe was found to contain more than 95% of the total gonadotrophic activity (Dodd *et al.*, 1982). We have raised an antibody to the partially purified gonadotrophin of *S. canicula*, and extracted a gonadotrophin from the buccal lobes of *H. colliei*. The former, whilst it neutralises the steroidogenic effect of dogfish gonadotrophin *in vivo*, does not cross-react with the ratfish hormone. Clearly, a degree of specificity has evolved in the two hormones over evolutionary time.

A structural feature of the hypophyseal complex of these fish that is of particular interest here is the vascularisation of the pituitary gland. It seems likely that the rostral and median lobes have a portal blood supply as in most other vertebrates, since there is a well-developed median eminence of two regions. But the ventral and buccal lobes are supplied directly from the internal carotid arteries. Thus it seems likely that any hypothalamic control of the activities of these lobes must be exerted *via* the peripheral circulation. There is no unequivocal direct evidence that gonadotrophin-releasing hormone (GnRH) is produced by the elasmobranch hypothalamus, though there is a good deal of indirect evidence (King and Millar, 1979, 1980). The latter authors found a higher-than-usual concentration of immunoreactive GnRH in elasmobranch systemic blood, a finding that may give some support to the possibility that it is delivered to the isolated lobe by a systemic route. In a different approach, we recently have shown that systemic injection of extracts of dogfish hypothalamus elevates circulatory sex steroid levels, as does synthetic mammalian GnRH (Jenkins and Dodd, 1980). Furthermore, hypothalamic extracts and synthetic GnRH induce ovulation in the dogfish, and the latter is equally effective in *Hydrolagus colliei.*

Jenkins and Dodd (1980) have shown, using radioreceptor assays of cytosol and autoradiography, that the hypothalamus of *S. canicula* contains oestrogen-specific receptors, though, unlike the situation in mammals, they are absent from the pituitary. Thus, an oestrogen feedback system is established in the dogfish, though it appears to be based mainly in the hypothalamus.

Evolutionary considerations

Three aspects of the role of hypothalamus and pituitary in reproduction in extant cartilaginous fishes call for comment in the context of evolution: the segregated gonadotrophic lobe of the pituitary, its non-portal blood supply, and the question of the gonadotrophic hormones and their releasers. Subdivisions of the adenophypophysis on the the basis of cell distribution is usual in aquatic vertebrates. The gonadotrophs in lampreys and most bony fishes are located in the proximal pars distalis, and the segregated lobes in the cartilaginous fishes increase the degree of separation. It is difficult to provide a reason for this regionalisation, though it is tempting to suggest that it may date back to the time when hypothalamic control of pituitary activity was less sophisticated and the blood supply to the pituitary may have been more directional than now. It is generally true that, in bony fishes, the rostral lobe contains prolactin-secreting cells and adrenocorticotrophic cells, both concerned with salt and water balance, whereas the proximal pars distalis contains the gonadotrophs, thyrotrophs and somatotrophs, all implicated in reproduction. Is it possible that earlier in evolution the lobes were controlled rather than the individual cells?

Fossil evidence seems to support the idea that a segregated ventral lobe was present in early elasmobranchs; a hypophyseal canal is present in early fossil skulls. The absence of a portal blood supply to the main gonadotrophic region of the pituitary in cartilaginous fishes calls for special comment, though it should be remembered that such a system is absent also in cyclostomes, and the position in teleosts is variable. It is of considerable interest that the coelacanth, *Latimeria chalumnae*, present day survivor of fish that lived 300 million years ago and which looked similar, has a segregated pituitary lobe that contains gonadotrophs and is vascularised by the internal carotid arteries. Both produce large yolky eggs, possibly over an extended period, and it may be that a hypothalamic portal system, whilst appropriate for discrete pulses at precise times, is inappropriate to support ovarian growth over an extended period; tonic secretion of gonadotrophin might be more effective.

Aspects of viviparity in Chondrichthyes

Fifty-four families of extant fishes bear living young and, of these, 40 are cartilaginous, comprising 99 genera and 420 species (see Wourms, 1981 for detailed and comprehensive review and for reference). Viviparity appears to have evolved independently and frequently during vertebrate evolution and in widely separated taxonomic groups; it cannot, therefore, be used to identify relationships. However, it is usually accepted as being an apomorphous (advanced) character, species that are oviparous belonging to less advanced families, though this may be an over-simplification. The only vertebrates in which viviparity has not been exploited are cyclostomes and birds. In the former, oviducts (Müllerian ducts), in which gestation could occur, are absent and in the latter, it would appear to be incompatible with flight, viviparous insects notwithstanding!

Viviparity first appears in the vertebrate series in chondrichthyan fishes, though none of the extant holocephalans is viviparous and it was believed, until recently, that viviparity had never evolved in this group. However, two specimens of a newly discovered fetal holocephalan, *Delphyodontos dacriformes*, from the Lower Carboniferous of Montana, have recently been described (Lund, 1980). These have the well developed slashing and piercing dentition characteristic of extant elasmobranch species which open egg capsules during intrauterine feeding (oophagy). Lund suggests that this palaeozoic holocephalan was viviparous and that the developing young were oophagous. He further suggests that viviparity may have been a significant adaptive feature in palaeozoic chondrichthyans in general.

In extant elasmobranchs, viviparity is usually aplacental, though a yolk-sac placenta has evolved in two families of sharks, the Carcharhinidae and the Sphyrnidae (Fig. 5), which are believed, on other grounds, to be advanced (Nakaya, 1975). In both grades, the dependence on the mother during gestation ranges from the provision of shelter, water and oxygen to almost total dependence, at least in the later stages of gestation (Wourms, 1981).

Internal fertilization is an essential concomitant of viviparity, and all extant elasmobranchs, both oviparous and viviparous, have the highly evolved pelvic apparatus, consisting of claspers and siphons described above, by which this is achieved. These structures, as we have seen, are of ancient lineage. Other essential adaptations for viviparity are: retention of the fertilised eggs in the oviduct (this appears to involve *inter alia*, the disappearance of cilia from the oviducal lumen); modification of the oviducts to accomodate gestation, including an enhanced secretory function; reduction in size and function of the shell gland, though it usually continues to secrete a membrane; and modification of a specific region of the oviduct to form the maternal region of the placenta in placental species (Fig. 5). These modifications vary in scope with the degree of maternal dependence. Some aplacental genera, like *Squalus, Scymnus* and *Centrophorus*, rely entirely on yolk for development and the oviducts are relatively little modified, but in most aplacental species the uterine cavity becomes compartmentalised (*Mustellus manazo*, Fig. 4) and the uterine mucosa becomes modified to secrete embryotrophe or uterine milk. In another form of intrauterine feeding, oophagy, unfertilised eggs are ovulated and these enter the oviducts and are eaten (Lohberger, 1919; Shann, 1923; Ranzi, 1934; Springer, 1948; Wourms, 1977,1981). Shann (1923) reports that in porbeagle sharks (*Lamna* spp.) immature eggs and ovarian tissues are shed and enter the oviducts to be eaten by the developing young which develop a distended 'yolk stomach' for digesting this food. Oophagy in the sand-shark, *Odontaspis taurus*, is accompanied by highly active feeding behaviour *in utero*. These adaptations, leading to a degree of maternal dependence, are widespread and varied, but it is those that lead to cellular contact between the tissues of the embryo and those of the mother in the formation of a placenta that are of particular interest. Placental viviparity has evolved rather infrequently, perhaps not surprisingly, since a good deal more is involved. As we have seen, it is found in only two families of sharks among elasmobranchs. In both, the placenta is formed by the apposition of the embryonic yolk sac and the oviducal mucosa. Interchange between blood systems of embryo and mother takes place across five layers, namely: maternal endothelium; maternal epithelium; egg case, or membrane, which may or may not be present; fetal (yolk-sac) epithelium; fetal endothelium (Schlernitzauer and Gilbert, 1966). Even in placental species, dependence on the mother varies from slight to almost complete. For example, in the sharks *Sphyrno tiburo* and *Mustelus canis*, several months of an ovoviviparous existance precede the formation of the placenta, and another species of *Mustelus*, namely *M. laevis*, is aplacental.

Wourms (1981) has provided an excellent review of recent work on the structure and physiology of the elasmobranch placenta. It is clear that it falls far short of its mammalian counterpart in both scope and efficiency, yet there is little doubt that it has an important role in gestation in at least some of the species in which it is present.

Evolutionary considerations

The overriding advantage of viviparity in its fully developed manifestation *i.e.* in the mammals, may be that the individual is required to invest virtually no reserves in the egg. Thus, there is no metabolic loss if the egg is not fertilised or for some other reason fails to develop. But, clearly, there are other advantages associated with viviparity which may have been the important ones in the early stages of the evolution of maternal dependence. A survey of reproduction in contemporary elasmobranchs appears to show that viviparity has enabled viviparous species to advance more rapidly than oviparous species. Protection of the developing young may have been another advantage of viviparity, although heavily yoked eggs were still produced in the early stages of its evolution. Then, perhaps, methods of feeding the developing young *in utero* evolved and, allied to the production of still fewer eggs with less yolk, a placenta was evolved through which nutriment could be provided to the viable embryo by a vascular route.

Considering the earliest stages in the evolution of viviparity in elasmobranchs, Nakaya's classification (1977) of oviparity in the Scyliorhinidae is interesting and it may indicate, in contemporary species, the nature of these stages in the evolution of viviparity. He subdivides oviparity: 'single' oviparity accomodates fish like *Scyliorhinus canicula* (Fig. 3a) and *Proscyllium haberari* (Fig. 3b) in which each oviduct contains only a single egg at any one time. In *S. canicula*, it is laid after only a few days in the oviduct and prior to the start of development, whereas in *P. haberari*, the embryo develops to an advanced stage prior to oviposition. Multiple oviparity is exemplified by another scyliorhinid, *Halaelurus burgeri* (Fig. 3c) in which several egg capsules are present in each oviduct in gravid females, each containing an embryo at a stage of development corresponding to the time at which the egg was ovulated. Ovulation is serial, and when the embryos in the posterior pair of purses are almost fully developed these are laid. It may be noted that, unlike the situation in *S. canicula*, the attachment tendrils are virtually absent in both *P. haberari* and *H. burgeri*, a further indication that the eggs must hatch soon after being laid. Multiple oviparity may give some indication of the steps by which species like *S. acanthias* evolved their present day aplacental viviparity, the thick collagenous protective purses being replaced by the thin membranous investment that surrounds the embryos of *S. acanthias* (Fig. 3d).

It seems that viviparity may well be an ancient reproductive adaptation in fishes, as suggested by Lund (1980). Rather few gravid fossils have been described, though this is perhaps not surprising and it seems likely that more will be discovered in the future. This view is fostered by the discovery that extant coelacanths are ovoviviparous (Smith *et al.*, 1975), an earlier fossil showing signs of pregnancy having been misinterpreted, the recent discovery by Beltan (1977) of a full-term gravid specimen of *Birgeria*, a bony fish closely related to the chondrosteans (sturgeons), and the description by Lund (1980) of fossilised fetal holocephalans.

Summary and speculations

It appears, in view of their long phylogenetic history, that cyclostomes would have special relevance in evolutionary studies but, as we have seen, the expectation is only partly fulfilled in the context of reproduction because both groups are clearly specialised. However, it is possible to speculate as to relationships between the two groups, and to make some suggestions as to the nature of reproductive structures and processes in the early vertebrates.

In modern cyclostomes, reproduction and its hormonal control show major differences both within the two groups and between them and other vertebrates. The degree to which these differences are long standing, or are due to more recent specialisations, is impossible to assess, though both groups show clear evidence of some degree of specialisation. The magnitude of the inter-group differences seems to support the conclusion, arrived at on the basis of other evidence, that their origin is diphyletic. Although it is probably unsafe to draw any wide-ranging conclusions as to the nature of early reproductive structures and functions from the evidence provided by cyclostomes, especially from myxinoids, certain inferences may be made. For example, it seems likely that basic ovarian structure has changed relatively little from the early days. However, although atresia was probably a feature of ovaries in the earliest stages of evolution, the development of functional corpora lutea from post- ovulatory follicles was certainly a later development. Vitellogenesis is clearly an ancient function and it probably has been a liver-based, oestrogen- stimulated process from the early days. Steroids are ancient and ubiquitous molecules, and both androgens and oestrogens were probably present in early cyclostomes, if in small amounts. The discovery of specific oestrogen receptors on liver cells in hagfish and the role of steroids in vitellogenesis must be regarded as supporting the view that these are ancient functions. Since secondary sex characters are not present in the hagfish, it is difficult to identify functions other than vitellogenesis in which steroids are involved in these animals. In lampreys, however, they are known to stimulate the fin hypertrophy that occurs at sexual maturity and they also may be associated with the sophisticated behaviour associated with spawning. The situation in lampreys, as in cartilaginous fishes, supports the widely accepted view that morphological secondary sex characters are somatic structures which came under the influence of sex steroids at some point during their evolution.

It might also have been supposed that cyclostomes would provide clues as to the origins and evolution of the pituitary gland and of its functional relations with the brain, but this expectation has not been realised. The hagfish 'pituitary' is endodermal in origin and, therefore, not the homologue of the adenohypophysis of other vertebrates, and it has neither a demonstrable role in reproduction nor is it under hypothalamic control. It is not possible to say whether these are structures and functions that have been lost, though this seems unlikely. We can conclude only that the myxinoids are highly specialised and provide no clues relating to the origins and evolution of the hypothalamo-hypophysial axis in vertebrate reproduction. The lampreys, on the other hand, have a well developed pituitary of three regions, reminiscent of the gland in teleosts. It has a role in reproduction, albeit a restricted one, and in steroidogenesis. There are neither vascular nor nervous connections between hypothalamus and pituitary, and it is not known how the marked reproductive cyclicity shown by lampreys is mediated. However, it is of considerable interest that GnRH is present in the lamprey brain. The route by which it reaches the pituitary is not known, though it must presumably travel either by a systemic route or by simple diffusion. The close spatial relationship between the hypothalamus and pituitary support the latter suggestion and this may well have been the primitive route.

The reproductive biology of contemporary cartilaginous fishes supports the above speculations and allows us to go further. The ovary is sophisticated, as sophisticated as that of a bird. We have already pointed to the close similarities between the ovary of the dogfish and that of the hen (Dodd, 1975). The size hierarchy of oocytes that are ovulated in pairs at precise intervals testifies to the potentialities of the vertebrate ovary and leads to the view that the major change that has occurred en route to the mammal ovary is the loss of yolk. Corpora lutea with endocrine functions may have been evolved in viviparous elasmobranchs. Secondary sex characters are well established and partly under steroid control and, as we have seen, many of the reproductive structures found in amphibians and amniotes are already well established in Chondrichthyes. These have either appeared convergently or were present in the chondrichthyan ancestor.

The pituitary gland is specialised in having a gonadotrophic lobe that is separated from the rest of the pituitary. The precise significance of this in terms of the evolution of the system is not clear and, as in the case of the cyclostomes, the question of hypothalamic control of the gonadotrophic lobe is unresolved. However, in the elasmobranchs there is a well developed median eminence of two regions, though there is no direct connection between this and the ventral lobe. Gonadotropin-releasing hormone is present in the elasmobranch hypothalamus; this and its ubiquity suggest that it is an ancient hormone with a long evolutionary history.

The widespread occurrence of viviparity in elasmobranchs is perhaps the most remarkable feature in the reproductive biology of these animals. It is a striking example of convergent evolution and its present predominance and the fossil record lead us to believe that it evolved early, as did adaptations for internal fertilization, a necessary concomitant.

Finally, the close similarity between reproduction in elasmobranchs and holocephalans gives support to the view, held on other grounds, that these are sister groups sharing a common ancestor. Differences between them, like the external openings of the oviducts and the structure and chemical composition of the egg cases can probably be discounted.

Literature cited

BALINSKY, B.I. 1981. An introduction to embryology, 5th ed. CBS College Publishing, Philadelphia, Penn.

BELTAN, L. 1977. La parturition d'un actinopterygien de l'Eotrias du nord-ouest de Madagascar. C. r. hebd. Seanc. Acad. Sci. (Paris) **284D**: 2223-2225.

BREDER, C.M., and D.E. ROSEN. 1966. Modes of reproduction in fishes. The Natural History Press, New York.

BUSSON-MABILLOT, S. 1967a. Structure ovarienne de la lamproie adulte (*Lampetra planeri* Bloch). I. Zone pellucide, morphogénèse et constitution chimique. J. Microsc. (Paris) **6**: 577-598.

BUSSON-MABILLOT, S. 1967b. Structure ovarienne de la lamproie adulte (*Lampetra planeri* Bloch). II. Les enveloppes de l'ovocyte: Cellules folliculaires et stroma ovarienne. J. Microsc. (Paris) **6**: 807-838.

CAPPETTA, H. 1980. Les sélaciens du Crétacé Superieur du Liban. I. Requins. Palaeontographica **168A**: 69-148.

CHIEFFI, G. 1967. The reproductive system of elasmobranchs: developmental and endocrinological aspects. pp. 553-580 *In* Gilbert, P.W., R.F. Mathewson, and D.P. Rall [eds.] Sharks, skates and rays. John Hopkins Press, Baltimore, Maryland.

CRIM, J.W., A. URANO, and A. GORBMAN. 1979a. Immunocytochemical studies of luteinising hormone-releasing hormone in brains of agnathan fishes. I. Comparisons of adult Pacific lamprey (*Entosphenus tridentata*) and the Pacific hagfish (*Eptatretus stouti*). Gen. comp. Endocrinol. **37**: 294-305.

CRIM, J.W., A. URANO, and A. GORBMAN. 1979b. Immunocytochemical studies of luteinising hormone-releasing hormone in brains of agnathan fishes. II. Patterns of immunoreactivity in larval and maturing western brook lamprey (*Lampetra richardsoni*). Gen. comp. Endocrinol. **38**: 290-299.

DODD, J.M. 1972. Ovarian control in cyclostomes and elasmobranchs. Amer. Zool. **12**: 325-339.

DODD, J.M. 1975. The hormones of sex and reproduction and their effects in fish and lower chordates: twenty years on. Amer. Zool. **15** (suppl. 1): 137-171.

DODD, J.M. 1977. The structure of the ovary in non-mammalian vertebrates. pp. 219-263 *In* Zuckerman, S. and B.J. Weir [eds.] The ovary. Academic Press, New York.

DODD, J.M. 1983. Reproduction in cartilaginous fishes (Chondrichthyes). pp. 31-95 *In* Hoar, W.S., D.J. Randall, and E.M. Donaldson [eds.] Fish physiology, vol. 9, part A. Academic Press, New York.

DODD, J.M. and J.P. SUMPTER. 1984. Fishes. p. 1-126 *In* Lamming, G.E. [ed,] Marshall's physiology of reproduction, 4th ed., vol. 1. Churchill Livingstone, Edinburgh.

DODD, J.M., and C.K. GODDARD. 1960. Some effects of oestradiol benzoate on the reproductive ducts of the female dogfish, *Scyliorhinus canicula*. Proc. Zool. Soc. (Lond.) **137**: 325-331.

DODD, J.M., P.J. EVENNETT, and C.K. GODDARD. 1960. Reproductive endocrinology in Cyclostomes and Elasmobranchs. Symp. Zool. Soc. (Lond.) **1**: 77-103.

DODD, J.M., M.H.I. DODD, J.P. SUMPTER, and N. JENKINS. 1982. Gonadotrophic activity in the buccal lobe (Rachendach-hypophyse) of the pituitary gland of the rabbitfish *Hydrolagus colliei* (Chondrichthyes: Holocephali). Gen. comp. Endocrinol. **48**: 174-180.

EVENNETT, P.J., and J.M. DODD. 1963. Endocrinology of reproduction in the river lamprey. Nature (Lond.) **197**: 715-716.

FÄNGE, R. and A. MATTISSON. 1981. The lymphomyeloid (haemopoietic) system of the Atlantic nurse shark, *Ginglymostoma cirratum*. Biol. Bull. **160**: 240-249.

GORBMAN, A. 1965. Vascular relations between the neurohypophysis and adenohypophysis of cyclostomes and the problem of hypothalmic neuroendocrine control. Arch. Anat. microsc. Morphol. exp. **54**: 163-194.

GORBMAN, A. 1983. Reproduction in cyclostome fishes and its regulation. pp. 1-29 *In* Hoar, W.S., D.J. Randall, and E.M. Donaldson [eds.] Fish physiology, vol.

9, pt. A. Academic Press, New York.
GORBMAN, A., and W.W. DICKHOFF. 1978. Endocrine control of reproduction in hagfish. pp. 29-57 *In* Gaillard, P.J. and H.H. Boer [eds.] Comparative endocrinology. Elsevier Press, Amsterdam.
HARDISTY, M.W. 1971. Gonadogenesis, sex-differentiation and gametogenesis. pp. 295-360 *In* Hardisty, M.W. and I.C. Potter [eds.] Biology of lampreys, vol. 11. Academic Press, New York.
HARDISTY, M.W. 1979. Biology of cyclostomes. Chapman and Hall, London.
HISAW, F.L., and F.L. HISAW, Jr. 1959. Corpora lutea of elasmobranch fishes. Anat. Rec. **135**: 269-277.
HOLMES, R.L., and J.N. BALL. 1974. The pituitary gland. Cambridge University Press, London.
JARVIK, E. 1968. Aspects of vertebrate phylogeny. *In* Ørvig, T. [ed.] Current problems of lower vertebrate phylogeny. Almqvist and Wiksell, Stockholm.
JENKINS, N., and J.M. DODD. 1980. Effects of synthetic mammalian gonadotrophin-releasing hormone and dogfish hypothalamic extracts on levels of androgens and oestradiol in the circulation of the dogfish (*Scyliorhinus canicula* L.). J. Endocrinol. **86**: 171-177.
KING, J.A., and R.P. MILLAR. 1979. Heterogeneity of vertebrate luteinising hormone-releasing hormone. Science **206**: 67-69.
KING, J.A., and R.P. MILLAR. 1980. Comparative aspects of luteinising hormone-releasing hormone structure and function in vertebrate phylogeny. Endocrinology **106**: 707-717.
KNOWLES, F., L.VOLLRATH, and P. MEURLING. 1975. Cytology and neuroendocrine relations of the pituitary of the dogfish, *Scyliorhinus canicula*. Proc. R. Soc. (Lond.) **191B**: 507-525.
KOBAYASHI, H. 1972. Median eminence of the hagfish and ependymal absorption in higher vertebrates. pp. 67-78 *In* Brain-endocrine interaction. Median eminence: structure and function. International Symposium, Munich. Karger, Basel.
LARSEN, L.O. 1969. Effects of hypophysectomy before and during sexual maturation in the cyclostome *Lampetra fluviatilis* (L.) Gray. Gen. comp. Endocrinol. **12**: 200-208.
LARSEN, L.O. 1974. Effects of testosterone and oestradiol on gonadectomised and intact male and female river lampreys (*Lampetra fluviatilis* L.). Gen. comp. Endocrinol. **24**: 305-313.
LARSEN, L.O. 1978. Hormonal control of sexual maturation in lampreys. p. 105-108 *In* Gaillard, P.J. and H.H. Boer [eds.] Comparative endocrinology. Elsevier Press, Amsterdam.
LEWIS, J.C., and D.B. McMILLAN. 1965. The development of the ovary of the sea lamprey (*Petromyzon marinus* L.). J. Morphol. **117**: 425-466.
LOHNBERGER, J. 1919. Ueber zwei riesige Embryonen von *Lamna*. Abh. Bayer. Akad. Wiss. *4*: 1-45.
LØVTRUP, S. 1977. The phylogeny of vertebrata. Wiley, London.
LUND, R. 1980. Viviparity and intrauterine feeding in a new holocephalan fish from the Lower Carboniferous of Montana. Science **209**: 697-699.
MATTY, A.J., K. TSUNEKI, W.W. DICKHOFF, and A. GORBMAN. 1976. Thyroid and gonadal function in hypophysectomised hagfish, *Eptatretus stouti*. Gen. comp. Endocrinol. **30**: 500-516.
NAKAYA, K. 1975. Taxonomy, comparative anatomy and phylogeny of Japanese

catsharks, Scyliorhinidae. Mem. Fac. Fish. Hokkaido Univ. **23**: 1-94.

NORRIS, H.W. 1941. The plagiostome hypophysis, general morphology and types of structure. Grinell, Iowa.

NOZAKI, M., and H. KOBAYASHI. 1979. Distribution of LHRH-like substance in the vertebrate brain as revealed by immunohistochemistry. Arch. Histol. Jap. **42**: 201-219.

PATZNER, R.A. 1978. Cyclical changes in the ovary of the hagfish *Eptatretus burgeri* (Cyclostomata). Acta Zool. (Stockh.) **59**: 57-61.

PATZNER, R.A., and ICHIKAWA. 1977. Effects of hypophysectomy on the testis of the hagfish *Eptatretus burgeri* Girard. Zool. Anz. **199**: 371-380.

RANZI, S. 1934. Le basi fisio-morfologiche dello svillupo embrionali dei selaci. Pubbl. Stz. zool. Napoli **13**: 331-437.

SCHAEFFER, B. 1967. Comments on elasmobranch evolution. *In* Gilbert, P.W., R.F. Mathewson, and D.P. Rall [eds.] Sharks, skates and rays. Johns Hopkins Press, Baltimore, Maryland.

SCHLERNITZAUER, D.A., and P.W. GILBERT. 1966. Placentation and associated aspects of gestation in the bonnethead shark *Sphyrna tiburo*. J. Morph. **120**: 219-231.

SHANN, E.W. 1923. The embryonic development of the porbeagle shark, *Lamna cornubica*. Proc. Zool. Soc. (Lond.) **11**: 161-171.

SMITH, C.L., C.S. RAND, B. SCHAEFFER, and J.W. ATZ. 1975. *Latimeria*, the living coelacanth is ovoviviparous. Science **190**: 1105-1106.

SPRINGER, S. 1948. Oviphagous embryos of the sandshark, *Carcharias taurus*. Copeia **1948**: 153-157.

STANLEY, H.P. 1963. Urogenital morphology in the chimaeroid fish *Hydrolagus colliei* (Lay and Bennett). J. Morph. **112**: 99-124.

STENSIÖ, E.A. 1968. The cyclostomes with special reference to the diphyletic origin of the Petromyzontida and Myxinoidea. pp. 13-71 *In* Ørvig, T. [ed.] Current problems of lower vertebrate phylogeny. Almqvist and Wicksell, Stockholm.

SUMPTER, J.P., N. JENKINS, and J.M. DODD. 1978. Gonadotrophic hormone in the pituitary gland of the dogfish (*Scyliorhinus canicula* L.): distribution and physiological significance. Gen. comp. Endocrinol. **36**: 275-285.

TSUNEKI, K., and A. GORBMAN. 1975a. Ultrastructure of the anterior neurohypophysis and the pars distalis of the lamprey, *Lampetra tridentata*. Gen. comp. Endocrinol. **25**: 487-508.

TSUNEKI, K., and A. GORBMAN. 1975b. Ultrastructure of the pars nervosa and pars intermedia of the lamprey, *Lampetra tridentata*. Cell Tissue Res. **157**: 165-184.

TSUNEKI, K., and A. GORBMAN. 1977. Ultrastructure of the ovary of the hagfish, *Eptatretus stouti*. Acta Zool. (Stockh.) **58**: 27-40.

TURNER, R.T., W.W. DICKHOFF, and A. GORBMAN. 1982. Estrogen binding to hepatic nuclei of Pacific hagfish, *Eptatretus stouti*. Gen. comp. Endocrinol. **45**: 26-29.

VU TAN TUE. 1972. Variations cycliques des gonades et du quelques glandes endocrines chez *Chimaera monstrosa* Linné (Pisces, Holocephali). Ann. Sci. Nat. Zool. Biol. Anim. **14**: 49-94.

WOURMS, J.P. 1977. Reproduction and development in chondrichthyan fishes. Amer. Zool. **17**: 379-410.

WOURMS, J.P. 1981. Viviparity: the maternal-fetal relationship in fishes. Amer. Zool. **21**: 473-515.

YU, J.Y-L., W. W. DICKHOFF, P. SWANSON, and A. GORBMAN. 1981. Vitellogenesis and its hormonal regulation in the Pacfic hagfish, *Eptatretus stouti*. Gen. comp. Endocrinol. **43**: 492-503.

ON UREA FORMATION IN PRIMITIVE FISHES

G.W. Brown, Jr. and Susan G. Brown

School of Fisheries
University of Washington
Seattle, Washington, U.S.A.

I can make urea without the necessity of a kidney . . .
Letter from Wöhler to Berzelius, Feb. 22, 1828 (Hurt, 1978).

Introduction

In 1828, Friedrich Wöhler obtained urea by heating ammonium cyanate, this being the first deliberate extracorporeal synthesis of an organic compound by man. A century passed before Krebs and Henseleit (1932) demonstrated the biosynthesis of urea by mammalian liver through a process they termed the "ornithine cycle". It is fitting and historically instructive to note that between these two scientific achievements Salkowski (1877-78) provided the lead article in Hoppe-Seyler's new journal, his *Zeitschrift für physiologische Chemie*, "On the process of urea formation in animals and the influence on this by ammonium salts." Now, somewhat more than a half-century since the discovery of the ornithine cycle, we are still working on the details of how it operates. This cycle, which we will refer to here as the ornithine-urea cycle (reasons for which will become evident later), has been, and continues to be, the framework for a legion of studies in comparative biochemistry and physiology.

As is commonly understood, the occurrence of arginine in most proteins suggests that a mechanism for arginine synthesis must have occurred early in biological time. Autotrophic organisms would need a mechanism for its synthesis. Indeed, the ornithine-urea cycle is the only biochemical mechanism we know of for the synthesis, *de novo*, of arginine. In the consumption of protein for nourishment, heterotrophic organisms can use the carbon atoms of the amino acids of the protein. It is the disposition of this nitrogen which has provoked the considerable interest of comparative biochemists and physiologists.

A rallying point for those working on intermediary metabolism in primitive fishes is that dealing with ammonia and urea. The finding that urea occurs in high concentration in the tissues of the elasmobranchs (Staedeler and Frerichs, 1858) opened the door to a succession of much later studies on the osmotic role played by this compound (for pertinent references see review of Cohen and Brown, 1960; Schmidt-Nielsen and Kerr, 1970; Goldstein and Forster, 1970; Watts and Watts, 1974; Grisolia *et al.*, 1976). The Dutch clinician, Hermann Boerhaave (1668-1738), a contemporary of Leeuwenhoek, Fahrenheit, Descartes, and Malpighii, is said to have been the first chemist to separate urea from the urine (see Novak, 1971).

Reactions of intermediary nitrogen metabolism

A number of enzymes of intermediary metabolism have been measured for primitive fish tissues. An extensive literature survey on enzymes and other biochemical attributes of fish, in general, is provided by Love (1970, 1980). It appears that most of the enzymes of intermediary nitrogen metabolism of primitive fish serve essentially the same roles as do those of other vertebrates. Janssens (1964), for example, studied the glutamic-pyruvic and glutamic-oxalacetic transaminases in the African lungfish, *Protopterus* spp. D-amino acid oxidase (Fickeisen and Brown, 1977) and L-amino acid oxidase (Salvatore *et al.*, 1965) appear to function in elasmobranchs and teleosts as they do in other vertebrates. The main distinction among the vertebrates in the area of intermediary nitrogen metabolism appears to revolve around the mode of elimination of nitrogenous waste products leading to uricotelism, ureotelism, or ammonotelism. A caution in the use and interpretation of the last three terms is in order. These terms have been used to describe both the *nature* of the nitrogenous waste products themselves (uric acid, urea, or ammonia) or to indicate the *mechanism* involved in supporting a certain type of nitrogenous waste product. For example, the term ureotelism commonly suggests that animals exhibiting it possess the ornithine-urea cycle. In using the literature, the reader must get the meaning of any of these terms from the context in which they are used.

This paper will deal primarily with the reactions and processes that support the formation of urea in primitive fishes.

Ornithine-urea cycle

The work of a number of laboratories allows depiction of the ornithine-urea cycle as shown in Fig. 1. Critical to an understanding of how ammonia was incorporated into the cycle was the synthesis of carbamoyl phosphate by Jones *et al.* (1955). The reactions for the synthesis of arginino-succinate and its conversion to arginine and fumarate were also not a part of the original formulation of the cycle by Krebs and Henseleit (1932).

A number of studies (for citations see Brown, 1964a) indicated that during development of Amphibia, arginase of the liver increased in activity. It remained for Brown *et al.* (1959) to show induction of the entire ornithine-urea cycle through increases in levels of all the enzymes of the cycle for the frog (*Rana catesbeiana*)

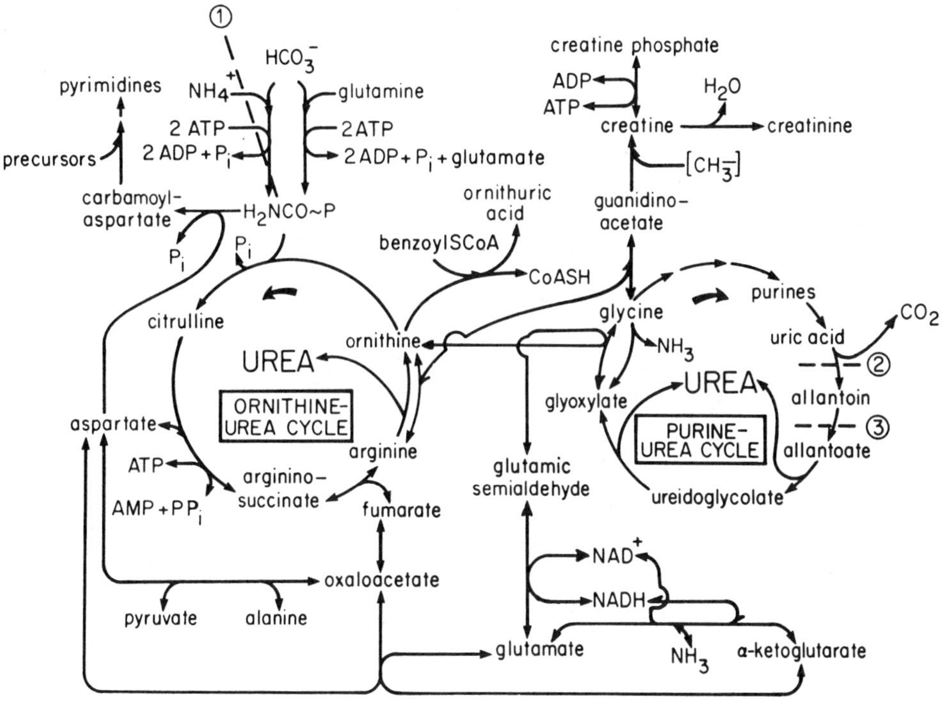

Fig. 1. Ornithine-urea and purine-urea cycles and some ancillary reactions. Dashed lines are drawn across enzymic steps presumably absent in 1) Aves, Squamata, Crocodilia, Teleostei, and possibly absent in Rhynchocephalia, Cladista, and Cyclostomi. In these groups carbamoyl phosphate may be synthesized only by the enzyme that does not require N-acetylglutamate or related compound; 2) Primates, Aves, Reptilia (all?); 3) Mammalia, Aves, Reptilia (all?). (From Brown, 1970)

as it proceeded through larval development. Having developed a systematic series of assays for ornithine-urea cycle enzymes for small amounts of liver tissues (Brown and Cohen, 1959), Brown and Cohen (1960) initiated a series of comparative studies to determine the distribution of cycle enzyme activities in various groups of vertebrates. The outgrowth of this study was a depiction of the occurrence or absence of the ornithine-urea cycle in relation to vertebrate phylogeny, as shown in the updated version of the original phylogenetic tree as it applies to fishes (see Fig. 2). Various taxonomic groups depicted were accompanied by a plus or a minus sign to indicate the presence or absence, respectively, of the ornithine-urea cycle in a given group.

A parenthesized mark indicated the postulated presence or postulated absence of the cycle. For example, the figure indicates that the cycle was possibly present (+) in evolution before emergence of the jawless fishes (Agnatha) but that by the

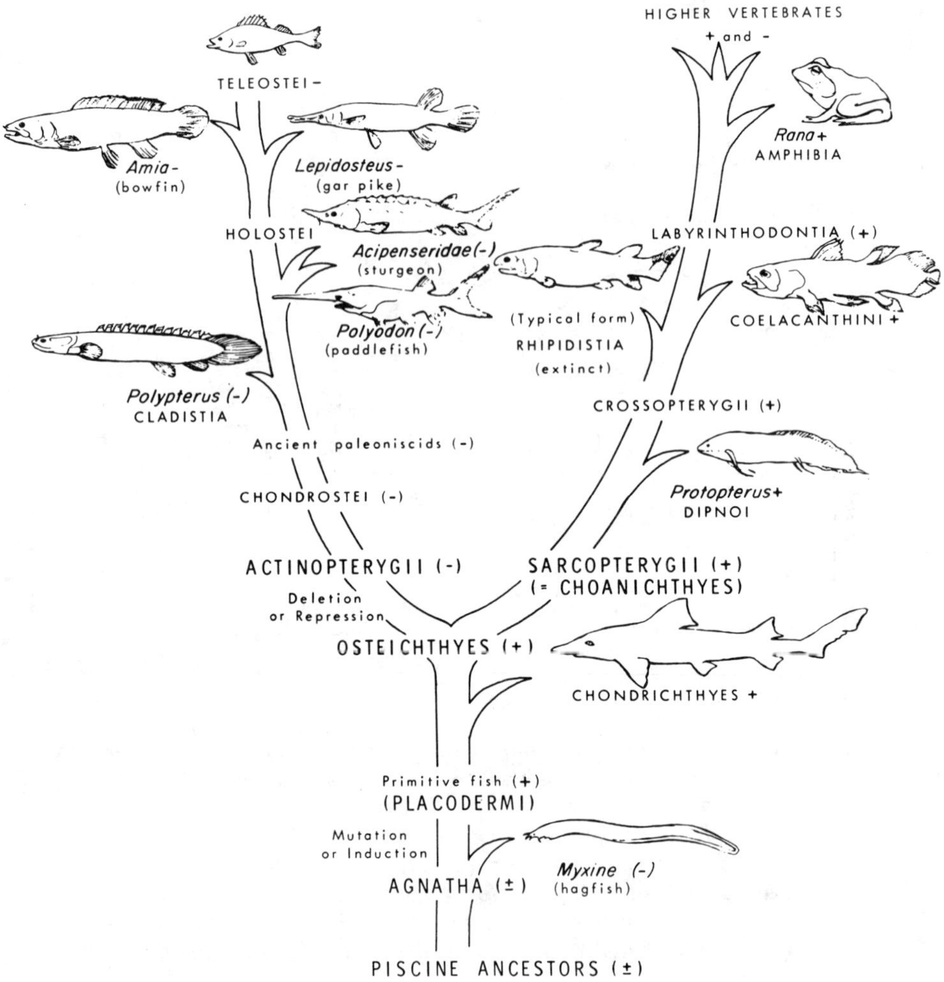

Fig. 2. Evolutionary tree of the vertebrates and occurrence of the ornithine-urea cycle. Format after the style of Romer. Presence of cycle, + ; absence, - ; presumed presence (+); presumed absence (-). Assignments based on the numerous studies cited in text. (From Brown and Brown, 1967)

time sharks arose the cycle was definitely active. In the Choanichthian (or Sarcopterygian) branch, the original tree (Brown and Cohen, 1960) shows activity was retained through the stem reptiles, was retained by mammals, but was lost by the time the reptiles had reached to the saurian reptiles and birds. Brown and Cohen used the term "deletion" to indicate the loss of one or more of the enzymes of the cycle, thinking first in genetic terms of the actual loss of enzyme proteins.

However, they pointed out that it could be interpreted to mean a loss of functional activity of the cycle as a physiologically important apparatus for urea biosynthesis, *i.e.* "as a lowering of enzyme activity to such a level that the urea cycle no longer functions to any significant extent as a system for the disposal of ammonia as urea." (Brown and Cohen, 1960).

The original phylogenetic chart indicated the presumed presence of a functioning cycle in the coelacanth, *Latimeria chalumnae*. This prediction was confirmed by our work (Brown and Brown, 1967), inferred by that of Pickford and Grant (1967), and clinched by that of Goldstein *et al.* (1973).

Synthesis of carbamoyl phosphate

The initial step in the synthesis of urea by the ornithine-urea cycle is that of the synthesis of carbamoyl phosphate (see Fig. 1). While synthesis of carbamoyl phosphate could readily be demonstrated in various Amphibia and Mammalia, initial attempts to demonstrate activity in the liver of elasmobranchs were uniformly unsuccessful (Baldwin, 1960; Brown and Cohen, 1960). The first clearcut demonstration of the synthesis of carbamoyl phosphate in elasmobranchs was provided from studies on sharks (Brown, 1964b) and confirmed by Watts and Watts (1966). But even those demonstrations were not definitive in determining the true nature of the enzyme catalyzing synthesis of carbamoyl phosphate. In Brown's work, ammonium ion was used as the $-NH_2$ donor (see below), and strangely, manganous instead of magnesium ion stimulated the reaction. Furthermore, the enzyme activity of the preparations deteriorated rapidly. The elegant studies of Anderson and coworkers in Duluth (Anderson, 1980; Anderson, 1981; Casey and Anderson, 1982; Casey and Anderson, 1983) on the nature of carbamoyl phosphate synthesis in fishes has shed new light on the problem. It is now known that synthesis of carbamoyl phosphate in the shark *Squalus acanthias* is by an enzyme termed CPSase III which required glutamine as the $-NH_2$ donor for maximum rate of synthesis of carbamoyl phosphate and which requires the cofactor, N-acetyl-L-glutamate, as well. Current terminology reserves the designation CPSase I for the enzyme of amphibian and mammalian liver that uses ammonia instead of glutamine, but which requires the same cofactor. The enzyme dealing with carbamoyl phosphate synthesis for pyrimidine formation is designated CPSase II. The characteristics of these three enzymes are summarized in Table I. Some enzyme levels are given in Table II.

Most of the works on fish where synthesis of carbamoyl phosphate has been studied are ones in which ammonia, not glutamine, was employed. Examination of those studies indicates that the carbamoyl phosphate synthetase activity is often at the lower limit of detection by the usual colorimetric assay procedures, and many were carried out without appropriate controls (*e.g.* use of boiled extract, absence of individual components, graded responses of additives).

We would be remiss here not to remark that Tramell and Campbell (1970) reported on a CPSase in a mitochondrial fraction of the land snail *Strophocheilus oblongus* which required L-glutamine and N-acetyl-L-glutamate. Aspartate transaminase (CPSase II of vertebrates) occurred in the cytosol.

Table I. Vertebrate carbamoyl phosphate synthetase

	CPSase I	CPSase II	CPSase III
$-NH_2$ donor	ammonia	glutamine	glutamine
cofactor	NAG	none	NAG
energy source	ATP	ATP	ATP

NAG = N-acetyl-L-glutamate

Table II. Ornithine-urea cycle enzyme activities

Fish	CPS*	OCT*	ARSS*	ARGINASE
		μmol $h^{-1}g$ liver^{-1} (25-37° C)		
Latimeria chalumnae[1]	4.75	8.24×10^3	10.0	3.00×10^4
Dasyatis americana[2]	6.5	1.44×10^4	21.6	3.47×10^4
Protopterus sp.[3]	30.5	1.68×10^3	6.6	3.48×10^4
Potamotrygon sp.[2]	0.36	1.68×10^3	9.4	4.31×10^3
Rana catesbeiana[4]	980	9.70×10^3	46.3	2.46×10^4

*CPS, carbomyl phosphate synthetase; OCT, ornithine carbomyltransferase; ARSS, argininosuccinate synthetase.

[1]Goldstein *et al.* (1973)
[2]Goldstein and Forster (1971)
[3]Janssens and Cohen (1966)
[4]Brown and Cohen (1960) (Bullfrog)

Nuclear DNA content of cells

The idea was advanced a number of years ago that the ornithine-urea cycle occurred only in those vertebrates that had a somatic cell (2N) DNA content of greater than about 5 picograms, and was absent in those with a DNA content of less than about 5 picograms (Brown, 1962). The prediction that invertebrates would not possess ornithine-urea cycle activity now seems to have been incorrect, for the cycle appears to be active in some invertebrates (see, for example, Campbell, 1965).

When tissues of the coelacanth became available for enzymic studies, the coelacanth was shown to have liver ornithine-urea cycle activity (Brown and Brown, 1967) and the DNA content of its erythrocytes was shown to be 7.22 picograms

(Cimino and Bahr, 1973, 1974) or 13.2 picograms (Thomson *et al.*, 1973). We are not clear why these values are so divergent. In any event, the cellular, nuclear DNA content of the coelacanth seems to be above the cutoff value of 5 picograms. There has been a gradual rise in cellular DNA content in the vertebrates during evolution. This association of high DNA level and occurrence of ornithine-urea cycle activity defies any immediate, simplistic explanation other than that the cellular content of the enzymes in the liver involved may bear some direct relationship to the amount of genetic information repeated. However, that may be merely a statement of fact and not an explanation. Hinegardner (1976) reports nuclear DNA as high as 10.2 picograms in some chondrosteans, and the occurrence of the ornithine-urea cycle in fishes of this group is not well documented. The relation between DNA content and the ornithine-urea cycle may be a red herring, but it is worth some further analysis and study.

Glutamine synthetase

Glutamine synthetase catalyzes the reaction:

$$\text{glutamate} + NH_3 + \text{ATP} \dashrightarrow \text{glutamine} + \text{ADP} + P_i \qquad (1)$$

High glutamine synthetase activity of liver is associated with the occurrence of an active ornithine-urea cycle in fishes (Webb and Brown, 1976, 1980). Anderson (1980, 1981) has shown that the liver of *Squalus acanthias* contains a CPSase III and that it, ornithine carbamoyl transferase (ornithine transcarbamoylase), and arginase are mitochondrial in location; the enzymes are synthesized outside the mitochondrion and imported to it. In mammals and amphibians, arginase is extramitochondrial. Further, the glutamine-dependent synthesis of carbamoyl phosphate profits from the presence of the high glutamine synthetase activity in the liver of elasmobranchs, for it is now known that this enzyme is also mitochondrial in nature (Casey and Anderson, 1982), it being associated with the enzyme for the synthesis of citrulline (see Fig. 1).

It should be noted that glutamine serves both for the synthesis of urea by the ornithine-urea cycle and for the incorporation of its amide nitrogen into purines. Ultimately, the amide nitrogen appears in urea in fishes through the operation of a purine-urea cycle (see Fig. 1 for this cycle).

Chondrichthyans

As indicated elsewhere in this paper, the operation of the ornithine-urea cycle in elasmobranchs is not questioned (see Table II for *Dasyatis americana*). The definitive work on arginase of an elasmobranch (*Mustelus canis*) is that of Campbell (1961).

Squalus acanthias, a urea-retainer with CPSase III, has a cell DNA content of 12.0 picograms. All other chondrichthyans studied have a DNA content above the 5 picogram level, except for *Hydrolagus colliei*, which is a urea-retainer; presumably it has a fully functioning ornithine-urea cycle, but it has a DNA content of only 3.2 picograms (Hinegardner, 1976).

Thorson *et al.* (1967) destroyed the great generalization that elasmobranchs, even freshwater sharks of Lake Nicaragua, maintain high concentrations of urea in their blood. *Potamotrygon* spp. maintain concentrations of urea in their blood at only 1/100th that of typical elasmobranchs. They do not concentrate urea when exposed to a saline medium (Thorson, 1970). They appear to lack the ability for tubular reabsorption of urea as in most other elasmobranchs (Goldstein and Forster, 1971). Studies by Goldstein and Forster (1971) indicate that enzymes of the ornithine-urea cycle are present in the liver of *Potamotrygon* spp., but at relatively low levels of activity. For example, carbamoyl phosphate synthetase activity was less than 1/10 that of two marine rays and less than 1/1000 the activity of the bullfrog, *Rana catesbeiana* (see Table II).

Dipnoans

See Table II for levels of ornithine-urea enzymes in *Protopterus*. Enzymes for synthesis of urea, albeit at relatively low levels compared with Amphibia, have been assayed in liver homogenates of the South American lungfish, *Lepidosiren paradoxa* (Funkhauser *et al.*, 1972). Operation of the ornithine-urea cycle was documented by showing that ^{14}C-bicarbonate was incorporated into urea through incubation with liver slices. Surprisingly, with the same species of lungfish, Carlisky and Barrio (1972) found that no ornithine carbamoyltransferase for the synthesis of citrulline could be detected in homogenates. Nor could they detect an arginase that hydrolyzed L-arginine. These workers claimed that substitution of the D-isomer for the L- isomer of arginine led to demonstration of a D-arginase activity. Yet their table indicates that it was DL-arginine that led to their demonstration of arginase activity, not the pure D-isomer of arginine. It is most disconcerting that analytical data (*e.g.* optical rotation) were not provided on the purported L-arginine sample for which no arginase activity could be shown or that no arginase activity was shown toward the sample with a known source of arginase active toward the L-isomer. We are at a loss to explain the findings of Carlisky and Barrio.

Janssens (1964) determined urea production from carbonate and ammonium ions by liver slices of *Protopterus annectens* in a system similar to that of Krebs and Henseleit (1932). Surprisingly, addition of ornithine to the medium did not enhance urea production by either control liver slices or those from the liver of an aestivating lungfish. It was the enhancement of urea production by catalytic amounts of ornithine that led to the discovery of the ornithine-urea cycle.

Coelacanth

It may be of interest that the first enzyme assayed in coelacanth liver was that for ornithine carbamoyltransferase (Brown and Brown, 1967). Levels of the enzymes of the ornithine-urea cycle are given in Table II. In view of the finding (see above) that glutamine is implicated in the reaction for the synthesis of carbamoyl phosphate in the shark, *Squalus acanthias*, assay for carbamoyl phosphate synthesis should now be conducted in the presence of glutamine and compared with production in the presence of ammonia. It seems workers will have to wait for the availability of more frozen liver from the Comoros before characterization of the relevant enzyme from coelacanth liver.

The unexpected yellow color that developed in a zero-time control for determination of citrulline in the ornithine carbamoyltransferase assay told us (Brown and Brown, 1967) that coelacanth liver had large quantities of urea in it. Upon pulling the citrulline assay tubes from the boiling water bath, GWB exclaimed "It's a shark!" Liver tissue was then analyzed for urea and was shown to have 1.7% urea by wet weight. In that same specimen, blood urea was 2.26% (Pickford and Grant, 1967). Taking into account the water content of liver, those two figures are comparable. Griffith *et al.* (1976) got about the same figure for the urea of bladder urine, namely, 2.33%.

Paleoniscids

The African bichir (*Polypterus senegalis*) is a living representative of ancient paleoniscid fishes that roamed fresh waters possibly as long as 300 $\times 10^6$ years ago. *Polypterus* is a member of a class of fishes that emerged and took an evolutionary route different from that of the rhipidistian and coelacanthian fishes with which the ancient paleoniscid fishes were contemporary. Few studies in the area of nitrogen metabolism are available on this group of fishes. Brown (1970) could not demonstrate the occurrence of ornithine carbamoyl transferase in the liver of *Polypterus senegalis*. The cellular DNA content of *Polypterus* spp. is reported to be 9.4 picograms, well above the cutoff of 5 picograms indicated for the occurrence of the ornithine-urea cycle in the section on cellular DNA content above. This argues against Brown's (1962) suggestion.

Chondrosteans

Extremely low activity was reported (Cvancara, 1974) for the synthesis of carbamoyl phosphate in liver of the shovel-nosed sturgeon (*Scaphirhynchus platorynchus*) and the paddlefish (*Polyodon spathula*). Values were around 1/1000 that of typical aquatic Amphibia and mammals. The significance of this low level of activity as it relates to operation of the ornithine-urea cycle is obscure. Few reports have appeared on nitrogen metabolism in chondrosteans other than those dealing with feeding and nutrition.

Holosteans

As with chondrostean fish, extremely low levels of activity for the synthesis of carbamoyl phosphate have been put forward. Activity for the liver of the short-nose gar *Lepisosteus platostomus* and the bowfin *Amia calva* are reported by Cvancara (1974), but at levels 1/100 that of typical Amphibia or mammals. The cellular DNA content of holostean fishes is reported to be less than 3 picograms (Hinegardner, 1976).

Teleosts

A number of studies have indicated the occurrence of some of the ornithine-urea cycle enzymes in teleosts (Mayhall and Brown, 1967; Huggins *et al.*, 1969; Read, 1971). Arginase has long been known to occur in the liver of teleosts (for references, see Watts and Watts, 1974). A definitive study on the occurrence of arginase was that of Hunter and Dauphinee (1924-25). It has been claimed, however, that all of the enzymes of the ornithine-urea cycle occur in teleostean liver (Huggins *et al.*, 1969; Read, 1971). First of all, the activities for at least one of the enzymes (usually that reported for synthesis of carbamoyl phosphate) typically have been of the order of 1/100 to 1/1000 the activity of the corresponding synthetic activity for adult aquatic frogs and mammals. In fact, the activities reported in experiments with teleosts (except for *Opsanus tau*, see below) are from experiments in which the colorimetric determination of product formed are at the lower limits of detection. Moreover, in most cases there are insufficient controls. In no case where a CPSase activity has been reported in teleosts has the stoichiometry of the reaction been reported nor has a comparison been made of activity of ammonia *vs.* glutamine as the $-NH_2$ donor (excluding, of course, the experiments of Anderson's group, see above). Even though it appears now that there may be some teleosts that exhibit a glutamine-dependent synthesis of carbamoyl phosphate, we have no example of studies with teleostean fishes that support demonstration of synthesis of arginine sufficient to satisfy dietary requirements. In fact, where studied, teleostean fishes all show a dietary requirement for arginine (Ketola, 1977). Hence the occurrence of a truly functional ornithine-urea cycle in teleosts is still questionable.

A number of years ago, Mayhall and Brown (1967) observed an unusually high value for ornithine carbamoyltransferase in liver extracts of the toadfish, *Opsanus beta*. A high level was also found for the related species, *Opsanus tau* (Read, 1971). When Paul Anderson was on sabbatical leave in our laboratory, he began a detailed study of the occurrence and nature of the glutamine and N-acetyl-L-glutamate dependent CPSase III. He (Anderson, 1980) subsequently showed that CPSase III occurred in liver of the shark *Squalus acanthias*. For a survey of the occurrence of this enzyme in marine teleosts we suggested that he include the midshipman (*Porichthyes notatum*) because it is the same family (Batrachoididae) as *Opsanus*, and because we had also noted the occurrence of a high ornithine carbamoyltransferase activity in the liver of the midshipman. Of the several teleost liver enzymes studied, the midshipman was the only one whose synthetase showed a greater activity for glutamine than for ammonia as the $-NH_2$ donor to carbamoyl phosphate. Its near relative, *Opsanus tau*, exhibits the highest ornithine-urea cycle activity for all the teleostean fishes so far studied (Read, 1971). The Batrachoididae may be a most unusual family of teleosts in exhibiting considerable activity for the enzymes of the ornithine-urea cycle. A further investigation of this unusual family is strongly indicated.

Vellas and Serfaty (1974) concluded from their work with the carp *Cyprinus carpio* that the urea produced by this fish appears to stem not from synthesis by the ornithine-urea cycle but from endogenous arginine and purines.

Casey and Anderson (1983) have isolated a CPSase III from the liver of the largemouth bass (*Micropterus salmoides*), and brought it to a high state of purity. It does not give any immunological cross-reaction with the antibody to the CPSase I from rat liver, suggesting that the two enzyme proteins are not closely related.

Agnatha

The Pacific lamprey, *Entosphenus tridentata*, exhibited liver enzyme activity (appx. 2 moles h^{-1} g^{-1} liver) for the synthesis of carbamoyl phosphate, about 1/100 that of typical Amphibia and mammals (Read, 1968). Again, this assay is at the lower level of detection by the usual colorimetric procedures. It is to be noted that the cell DNA content of nine species of lampreys ranges from 2.2 (*Ichthymoyzon gagei*) to 3.6 (*Petromyzon marinus*) (Robinson *et al.*, 1975). Only a CPSase activity and an arginase activity could be demonstrated with liver of the hagfish, *Bdellostoma cirrhatum* (Read, 1975). This fish has a cell DNA content of 5.6 picograms (Hinegardner, 1976), just at about the 5 picogram cutoff point indicated above for occurrence or absence of the ornithine-urea cycle in a number of vertebrates.

Amphibia

Amphibia are, of course, not fishes, but they are an upward extension of evolution from the fishes and are a transitional habitat group, as their name implies. The level of ornithine-urea cycle activity in Amphibia is correlated with the nature of their environment and ontogenic development (Brown, 1964a); cycle activity and the ratio of urea to ammonia excreted increase during larval development of frogs and as Amphibia show a greater independence of a watery environment (Brown and Cohen, 1960). Imagine the surprise, then, to find that certain xerophilous frogs have turned to the mode of nitrogen excretion found in saurian reptiles (lizards, snakes) and excrete most of their waste nitrogen as uric acid (!) (Loverage, 1970; Shoemaker and McClanahan, 1975). In this connection, Moyle (1949) showed many years ago that *turtles* select various combinations from among ammonia, urea, and uric acid as excretion products, depending upon availability of water in their environment.

Purine-urea cycle

A purine cycle has been proposed as operative in plants (Schlee and Reinbothe, 1963) and in fishes (Brown *et al.*, 1966). To distinguish this cycle from the ornithine-urea cycle, we have used the term purine-urea cycle. Before the conception of a purine-urea cycle, all steps but one of such a cycle had been characterized (see Brown, 1964a; Watts and Watts, 1974) and the purinolytic phase had been observed operating in amphibians, teleosts, elasmobranchs, and lungfish. However, there was not an appreciation that purine synthesis and degradation could be regarded as a cyclic process. The kingpin reaction completing the purine-urea cycle is that catalyzed by ornithine δ-aminotransferase which can convert glyoxylate to glycine (see Fig. 1) to begin the cycle anew:

$$\text{glyoxylate + ornithine ---> glycine + glutamic semialdehyde} \quad (2)$$

This reaction locks the ornithine-urea cycle and the purine cycles together in organisms where they both occur. Even in teleosts (which are presumed not to have a complete or fully-functioning ornithine-urea cycle), arginase can serve to make available part of the molecule of arginine, in the form of ornithine, for the synthesis of glycine. Further, the glutamic semialdehyde produced can be seen as being converted to glutamic acid through oxidation. The ornithine can also be converted to proline. In these ways, most of the original arginine molecule can be pushed back into the main stream of intermediary nitrogen metabolism. Also, the presence of this enzyme could play a role as a regulatory mechanism for both of the cycles. The enzyme occurs in all fishes studied (Wekell and Brown, 1973).

At one time it was thought that some fishes did not possess allantoicase and that the cycle terminated in some fishes at the level of allantoic acid. But Goldstein and Forster (1965) put this idea to rest; all fishes they studied could break down uric acid to urea and glyoxylic acid. The purine-urea cycle is continuous only to uric acid in primates, birds, and saurian reptiles, but presumably it is complete in all fishes, Amphibia, and chelonian reptiles. (But see immediately below).

Studies by Cvancara (1969) with freshwater fishes support the idea that uricolysis accounts for substantial urea production. However, Carlisky and Barrio (1972) found little or no urea was formed by the liver of the South American lungfish, *Lepidosiren paradoxa.* They studied the purine pathway by use of L-serine-3-^{14}C. The reactions of purine synthesis should lead to incorporation of that isotope into the ureido carbons of uric acid and into the carbon of urea.

Some levels for activity of the purinolytic portion of the purine-urea cycle for liver of the African lungfish are given in Table III. Studies with *Protopterus aethiopicus* by Brown *et al.* (1966) led them to suggest that some activities of the purine-urea cycle in the lungfish are sufficiently high to support a urea formation that may exceed the rate of urea synthesis by way of the ornithine-urea cycle. Forster and Goldstein (1966) criticized this position on the basis of their studies with ^{14}C-labelled bicarbonate (for measurement of ornithine-urea cycle activity) and with ^{14}C-labelled (carbon 3) serine (for measurement of purine-urea cycle activity). However, 1) the degree of the incorporation into urea by the two pathways will be affected by isotope dilution in various intermediate pools, and 2) the resulting incorporations into urea are from exogenously-administered starting compounds which may not be taken up by cells to the same extent and may be delivered at different rates to the sites of reaction in cellular components. These two points argue against making a comparison of the two routes of urea synthesis by the methodology employed by Forster and Goldstein (1966).

Table III. Purine degradation enzymes in the African lungfish, *Protopterus aethiopicus**

Enzyme	Activity μmol h^{-1} g^{-1} liver
uricase	76.2
allantoinase	382
allantoicase	75

*After Brown *et al.* (1966)

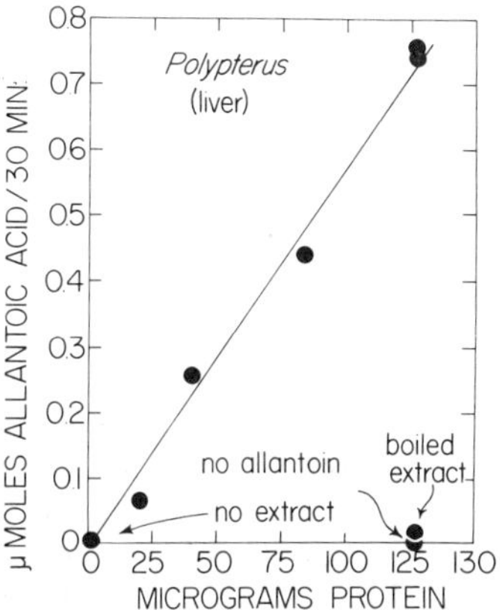

Fig. 3. Liver allantoinase of *Polypterus senegalis*. From Brown (1970).

It should be borne in mind that birds and saurian reptiles have achieved a rate of synthesis along the anabolic portion of the purine-urea cycle to provide for the bulk of their waste nitrogen in the form of uric acid which would otherwise be excreted as urea by most Amphibia and mammals.

Uricase has been demonstrated to occur in the liver of the shovel-nose sturgeon *Scaphirhynchus platorynchus* and other species of sturgeon and teleosts studied (Cvancara, 1969). Allantoinase is found in liver of *Polypterus senegalis* (Fig. 3).

Genetic aspects and adaptation

It is clear that the ornithine-urea cycle enzymes in Amphibia do not become fully expressed (when they do) until the adult stage (Brown, 1964a). This suggests an alternative to the idea of an actual loss of the ornithine-urea cycle enzyme proteins by an outright deletion. There could be mere suppression of such activities in vertebrates that do not appear to have a physiologically functioning ornithine-urea cycle, as in the teleosts, for example. We have indicated that residual ornithine-urea cycle activities have been demonstrated in teleosts even in situations where low activity is shown for CPSase. The presence of such residual ornithine-urea cycle activities in various tissues of various organisms may receive some explanation in the recent findings of Rosenberg *et al.* (1983). In spf^{ash} mutant mice they found that two distinct forms of carbamoylphosphate transferase precursor polypeptides are produced. One is normal in size, the other is elongated. They are imported and processed by the mitochondria. But only the normal one, having only 5-10% of the usual tissue activity, is assembled into the active form of the enzyme. Hence, the genetic aspect of control of a level of enzyme activity may be exerted in ways other than by a simple deletion of the original gene for cycle enzyme activity. A variety of types of genetic alterations may come into play during evolution to delete all or partial activity of the ornithine-urea cycle or to reinstate activity. That is really what the original phylogenetic chart (Brown and Cohen, 1960) was meant to depict -- a rise and fall (loss equals deletion, even) to yield the current distribution of enzyme activities among the vertebrate groups. The phylogenetic chart serves and aids in organizing and synthesizing information relating to the occurrence of the ornithine-urea cycle in the various vertebrate groups. It aids further in leading to suggestions as to the direction of further lines of inquiry.

Now a striking observation is provided by Horowich *et al.* (1984). They find that a 25% matching exists between the amino acid sequence of mature human ornithine carbamoyltransferase subunit and that of the aspartic carbamoyltransferase of *Escherichia coli.* Aspartic carbamoyltransferase is CPSase II. This finding strongly points to a primitive molecule that has been exploited to serve more than one function. Synthesis of arginine for proteins and pyrimidines for nucleic acids must have been around at the beginning of biological time, since these are crucial biochemical entities for life on earth as we know it.

We see how adaptable organisms are, to carry on, remove, or resurrect metabolic devices to aid in their further evolution, to support pathways for special tasks, and to provide an economy for coping with environmental changes and stresses, as well as to provide for the many ordinary biochemical chores associated with life's processes.

Studies with primitive fish provide us with information about them in particular, but also about processes which have become important to organisms further along the evolutionary road.

Literature Cited

ANDERSON, P.M. 1980. Glutamine- and L-acetyl-glutamate-dependent carbamoyl phosphate synthetase in elasmobranchs. Science **208**: 291-293.

ANDERSON, P.M. 1981. Purification and properties of the glutamine- and N-acetyl-L-glutamate-dependent carbamoyl phosphate synthetase from liver of *Squalus acanthias*. J. biol Chem. **256**: 12228-12238.

BALDWIN, E. 1960. Ureogenesis in elasmobranch fishes. Comp. Biochem. Physiol. **1**: 24-37.

BROWN, G.W., JR. 1962. Urea cycle and cellular deoxyribonucleic acid content. Nature **194**: 1279-1280.

BROWN, G.W., JR. 1964a. Metabolism of Amphibia. pp. 1-98 *In* Moore, J.A. [ed.] Physiology of the Amphibia. Academic Press, New York.

BROWN, G.W., JR. 1964b. Urea synthesis in elasmobranchs. pp. 407-416 *In* Leone, C.A. [ed.] Taxonomic biochemistry and serology. Ronald Press, New York.

BROWN, G.W., JR. 1970. Some evolutionary aspects of urea biosynthesis. pp. 3-14 *In* Schmidt-Nielsen, B., and D.W.S. Kerr [eds.] Urea and the kidney. Excerpta Medica Foundation, Amsterdam.

BROWN, G.W., JR., and S.G. BROWN. 1967. Urea and its formation in coelacanth liver. Science **155**: 570-573.

BROWN, G.W., JR., and P.P. COHEN. 1959. I. Methods for the quantitative assay of urea cycle enzymes in liver. J. biol. Chem. **234**: 1769-1774.

BROWN, G.W., JR., and P.P. COHEN. 1960. Comparative biochemistry of urea synthesis. 3. Activities of urea-cycle enzymes in various higher and lower vertebrates. Biochem. J. **75**: 82-91.

BROWN, G.W., JR., W.R. BROWN, and P.P. COHEN. 1959. Comparative biochemistry of urea synthesis. II. Levels of urea cycle enzymes in metamorphosing *Rana catesbeiana* tadpoles. J. biol. Chem. **234**: 1775-1780.

BROWN, G.W., JR., J. JAMES, R.J. HENDERSON, W.N. THOMAS, R.O. ROBINSON, A.L. THOMPSON, E. BROWN, and S.G. BROWN. 1966. Uricolytic enzymes in the liver of the dipnoan *Protopterus aethiopicus*. Science **153**: 1653-1654.

CAMPBELL, J.W. 1961. Studies on tissue arginase and ureogenesis in the elasmobranch, *Mustelus canis*. Arch. Biochem. Biophys. **93**: 448-455.

CAMPBELL, J.W. 1965. Arginine and urea biosynthesis in the land planarian: its significance in biochemical evolution. Nature **208**: 1299-1301.

CARLISKY, N.J., and A. BARRIO. 1972. Nitrogen metabolism of the South American lungfish, *Lepidosiren paradoxa*. Comp. Biochem. Physiol. **41B**: 857-873.

CASEY, C.A., and P.M. ANDERSON. 1982. Subcellular location of glutamine synthetase and urea cycle enzymes in liver of the spiny dogfish (*Squalus acanthias*). J. biol. Chem. **257**: 8449-8453.

CASEY, C.A., and P.M. ANDERSON. 1983. Glutamine- and N-acetyl-L-glutamate- dependent carbamoyl phosphate synthetase from *Micropterus salmoides*. J. biol. Chem. **258**: 8723-8732.

CIMINO, M.C., and G.F. BAHR. 1973. The nuclear DNA content and chromatin ultrastructure of the coelacanth, *Latimeria chalumnae*. J. Cell Biol. **59**: 55A.

CIMINO, M.C., and G.F. BAHR. 1974. The nuclear DNA content and chromatin ultrastructure of the coelacanth *Latimeria chalumnae*. Exp. Cell Res. **88**: 263-272.

COHEN, P.P., and G.W. BROWN, JR. 1960. Ammonia metabolism and urea biosynthesis. pp. 161-244 *In* Florkin, M., and H.S. Mason [eds.] Comparative biochemistry, vol. 2. Academic Press, New York.

CVANCARA, V.A. 1969. Comparative study of liver uricase activity in fresh-water teleosts. Comp. Biochem. Physiol. **28**: 725-732.

CVANCARA, V.A. 1974. Liver carbamyl phosphate synthetase in the primitive fresh-water bony fishes (Chondrostei, Holostei). Comp. Biochem. Physiol. **49B**: 785-787.

FICKEISEN, D.H., and G.W. BROWN, JR. 1977. D-Amino acid oxidase in various fishes. J. Fish Biol. **10**: 457-465.

FORSTER, R.P., and L. GOLDSTEIN. 1966. Urea synthesis in the lungfish: relative importance of purine and ornithine cycle pathways. Science. **153**: 1650-1652.

FUNKHOUSER, D., L. GOLDSTEIN, and R.P. FORSTER. 1972. Urea biosynthesis in the South American lungfish, *Lepidosiren paradoxa*: relation to its ecology. Comp. Biochem. Physiol. **41A**: 439-443.

GOLDSTEIN, L., and R.P. FORSTER. 1965. The role of uricolysis in the production of urea by fishes and other aquatic vertebrates. Comp. Biochem. Physiol. **14**: 567-576.

GOLDSTEIN, L., and R.P. FORSTER. 1970. Nitrogen metabolism in fishes. pp. 495-578 *In* Campbell, J.W. [ed.] Comparative biochemistry of nitrogen metabolism, vol. 2. Academic Press, London

GOLDSTEIN, L., and R.P. FORSTER. 1971. Urea biosynthesis and excretion in freshwater and marine elasmobranchs. Comp. Biochem. Physiol. **39B**: 415-421.

GOLDSTEIN, L., S. HARLEY-DeWITT, and R.P. FORSTER. 1973. Activities of ornithine-urea cycle enzymes and of trimethylamine oxidase in the coelacanth, *Latimeria chalumnae*. Comp. Biochem. Physiol. **44B**: 357-362.

GRIFFITH, R.W., B.L. UMMINGER, B.F. GRANT, P.K.T. PANG, L. GOLDSTEIN, and G.E. PICKFORD. 1976. Composition of bladder urine of the coelacanth, *Latimeria chalumnae*. J. exp. Zool. **196**: 371-380.

GRISOLIA, S, R. BAGUEANA, and F. MAYOR. [eds.] 1976. The urea cycle. John Wiley and Sons, New York. 579 pp.

HINEGARDNER, R. 1976. The cellular DNA content of sharks, rays and some other fishes. Comp. Biochem. Physiol. **55**: 367-370.

HORWICH, A.L., W.A. FENTON, K.R. WILLIAMS, F. KALOUSEK, J.P. KRAUS, R.F. DOOLITTLE, W. KONIGSBERG, and L.E. ROSENBERG. 1984. Structure and expression of a complementary DNA for the nuclear coded precursor of human mitochondrial ornithine transcarbamylase. Science **224**: 1068-1074.

HUGGINS, A.K., G. SKUTSCH, and E. BALDWIN. 1969. Ornithine-urea cycle enzymes in teleostean fish. Comp. Biochem. Physiol. **28**: 587-602.

HUNTER, A., and J. DAUPHINEE. 1924-25. Quantitative studies concerning the distribution of arginase in fishes and other vertebrates. Proc. R. Soc. (Lond.) **B17**: 227-242.

HURT, H. 1978. *In* Organic division dedicates program to Friedrich Wöhler. Chem. Eng. News. **56**: 19.

JANSSENS, P.A. 1964. The metabolism of the aestivating African lungfish. Comp. Biochem. Physiol. **11**: 105-117.

JANSSENS, P.A., and P.P. COHEN. 1966. Ornithine-urea cycle enzymes in the African lungfish, *Protopterus aethiopicus*. Science **152**: 358-359.

JONES, M.E., L. SPECTOR, and F. LIPMANN. 1955. Carbamyl phosphate, the carbamyl donor in enzymatic citrulline synthesis. J. Amer. Chem. Soc. **77**: 819-820.

KETOLA, G. 1977. Amino acids. pp. 411-412 *In* Rechcigl, M., Jr. [ed.] CRC handbook series in nutrition and food. Section D: nutrition requirements, vol. 1. CRC Press. Cleveland, Ohio. **1**: 411-412.

KREBS, H.A., and K. HENSELEIT. 1932. Untersuchungen über Harnstoffbildung im Tierkörper. Z. physiol. Chem. **210**: 33-66.

LOVE, R.M. 1970. Chemical biology of fishes. Academic Press, New York. 547 pp.

LOVE, R.M. 1980. Chemical biology of fishes. vol. 2. Academic Press, New York. 943 pp.

LOVERAGE, J.P. 1970. Observations on nitrogenous excretion and water relations of *Chiromantis xerampelina* (Amphibia, Anura). Arnoldia (Rhodesia) **5**: 1-6. Biol Abst. **52**: 8726. (1971) No. 87465.

MAYHALL, W.S.T., and G.W. BROWN, JR. 1967. Ornithine carbamoyltransferase activity in toadfish liver. Texas Rep. Biol. Med. **25**: 488-489.

MOYLE, V. 1949. Nitrogenous excretion in chelonian reptiles. Biochem. J. **44**: 581-584.

NOVAK, A. 1971. Boerhaave: Three chairs to oblivion. Bioscience **21**: 479-482.

PICKFORD, G.E., and F.B. GRANT. 1967. Serum osmolality in the coelacanth, *Latimeria chalumnae*: urea retention and ion regulation. Science **155**: 568-570.

READ, L.J. 1968. A study of ammonia and urea production and excretion in the freshwater-adapted form of the Pacific lamprey, *Entosphenus tridentatus*.

Comp. Biochem. Physiol. **26**: 455-466.

READ, L.J. 1971. The presence of high ornithine-urea cycle enzyme activity in the teleost *Opsanus tau*. Comp. Biochem. Physiol. **39B**: 409-413.

READ, L.J. 1975. Absence of ureogenic pathways in liver of the hagfish *Bdellostoma cirrhatum (Eptatretus cirratum)*. Comp. Biochem. Physiol. **51B**: 139-141.

ROBINSON, E.S., I.C. POTTER, and N.B. ATKIN. 1975. The nuclear DNA content of lampreys. Experientia. **31**: 912-913.

ROSENBERG, L.E., F. KALOUSEK, and M.D. ORSULAK. 1983. Biogenesis of ornithine transcarbamylase in spf^{ash} mutant mice: two cytoplasmic precursors, one mitochondrial enzyme. Science **222**: 426-428.

SALKOWSKI, E. 1877-1879. Über den Vorgang der Harnstoffbildung im Tierkörper und den Einfluss der Ammoniaksalze auf denselben. Z. Physiol. Chem. **1**: 1-59.

SALVATORE, F., V. ZAPPIA, and C. COSTA. 1965. Comparative biochemistry of deamination of L-amino acids in elasmobranch and teleost fish. Comp. Biochem. Physiol. **16**: 303-309.

SCHLEE, D., and H. REINBOTHE. 1963. Über eine funktionelle Inversion der C-Atome von Glycine im Purinstoffwechsel. Phytochemistry. **2**: 231-236.

SCHMIDT-NIELSEN, B., and D.W.S. KERR. [eds.] 1970. Urea and the kidney. Excerpta Medica Foundation. Amsterdam. 494 pp.

SHOEMAKER, V.H., and L.L. McCLANAHAN, JR. 1975. Evaporative water loss, nitrogen excretion and osmoregulation in phyllomedusine frogs. J. comp. Physiol. **100**: 331-345.

STAEDELER, G., and FR. TH. FRERICHS. 1858, X. Über das Vorkommen von Harnstoff, Taurin und Scyllit in den Organen der Plagiostomen. J. Prakt. Chem. **73**: 48-55.

THOMSON, K.S., J.G. GALL, and L.W. COGGINS. 1973. Nuclear DNA content of coelacanth erythrocytes. Nature **241**: 126.

THORSON, T.B. 1970. Freshwater stingrays, *Potamotrygon* spp.: failure to concentrate urea when exposed to saline medium. Life Sci. **9**: 893-900.

THORSON, T.B., C.M. COWAN, and D.E. WATSON. 1967. *Potamotrygon* spp.: elasmobranchs with low urea content. Science **158**: 375-377.

TRAMELL, T.B., and J.W. CAMPBELL. 1970. Carbamyl phosphate synthesis in a landsnail, *Strophocheilus oblongus*. J. biol. Chem. **245**: 6634-6641.

VELLAS, F., and A. SERFATY. 1974. L'ammoniaque et l'urée chez un téléostéen d'eau douce: La carp (*Cyprinus carpio* L.). J. Physiol. (Paris) **68**: 591-614.

WATTS, D.C., and R.L. WATTS. 1966. Carbamoyl phosphate synthetase in the Elasmobranchii: osmoregulatory function and evolutionary implications. Comp. Biochem. Physiol. **17**: 785-798.

WATTS, R.L., and D.C. WATTS. 1974. Nitrogen metabolism in fishes. pp. 369-466 *In* Florkin, M., and B.T. Scheer [eds.] Chemical zoology, vol. 8. Deuterostomians, cyclostomes and fishes. Academic Press, New York.

WEBB, J.T., and G.W. BROWN, JR. 1976. Some properties and occurrence of glutamine synthetase in fish. Comp. Biochem. Physiol. **54B**: 171-175.

WEBB, J.T., and G.W. BROWN, JR. 1980. Glutamine synthetase: assimilatory role in liver as related to urea retention in marine Chondrichthyes. Science **208**: 293-295.

WEKELL, M.M.B., and G.W. BROWN, JR. 1973. Ornithine aminotransferase of fishes. Comp. Biochem. Physiol. **46B**: 779-795.

SOME ASPECTS OF HORMONAL REGULATION OF METABOLISM IN AGNATHANS

Erika Plisetskaya

Department of Zoology
University of Washington
Seattle, Washington

Introduction

A short paper by Barrington, concerning the morphology of the endocrine pancreatic organ in the larval lamprey and its assumed influence on plasma blood sugar, appeared in 1942. For about twenty years this pioneer effort was not followed by additional research on the metabolic effects of the hormones in cyclostomes. In the early sixties, almost simultaneously and independently of each other, zoologists from Austria, the USSR, Sweden and Great Britain initiated further work in this research area on the representatives of both groups of the most ancient living vertebrates, lampreys and hagfish. The effects of hormones on blood glucose and hepatic and muscle glycogen content came under study first (Falkmer, 1962; Leibson *et al.*, 1963; Schirner, 1963a, b; Falkmer and Windbladh, 1964; Plisetskaya, 1964; Plisetskaya *et al.*, 1964; Bentley and Follet, 1965b; Matty, 1965; Plisetskaya, 1965). From this point, our knowledge of the hormonal control of metabolism in agnathans has been steadily growing.

The sheer number of publications and exhaustive reviews in this field during the last ten years (Plisetskaya, 1975, 1980; Hardisty, 1979; Epple *et al.*, 1980; Larsen, 1980; Murat *et al.*, 1981; Youson, 1981; Hardisty and Baker, 1982; Rovainen, 1982; Hardisty and Rovainen, 1982; Plisetskaya *et al.*, 1983c) makes it impossible to do more here than to summarize them. Furthermore, discussion of the hormonal effects on nonmetabolic functions in cyclostomes must be left to other chapters in this volume.

My task is to outline certain metabolic events, and their hormonal regulation, which seems to reflect the phylogenic position of agnathans, or are relevant to their way of life.

Stores of energy

Energy production appears to be a relatively uniform phenomenon in different animal species. The intermediary pathways of glycolysis, the citric acid cycle, as well as phosphorylation coupled to oxidation in the respiratory chain, creating the energy of adenosine triphosphate, are basic for living organisms. Cyclostomes and fishes store carbohydrate and fat between feedings, as do all other animals. Although fat, and even protein, can be mobilized under normal conditions, the immediate source of energy for vigorous and rapid movement is glycogen, accumulated for easy availability in muscles. The energetically richest and lightest substrate, the lipids, are utilized during long migrations, or during hibernation (cf. Drummond and Black, 1960; Hochachka and Somero, 1973).

Stores of hepatic glycogen are regarded as reservoirs for maintaining constant plasma glycemic levels, which are important for providing the central nervous system with essential fuel. A striking feature, which is characteristic for lampreys and hagfish, and different from other fishes (elasmobranchs or teleosts), is the moderate content of glycogen in their livers.

The values shown in Fig. 1 are in good agreement with the data reported by others (Hardisty *et al.*, 1975; Inui and Gorbman, 1977; O'Boyle and Beamish, 1977). The assumption that the liver of neither naturally fasting lampreys during their spawning migration, nor actively feeding hagfish and ammocoetes, is a primary organ for carbohydrate metabolism has been supported by experiments on hepatectomized lampreys and hagfish (Larsen, 1978; Inui and Gorbman, 1978). No substantial shifts in glycemic levels followed such surgery. Moreover, the plasma amino-nitrogen levels remained unchanged, indicating that the hagfish liver is also less engaged in amino acid metabolism than is the liver of other vertebrates.

Finally, glucose-6-phosphatase activity in the lamprey and hagfish liver appear to be low, as compared with the activity of the same enzyme in the kidney and in the brain (Inui and Gorbman, 1978; Murat *et al.*, 1979).

Our data concerning the glucose-6-phosphatase activity in different organs of Pacific hagfish, Pacific lamprey and, for comparison, of Atlantic salmon (juveniles) are shown in Table I.

Morphological and biochemical studies on ammocoetes, reviewed extensively by Youson (1981), suggest that, in the larval stage, the lamprey liver performs more functions (like glycogenolysis, gluconeogenesis, *etc.*) attributed to the livers of other vertebrates. The same is true for young feeding lampreys (cf. Beamish *et al.*, 1979).

In contrast to the liver, skeletal muscles of lamprey and hagfish are the main storage not only for carbohydrate, but, in lamprey, also for fat. Muscle makes up about 70% of the lamprey's total body weight. Because glycogen concentrations in lamprey muscles are about twice as high as those in the liver and, additionally, fat cells form layers between and around each bundle of muscle fibers, we must agree with Bentley and Follett (1965a, b) that muscles, not liver, are the main energy reserve in these animals. As for the hagfish, the concentration of glycogen in their

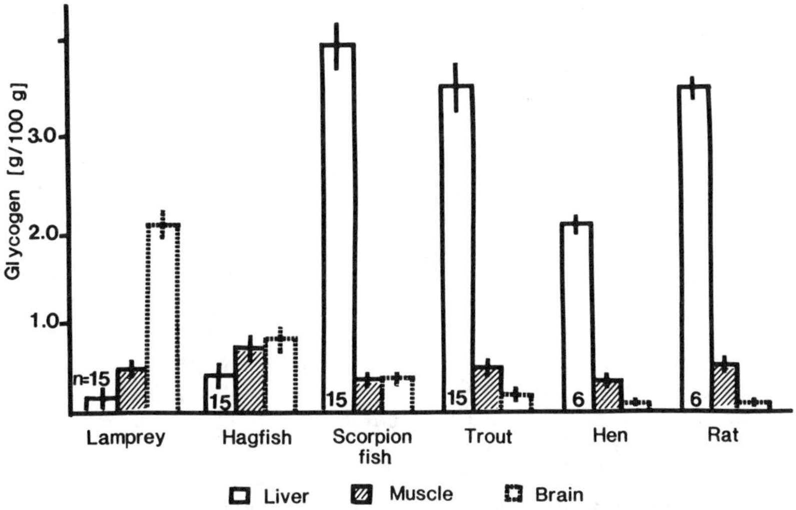

Fig. 1. The comparative amounts of glycogen in the liver, brain, and muscles of some vertebrates (according to Plisetskaya, 1975, and unpublished data). Lamprey, *Lampetra fluviatilis*; hagfish, *Eptatretus stouti*; scorpion fish, *Scorpaena porcus*; trout, *Salmo irideus*; hen, *Gallus* sp.; rat, *Rattus norvegicus*.

Table I. Glucose-6-phosphatase activity in different organs of Lampreys, Hagfish, and Salmon (μm P g^{-1} protein min^{-1}) (according to Plisetskaya, unpublished)

Species	Liver (n)	Brain (n)	Kidney (n)
Hagfish *Eptatretus stouti*	3.7 ± 0.40 (6)	11.80 (2)	12.3 ± 0.98 (5) 10.5 ± 1.88 (4)
Lamprey *Entosphenus tridentatus*	4.7 ± 1.65 (9) undetectable (7)	8.5 ± 0.70 (5)	5.2 ± 0.56 (4)
Salmon *Salmo salar*	21.5 ± 1.43 (7) 20.1 ± 2.30 (8)	4.0 ± 0.43 (6)	1.75 (2) undetectable (4)

muscles is about twice as high as that in the liver (Emdin, 1982; Plisetskaya, unpublished). Myxines have additional stores of lipid in the liver, around the intestine and in the visceral peritoneum. However, the liver lipids do not seem to be easily mobilized during at least one month of starvation (Emdin, 1982).

In lampreys the muscles, instead of liver, seem to be the principal site of conversion of glycerol to glycogen and glucose (Savina and Vilkova, 1976; Savina and Plisetskaya, 1976; Savina and Wojtczak, 1977). Thus, large quantities of fat, which anadromous lampreys, like other migrating animals, store before their spawning run, are converted to free fatty acids and glycerol, providing not only fuel for functioning muscles, but also some quantities of glycogen.

Gluconeogenesis from proteins is the ultimate energetic resource in the lamprey, taking place in the final stage of the spawning migration, though both participating enzymes, aspartate- and alanine-amino-transferase are present in lamprey muscles (Serebrenikova and Lyzlova, 1977).

Since the glycemic levels in hagfish and lampreys seem to be constant, it may be assumed that glycogen stored or synthesized from glycerol in skeletal muscles of fasting lampreys can be broken down to glucose and enter the blood stream. Glucose-6-phoshatase, which acts either in glycolytic or gluconeogenic pathways, splitting glucose from glucose-6-phosphate, is absent from both lamprey and hagfish muscle (Inui and Gorbman, 1977; Plisetskaya, unpublished). Nevertheless, another enzyme, γamylase, which catalyzes the splitting of glucose from glycogen, occurs in lamprey skeletal muscle and obviously can fulfill a similar role (Plisetskaya and Zheludkova, 1973). The kidney also may be a source of glucose during lipid mobilization (Murat *et al.*, 1979).

The unusually high content of glycogen in the lamprey brain is measurable at the very beginning of the spawning migration (Plisetskaya, 1968). The concentration of glycogen in the brain of fresh-caught hagfish is relatively high also (Fig. 1). It has been shown that the addition of glucose to incubation media, which generally has an immediate and strong stimulatory effect on the respiration of vertebrate brain, does not affect the respiration of lamprey brain (Plisetskaya, 1967) (Fig. 2). Neither a physiological concentration of glucose (0.5 mg/ml) nor a high concentration (2.0 mg/ml) increased respiration in lamprey brain, whereas in chicken the respiration was increased two-fold by a physiological (for chicken) concentration of glucose (2 mg/ml).

Thus, it is possible that the lamprey brain, endowed with an endogenous carboyhydrate store, is relatively autonomous with respect to carbohydrates. According to Rovainen (Rovainen, 1970, 1979, 1982; Rovainen *et al.*, 1969, 1971) the glycogen in the lamprey brain is located mainly in the supportive tissues, namely meningeal cells. Moreover, Rovainen and collaborators demonstrated that the meninges of both adult and larval lampreys have an unusual ability for release of glucose, which can be metabolized in the brain. Peculiar meningeal cells, so-called "round" or "arachnoid" cells, contain fat and glycogen. Their ultrastructure, according to Rovainen *et al.* (1971), indicates that they are storage sites for lipids and carbohydrates, capable of rapid metabolic activity, and they are able to secrete or take up substances at their surfaces. It has been reported also that the glial cells

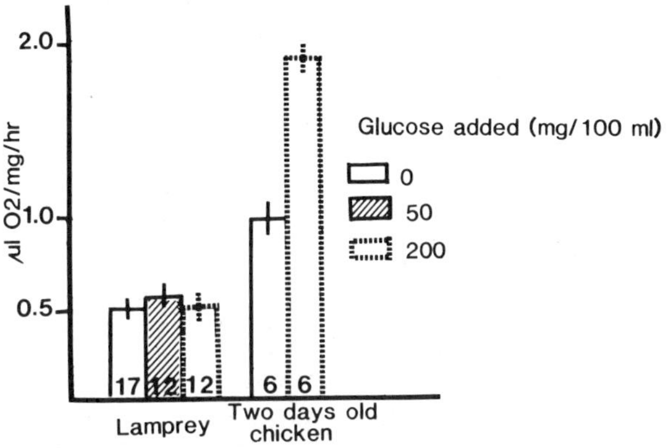

Fig. 2. The effect of added glucose on the respiratory rates (μ l O_2 mg^{-1} hr^{-1}) in lamprey and chicken brain. Numbers at the base of each column indicate the number of samples assayed.

form "anchoring" fibrils which extend into the meningeal tissues (Nakao, 1979). The activity of glucose-6-phosphatase, the enzyme which liberates gucose, is high in both lamprey and hagfish brains (Table I), and, assayed more precisely, in the meningeal tissues of the lamprey brain (Rovainen, 1970; Ogorodnikova and Fotina, 1977). This activity is sufficient to account for the observed rates of glucose release: 100 mmol $kg^{-1}hr^{-1}$ (Rovainen, 1970). Experiments with isolated ammocoete heads have demonstrated that the concentration of glucose increased in both meningeal tissues and the nervous tissue. Isolated brains cleared of membranes and incubated separately, show no such elevation of glucose; therefore, it has been suggested that glucose produced in the meninges probably moves to the nerve cells of the brain, supporting their metabolism during stress conditions or long periods of natural fasting (Rovainen *et al.*, 1971). It also explains why the respiration of the lamprey brain isolated together with the supportive tissues was not affected by added glucose (Plisetskaya, 1967; Leibson and Plisetskaya, 1968). Hagfish, which have been feeding actively in nature, can survive in captivity for many months without food. This ability seems to be an adaptation to the irregularity of food supply at the sea bottom at depths more than 100 m. Though the metabolism of glucose in the hagfish brain has never been studied like that of the lamprey, we can assume from its high glycogen content, and high glucose-6-phosphatase activity, as well as from its resistance to insulin hypoglycemia, that the metabolic pathways in hagfish brain have features that resemble those of larval and adult lampreys.

In cyclostomes, as in some other fish species that consume mostly protein and lipids, the metabolism of nervous tissue also may be supported by ketone bodies (ß-hydroxybutyrate and presumably acetoacetate) (De Roos *et al.*, 1985). However, as far as we know at this time, the activities of enzymes that participate in the metabolism of ketone bodies, like acetoacetyl-CoA-deacylase, are low in the lamprey (Phillips and Hird, 1979).

Levels of metabolites in male and female lampreys during the spawning migration and spawning

A feature which cyclostomes share with many other fishes is the distinct sexual difference in the content of certain metabolites. The differences in proximate composition of the bodies of male and female anadromous sea lamprey, *Petromyzon marinus*, including the composition of gonads, were reported by Lowe *et al.* (1973) and Beamish *et al.* (1979). Here we will point out only some particularities revealed in our own studies. Glycogen levels in the liver of male Baltic lamprey, *Lampetra fluviatilis*, are significantly higher than in females when they enter freshwater and for some months after that time (Hardisty *et al.*, 1975; Plisetskaya, 1975; Plisetskaya and Murat, 1980). The activity of the key enzyme engaged in glycogen synthesis, glycogen-synthetase, is also significantly higher in the male liver at that period (Plisetskaya, 1975). The situation changes as spawning approaches. At this time a higher glycogen content, obviously formed at the expense of gluconeogenesis from lipids, has been observed in female lampreys (Plisetskaya and Murat, 1980) (Table II).

Plasma circulating levels of free fatty acids are slightly higher in females than in males during the river period of their life before reproduction. Probably this indicates a more intensive lipolysis (Plisetskaya, 1975, 1980). Our recent assays (Sower *et al.*, 1985) have demonstrated that, at spawning grounds, the females of another lamprey species, the landlocked marine lamprey, *Petromyzon marinus*, still have a comparatively high level of free fatty acids circulating in blood; whereas in males these levels have decreased substantially (Table II). The plasma proteins, on the other hand, have dropped in females and remain approximately unchanged in males. These metabolic changes reflect the decline in the lipids in male liver, and protein in female liver at spawning time, as reported by Beamish *et al.* (1979).

Are the metabolic peculiarities described above in lampreys and hagfish influenced by the hormones or only by the regulatory systems directly related to substrate concentrations? The second assumption is shared by many (cf. Larsen, 1980; Savina and Derkachev, 1983), and the recent publication of Savina and Derkachev (1983) illustrates this line of thought. They reported that the potential activity of one of the gluconeogenic enzymes, pyruvate carboxylase, in wintering adult lampreys is similar to that in mammalian liver; however a deficit of mitochondrial ATP inhibits the gluconeogenic process at that particular season. More specifically, the low energy state of the liver cells in lampreys is caused by the inhibition of adenine nucleotide translocase by long-chain fatty acids and/or their acyl-CoA derivatives. In turn, the accumulation of fatty acids has been caused by "unbalanced oxidation" under conditions of low water temperature in winter. The warming of water in an experiment, or during natural seasonal changes, initiates an enhanced utilization of fatty acid. The translocase inhibition disappears and a rapid increase in ATP levels and in the NAD/NADH ratio in liver cells takes place. Both the intensity of gluconeogenesis and of the accumulation of glycogen are consequently enhanced. The authors conclude that glucose synthesis in lamprey liver seems to be an oscillatory process based on a cyclic "switch on-switch off" mechanism triggered by seasonal changes in water temperature.

Table II. Liver glycogen and plasma fatty acids in male and female lampreys. (According to Plisetskaya, 1975; Plisetskaya and Murat, 1980; Sower *et al.*, 1985).

Sex	Season	Liver Glycogen (mg/100 g)	Liver glycogen Synthetase (I-form) (μm UDF/100 mg)	Plasma FFA (μEq/ml)
		Lampetra fluviatilis		
Male	October	236 ± 2.1 (24)	0.34 ± 0.03 (6)	
Female		150 ± 2.0 (15)	0.21 ± 0.03 (6)	
Male	December	286 ± 4.3 (10)		0.88 ± 0.03 (30)
Female		171 ± 3.5 (10)		1.02 ± 0.06 (28)
Male	May (one month	152 ± 9.1 (4)		
Female	before spawning)	227 ± 7.0 (14)		
Male	May (one week	149 ± 1.1 (9)		
Female	before spawning)	513 ± 4.6 (14)		
Male	June (after	75 ± 2.2 (8)		
	spawning)	traces (2)		
		Petromyzon marinus		
Male	July			0.35 ± 0.09 (7)
Female	(one week before spawning)			0.59 ± 0.06 (9)
Male	Spawning			
Female				0.68 ± 0.02 (5)

It is difficult to deny the important role which metabolites themselves can play in regulation of metabolic pathways. Nevertheless, changes of plasma levels of hormones also are occurring at that time; and in view of the known properties of these hormones, their roles in the metabolic events observed must be considered. Cyclic changes in hormonal levels are probably influenced by the same stimulus: the change of the water temperature, resulting in a complex interaction between hormones and substrates, which in turn direct the metabolic flow.

Hormonal effects on metabolism in agnathans

New techniques have made it possible to measure plasma levels and organ content of many hormones which are assumed to participate in regulation of metabolism in agnathans (*e.g.* thyroid hormones, catecholamines, and glucocorticoids).

Except for hagfish insulin, no appropriate quantitative assays are available at this time for peptide pancreatic hormones. Emdin and Steiner (1980), using their homologous assay for hagfish insulin, found that the circulating levels are ten times higher than were measured in lampreys by employment of heterologous radioimmune systems that included mammalian or even fish components (Plisetskaya and Leibush, 1972; Plisetskaya, unpublished).

It is now clear that the doses of hormones, which were administered to agnathans in the earlier studies, were far in excess of physiological concentrations. In this review emphasis will be given to studies in which low doses of hormones were injected, or in which deficiencies in hormonal concentration were caused either by prolonged fasting, or by adminstration of antisera, or by extirpation of an endocrine gland.

In Atlantic hagfish, *Myxine glutinosa*, after one month of fasting, insulin levels declined 50%, though they still remained about five times higher than in the lamprey (Emdin, 1982; Plisetskaya *et al.*, 1976). Purified lamprey insulin will be obligatory for further studies on carbohydrate and lipid metabolism in lampreys at different stages of their life cycle.

Even though plasma levels of insulin in different phases of the life cycle cannot yet be compared quantitatively, we still can compare them qualitatively to trace any possible relative changes. Recently we made such a comparison between the plasma circulating levels of insulin in the Baltic lamprey (*Lampetra fluviatilis*) and the landlocked marine lamprey (*Petromyzon marinus*) during the final maturation and spawning periods. Some interesting similarities were revealed (Fig. 3).

The Baltic lampreys in the Leningrad area, after entering the river, remain in fresh water from October until May-June. Vitellogenesis progresses slowly and is completed by the following March or early April (Plisetskaya *et al.*, 1976; Murat *et al.*, 1981). The start of spawning depends on the water temperature. To the contrary, histological examination of the ovaries of *Petromyzon marinus* made by Stacia Sower indicated that vitellogenesis has been virtually completed when they enter the river after the parasitic lake stage of their life. If we compare plasma insulin levels in these two species of lampreys at equivalent phases of their terminal freshwater existence (Fig. 3), these levels follow the same progressive pattern, reflecting an apparent similarity in physiological conditions of lamprey and probably a similar influence of insulin on metabolic processes. The sharp drop in insulin levels just before or during spawning obviously can be a part of a mechanism leading the metabolic processes into catabolism, and enhancing the spending of the remaining energy resources, which include even protein in muscles (Ivanova-Berg and Sokolova, 1959; Bentley and Follet, 1965a; O'Boyle and Beamish, 1977). The constantly low level of insulin is obviously responsible for the hyperglycemia at the time of spawning (Larsen 1976, 1980).

A state of acute insulin insufficiency can be produced experimentally by administration of anti-insulin serum to animals just entering the river mouth

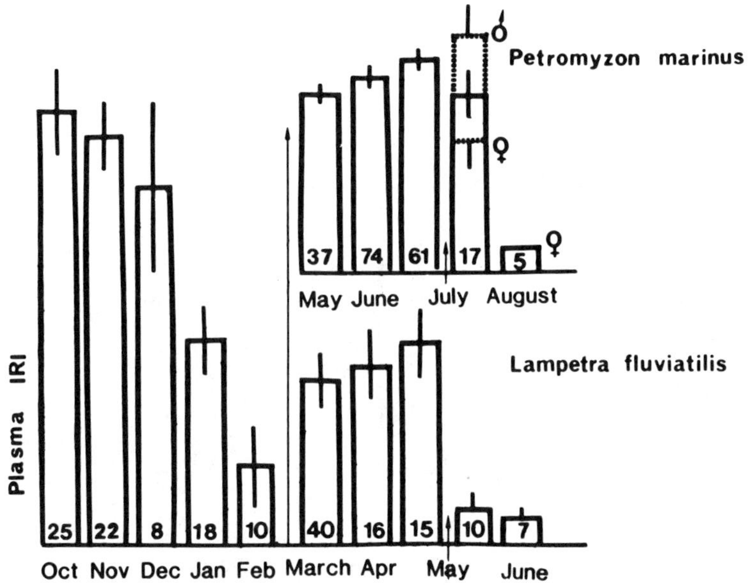

Fig. 3. Relative changes in plasma circulating levels of insulin in *L. fluviatilis* and *P. marinus* (from Sower, Plisetskaya and Gorbman, 1985). The columns represent plasma levels of insulin in their relation to the lowest level at spawning time. The number of plasma samples is indicated at the bases of the columns. The long arrow indicates completion of vitellogenesis. Shorter arrows indicate spawning.

(Plisetskaya and Leibush, 1972; Plisetskaya *et al.*, 1976). The results of such a procedure are presented in Fig. 4. The administration of anti-insulin serum to the Atlantic hagfish, *M. glutinosa*, had no effect (Falkmer and Wilson, 1967), whereas in our experiments on Pacific hagfish, *E. stouti*, the same treatment caused an elevation of plasma glucose, free fatty acids, and amino-nitrogen levels. The decline in plasma protein levels was insignificant (Plisetskaya *et al.*, 1983b). The extirpation of the islet tissue also has different effects on lampreys and on Atlantic hagfish. In lampreys, total isletectomy was followed by a decline in plasma circulating levels of insulin-like activity, and a hyperglycemia up to 5-7 times above normal glycemic levels. After surgery, the animals were unable to remove the glucose load (Hardisty *et al.*, 1975; Zelnik *et al.*, 1977). On the contrary, isletectomy performed on *M. glutinosa* did not affect either glycemic levels or the rate of elimination of the glucose load (Falkmer and Matty, 1966). The same surgery performed by Matty on Pacific hagfish was associated with some hyperglycemia (Matty and Gorbman, 1978). It appears that the Pacific hagfish is sensitive to insulin (Inui and Gorbman, 1977) and more dependent on it for regulation of its carbohydrate metabolism than its Atlantic counterpart. Could this be the reason for an absence of shifts in plasma glucose or plasma fatty acids in *M. glutinosa* injected by Emdin (1982) with an insulin from the same species?

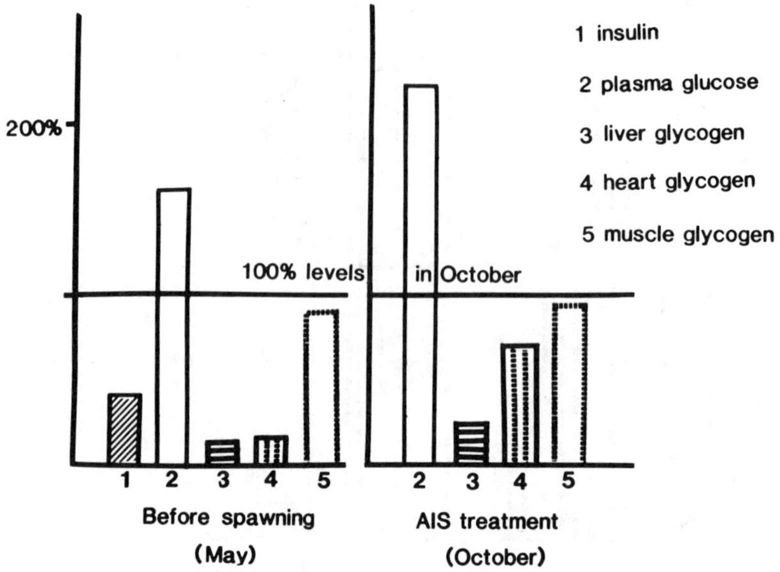

Fig. 4. Comparison of some metabolic indices in Baltic lampreys at the end of their spawing run (May) when they experience chronic insulin insufficiency, and after the treatment of the lampreys with anti-insulin serum at the beginning of their spawning run (October). The levels in untreated lampreys at the beginning of the run are considered as 100%. (According to Plisetskaya and Leibush, 1972; Larsen, 1976; Plisetskaya, 1980).

A puzzling finding in mature Baltic lampreys some months before spawning is a "metabolic surge" which appears after a long period of complete fasting. In Baltic lampreys that period may be as long as five months. It takes place at the time when vitellogenesis is completed; and it coincides, at least in Baltic lampreys, with the elevation of water temperature (Plisetskaya *et al.*, 1976). As was mentioned above, it seems to be a time of intensification of gluconeogenesis (Savina and Derkachev, 1983) which results in redistribution of glycogen in male and female livers (Plisetskaya and Murat, 1980). The precise role of insulin, at the time when the gluconeogenic processes prevail, is not clear. In fact, insulin or insulin-like substances have not been measured separately in males and females except at spawning time (Sower *et al.*, 1985) (Fig. 3). If we compare lampreys with their so-called ecological parallels, Pacific salmon (Berg, 1935), we see here also that differences appear between the two sexes in the plasma insulin profiles (Bondareva *et al.*, 1980). In female salmon, insulin levels drop continually until spawning; in males they are unchanged, or even increase, as the spawning time approaches. We may assume that lowered insulin levels, along with elevated levels of some other (steroid?) hormones, will lead to enhanced gluconeogenesis in female lampreys, possibly to support the more severe physiological demands of ovogenesis. The elevation of liver glycogen in females fits in with this interpretation. Another role which we can conceive for insulin may be to protect energy stores, especially muscle glycogen and protein, from premature exhaustion. In their work on carp, Castilla and Murat (1975) observed that insulin seems to preserve muscle glycogen, which has been made available as a result of intensive gluconeogenesis (Savina and Plisetskaya, 1976; Savina and Wojtczak, 1977). Immediately after vigorous motor activity at the time of spawning, both plasma insulin levels and glycogen content in skeletal muscles decline abruptly.

Many questions dealing with the role of insulin in agnathans are still to be addressed. One of them is the question of the role of this hormone in larval lampreys and during metamorphosis when the larvae stop feeding and many important metabolic changes in the liver take place (cf. Youson, 1981).

The primary hormones stimulating gluconeogenesis in vertebrates are the glucocorticoids and "the hormone of hunger," glucagon. These hormones are either absent, or present in extremely low quantities in agnathans (Buus and Larsen (1975); Weisbart and Idler (1970); Weisbart and Youson (1977); Weisbart *et al.* (1980); Katz *et al.* (1982). We can only guess that some steroids of gonadal origin (cf. Weisbart and Youson, 1977) may take over the role of corticosteroids in enhancing gluconeogenesis in cyclostomes. The injection of mammalian ACTH increases the steroid levels found in hagfish plasma (Weisbart *et al.*, 1980). As reported by Eastman and Portanova (1982), Baker and Buckingham (1983) and Buckingham *et al.* (1985), corticotropin-like bioactivity is present in the pituitaries, and to a lesser extent in the brain, of both lampreys and hagfish. The question still remains unsolved about the physiological meaning of these findings, as well as about any relations of these pituitary activities to the steroid-producing tissues. One could also consider the possibility that some unusual, still unidentified corticoids exist, which could be as specific for agnathans as 1α-hydroxy-corticosterone is specific for elasmobranchs (Idler and Truscott, 1966). In contrast to the situation in adult lampreys, higher plasma levels of glucocorticosteroids were discovered by Dashow *et al.* (1984) in ammocoetes of *P. marinus*. Even with the reservations which we share with these authors, we must assume that higher levels of glucocorticoids circulating in plasma may have a metabolic effect on ammocoete liver. Appropriate studies remain to be done.

Glucagon-like immunoreactivity has been found in extracts of agnathan intestine and the so-called "cranial" pancreatic islets, though it is possible that the latter activity was due to contamination by gut tissue (Zelnik *et al.*, 1977). The presence of a glucagon-like substance in the blood of Pacific hagfish has been reported by Stewart *et al.* (1978). The administration of different doses of mammalian glucagon to lampreys was ineffective, or had an insulin-like effect, at least with respect to plasma glucose, plasma fatty acids, tissue glycogen, and glycogen-synthetase activity (Plisetskaya and Mazina, 1969; Plisetskaya, 1975; Plisetskaya and Murat, 1980). The "paradoxical" effect has been considered to be an indirect one, *via* enhanced insulin secretion. High doses of mammalian glucagon elevated insulin levels in lampreys (Plisetskaya *et al.*, 1976); nevertheless, treatment of lampreys with antimammalian glucagon serum, though it raised the plasma fatty acid level, did not decrease plasma immunoreactive insulin (Plisetskaya, 1980).

Since either circulating levels (if any), or amino-acid sequence of glucagon in agnathans are unknown, no experiments with physiological doses of that hormone have been made.

The importance of administering physiological doses of a hormone was clearly demonstrated in experiments with epinephrine. This presumably hyperglycemic and hyperlipemic factor (at least in the lampreys), when used in pharmacological doses, had also an inhibitory effect on enzymes like glycogen-synthetase in liver and muscles (Plisetskaya, 1975).

Recently, the circulating levels of catecholamines in lamprey and hagfish blood have been measured using a modern technique (Dashow *et al.*, 1982; Dashow and Epple, 1983; Plisetskaya *et al.*, 1984). The basal levels in lamprey appeared to be slightly lower than levels measured by earlier methods (Mazeaud, 1969; Plisetskaya and Prosorovskaya, 1971). Stressful experimental conditions evoked a tremendous rise in these levels, as reported by numerous investigators (Plisetskaya and Prosorovskaya, 1971; Dashow and Epple, 1983; Plisetskaya *et al.*, 1984). The elevation of catecholamine levels coincides with high concentrations of plasma glucose and fatty acids.

There are differences in plasma catecholamine levels in lampreys, *P. marinus*, of the two sexes, namely 1.4 ng/ml in females and 0.7 ng/ml in males (Mazeaud, 1969). This seems to be in good agreement with lower liver glycogen concentration, as well as lower glycogen-synthetase activity and higher level of plasma fatty acids in females of *L. fluviatilis* (Plisetskaya, 1975; Table II). Catecholamines may be assumed to play some role in enhancing gluconeogenesis. In the carp, an activation of gluconeogenesis by epinephrine was reported by Murat (1976). Moreover, Dashow *et al.* (1982) and Dashow and Epple (1983) measured plasma epinephrine levels in early migrants of *P. marinus* and in lampreys close to spawning. Levels in the second group appear to be 1-2 orders of magnitude higher. However, recently some puzzling results have come from Epple's laboratory (Dashow and Epple, 1983). They reported that epinephrine in doses up to 5 ng/g do not cause hyperglycemias in lampreys. We have repeated the experiment with Pacific hagfish and obtained the same results (Fig. 5). Plasma glucose was not elevated after low doses of epinephrine, whereas high doses were hyperglycemic. Must we agree with Dashow and Epple's (1983) suggestion that the action of catecholamines in agnathans is restricted to cardiovascular, respiratory and osmoregulatory, but not metabolic effects? Furthermore, are the parallel changes in epinephrine titres and some metabolic indices, either in nature or under experimental conditions, just an occasional coincidence? It is difficult to believe this, but at the moment there is no experimental proof of a metabolic effect of physiological doses of epinephrine on agnathans.

If the role of epinephrine as a lipolytic hormone is questionable, is there any other candidate for such a role? Arginine-vasotocin has been reported to have a lipolytic action in lampreys (John *et al.*, 1977) but little further detail is yet available with respect to this proposal. Recently we have investigated whether thyroid hormones, especially triiodothyronine (T_3), participate in regulation of any metabolic pathways in cyclostomes directly or permissively (Plisetskaya *et al.*, 1983a,b, 1984).

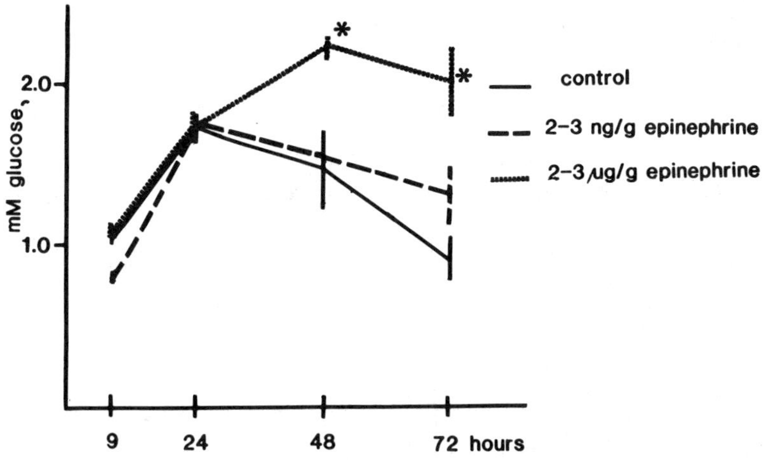

Fig. 5. Plasma glucose levels in hagfish after the injection of epinephrine. (According to Plisetskaya *et al.*, 1984).

The role of thyroid hormones in intermediary metabolism in agnathans is a virtually untouched field of investigation. In earlier work, since normal plasma levels of thyroid hormone, triiodothyronine (T_3), were unknown, there was no rational choice of dosage of T_3 to be used. The transient decrease of plasma T_3 which accompanies acute, experimentally-produced insulin deficiency argues for a functional relationship. Furthermore, in fresh-caught hagfish there is a negative correlation: the individuals with higher plasma circulating levels of T_3 have lower glycemic levels (Plisetskaya *et al.*, 1983a,b). Both observations lead us to conclude that thyroid hormones may act under some conditions through stimulation of insulin secretion (cf. Murat and Serfaty, 1970). Experimental verification of a thyroid-insulin relationship is needed.

One likely role of thyroid hormones in regulation of intermediary metabolism in agnathans seems to be in lipid metabolism. In our experiments on hagfish (*Eptatretus stouti*) fasted for some months, 1 ng/g of T_3, the lowest dose used, was accompanied by a strong lipolytic effect. After implanting hagfish with a silastic capsule containing the goitrogen, 6- propylthiouracil, the opposite effect, namely a drop in plasma free fatty acids, has been observed. In accordance with current information, growth hormone, prolactin and glucagon have no demonstrable role in regulation of lipid metabolism in cyclostomes (Hardisty and Baker, 1982). Our results (Plisetskaya *et al.*, 1984) suggest that the lipolytic effect of T_3 is also independent of catecholamines. Though T_3 treatment elevated circulating epinephrine levels more than an injection of saline, physiological doses of epinephrine have no effect on plasma levels of free fatty acids.

In spite of such evidence, it is difficult to consider T_3 to be an important hormone directly regulating lipid metabolism, since it requires as long as 24-48 hours to exert its maximum response. We can only speculate that the slow development of the T_3 lipolytic effect is the resultant of a combined lipolytic and lipogenic effect of thyroid hormones (Bernal and De Groot, 1980). Recently, the stimulating effect of T_3 at particular concentrations on several essential enzymes, involved in the synthesis and the esterification of fatty acids, was reported in mammals (Gharbi-Chihi *et al.*, 1983).

The circulating levels of thyroid hormones are much higher in lamprey larvae than in adult lampreys (Wright and Youson, 1980; Lintlop and Youson, 1983a). These high levels of the hormones imply an important involvement in satisfying the special metabolic requirements of larvae (Lintlop and Youson, 1983a). At this time we know only that the rise of plasma T_4 levels in spring, dependent on or correlated with, a rise in water temperature, and decline of T_4 level in late summer, are in parallel with an accumulation and depletion of fat (O'Boyle and Beamish, 1977; Youson *et al.*, 1979). At the same time, plasma T_3 levels are inversely correlated with the changes of the ambient temperature. Thus, the highest level of T_3 coincides with lipid depletion, whereas, the lowest coincides with lipid accumulation. This seems to indicate tentatively a lipolytic effect of T_3 at this stage of lamprey development (cf. Plisetskaya *et al.*, 1983c).

It remains for future investigations to decide definitively whether hormones, like insulin or somatostatin, participate in the regulation of metabolism in larval lampreys. Somatostatin has been shown to inhibit insulin release in hagfish (Stewart *et al.*, 1978) as it does in other vertebrates. Recently we (Sheridan *et al.*, 1985) have demonstrated a strong lipolytic action of salmon somatostatin in juvenile salmon, similar to the reported action of somatostatin in lampreys (Plisetskaya, 1980). Theoretically, we can expect to find an enhanced metabolic role (and elevated levels) of somatostatin during fasting periods in the life cycle of lampreys: either during metamorphosis or spawning migration. The hormone, which inhibits insulin secretion, may be involved in regulation of metabolism, substituting in this way for the absent glucagon. One of the indirect proofs of this statement may be seen in the activation and hyperplasia of B-cells in both lamprey and Pacific salmon close to the spawning period, which is not reflected in accompanying circulating levels of plasma insulin (Poljakova and Plisetskaya, 1977). There are two possibilities to be considered: the higher utilization of insulin, or the inhibition of its secretion. The metabolic situation at spawning time inclines one to favor the second explanation.

Further experiments employing purified lamprey somatostatin, which is not yet available, supplemented by evaluation of secretory potencies for both hormones in male and female lampreys, may provide answers to such questions.

Hormonal receptors in agnathans

Studies of hormonal regulation in agnathans mostly have been concerned with postreceptor events. Lintlop and Youson (1983a,b) have reported that tissue binding capacities for T_3 diminish progressively in metamorphosing individuals, young parasitic adults, and in upstream migrants in parallel with the diminishing circulating levels of the same hormone. Such results bring into question the physiological significance of thyroid hormones at the very end of the spawning run of lampreys.

Somewhat more is known about the receptors for insulin, both in hagfish and lampreys. The subunit structure of the insulin receptor in *Myxine* liver appears to be similar to that of the mammalian insulin receptor (Czech and Massague, 1982). Hagfish insulin receptor shows not only structural, but also functional similarity to mammalian receptor with respect to the absolute and relative affinities for insulins of different vertebrate species. The rank order of preference for various insulins was very similar: chicken>pig>hagfish for the receptors in *Myxine* blood cells (Muggeo *et al.*, 1979a) or pig>salmon>hagfish for the receptors in the lamprey brain (Leibush, 1983). These assays support the conclusion that the insulin receptor is functionally better conserved in the course of evolution than the insulins themselves (Muggeo *et al.*, 1979a).

Nevertheless, Muggeo *et al.* (1979b) observed that hagfish insulin, though weakest in relative bioactivity, was more potent in binding to the hagfish receptor than to the mammalian receptor. For all other insulins studied so far (*e.g.* mammalian, chicken), the receptor affinities for the hormones were equal regardless of the species source of the receptor. For species like hagfish, whose insulin has a relatively low affinity for the receptor, there is usually compensation by high levels of plasma circulating hormone (Emdin and Steiner, 1980), high concentration of receptors on the target cells (Muggeo *et al.*, 1979a,b), and/or increased sensitivity of receptor to insulin, *i.e.* lower inhibition constant (Leibush and Bondareva, 1981). The presence of insulin receptors in liver and erythrocytes of *M. glutinosa* raises several additional questions. If hagfish insulin binds to its receptor in liver, and presumably in other organs as well, why was the injection of exogenous insulin in Emdin's experiment (Emdin, 1982) ineffective? In such a case, is a failure in postreceptor mechanisms responsible for the lack of a physiological action? Could there be a difference in hormone-receptor interactions between Atlantic and Pacific hagfish, explaining the absence of metabolic consequences after isletectomy and following the treatment with anti-insulin serum in *M. glutinosa*, but their presence in *E. stouti*?

Another exciting current question deals with the evolution of the insulin molecule, its phylogenic appearance, and its function in the cyclostome brain.

As discussed above, in meningeal tissues of lampreys, and to a lesser degree in hagfish brain, there are stores of glycogen accompanied by some appropriate gluconeogenic enzymes (Plisetskaya, 1968; Rovainen, 1979, 1982). Leibush (1983), when reporting the presence of insulin receptors in lamprey brain, did not specify the brain tissue in which they were located, but data dealing with insulin receptors in mammalian glial cells already have appeared (Clarke *et al.*, 1984). These latter authors report specific insulin binding sites, with appropriate receptor characteristics, in the glial cells of the rat brain. They demonstrated that the binding of insulin to these receptors stimulates 2-deoxy-d-glucose uptake into the brain cells.

Similar events may be anticipated in the lamprey brain. However, a related question is whether brain insulin is of islet or of brain origin.

The presence of considerable glycogen stores in the neurons of some invertebrates, like molluscs, and lower chordates, like lancelets, has been known for a long time (Gage, 1917). Similarly, rich stores were found in the brains of some embryonic mammals and in the course of winter hibernation (cf. Wolff, 1968; Oksche *et al.*, 1969). Such energy-yielding stores in the nervous system endow the brain or the nervous ganglia with a degree of autonomy. In the course of vertebrate evolution, most neurons have lost their ability to store glycogen. This shift has been accompanied by an increasing intensity of metabolism. As part of this evolutionary scenario, the nervous system has to depend fully on blood glucose as an essential fuel (Shabadash, 1949).

We can assume that at the earliest stages of evolution, when the nerve cells still are storing glycogen, they also produce the regulatory hormonal peptides for directing the utilization or processing of carbohydrates. In fact, insulin and insulin-like substances have been found in the nerve cells of insects and molluscs, together with many other brain and gut peptides (cf. Thorpe and Duve, 1984; Le Roith *et al.*, 1981, 1983). Moreover, by both immunocytochemical and biochemical methods, insulin was detected in the brain of newborn rats; its sharp decline during the first 20 days of postnatal development was described (Bernstein *et al.*, 1984). Furthermore, it seems reasonable to assume that, at least in lower vertebrates, whose neurons are able to support their energetic demands by metabolizing endogenous glycogen (and possibly ketone bodies), insulin or other regulatory peptides have to be within the blood-brain barrier to be effective.

Definitive evidence is still not available to decide whether insulin found in the brain was produced there along with other characteristic brain peptides (cf. Steiner *et al.*, 1984). Nevertheless, it may be predicted tentatively, that if any vertebrates retain the ability to synthesize insulin in their neurons, agnathans should be among them. It is puzzling that Falkmer (1984) reports recently, that neither lamprey nor hagfish brain contain insulin indentifiable immunocytochemically or radioimmunologically. This is in some contrast to Falkmer *et al.* (1984) separately claiming the opposite. Clearly this question must be reinvestigated, not only in adult lampreys, but also in lamprey larvae. If, indeed, there is no insulin in the lamprey brain, then the presence of "neuronal" insulin in invertebrates becomes enigmatic. This would mean that "neuronal" insulin was characteristic of some invertebrates, disappeared from that tissue during evolution, and reappeared in vertebrates at some time later than the agnathans, since it is demonstrable in mammals (cf. Bernstein *et al.*, 1984). What is the function of insulin receptors in the lamprey brain? These are important questions that deserve early investigative attention.

Another related question is the molecular nature of "neuronal" insulin. We know that it is very difficult to measure the agnathan's insulin by use of heterologous RIA's, because of the low crossreactivity not only with antisera raised against mammalian insulin, but also against fish insulin (Emdin and Steiner, 1980; Plisetskaya, Dickhoff, Paquette, Gorbman, unpublished).

This difficulty might be predicted from the known primary sequences of the insulins, since mammalian and fish insulins are probably closer to each other than they are to hagfish insulin, which evolved long before fish and mammalian lines diverged from the vertebrate stem (Peterson *et al.*, 1975). Having said this, another puzzle appears in the ability of the insulin-like substances of insects, or even of unicellular organisms, to crossreact in RIA's with antisera raised against mammalian hormone (Le Roith *et al.*, 1981; Thorpe and Duve, 1984). Have the mammalian or chicken types of insulins a prototype structure that is close to that of an ancestral molecule? Has there been a reversion to (or preservation of) a primordial insulin that is now reflected in the fact that avian and mammalian insulins have the highest affinity for insulin receptor of any vertebrate investigated, including cyclostomes? There is no definite conclusion yet whether a bovine type of insulin was really detected in the brain of the guinea pig (cf. Le Roith *et al.*, 1983). Will the insulin of the agnathan brain, if ever found, look like a hagfish islet hormone or like mammalian-type insulin?

We may anticipate that the near future (in less time than the 20 years that have elapsed since the beginning of our studies) will bring us many profound and fascinating discoveries, which will give a better understanding of hormonal regulation of metabolism in agnathans.

Acknowledgements

The experimental work providing the data for this review was partly supported by grants from the U.S. National Science Foundation (PCM 8215041 and DCB 8415957). The author is deeply indebted to Dr. Aubrey Gorbman for his invaluable help in preparing the manuscript.

Literature Cited

BAKER, B.I., and J.C. BUCKINGHAM. 1983. A study of corticotrophic and melanotrophic activities in the pituitary and brain of the lamprey, *Lampetra fluviatilis*. Gen. comp. Endocrinol. **52**: 283-290.

BARRINGTON, E.J.W. 1942. Blood sugar and the follicles of Langerhans in the ammocoete larva. J. exp. Biol. **19**: 45-55.

BEAMISH, F.W.H., I.C. POTTER, and E. THOMAS. 1979. Proximate composition of the adult anadromous sea lamprey, *Petromyzon marinus*, in relation to feeding, migration and reproduction. J. Anim. Ecol. **48**: 1-19.

BENTLEY, P.J., and B.K. FOLLETT. 1965a. Fat and carbohydrate reserves in the river lamprey during spawning migration. Life Sci. **4**: 2003-2007.

BENTLEY, P.J., and B.K. FOLLETT. 1965b. The effects of hormones on the carbohydrate metabolism of the lamprey, *Lampetra fluviatilis*. J. Endocrinol. **31**: 127-137.

BERG, L.S. 1935. Ecological parallels between Petromizonidae and Salmonidae. Dokl. Akad. Nauk. **3**: 91-93. (In Russian).

BERNAL, J., and L.J. DE GROOT. 1980. Mode of action of thyroid hormones. pp. 123-143 *In* De Visscher [ed.] The thyroid gland. Raven Press, New York.

BERNSTEIN, H.G., A. DORN, M. REISER, and M. ZIEGLER. 1984. Cerebral insulin-like immunoreactivity in rats and mice. Drastic decline during postnatal ontogenesis. Acta histochem. **74**: 33-36.

BONDAREVA, O.M., L.P. SOLTITSKAYA, and YU. I. RUSACOV. 1980. Immunobiological peculiarities of insulin in the salmon, *Oncorhynchus gorbuscha*, and a species-specific system for its assay. Zh. evol. Biokhim Fiziol. **16**: 518-521. (in Russian).

BUCKINGHAM, J.C., J.H. LEACH, E. PLISETSKAYA, S.A. SOWER, and A. GORBMAN. 1985. Corticotrophin-like bioactivity in the pituitary gland and brain of the Pacific hagfish, *Eptatretus stouti*. Gen. comp. Endocrinol. **57**: 434-437.

BUUS, O., and L.O. LARSEN. 1975. Absence of known corticosteroids in blood of river lampreys (*Lampetra fluviatilis*) after treatment with mammalian corticotropin. Gen. comp. Endocrinol. **26**: 96-99.

CASTILLA, C., and J.C. MURAT. 1975. Effets de l'insuline sur le metabolisme proteique dans le foie de Carpe. C.r. Seanc. Soc. Biol. **169**: 1605-1609.

CLARKE, D.W., F.T. BOYD, JR., M.S. KAPPY, and M.K. RAIZADA. 1984. Insulin binds to specific receptors and stimulates 2-deoxy-D-glucose uptake in cultured glial cells from rat brain. J. biol. Chem. **259**: 11672-11675.

CZECH, M.P., and J. MASSAGUE. 1982. Subunit structure and dynamics of the insulin receptor. Fed. Proc. **41**: 2719-2723.

DASHOW, L., and A. EPPLE. 1983. Effects of exogenous catecholamines on plasma catecholamines and glucose in the sea lamprey, *Petromyzon marinus*. J. comp. Physiol. B. **152**: 35-42.

DASHOW, L, A. EPPLE, and B. NIBBIO. 1982. Catecholamines in anadromous lampreys: baseline levels and stress-induced changes, with a note on cardiac cannulation. Gen. comp. Endocrinol. **46**: 500-504.

DASHOW, L., Y. KATZ, M.S. TRACHTMAN, and A. EPPLE. 1984. Plasma steroids in the ammocoete of *Petromyzon marinus*. Gen. comp. Endocrinol. **55**: 361-366.

DE ROOS, R., C.C. DE ROOS, C.S. WERNER, and H. WERNER. 1985. Plasma levels of glucose, alanine, lactate and ß-hydroxy-butyrate in the unfed spiny dogfish shark (*Squalus acanthias*) after surgery and following mammalian insulin infusion. Gen. comp. Endocrinol. **58**: 28-43.

DRUMMOND, G.I., and E.C. BLACK. 1960. Comparative physiology: fuel of muscle metabolism. Ann. Rev. Physiol. **22**: 169-190.

EASTMAN, Y.T., and R. PORTANOVA. 1982. ACTH activity in the pituitary and brain of the least Brook lamprey, *Lampetra aepyptera*. Gen. comp. Endocrinol. **47**: 346-350.

EMDIN, S.O. 1982. Effects of hagfish insulin in the Atlantic hagfish, *Myxine glutinosa*. Gen. comp. Endocrinol. **47**: 414-425.

EMDIN, S.O., and D.F. STEINER. 1980. A specific antiserum against insulin from the Atlantic hagfish, *Myxine glutinosa*: characterization of the antiserum, its use in a homologous radioimmunoassay, and immunofluorescent microscopy. Gen. comp. Endocrinol. **42**: 251-258.

EPPLE, A., J.E. BRINN, and J.B. YOUNG. 1980. Evolution of pancreatic islet function. pp. 269-321 *In* Pang, P.K.T., and A. Epple [eds.] Evolution of vertebrate endocrine systems. Texas Tech. Press, Lubbock.

FALKMER, S. 1962. Experimental studies on the cells of the pancreas-like organ of *Myxine glutinosa*. Rep. Third. Scand. Confer. Cell Res. p. 28.

FALKMER, S. 1984. Phylogenetical aspects on the brain-gut axis, with special reference to islet hormones in invertebrates and lower vertebrates. Kobayashi, H., H.A. Bern and A. Urano [eds.] Proc. 9th Inter. Symp. Neurosecr. Japan Sci. Soc. Press, Tokyo (in press).

FALKMER, S., M. EL-SALHY, and M. TITLBACH. 1984. Evolution of the neuroendocrine system in vertebrates. pp. 59-87 *In* Falkmer, S., R. Hakanson, and F. Sundler [eds.] Evolution and tumour pathology of the neuroendocrine system. Elsevier, Amsterdam.

FALKMER, S., and A.J. MATTY. 1966. Blood sugar regulation in the hagfish, *Myxine glutinosa*. Gen. comp. Endocrinol. **6**: 334-346.

FALKMER, S., and S. WILSON. 1967. Comparative immunology and biology of insulin. Diabetologia. **3**: 519-528.

FALKMER, S., and L. WINBLADH. 1964. An investigation of the pancreatic islet tissue of the hagfish (*Myxine glutinosa*) by light and electron microscopy. p. 17 *In* The structure and metabolism of the pancreatic islets. Pergamon Press, Oxford.

GAGE, S.H. 1917. Glycogen in the nervous system of vertebrates. J. comp. Neurol. **27**: 451-465.

GHARBI-CHIHI, J., J. BISMUTH, S. LISSITZKY, and J. TORRESANI. 1983. The effect of triiodothyronine on fatty acid synthetase activity and content in differentiating ob-17 preadipocites. Biochim. biophys. Acta. **750**: 282-290.

HARDISTY, M.W. 1979. The biology of cyclostomes. Chapman and Hall, London.

HARDISTY, M.W., and B.I. BAKER. 1982. Endocrinology of lampreys. pp. 1-115 *In*: Hardisty, M.W, and I.C. Potter [eds.] The biology of lampreys. Academic Press, London.

HARDISTY, M.W., and C.M. ROVAINEN. 1982. Morphological and functional aspects of the muscular system. pp. 137-231 *In* Hardisty, M.W., and I.C. Potter [eds.] The biology of lampreys. Academic Press, London.

HARDISTY, M.W., P.R. ZELNIK, and I.A. MOORE. 1975. The effects of subtotal and total isletectomy in the river lamprey, *Lampetra fluviatilis*. Gen. comp. Endocrinol. **27**: 179-192.

HOCHACHKA, P.W., and C.N. SOMERO. 1973. Strategies of biochemical adaptation. W.B. Saunders Company, Philadelphia.

IDLER, D.R., AND B. TRUSCOTT. 1966. 1 α-hydroxycorticosterone from cartilaginous fish: a new adrenal steroid in blood. J. Fish. Res. Bd. Can. **23**: 615-619.

INUI, Y., and A. GORBMAN. 1977. Sensitivity of Pacific hagfish *Eptatretus stouti* to mammalian insulin. Gen. comp. Endocrinol. **33**: 423-427.

INUI, Y., and A. GORBMAN. 1978. Role of the liver in regulation of carbohydrate metabolism in hagfish *Eptatretus stouti*. Comp. Biochem. Physiol. **60A**: 181-183.

IVANOVA-BERG, M.M., and M.M. SOKOLOVA. 1959. Seasonal changes of the blood content in the river lamprey (*Lampetra fluviatilis* L.) Vopr. Ikhtiol. **13**: 156-162. (in Russian).

JOHN, T.M., E. THOMAS, J.C. GEORGE, and F.W.H. BEAMISH. 1977. Effect of vasotocin on plasma free fatty acid level in the migrating anadromous sea lamprey. Arch. int. Physiol. Biochim. **85**: 865-970.

KATZ, Y., L. DASHOW, and A. EPPLE. 1982. Circulating steroid hormones of anadromous sea lampreys under various experimental conditions. Gen. comp. Endocrinol. **29**: 1-13.

LARSEN, L.O. 1976. Blood glucose levels in intact and hypophysectomized river lampreys (*Lampetra fluviatilis* L.) treated with insulin, "stress", or glucose, before and during the period of sexual maturation. Gen. comp. Endocrinol. **29**: 1-13.

LARSEN, L.O. 1978. Sub-total hepatectomy in intact or hypophysectomized river lampreys (*Lampetra fluviatilis* L.). Effect on regeneration, blood glucose regulation and vitellogenesis. Gen. comp. Endocrinol. **35**: 197-204.

LARSEN, L. 1980. Physiology of adult lampreys with special regard to natural starvation, reproduction and death after spawning. Can. J. Fish. Aquat. Sci. **37**: 1762-1779.

LEIBSON, L., and E.M. PLISETSKAYA. 1968. Effect of insulin on blood sugar level and glycogen content in organs of some cyclostomes and fish. Gen. comp. Endocrinol. **11**: 381-392.

LEIBSON, L.Y., E.M. PLISETSKAYA, and E.M. STABROVSKY. 1963. Effect of insulin on carbohydrate metabolism in cyclostomes and elasmobranch fish. Fiziol. Zh. USSR. **49**: 583-588. (in Russian).

LEIBUSH, B.N. 1983. Insulin receptors of the brain in evolution of vertebrates. Zh. evol. Biokhim. Fiziol. **19**: 403-413. (in Russian).

LEIBUSH, B.N, and V.M. BONDAREVA. 1981. Insulin receptor of the plasma membrane of liver cells in the scorpion fish, *Scorpaena porcus*, in comparison with the receptor in mammals. Zh. evol. Biokhim. Fiziol. **17**: 141-147. (in Russian).

LE ROITH, D., S.A. HENDRICKS, M.A. LESNIAK, S. RISHI, K.L. BECKER, J. HAVRANKOVA, J.L. ROSENZWEIG, M.J. BROWNSTEIN, and J. ROTH. 1983. Insulin in brain and other extrapancreatic tissues of vertebrates and nonvertebrates. Adv. Metab. Disorders **10**: 303-340.

LE ROITH, D., M.A. LESNIAK, and J. ROTH. 1981. Insulin in insects and annelids. Diabetes **30**: 70-76.

LINTLOP, S., and J.H. YOUSON. 1983a. Concentration of triiodothyronine in the sera of the sea lamprey, *Petromyzon marinus*., and the brook lamprey, *Lampetra lamottenii*, at various phases of the life cycle. Gen. comp. Endocrinol. **49**: 187-194.

LINTLOP, S.P., and J.H. YOUSON. 1983b. Binding of triiodothyronine to hepatocyte nuclei from sea lampreys, *Petromyzon marinus* L., at various stages of the life cycle. Gen. comp. Endocrinol. **49**: 428-436.

LOWE, D.R., F.W.H. BEAMISH, and I.C. POTTER. 1973. Changes in the proximate body composition of the landlocked sea lamprey *Petromyzon marinus* L. during larval life and metamorphosis. J. Fish Biol. **5**: 673-682.

MATTY, A. 1965. Hormonal control of carbohydrate metabolism in *Myxine glutinosa*. Gen. comp. Endocrinol. **5**: 701.

MATTY, A., and A. GORBMAN. 1978. The effects of isletectomy and hypophysectomy on some blood plasma constituents of the hagfish, *E. stouti*. Gen. comp. Endocrinol. **54**: 94 (Abstract).

MAZEAUD, M. 1969. Adrénalinémie et noradrénalinémie chez la Lamproie marine (*Petromyzon marinus* L.). C. r. Seanc. Soc. Biol. **163**: 349-352.

MUGGEO, M, B.H. GINSBERG, J. ROTH, D.M. NEVILLE, P. DE MEYTS, JR., and C.R. KAHN. 1979a. The insulin receptor in vertebrates is functionally more conserved during evolution than insulin itself. Endocrinology. **104**: 1393-1402.

MUGGEO, M., E. VAN OBBERGHEN, C.R. KAHN, J. ROTH, B.H. GINSBERG, P. DE MEYTS, S.O. EMDIN, and S. FALKMER. 1979b. The insulin receptor and insulin of the Atlantic hagfish. Diabetes. **28**: 175-181.

MURAT, J.C. 1976. Recherches sur la mobilisation des glucides tissulaires chez la Carpe. Thése Doct. Etat. Toulouse.

MURAT, J.C., E.M. PLISETSKAYA, and L.P. SOLTITSKAYA. 1979. Glucose-6-phosphatase activity in kidney of the river lamprey (*Lampetra fluviatilis* L.). Gen. comp. Endocrinol. **39**: 115-117.

MURAT, J.C., E.M. PLISETSKAYA, and N.Y.S. WOO. 1981. Endocrine control of nutrition in cyclostomes and fish. Comp. Biochem. Physiol. **68A**: 149-158.

MURAT, J.C., and A. SERFATY. 1970. Au sujet d'un effet hypoglycémiante de la thyroxine chez la Carpe, *Cyprinus carpio* L. C. r. Seanc. Soc. Biol. **164**: 1842-1845.

NAKAO, T. 1979. Electron microscopic studies on the lamprey meninges. J. comp. Neurol. **183**: 429-453.

O'BOYLE, R.N., and F.W.H. BEAMISH. 1977. Growth and intermediary metabolism of larval and metamorphosing stages of the landlocked sea lamprey, *Petromyzon marinus* L. Environ. Biol. Fish. **2**: 103-120.

OGORODNIKOVA, L.G., and E.B. FOTINA. 1977. Glucose-6-phosphatase activity in the pia mater of some vertebrates. Zh. evol. Biokhim. Fiziol. **13**: 340-343. (in Russian).

OKSCHE, A., H. KIRSCHSTEIN, and M. VAUPEL VON HARNACK. 1969. Vergleichende ultrastruktur Studien an glykogenreichen *Plexus chorioidei* (Embryonalzustand, Winterschlaf). Z. Zellforsch. **94**: 232-251.

PETERSON, J.D., D.F. STEINER, S.O. EMDIN, and S. FALKMER. 1975. The amino acid sequence from a primitive vertebrate, the Atlantic hagfish (*Myxine glutinosa*). J. biol. Chem. **250**: 5183-5191.

PHILLIPS, J.W., and F.J.R. HIRD. 1977. Ketogenesis in vertebrate livers. Comp. Biochem. Physiol. **57B**: 133-138.

PLISETSKAYA, E.M. 1964. Hormonal regulation of carbohydrate metabolism in cyclostomes and fish. Adv. Mod. Biol. **57**: 128. (in Russian).

PLISETSKAYA, E.M. 1965. Effects of insulin and epinephrine on glycaemic levels and glycogen content in liver and muscles of larval lampreys. Zh. evol. Biokhim. Fiziol. **1**: 213-219. (in Russian).

PLISETSKAYA, E.M. 1967. Respiration and glycogen content in lamprey brain. pp. 149-155 *In* Kreps, E.M. [ed.] Evolutionary neurophysiology and neurochemistry. Nauka, Leningrad. (in Russian).

PLISETSKAYA, E.M. 1968. Brain and heart glycogen content in some vertebrates and the effect of insulin. Endocr. Exp. **2**: 251-262.

PLISETSKAYA, E.M. 1975. Hormonal Regulation of Carbohydrate Metabolism in Lower Vertebrates. Nauka, Leningrad. (in Russian).

PLISETSKAYA, E.M. 1980. Fatty acid levels in blood of cyclostomes and fish. Environ. Biol. Fish. **5**: 273-290.

PLISETSKAYA, E.M., W.W. DICKHOFF, and A. GORBMAN. 1983a. Plasma thyroid hormones in cyclostomes. Do they have a role in regulation of glycemic levels? Gen. comp. Endocrinol. **49**: 97-107.

PLISETSKAYA, E.M., L.G. LEIBSON, and E.M. STABROVSKI. 1964. Effect of epinephrine on carbohydrate metabolism in cyclostomes and elasmobranch fish. Fiziol. Zh. SSSR. **50**: 117-112. (in Russian).

PLISETSKAYA, E.M., and B.N. LEIBUSH. 1972. Insulin-like activity and immunoreactive insulin in the blood of the lamprey, *Lampetra fluviatilis* L. Zh. evol. Biokhim. Fiziol. **8**: 499-505. (in Russian).

PLISETSKAYA, E., B. LEIBUSH, and V. BONDAREVA. 1976. The secretion of insulin and its role in cyclostomes and fishes. pp. 251-269 *In*: Grillo, T.A.I., and A. Epple [eds.] The evolution of pancreatic islets. Pergamon Press, Oxford.

PLISETSKAYA, E.M., and T.I. MAZINA. 1969. The effects of the hormones on nonesterified fatty acids in blood of the Baltic lamprey (*Lampetra fluviatilis* L.). Zh. evol. Biokhim. Fiziol. **5**: 457-463. (in Russian).

PLISETSKAYA, E., and J.C. MURAT. 1980. Interventions endocriniennes dans la régulation du métabolisme nutritionnel chez les poissons. pp. 323-336 *In*: Fontaine, M. [ed.] Nutrition des poissons. Centre National de la Recherce Scientifique, Paris.

PLISETSKAYA, E.M., and M.P. PROSOROVSKAYA. 1971. Catecholamines in the heart muscle of the lamprey, *Lampetra fluviatilis*, during insulin hypoglycemia. Zh. evol. Biokhim. Fiziol. **7**: 101-103. (in Russian).

PLISETSKAYA, E.M., A.A. RICH, W.W. DICKHOFF, and A. GORBMAN. 1984. A study of triiodothyronine-catecholamine interactions: their effect on plasma fatty acids in Pacific hagfish *Eptatretus stouti*. Comp. Biochem. Physiol. **78A**: 767-772.

PLISETSKAYA, E., S.A. SOWER, and A. GORBMAN. 1983b. The effect of insulin insufficiency on plasma thyroid hormones and some metabolic constituents in Pacific hagfish, *Eptatretus stouti*. Gen. comp. Endocrinol. **49**: 315-319.

PLISETSKAYA, E., N.Y.S. WOO, and J.C. MURAT. 1983c. Thyroid hormones in cyclostomes and fish and their role in regulation of intermediary metabolism. Comp. Biochem. Physiol. **74A**: 179-187.

PLISETSKAYA, E.M., and Z.P. ZHELUDKOVA. 1973. The effect of epinephrine on the γ-amylase activity in the liver and muscles of the lamprey *Lampetra fluviatilis* Zh. evol. Biokhim. Fiziol. **9**: 611-613. (in Russian).

POLJAKOVA, T.I., and E.M. PLISETSKAYA. 1977. Cytological and functional characteristics of pancreatic islets in lampreys in different stages of their life cycle. Tsitologiya. **19**: 1238-1244.

ROVAINEN, C.M. 1970. Glucose production by lamprey meninges. Science. **167**: 889-890.

ROVAINEN, C.M. 1979. Neurobiology of lampreys. Physiol. Rev. **59**: 1007-1077.

ROVAINEN, C.M. 1982. Neurophysiology. pp. 1-136 *In* Hardisty, M.W., and I.C. Potter [eds.] The biology of lampreys. Academic Press, London.

ROVAINEN, C.M., O.H. LOWRY, and J.V. PASSONNEAU. 1969. Levels of metabolites and production of glucose in the lamprey brain. J. Neurochem. **16**: 1451-1458.

ROVAINEN, C.M., G.E. LEMCOE, and A. PETERSON. 1971. Structure and chemistry of glucose-producing cells in meningeal tissue of the lamprey. Brain Res. **30**: 99-118.

SAVINA, M.V., and E.F. DERKACHEV. 1983. Switch on and switch off phenomenon of liver gluconeogenic function on lamprey (*Lampetra fluviatilis* L.) under the influence of season and temperature. Comp. Biochem. Physiol. **75B**: 531-540.

SAVINA, M.V., and E.M. PLISETSKAYA. 1976. Synthesis of glycogen from glycerol in isolated tissues of the river lamprey, *Lampetra fluviatilis*. Zh. Evol. Biokhim. Fiziol. **12**: 282-284. (in Russian).

SAVINA, M.V., and V.A. VILKOVA. 1976. Gluconeogenesis from glycerine in organs of the lamprey *Lampetra fluviatilis* during the prespawning period. Zh. Evol. Biokhim. Fiziol. **12**: 174-176. (in Russian).

SAVINA, M.V., and A.B. WOJTCZAK. 1977. Enzymes of gluconeogenesis and the synthesis of glycogen from glycerol in various organs of the lamprey (*Lampetra fluviatilis*). Comp. Biochem. Physiol. **57B**: 185-190.

SCHIRNER, H. 1963a. Unveränderter Blutzuckerspiegel nach Entfernung der Inselgewebes bei *Myxine glutinosa.* Naturwissenschaften. **50**: 127.

SCHIRNER, H. 1963b. The pancreas. pp.481-487 *In* The Biology of *Myxine*. Universitetsforlaget, Oslo.

SEREBRENIKOVA, T.P., and E.M. LYZLOVA. 1977. Some characteristics of molecular evolution of glycogen phosphorylase and aminotransferases of vertebrate muscle tissue. Zh. Evol. Biokhim. Fiziol. **13**: 106-113. (in Russian).

SHABADASH, A.L. 1949. The histochemistry of glycogen in the normal nervous system. Medgis, Moskwa. (in Russian).

SHERIDAN, M.A., E.M. PLISETSKAYA, H.A. BERN, and A. GORBMAN. 1985. Effects of somatostatin and urotensin II on lipid and carbohydrate metabolism in coho salmon. FEBS Letters. 44:632.

SOWER, S.A., E. PLISETSKAYA, and A. GORBMAN. 1985. Changes in plasma steroid and thyroid hormones and immunoreactive insulin during final maturation and spawning of the sea lamprey, *Petromyzon marinus*. Gen. comp. Endocrinol. **58**: 259-269.

STEINER, D.F., S.J. CHAN, K. DOCHERTY, S.O. EMDIN, G.G. DODSON, and S. FALKMER. 1984. Evolution of polypeptide hormones and their precursor processing mechanisms. pp. 203-223 *In* Falkmer, S., R. Hakanson, and F. Sundler. [eds.] Evolution and tumour pathology of the neuroendocrine system. Elsevier, Amsterdam.

STEWART, J.K., C.J. GOODNER, D.J. KOERKER, A. GORBMAN, J. ENSINCK, and M. KAUFMAN. 1978. Evidence for a biological role of somatostatin in the Pacific hagfish, *Eptatretus stouti*. Gen. comp. Endocrinol. **36**: 408-414.

THORPE, A., and H. DUVE. 1984. Insulin- and glucagon-like peptides in insects and molluscs. Molec. Physiol. **5**: 235-260.

WEISBART, M., W.W. DICKHOFF, A. GORBMAN, and D.R. IDLER. 1980. The presence of steroids in the sera of the Pacific hagfish, *Eptatretus stouti* and the sea lamprey, *Petromyzon marinus*. Gen. comp. Endocrinol. **41**: 506-519.

WEISBART, M., and D.R. IDLER. 1970. Re-examination of the presence of corticosteroids in two cyclostomes, the Atlantic hagfish (*Myxine glutinosa* L.) and the sea lamprey (*Petromyzon marinus* L.). J. Endocrinol. **46**: 29-43.

WEISBART, M., and J.H. YOUSON. 1977. *In vivo* formation of steroid from (1,2,6,7-^{3}H) progesterone by the sea lamprey, *Petromyzon marinus* L. J. Ster. Biochem. **8**: 1249-1252.

WOLFF, H. 1968. Histochemische und elektronenmikroskopische Beobachtungen uber die Glykogenverteilung im Hypothalamus einiger Winterschlafer. (mit quantitativen Bemerkungen). Z. Zellforsch. **88**: 228-261.

WRIGHT, G.M., and J.H. YOUSON. 1980. Variation in serum levels of thyroxine in anadromous larval lampreys, *Petromyzon marinus* L. Gen. Comp. Endocrinol. **41**: 321-324.

YOUSON, J.H. 1981. The liver. pp. 263-332 *In* Hardisty, M.W., and I.C. Potter [eds.] The biology of lampreys. Academic Press, London.

YOUSON, J.H., J. LEE, and I.C. POTTER. 1979. The distribution of fat in larval, metamorphosing, and young adult anadromous sea lampreys, *Petromyzon marinus* L. Can. J. Zool. **57**: 237-246.

ZELNIK, P.R., D.J. HORNSEY, and M.W. HARDISTY. 1977. Insulin and glucagon-like immunoreactivity in the river lamprey (*Lampetra fluviatilis*). Gen. comp. Endocrinol. **33**: 53-60.

HAGFISH INSULIN: EVOLUTION OF INSULIN

Stefan O. Emdin

Department of Surgery
University of Umea
Umea, Sweden

Donald F. Steiner and Sju Jin Chan

Department of Biochemistry
University of Chicago
Chicago, Illinois 60637

Sture Falkmer

Department of Tumor Pathology
Karolinska Hospital
Stockholm Sweden

Introduction

Insulin plays a profound metabolic role in vertebrates and possibly also in many invertebrate species. Insulin regulates transport and metabolism of carbohydrates and amino acids, stimulates biosynthesis of lipids and proteins. Thus, insulin has major effects upon nutrition, both at the cellular level and at the level of integrating the anabolic needs of an organism. The evolution of the insulin molecule and its receptors-effectors is an interesting problem of potential relevance.

With the elucidation by Sanger and associates (Ryle *et al.*, 1955; Sanger, 1959) of the unique double-chain structure and the amino acid sequence of the insulin molecule, one of the cornerstones for molecular biology was put in place, and the way was cleared for crystallographic analysis of insulin. The three-dimensional elucidation of insulin's structure (Adams *et al.*, 1969; Hodgkin, 1974) provided a clear basis for understanding the conservation of certain primary structural features in the insulin molecule throughout all of vertebrate evolution. The discovery of proinsulin (Steiner, 1967) and later pre-proinsulin (Chan *et al.*, 1979) gave additional insight into evolutionary widespread cellular mechanisms of protein processing. Recently, the advances made in the field of molecular genetics have provided a basis for studying the evolutionary origins of peptide hormones. It has been made possible to examine in detail the genes encoding the hormone precursors from which the hormones are ultimately derived by post-translational proteolysis.

Islet organization

In invertebrates the equivalent of the vertebrate gastro-entero-pancreatic system is confined to the digestive tract mucosa only. In vertebrates the evolution of the endocrine pancreas is a step-wise process. The first pancreatic islet organ is formed at the level of the cyclostomes. This endocrine organ is completely devoid of exocrine tissue and it is closely associated with the gut mucosa and the bile-duct. In the Atlantic hagfish, *Myxine glutinosa*, the islet organ appears as a whitish swelling surrounding the common bile duct as it enters the gut (Fig. 1). The hagfish islet contains mostly B cells and some somatostatin-producing D cells. The glucagon and pancreatic polypeptide (PP) producing cells are dispersed endocrine cells in the gut mucosa. Thus, the cyclostomes appear to have a two hormone endocrine pancreas. The next step towards the ultimate four hormone islet is found at the level of cartilaginous holocephalan fish. Thus, in the Atlantic and Pacific ratfish, *Chimaera monstrosa* and *Hydrolagus colliei*, respectively, an actual mixed endocrine-exocrine gland is present. In the islets, insulin, glucagon- and somatostatin-producing cells are found. PP-producing cells are still mostly situated in the gut mucosa. There is yet no structural information available about insulin from holocephalan species. In elasmobranchian cartilaginous fish a distinct stomach and duodenum appear for the first time in vertebrate evolution. The endocrine pancreas has now become a four hormone islet. The primary sequence of insulin from the spiny dogfish, *Squalus acanthias*, is now known (Bajaj *et al.*, 1983). After these three major steps to a four hormone islet parenchyma, no radical changes of islet organization occur during vertebrate evolution (Van Norden and Falkmer, 1980).

Analyzing insulin evolution, we have focused on one species representing the earliest vertebrates extant, the Atlantic hagfish. We will discuss how its insulin, which diverged from that of gnathostomian vertebrates some five to six hundred million years ago, is processed, secreted and handled.

Insulin in the Atlantic hagfish

The way the hagfish manufactures its insulin is in many ways similar to that of all other vertebrate species investigated. The hagfish insulin gene contains two introns in the same regions on the gene as found in higher vertebrates (Steiner *et al.*, 1984). The sequence of hagfish pre-proinsulin (Fig. 2) shows that the over-all organization is similar to higher vertebrate pre-proinsulins (Chan *et al.*, 1981). Hence, the N-terminal extension, *viz.* the pre-peptide, is 26 amino acid residues long and has a generally hydrophobic character, and is believed to serve as an initiator of ribosomal binding to microsomal membranes and then to guide the pre-proinsulin molecule into the endoplasmic reticulum. Once inside this compartment

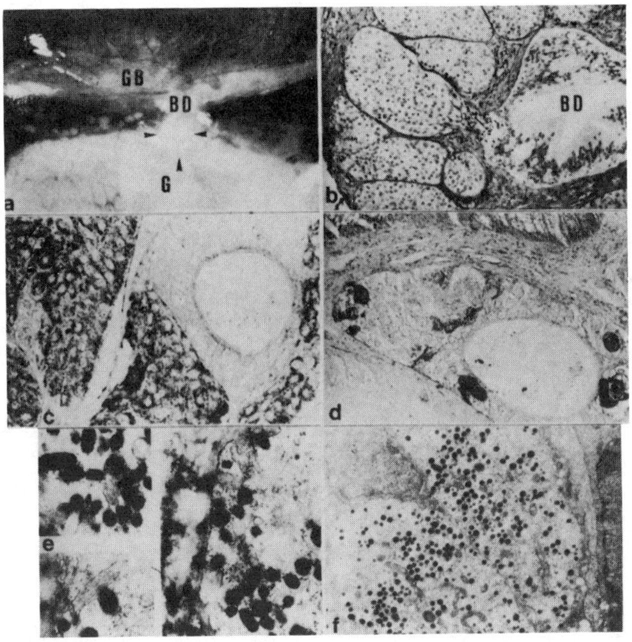

Fig. 1. The islet organ of the Atlantic hagfish. a) The islet organ (arrows) appears as a swelling around the bile-duct (*BD*) as it enters the gut (*G*). *GB*, gall bladder. b) Transverse section of the bile-duct, surrounded by nests of islet cells, some of them budding out from the bile-duct epithelium. c) Islet lobules immunostained to show insulin and d) somatostatin. e) Electron micrographs of the secretory granules of the insulin and f) somatostatin cells. The insulin granules are rather pleomorphic and dense, whereas somatostatin granules are spherical. e) x 23,000 approx., f) x 9,000 approx.

the N-terminal extension is proteolytically cleaved. The proinsulin molecule is then free to fold and its disulfide-bonds are formed.

The conversion of proinsulin to insulin and C-peptide by proteolytic cleavage is believed to start inside the Golgi apparatus and to be completed inside the secretory granules. By pulse-chase experiments (Emdin and Falkmer, 1977) and subcellular fractionation we have shown that hagfish proinsulin conversion is indeed initiated inside the Golgi and continued within the storage granules. As can be expected, hagfish proinsulin biosynthesis and conversion is temperature dependent (Emdin and Falkmer, 1977). The process as a whole is sluggish, and at 11°C the half-time of conversion is about ten times slower in the hagfish than in the rat at 37°C. It takes a minimum of 20 h at 11°C before any newly converted insulin is released. Since another 20 h are needed to synthesize and convert pre-proinsulin into insulin,

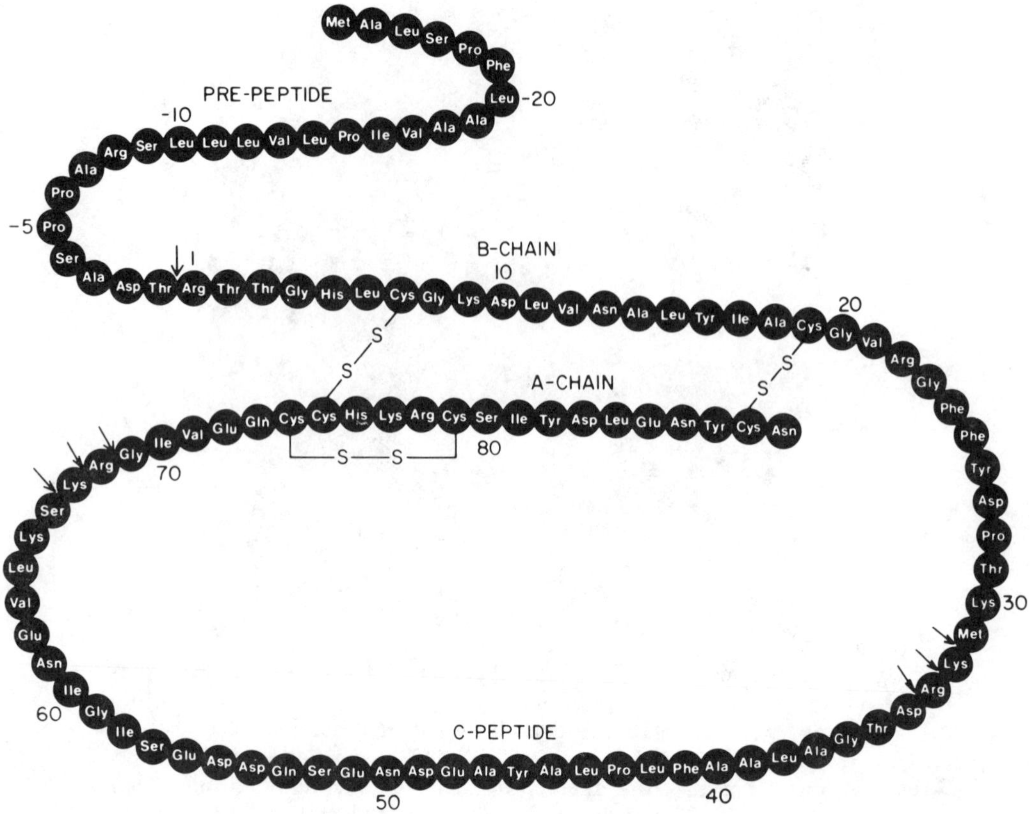

Fig. 2. Primary structure of hagfish pre-proinsulin derived from the nucleotide sequence of a cDNA clone corresponding to the mRNA sequence (Chan *et al.*, 1981). Arrows indicate points of processing required to generate mature hagfish insulin from the precursor. Reproduced from Steiner *et al.*, 1984, with permission.

a total of 40 h is needed before newly processed insulin ultimately reaches the circulation (Emdin and Falkmer, 1977).

Glucose is a positive modulator of insulin biosynthesis in higher animals (Steiner *et al.*, 1972), which seems logical. On this point the hagfish differs from other animals studied, since we have not been able to enhance proinsulin biosynthesis by administered glucose, or a number of other nutrients or chemical substances (Emdin and Falkmer, 1977). This is perhaps understandable against the background that any insulinotropic agent will need about 40 h before it can contribute to peripheral insulin needs. Possibly the rate of proinsulin biosynthesis is constant for a given temperature, and the pool of mature granules that are not secreted disintegrate and their C-peptide contents are degraded. Such insulin degradation inside the B cell has been demonstrated in cultured rat islets (Halban and Wollheim, 1980). The hagfish insulin C-peptide is normally degraded within the islet parenchyma since only about 10 percent of the C-peptide is recovered after purification when compared with insulin on a molar basis (Emdin, unpublished). It is known that a certain fraction of the rat C-peptide is normally degraded inside the B cell (Tager *et al.*, 1973).

The conversion of hagfish, as well as all other proinsulins, into mature insulin is accomplished by proteolytic cleavage occurring at particular pairs of basic residues (Steiner *et al.*, 1984). This appears to be a widespread cellular phenomenon for conversion of proproteins into mature products. This suggests that the modified tryptic-like conversion mechanism for proproteins, requiring paired basic residues, is an ancient machinery which antedated the appearance of the vertebrates. Moreover, complete conversion of the hagfish proinsulin to insulin and C-peptide requires the succesive actions of both a trypsin-like endoprotease as well as a carboxypeptidase B-like exopeptidase. The C-peptide is known to "accept" a high number of point mutations. It is therefore not surprising that the hagfish C-peptide does not show any resemblance to C-peptides of higher vertebrates (Chan *et al.*, 1981). The lack of conserved structural features in the C-peptide region is consistent with the proposed role of the C-peptide in converting the bimolecular reaction of chain combination for sulfhydryl oxidation to a more efficient and concentration-independent monomolecular reaction, without necessarily imposing any constraints on the folding process itself (Steiner, 1978). The length of the C-peptide, about 30 amino acid residues, is best explained by proposing that secretory protein precursors must maintain a minimum overall chain length in order to be efficiently segregated *via* vectorial discharge into the cisternae of the rough endoplasmic reticulum, and the C-peptide serves here essentially as a spacer with little restraint on the amino acid sequence (Patzelt, *et al.*, 1978).

We have studied hagfish insulin secretion *in vitro* using a homologous radioimmunoassay for hagfish insulin (Emdin and Steiner, 1980; Emdin, 1982a). As in most other animals studied, it was found that glucose stimulated insulin release with a half-maximal response around 3 mM glucose (Emdin, 1982a). A stimulatory effect was seen already at 1 mM and the maximum response was recorded at 5 mM (Emdin, 1982a). Overall a three-fold stimulation of insulin release, induced by glucose, was recorded. These glucose levels correspond to the levels seen in fasting and fed hagfish (Emdin, 1982b). It was also found that omission of calcium markedly inhibited the glucose-induced insulin release (Emdin, 1982a). This phenomenon is also well known in higher vertebrates (Dahl and Henquin, 1978). The time of full onset and cessation of glucose-induced insulin release was about 20 minutes. This may seem long when compared with the almost instantaneous release observed in higher mammals. However, the architecture of the islet offers an explanation. The individual follicles of B cells are avascular and are surrounded by a thick connective tissue capsule which a loose net of capillaries traverses. Thus, after exocytosis, the insulin released must diffuse a considerable distance. When compared with the 40 h needed for *de novo* synthesized insulin to be released (see above), the time of onset of glucose-induced release is not long. It was found also (Emdin, 1982a) that amino acids did not stimulate insulin-release in the hagfish. This is in contrast to most higher animals, including teleost fish. It has been suggested that, under physiological conditions, amino acids not only stimulate insulin release in higher animals but also stimulate glucagon secretion (see Gerich *et al.*, 1976 for references). Hence, it is possible that amino acids primarily control hormonal release from A cells rather than from B cells. As has been pointed out earlier, the hagfish lacks glucagon-producing islet cells and it does not respond with hyperglycemia when injected with huge doses of mammalian glucagon (Falkmer and Matty, 1966). We have speculated that the insulin secretory response to amino acids evolved only when glucagon and insulin cells came in close contact with each other (Emdin, 1982a).

Hagfish can cope effectively with starvation for several months (Inui *et al.*, 1978). How they adapt to starvation, and how their energy requirements are met, are essentially unknown. Data from the Pacific hagfish indicate that the liver is of relatively minor importance, since hepatectomized animals survive for at least a month without alterations of blood glucose and plasma amino-nitrogen levels (Inui and Gorbman, 1978). When Atlantic hagfish were starved for a month at 4-6°C it was found that, in comparison with the data obtained from newly caught and fed hagfish, the blood glucose and the plasma insulin values fell from 1.9 to 0.8 mM and 2.2 to 1.1 nM, respectively (Emdin, 1982b). Additional data are presented in Table I. If starved hagfish were loaded with glucose, the insulin values rose to 1.9 nM within 3 h, demonstrating that glucose stimulated insulin release not only *in vitro* but also *in vivo*, and to a level corresponding to the one seen in fish fed *ad libitum* (Emdin, 1982b). It was also observed that during starvation most of the liver and skeletal glycogen was consumed, whereas the content of protein and triglycerides was far more stable. Lowering of the levels of amino-nitrogen, triglycerides and free fatty acids was also observed in this experiment. The results indicate that glycogenolysis in skeletal muscle is the most important source of energy during starvation for one month (see article by Plisetskaya in this volume).

Insulin's role in the metabolism of lower vertebrates, in contrast with the situation in mammals, still is incompletely known. There is evidence, however, from experiments in teleosts fish, that similarities in hormonal function exist (Thorpe, 1976). In the Pacific hagfish it has been observed that insulin stimulates protein synthesis in skeletal muscle (Inui *et al.*, 1978).

By studying the metabolism of radioactively labeled metabolites (Emdin, 1982b) it was found that hagfish insulin (0.1 μg/g body weight) induced an approximately two-fold stimulation of the specific activity of hagfish skeletal muscle glycogen and protein, using either ^{14}C-glucose or ^{14}C-leucine. In addition, with ^{14}C-glucose an enhanced incorporation of label into neutral lipids was observed. In the hagfish liver, hagfish insulin increased the incorporation of radioactivity from ^{14}C-leucine, but not ^{14}C-glucose, into protein. Moreover, hagfish insulin did not affect the radioactivity of either liver lipids or glycogen, using either of the two isotopes. It was suggested that insulin's physiological role in the hagfish skeletal muscle is similar to what has been observed in higher animals, although the quantitative effects appeared smaller in the cyclostome (Emdin, 1982b). In another experiment with the above radioactive tracers (Emdin, 1982b) animals were pretreated with glucose and amino acids for three days before the isotopes were injected. The given glucose increased the serum insulin values to about 2nM. Moreover, these endogenously elevated insulin levels were high enough to evoke stimulatory effects on the incorporation of label into muscle. Hence, it seems as if glucose is able to

Table I. Mean contents of glycogen, protein, and triglycerides in the liver, skeletal muscle, and serum of fed hagfish, and of hagfish after one month of starvation at 4-6°C.

Tissue	Substance[a]		Contents ± SEM (sample size) Fed	Starved	P<
Liver	Glycogen	(µg/mg)	4.38 ± 0.52 (43)	0.33 ± 0.03 (36)	0.005
	Protein	(µg/mg)	84.93 ± 3.45 (43)	56.55 ± 4.22 (44)	0.005
	Triglycerides	(µg/mg)	4.15 ± 0.20 (35)	3.28 ± 0.21 (39)	0.005
Muscle	Glycogen	(µg/mg)	8.04 ± 0.64 (43)	0.31 ± 0.03 (33)	0.005
	Protein	(µg/mg)	114.95 ± 2.95 (43)	135.63 ± 2.81 (41)	0.005
	Triglycerides	(µg/mg)	1.45 ± 0.24 (28)	2.11 ± 0.22 (39)	0.005
Serum	Glucose	(mM)	1.89 ± 0.12 (35)	0.76 ± 0.11 (33)	0.005
	a-NH_2N	(mg/l)	84.10 ± 13.2 (40)	56.70 ± 4.50 (40)	0.05
	Triglycerides	(g/l)	8.26 ± 0.24 (31)	4.08 ± 0.34 (32)	0.005
	FFA	(µEq/l)	222.00 ± 14.2 (41)	129.80 ± 9.00 (39)	0.005
	Insulin	(nM)	2.16 ± 0.20 (40)	1.10 ± 0.12 (38)	0.005

[a] Tissue wet weight throughout

stimulate insulin secretion about two-fold, and that this elevated insulin level enhances lipid, protein and glycogen synthesis in skeletal muscle, whereas the liver remains relatively unaffected by the hormone. The general picture of insulin's effect in the Atlantic hagfish is that of a slow reacting animal with a narrow spectrum of metabolic adaptions. Regardless of this, the physiological role of insulin in the hagfish is still poorly known and a large number of important points have not yet been studied at all in any myxinoid species.

The structure of hagfish insulin

The study of the primary structure of hagfish insulin and a number of insulins from mammals, birds and fish shows that insulin is a polypeptide hormone that has undergone surprisingly few alterations during vertebrate evolution (Chan *et al.*, 1981). Nonetheless, hagfish insulin is one of the most highly substituted, naturally occurring insulins. There are altogether 19 amino acid residues out of 51 different from those of pig insulin, and 16 of these, mostly located in the B chain, have previously not been observed in these positions (Chan *et al.*, 1981). Surveying these differences, it is noteworthy that hagfish insulin does not appear to be readily related to insulins of mammals, birds or fish. On the other hand, of the so-called invariant residues, *i.e.* those that are present in all species so far investigated, all these have been demonstrated also in hagfish insulin, with one minor exception (Chan *et al.*, 1981). Sequence data shows that the residues important in stabilizing the insulin monomer and dimer are all conserved in hagfish insulin as they have been conserved in most species throughout evolution. This idea is substantiated by the observation that the dimerisation constants of hagfish and pig insulins are similar at neutral pH (Bruce H. Frank, personal communication). However, the sequence of hagfish insulin implies that Zn-coordination and hexamer formation is unlikely (Chan *et al.*, 1981). This similarity in structure, and preservation of certain parts of the sequence in the region of the hormone considered to be involved in expression of biological activity, prompted the study of Zn-free hagfish insulin crystals (Cutfield *et al.*, 1979; Falkmer and Emdin, 1981). Despite the differences in sequence and aggregation, pig and hagfish insulin have closely similar three-dimensional structures (Cutfield *et al.*, 1979; Falkmer and Emdin, 1981). The similarities extend beyond the general folding of the backbone, and many of the side chains are in the same positions. The only considerable differences in structure were found at the two ends of the B chain, where the residues in pig insulin are involved in hexamer formation. Their structural alteration in the hagfish insulin molecule is therefore understandable. A comparison of the two molecules is shown in figure 3. At one end of the B chain (residues B 28-31) the hagfish insulin takes a different path in the crystal structure, which probably reflects the change of primary structure in this region. In 2Zn pig insulin the two molecules in the dimer exhibit differences in conformation (Blundell *et al.*, 1972), and even more so in 4Zn pig insulin (Cutfield *et al.*, 1981). The structure of hagfish insulin is closely related to the pig insulin molecule 2 (Falkmer and Emdin, 1981). In fact, the tertiary structure of hagfish insulin is more similar to the pig insulin molecule 2 than were pig insulin molecules 1 and 2 to each other. The strict conservation of the structure of the dimer-forming residues in hagfish and pig 2Zn and 4Zn insulins imply that this stable region of the dimer is preserved in solution, perhaps also in the free monomer.

Hagfish insulin's behaviour in mammalian test systems

Despite the great structural similarities between hagfish and pig insulins in the crystalline state, there are substantial differences in the biological activities in mammalian test systems. In the free rat fat cell assay hagfish insulin has 5 percent biological activity when compared with pig insulin (Emdin *et al.*, 1977). In this study, it was also shown that the binding of hagfish insulin to the receptor was about 25 percent. Hagfish insulin was the first insulin to display a difference between receptor binding and activity (Emdin *et al.*, 1977). Hagfish insulin therefore can be defined as a partial insulin antagonist on the receptor, but on the whole cell as a full agonist due to the presence of a large number of spare receptors on the rat fat cell. Analysis of the rates of iodinated hagfish insulin association and dissociation from

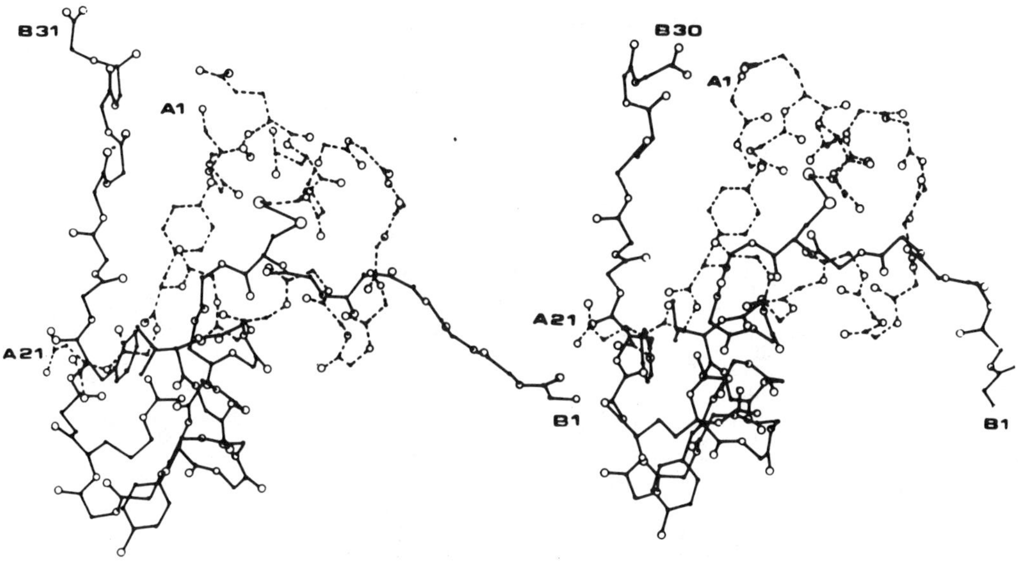

Fig. 3. A comparison of the atomic positions of the A and the B chains in hagfish insulin (left) and 2 Zn pig insulin molecule 2 (right) viewed parallel to the two folded axis. Side chains for the residues implicated in activity are shown. Reproduced from Cutfield *et al.* 1979, with permission.

the rat fat cell insulin receptor showed that the hagfish insulin dissociated and - even more so - associated slower than pig insulin did (Emdin *et al.*, 1980). It is tempting to speculate that the evolution beyond the hagfish has led to insulins being more efficient per unit of binding, thus activating a greater number of glucose carriers. This would cause an increase in sensitivity, but not necessarily an increase in the maximum response.

Most of the studies on the biological effects of hagfish insulin have been made with isolated rat fat cells, but there is additional information on its behaviour in other test systems in Table II.

Structure and activity: a problem

Hagfish insulin has all the residues implemented for high biological activity (Blundell *et al.*, 1972; Pullen *et al.*, 1976), and a structure in the crystal which is remarkably similar to the 2Zn pig insulin molecule 2. Yet, hagfish insulin must possess structural changes that add up to the small energy drop needed to go from full binding and activity down to 5-25 percent (Cutfield *et al.*, 1979). Clearly minute conformational changes could produce the reduction in binding affinity and biological activity seen in hagfish insulin. It is also possible that a certain molecular flexibility, rather than a specific residue or conformation, is of importance in expression of binding and action. Pig insulin can undergo substantial

Table II. Hagfish insulin: summary of biological behaviour relative to pig insulin.

	Percent or Molarity	References
Rat fat cells:		
Biological activity	4-7%	Emdin *et al*. (1977) Muggeo *et al*. (1979b)
Receptor binding as inhibition of trace pig insulin binding	23%	Emdin *et al*. (1977)
Receptor binding as trace hagfish insulin binding	25%	Emdin *et al*. (1980)
Inhibition of trace degradation by the membrane protease	12 nM (hagfish) 130 nM (pig)	Emdin *et al*. (1977)
Rat liver cells:		
Receptor binding	3-7%	Gammeltoft *et al*. (1978) Terris and Steiner (1975)
Inhibition of trace degradation by the membrane protease	15 nM (hagfish) 120 nM (pig)	Gammeltoft *et al*. (1978)
Degradation velocity	4%	Terris and Steiner (1975)
Hagfish erythrocytes:		
Receptor binding	25%	Muggeo *et al*. (1979b)
Human IM 9 lymphocytes:		
Receptor binding	23%	Emdin *et al*. (1980)
Ability to induce negative co-operativity	5%	Muggeo *et al*. (1979b)
Cultured human fibroblasts:		
Stimulation of thymidine incorporation	8%	King and Kahn (1981)

rearrangement in going from 2Zn to 4Zn structure (Cutfield *et al*., 1981). The importance of molecular flexibility is hard to study experimentally.

Since any biological function is at least bimolecular, it follows that its evolution is at least dual. Ideally, the evolution of a hormone should include also the evolution of its effector system. It has been shown that the insulin receptor evolves even more slowly than the homologous insulin, and the affinity of a given receptor for a given insulin is independent of the kind of insulin that is endogenous in that organism (Muggeo *et al.*, 1979a). Studies of hagfish erythrocyte insulin receptors (Muggeo *et al.*, 1979b) showed that these had similar absolute affinity and rank order of preference for insulin and insulin analogues as had receptors from higher vertebrates. Hence, the affinity of hagfish insulin was 25 percent of that of pig insulin.

Some remarks on hagfish insulin's evolution

The situation can be described from different viewpoints. In terms of molecular structure there is a remarkable conservatism throughout the evolution of the insulin molecule. The fact that pig and hagfish insulin are still so similar in their chemical and structural features shows that the primary and tertiary structures must exist under strict structural and functional constraints, even though evolution beyond the hagfish has led to more efficient insulins. On the other hand, the processing, secretion and utilization of hagfish insulin in the hagfish displays differences at several points; proinsulin biosynthesis is not modulated; secretion is not stimulated by amino acids; the liver seems to be of relatively minor importance, and the overall quantitative importance of insulin's peripheral effects also appears less obvious than in higher mammals. Hence, the hagfish is relatively less developed in these respects. The conservatism discussed above makes it reasonable to assume that the entire insulin processing machinery and at least some of insulin's peripheral effects antedated the appearance of the vertebrates.

Some general aspects on insulin evolution

As we and others have suggested (Steiner, 1969; Adelson, 1971; De Haen *et al.*, 1976; Hales, 1978; Chan *et al.*, 1981), it is likely that the ancestral precursors of many endocrine regulatory peptides were cellular proteins with different functions. These proteins became involved, in an incidental way, either directly or through their proteolytic break-down products, in some aspects of trans-membrane signalling or intercellular communication in eucaryotic organisms. Thus, the possible derivation of the insulin superfamily of related peptides (insulin, insulin-like growth factor, relaxin and perhaps nerve growth factor) from serine proteases (De Haen *et al.*, 1976; Chan *et al.*, 1981) might be viewed as reflecting the normal function of these proteases in a primitive digestive milieu, where an insulin-like product could have been generated proteolytically and absorbed into the blood. A related possibility would be that these proteases were secreted as end-products of lysosomal digestion in more primitive organisms and may have acted on nearby cells by degrading some surface components, thereby activating intracellular activities (Steiner *et al.*, 1980). On the other hand, these ancestral proteases may have acted without being secreted, by affecting the uptake of nutrients directly from phagocytic or lysosomal vacuoles into the cytosol compartment (Hales, 1978). Other proposals have been promulgated recently, arguing that peptides such as insulin arose as such in early unicellular organisms (Roth *et al*, 1982). It is perhaps not inconceivable that active centers of some small peptide hormones arose through chemical condensation during a pre-biotic period, although at this time there is no evidence on this point.

Using hagfish insulin as an example, we can see that the tertiary structure of functionally-related proteins is more highly conserved than the amino acid sequence. Also, the evolution of insulin's precursor has undergone only minute changes of perhaps minor importance. It is noteworthy that the characteristic pairs of basic residues are present on either side of the C-peptide in all proinsulins studied. This indicates that the precursor processing mechanisms for prohormones was evolutionarily "old" at the time of divergence of the hagfish from the main line of vertebrate evolution. Studies with endocrine precursor peptides of *Aplysia* (Schueller *et al*, 1982), as well as from yeast (Kurjan and Herskowitz, 1982), indeed confirm that proprotein processing mechanisms are of ancient evolutionary origin. This suggests that the basic segregation mechanism for secretory proteins *via* signal peptides is a very ancient mechanism. On the other hand, proprotein processing seems to be more characteristic of eucaryotic cells, particularily the use of paired basic residues to mark sites of processing. The origins of this mechanism may in some respects be viewed as parallel with the development of split genes in eucaryotes, and this connection may be significant, since gene splicing may have played an important role as an evolutionary mechanism in generating some of the genes for prohormones (see below).

It is likely that the members of the insulin superfamily of related peptides all arose from an ancestral proinsulin-like protein which may have been a serine protease (Chan *et al.*, 1981). With the advent of recombinant DNA technology it has become possible again to examine whether a serine protease could have generated the insulin superfamily. The results are indeed promising in the case of insulin, but by no means conclusive. Both the insulin and relaxin genes have introns within their C-peptide coding regions, suggesting a possible mechanism for the generation of a proinsulin-like peptide from a putative ancestral serine protease gene essentially by processing out the intervening coding region during transcription as though it were part of an intron, perhaps due to an error in RNA processing leading to the use of alternative splicing sites, as illustrated in figure 4 (Roth *et al.*, 1982). There is additional evidence to support this idea. The sequence of the connecting segment of porcine relaxin shows limited, but significant, homology with the corresponding central regions of serine proteases as expected if prorelaxin is an intermediate stage in the evolution of the serine gene product towards a proinsulin-like or insulin-like growth factor-like molecule (Steiner, 1983). The insulin gene's C-peptide intron is evolutionarily stable, being present in essentially the same position even in the hagfish gene. The serine protease genes (Craik *et al.*, 1983) are made up of several exons arranged so that the insulin B-like and A-like sequences are each on separate exons separated by a long nucleotide sequence which contains additional introns and exons (Fig. 4).

Accordingly, the origin of the insulin superfamily might have occurred through alterations in the processing of the mRNA of an ancestral protease gene, thereby giving rise, as a coincidental event, to small amounts of pre-proinsulin-like mRNA. Similar alternative splicing mechanisms have been found recently in several endocrine systems, where they led to the production of novel or altered hormonal products (Amara *et al.*, 1982; Gammeltoft *et al.*, 1978). Co-secretion of this insulin-like peptide, along with digestive enzymes, in some primitive gut cell may have been advantageous in several ways. If so, the gene encoding this particular RNA processing variant could then undergo duplication and subsequent mutational

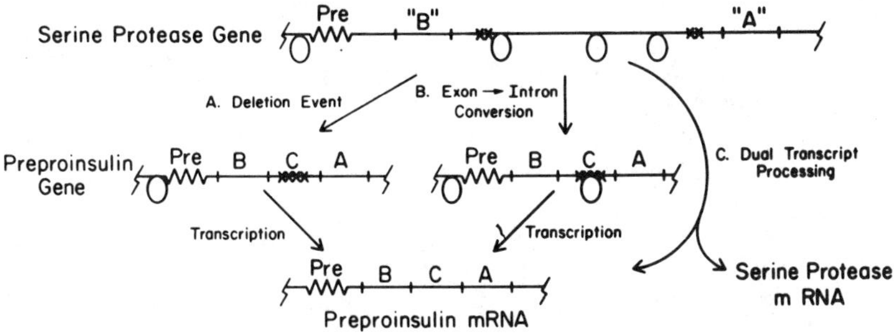

Fig. 4. A plausible scheme for the evolutionary origin of the gene for insulin via several genetic mechanisms. Classically, one would expect the gene to duplicate first and the additional copy then to be free to undergo reorganisation (*A*). An alternative possibility, based on our knowledge of gene structure, would be that a single serine protease gene may have given rise to two or more different functional mRNAs through alternative splicing of its initial transcript, as is known to occur in several systems (*C*). Translation of the major transcript would yield the expected products, while translation of the "modified" mRNAs could generate new products. If advantageous and useful these could become "locked in" genetically by duplication of the parental gene and further modification of one copy so as to generate only or mainly the alternative product (*B*). In the above example, certain exons from the central region of the protease gene could thus be processed differently to generate either proinsulin and IGF-like or prolaxin-like peptides. Reproduced from Steiner *et al.*, 1984.

changes, leading to the predominant expression of insulin-like rather than serine protease-like material under separate genetic control. By such a mechanism a "new" cell type could ultimately arise, with the exclusive task of elaborating this important product. In such a way, a cycle of evolution would be completed, beginning with the generation of a new gene product cut from older genetic "cloth" and culminating in the development of a new endocrine cell - the insulin producing cell.

Literature Cited

ADAMS, M.J., T.L. BLUNDELL, E.J. DODSON, G.G. DODSON, M. VIJAYAN, E.N. BAKER, M.M. HARDING, D.C. HODGKIN, B. RIMMER, and S. SHEAT. 1969. Structure of rhombohedral 2-zinc insulin crystals. Nature **224**: 491-495.

ADELSON, J.W. 1971. Enterosecretory proteins. Nature **229**: 321-325.

AMARA, S.G., V. JONAS, M.G. ROSENFELD, E.S. ONG, and R.M. EVANS. 1982. Alternate RNA processing in calcitonin gene expression generates mRNA encoding different polypeptide products. Nature **298**: 240-244.

BAJAJ, M., T.L. BLUNDELL, J.E. PITTS, S.P.WOOD, M.A. TATNELL, S. FALKMER, S.O. EMDIN, L.K. GOWAN, H. CROW, C. SCHWABE, A. WOLLMER, and W. STRASSBURGER. 1983. Dogfish insulin. Eur. J. Biochem. **135**: 535-542.

BLUNDELL, T., G. DODSON, D. HODGKIN, and D. MERCOLA. 1972. Insulin: the structure in the crystal and its reflection in chemistry and biology. Adv. Prot. Chem. **26**: 279-402.

CHAN, S.J., S.O. EMDIN, S.C.M. KWOK, J.M. KRAMER, S. FALKMER, and D.F. STEINER. 1981. Messenger RNA sequence and primary structure of preproinsulin in a primitive vertebrate, the Atlantic hagfish. J. Biol. Chem. **256**: 7597-7602.

CHAN, S.J., S.C.M. KOK, and D.F. STEINER. 1981. The biosynthesis of insulin: some genetic and evolutionary aspects. Diabetes Care **4**: 4-10.

CHAN, S.J., B.J. NOYES, K.L. AGARWAL, and D.F. STEINER. 1979. Construction and selection of recombinant plasmids containing full length cDNAs corresponding to rat insulins I and II. Proc. Nat. Acad. Sci. USA. **76**: 5036-5040.

CUTFIELD, J.F., S.M. CUTFIELD, E.J. DODSON, G.G. DODSON, S.O. EMDIN, and C.D. REYNOLDS. 1979. Structure and biological activity of hagfish insulin. J. Mol. Biol. **132**: 85-100.

CUTFIELD, J.F., S.M. CUTFIELD, E.J. DODSON, G.G.DODSON, C.D. REYNOLDS, and D. VALLELY. 1981. Similarities and differences in the crystal structures of insulin. pp. 527-546 *In* Dodson, G., G.P. Glusker, and D. Sayre [eds.] Structural studies of molecules of biological interest. Clarendon Press, Oxford.

CRAIK, C.S., W.J. RUTTER, and R. FLETTERICK. 1983. Splice junctions: association with variations in protein structure. Science **220**: 1125-1129.

DAHL, G., and J. C. HENQUIN. 1978. Cold-induced insulin release *in vitro*; evidence for exocytosis. Cell Tiss. Res. **194**: 387-398.

DE HAEN, C., E. SWANSON, and D.C. TELLER. 1976. The evolutionary origin of proinsulin: amino acid sequence homology with trypsin related serine proteases detected and evaluated by new statistical methods. J. Mol. Biol. **106**: 639-661.

EMDIN, S.O. 1982a. Effects of hagfish insulin in the Atlantic hagfish, *Myxine glutinosa*: *in vivo* metabolism of ^{14}C-glucose and ^{14}C-leucine, and studies on starvation and glucose loading. Gen Comp. Endocrinol. **47**: 414-425.

EMDIN, S.O. 1982b. Insulin release in the Atlantic hagfish, *Myxine glutinosa, in vitro*. Gen. Comp. Endocrinol. **48**: 333-341.

EMDIN, S.O., and S. FALKMER. 1977. Phylogeny of insulin: some evolutionary aspects of insulin production with particular regard to the biosynthesis of insulin in *Myxine glutinosa*. Acta Paediatr. Scand. Suppl. **270**: 15-23.

EMDIN, S.O., S. GAMMELTOFT, and J. GLIEMANN. 1977. Degradation, receptor binding affininity, and potency of insulin from the Atlantic hagfish, *Myxine glutinosa*, determined in isolated rat fat cells. J. Biol. Chem. **252**: 602-608.

EMDIN, S.O., O. SONNE, and J. GLIEMANN. 1980. Hagfish insulin: the discrepancy between binding affinity and biological activity. Diabetes **29**: 301-303.

EMDIN, S.O., and D.F. STEINER. 1980. A specific antiserum against insulin from the Atlantic hagfish, *Myxine glutinosa*: characterization of the antiserum, its use in a homologous radioimmunoassay, and immunofluorescent microscopy. Gen. Comp. Endocrinol. **42**: 251-258.

FALKMER, S., and S.O. EMDIN. 1981. Insulin evolution. pp. 420-440 *In* Dodson, G., J. P. Glusker, and D. Sayre [eds.] Structural studies of molecules of biological interest. Clarendon Press, Oxford.

FALKMER, S., and A.J. MATTY. 1966. Blood sugar regulation in the hagfish. Gen. Comp. Endocrinol. **6**: 334-346.

GAMMELTOFT, S., L. OSTERGAARD-KRISTENSEN, and L. SESTOFT. 1978. Insulin receptors in isolated rat hepatocytes: reassessment of binding properties and observations of the inactivation of insulin at 37°C. J. Biol. Chem. **253**: 8406-8413.

GERICH, J.E., M.A. CHARLES, and G.M. GRODSKY. 1976. Regulation of pancreatic insulin and glucagon secretion. Ann. Rev. Physiol. **38**: 353-388.

HALBAN, P., and C.B. WOLLHEIM. 1980. Intracellular degradation of insulin stores by rat pancreatic islets *in vitro*. J. Biol. Chem. **255**: 6003-6006.

HALES, C.N. 1978. Proteolysis and the evolutionary origin of polypeptide hormones. FEBS Letters **94**: 10-16.

HODGKIN, D.C. 1974. Insulin, its chemistry and biochemistry. Proc. Roy. Soc. **A338**: 251-275.

INUI, Y., and A. GORBMAN. 1978. Role of the liver in regulation of carbohydrate metabolism in hagfish, *Eptatretus stouti*. Comp. Biochem. Physiol. **60A**: 181-183.

INUI, Y., J.Y.-L. YU, and A. GORBMAN. 1978. Effect of bovine insulin on the incorporation of (^{14}C)-glycine into protein and carbohydrate in liver and muscle of hagfish, *Eptatretus stouti*. Gen. Comp. Endocrinol. **36**: 133-141.

KING, G.L., and C.R. KAHN. 1981. Non-parallel evolution of metabolic and growth promoting functions of insulin. Nature **292**: 644-646.

KURJAN, J., and I. HERSKOWITZ. 1982. Structure of a yeast pheromone gene MF α : a putative α-factor precursor contains four tandem copies of mature α-factor. Cell **30**: 933-938.

LEROITH, D., S. HENDRICKS, M.A. LESNIAK, S. RISHI, K.L. BECKER, J. HAVRANKOBA, J.L. ROSENZWEIG, M.J. BROWNSTEIN, and J. ROTH. 1983. Insulin in brain and other extrapancreatic tissues of vertebrates and non-vertebrates. Adv. in Metab. Disord. **10**: 303-340.

MILLER, W.M., and N.L. EBERHARDT. 1983. Structure and evolution of the growth hormone gene family. Endocrine Rev. **4**: 97-130.

MUGGEO, M., B.H. GINSBERG, J. ROTH, C.R. KAHN, P. DEMEYTS, and D.M. NEVILLE JR. 1979. The insulin receptor in vertebrates is functionally more conserved during evolution than insulin itself. Endocrinology. **104**: 1393-1402.

MUGGEO, M., E. VAN OBBERGHEN, C.R. KAHN, J. ROTH, G.H. GINSBERG, P. DEMEYTS, S.O. EMDIN, and S. FALKMER. 1979. The insulin receptor and insulin of the Atlantic hagfish: extraordinary conservation of binding specificity and negative cooperativity in the most primitive vertebrate. Diabetes **28**: 175-181.

PATZELT, C., S.J. CHAN, J. DUGUID, G. HORTIN, P. KEIM, R.L. HEINRIKSON, and D.F. STEINER. 1978. Biosynthesis of polypeptide hormones in intact and cell free systems. pp. 69-78 *In* S. Magnusson [ed.] Regulatory proteolytic enzymes and their inhibitors. Proc. vol. 47, Symp. A6. Pergamon Press, N.Y.

PULLEN, R.A., D.G. LINDSAY, S.P. WOOD, I.J. TICKLE, T.L. BLUNDELL, A. WOLLMER, G. KRAIL, D. BRANDENBURG, H. ZAHN, J. GLIEMANN, and S. GAMMELTOFT. 1976. Receptor binding region of insulin. Nature **259**: 369-373.

ROTH, J., D. LEROITH, J. SHILOACH, J.L. ROSENZWEIG, M.A. LESNIAK, and J. HAVRANKOVA. 1982. Sem. Med. Beth Israel Hospital, Boston **306**: 523-527.

RYLE, A.P., F. SANGER, L.F. SMITH, and R. KITAI. 1955. The disulphide bonds of insulin. Biochem. J. **60**: 541-556.

SANGER, F. 1959. Chemistry of insulin. Science **129**: 1340-1344.

SCHUELLER, R.H., J.F. JACKSON, L. McALLISTER, J. SCHWARTZ, E.R. KANDEL, and R. AXEL. 1982. A family of genes that codes for ELH, a neuropeptide eliciting a stereotyped pattern of behavior in *Aplysia.* Cell **28**: 707-719.

STEINER, D.F. 1967. Evidence for a precursor in the biosynthesis of insulin. Trans. N.Y. Acad. Sci. Ser. II, **30**: 60-68.

STEINER, D.F. 1969. Proinsulin and the biosynthesis of insulin. Rec. Progr. Horm. Res. **25**: 207-268.

STEINER, D.F. 1978. On the role of the proinsulin C-peptide. Diabetes **27**: Suppl. 1, 145-148.

STEINER, D.F. 1983. The biosynthesis of insulin: genetic, evolutionary and pathophysiologic aspects. The Harvey Lectures, series **78**: 191-228.

STEINER, D.F., S.J. CHAN, K. DOCHERTY, S.O. EMDIN, G.G. DODSON, and S. FALKMER. 1984. Evolution of polypeptide hormones and their precursor processing mechanisms. pp. 203-223 *In* Falkmer, S., R. Håkansson, and F. Sundler [eds.] Evolution and tumour pathology of the neuroendocrine system. Elsevier, Amsterdam.

STEINER, D.F., W. KEMMLER, J.L. CLARK, P.E. OYER, and A.H. RUBINSTEIN. 1972. The biosynthesis of insulin. pp. 175-198 *In* Steiner, D.F., and N. Freinkel [eds.] Handbook of physiology: Sect. 7. vol 1: The endocrine pancreas. Williams and Wilkins, Baltimore.

STEINER, D.F., C. PATZELT, S.J. CHAN, P.S. QUIN, H.S. TAGER, D. NIELSEN, Å. LERNMARK, B.E. NOUYES, K.L. AGARWAL, K.H. GABBAY, and A.H. RUBINSTEIN. 1980. Formation of biologically active peptides. Proc. Roy. Soc. **210**: 45-59.

TAGER, H.S., S.O. EMDIN, J.L. CLARK, and D.F. STEINER. 1973. Studies on the conversion of proinsulin to insulin II. J. Biol. Chem. **248**: 3476-3482.

TERRIS, S., and D. F. STEINER. 1975. Binding and degradation of ^{125}I-insulin by rat hepatocytes. J. Biol. Chem. **250**: 8389-8398.

THORPE, A. 1976. Studies on the role of insulin in teleost metabolism. pp. 271-284 *In* Grillo, T.A.I., L. Leibson, and A. Epple [eds.] The evolution of pancreatic islets. Pergamon Press, Oxford.

VAN NORDEN, S., and S. FALKMER. 1980. Gut-islet endocrinology - some evolutionary aspects. Invest. Cell Path. **3**: 21-36.

EVOLUTION OF GASTRO-ENTERO-PANCREATIC ENDOCRINE SYSTEMS IN LOWER VERTEBRATES

Michael C. Thorndyke

Dept. Zoology, University of London
Royal Holloway and Bedford New College
Egham, Surrey TW20 0EX, U.K.

Sture Falkmer

Dept. of Tumor Pathology
Karolinska Hospital
Stockholm, Sweden

Introduction

Although the title of this chapter uses the term endocrine, the division between the endocrine and nervous systems in vertebrates, particularly with regard to neurohormonal peptides, is now so small as to be virtually non- existent. For this reason it is impossible to consider the gut endocrine system in isolation, and necessarily this chapter will include, where relevant, due appreciation of neuronal peptides. In recent years increasing attention has been focussed upon the regulatory mechanisms in the vertebrate gut and their evolutionary interrelationships. The common feature which has emerged from these studies is that of the fundamental role of the peptide regulator. Peptide hormones have long been acknowledged to play an important part in gastrointestinal control mechanisms following the discovery of secretin over 80 years ago (Bayliss and Starling, 1903). Since this time, knowledge of gastro-entero-pancreatic (GEP) endocrine systems has evolved in a somewhat staccato fashion, bursts of activity frequently resulting from the appearance of new technical methods. The availability of immunochemical techniques has been a key development in recent years while currently, recombinant DNA technology has heralded a new era in GEP hormone research.

The most important concept to manifest itself in the last ten years has been the recognition that peptides are not restricted to classic gut endocrine cells but are, in addition, important components of the autonomic nervous system which innervates the gut (Grossman, 1979). With the realisation that peptides are not only located in the peripheral parts of the nervous system but also may be found centrally, the idea of duality has been extended with the development of the so called Brain-Gut Axis. Although this principle derives to a large extent from mammalian studies, the origins of the chordate brain-gut axis may be found in the immediate deuterostome protochordate ancestors of vertebrates, the urochordates and cephalochordates. From here patterns of development and sophistication may be traced through the vertebrate series.

Notwithstanding the significant progress made in recent years, it is crucial to be aware of the restraints with which we are faced. Pre-eminently, it is important to remember that we can only deal with living species. Peptide hormones are not fossilized, undoubtedly living species are likely to have become both specialised and highly adapted, and it may be difficult to relate present findings to a truly primitive condition. Furthermore the study of the molecules alone can lead to all kinds of convolutions, for example, the frog skin peptide caerulein, a member of the gastrin/cholecystokinin (gastrin/CCK) family has been suggested as being ancestral to both these moieties (Larsson and Rehfeld, 1977). More recent evidence suggests this may be a specific adaptation in certain amphibians and its presence restricted to the skin in these animals (Dimaline, 1982). Despite these limitations, however, the careful use of a variety of techniques, including immunochemical, physiological and biological assays, can contribute substantially to our understanding of the evolution of GEP neurohormonal endocrine systems.

Criteria for analysis

The majority of studies on peptide evolution depend upon immunochemical techniques of one kind or another. These are usually of two types: (i) detection of presence and cellular origin of peptide by immunocytochemistry (ICC) (Polak and Van Noorden, 1985); (ii) identification of hormones in tissue extracts and/or serum by radioimmunoassay (RIA). There are a number of problems associated with these approaches, among them that of cross reactivity and specificity of antibody-antigen binding. This is particularly pertinent since studies in lower vertebrates frequently utilize antibodies raised against mammalian peptides. Given the accepted view that the antigenic determinants for peptides are of the order of 4-8 amino acid residues at the most, it is clear that both false negatives and false positives are possible. In this way it would be possible to localise an antigen that has, in fact, only limited chemical similarity and perhaps none biologically, to the original antigen. Thus one might achieve a "positive" location of a totally unrelated peptide or small protein (Jornvall, 1984; Rehfeld, 1984). In a similar way, only subtle differences in the native peptide antigen may render it unresponsive to heterologous antisera. Despite these problems, with the judicious use of controls, such as pre-absorption of antisera with known antigen, together with the use of panels of antisera, each specific for an appropriate region or residue of the known peptide, some advances can be made. RIA is least open to misinterpretation since, following extraction, suitable fractionation and allied chromatographic techniques can be utilized to further define similarities and/or discrepancies between molecules. A more recent approach has been the use of cDNA probes to detect those genes and mRNA molecules responsible for directing synthesis of the peptide and its precursors. Once again, with notable exceptions (e.g. insulin - See Emdin, this volume), probes are based upon mammalian genes and to a certain extent may be open to the specificity problems associated with immunological methods. The use of different nucleotide probes is one way around this difficulty (Rehfeld, 1984).

More traditional methods of hormone identification have involved bioassay and indeed the original discovery of secretin was based upon bioassay. Classic mammalian preparations such as pancreatic secretion in cat or rat, and gall bladder contraction in guinea pig or rabbit (*in vivo* or *in vitro*) have frequently been used to detect the presence of CCK-like and secretin-like molecules in lower vertebrates (Nilsson, 1970; Vigna, 1979). While these are useful indicators of biological activity, they tend to be less sensitive than RIA and may also suffer from the same limitations in terms of specificity of response. For example, the amphibian stomach apparently produces a CCK-like peptide which does not stimulate gastric acid secretion in typical mammalian assays. On the other hand, in frogs, mammalian gastrin is an ineffective agonist for gastric acid secretion, while CCK is quite potent (Negri and Erspamer, 1973). This brings to light additional methods of investigation, that of demonstrating hormonal response in a lower vertebrate with the application of mammalian peptides. Once again the studies noted above highlight the problems and dangers associated with the expectation of a certain response from a certain peptide based upon its activity in mammals. The only reliable bioassay is that of assay of lower vertebrate peptides on their own systems. This has only been carried out on relatively few occasions (see Emdin, Vigna, this volume). Straightforward chemical methods are also available and have been used with success in mammalian studies. Outstanding work at the Karolinska Institute, Stockholm (Tatemoto and Mutt, 1980) has developed a novel chemical assay based upon the identification of peptides in tissue extracts by means of their characteristic C-terminal amidation. In this way a number of new peptides have been identified in mammals (Tatemoto and Mutt, 1981). As yet these techniques have not been applied to lower vertebrates.

Finally, it is worth noting that workers in this field are not only beset by investigative problems such as those outlined above; they also labour under difficulties of nomenclature which are of their own making. Hence the semantic use of peptide names has dogged research in this field where some hormones have been named after their first discovered function (secretin), or from their organ of first isolation (insulin). Others receive names based upon their chemistry and structural features (PHI). The crux of the problem is that while a peptide may have certain function in one species, it may not have this function in another species. For example, what is the significance of the name cholecystokinin in the rat, which has no gall bladder? The danger here is that it is all too easy to enter this field with preconceived ideas as to possible or even probable functions of peptides in lower species. It is crucial to remember that hormones do not evolve in isolation; receptors and target organs are exposed to the same selective pressures as the hormones themselves and we must expect changes here as well. With the emergence of the concept of a brain-gut axis for neurohormonal peptides, where the same peptide may be present in the brain, gut endocrine cells and gastrointestinal neurones of the same species, it is all the more important to have an open-minded approach. Against this background, however, distinctive patterns of GEP neurohormonal evolution have emerged and some of these are discussed below as well as elsewhere in this volume.

The brain-gut axis in protochordates

There can now be little doubt that the origin of many, if not all, neurohormonal peptides may be traced back to primitive invertebrate nervous systems and this idea has been the subject of a number of recent reviews (Van Noorden, 1984; Thorndyke, 1985). Our present concern, however, is for the vertebrates and their most immediate ancestors. The closest surviving invertebrate relatives of the vertebrates are the protochordates, a rather loose assemblage of animals which includes the urochordates (tunicates) and cephalochordates (lancelets). Here the intrinsic elements of the brain-gut axis and presumptive islet peptides are already present. A number of studies, in the main relying heavily upon immunocytochemistry and radioimmunoassay, have established the presence of a wide range of peptide hormones both in the gut epithelium as well as in neuronal cell bodies and fibres of the simple neural ganglion (Bevis and Thorndyke, 1978, 1979; Fritsch *et al.*, 1982; Thorndyke, 1982). Thus peptides have been detected using antisera raised against ACTH, calcitonin, substance P, neurotensin, bombesin, secretin, endorphin, gastrin/CCK, VIP and others. Gastrin/CCK-like activity is especially noteworthy since it appears to be a major component of the central nervous system in these animals (Fig. 1) as well as being present in gut endocrine cells (Fritsch *et al.*, 1982) and gut extracts (Larson and Vigna, 1983; Dimaline and Thorndyke, 1981 unpublished observations).

Recently, gastrin/CCK-like activity has been confirmed in tissue extracts from the neural complex in *Ciona* where it seems to be a CCK-like molecule rather than gastrin-like (Dockray and Thorndyke, unpublished observations). Furthermore, in one of the few physiological studies to be attempted in tunicates, using the solitary ascidian *Styela clava*, both CCK_8 and CCK_{33} were shown to be effective stimulants of secretory activity in the presumptive pre-pancreatic zymogen cells characteristic of these animals (Bevis and Thorndyke, 1981; Thorndyke and Bevis, 1984). A final piece of evidence in support of this early emergence of a potential CCK-like factor as a zymogen cell secretogogue comes from a short series of experiments where the extracted *Styela* peptide was assayed in its animal of origin. Here the partially purified *Styela* gut extract proved a most effective agonist, with a potency considerably greater than CCK (Fig. 2).

One of the most interesting and significant concepts to emerge from mammalian peptide studies in recent years has been the idea of tissue-specific mRNA processing. According to this hypothesis, alternative processing of the mRNA derived from a peptide coding gene may result in the production of a variety of mRNAs, each coding for a particular peptide. In this way it has been shown that mRNA transcribed from the calcitonin gene in thyroidal 'C' cells produced calcitonin, whereas in neural tissues transcribed mRNA encodes a novel neuropeptide, calcitonin gene-related peptide (CGRP) (Rosenfeld *et al.*, 1983). Current evidence from protochordates (S.I. Girgis, P.J.R. Bevis, I. Macintyre and M.C. Thorndyke unpublished observations) indicates what is apparently a startling cross species example of this phenomenon. Immunocytochemical and RIA investigation of the neural complex in *Styela clava* and *Ciona intestinalis* indicate that in *Ciona*, CGRP immunoreactive material predominates over calcitonin, whereas in *Styela* the opposite applies, here calcitonin appears in much higher concentrations than CGRP (Fig. 3). Thus, one might suggest that in one species

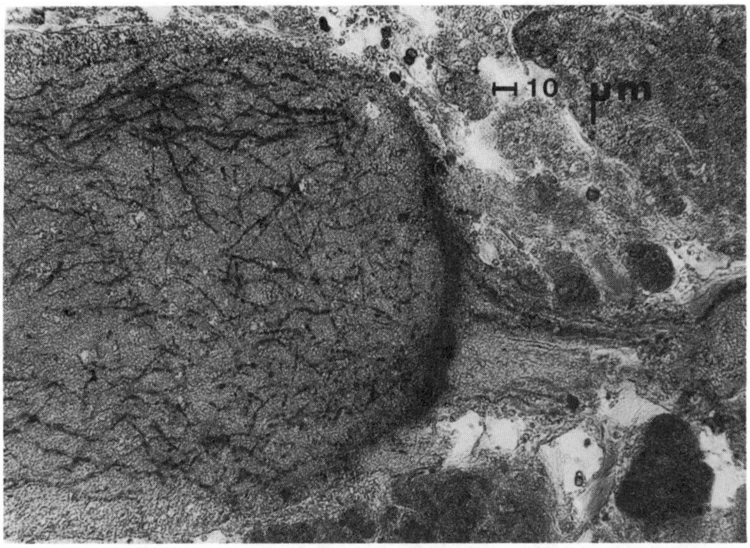

Fig. 1. Gastrin/CCK-like immunoreactive neurones in the neural ganglion of the ascidian *Ascidiella aspersa*, PAP method. Photomicrograph kindly provided by Greg O'Neil from unpublished work.

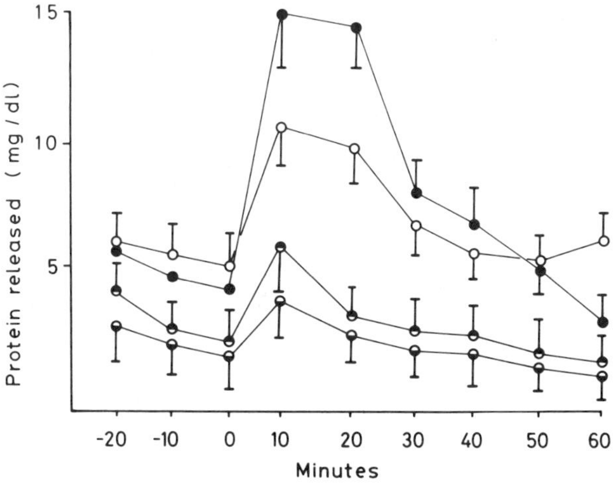

Fig. 2. Response of perfused *Styela clava* stomach to CCK_{33} and caerulein compared with that obtained using partially purified homologous stomach extracts. ◓ CCK_8 100 μg (2.55 x 10^{-8} moles); ◒ caerulein 100 μg (7.4 x 10^{-8} moles); ● *Styela* gut extract, 1.0 μg; ○ *Styela* gut extract 0.5 μg. Mean ± SD. Methods according to Bevis and Thorndyke (1981).

(*Ciona*) the calcitonin gene transcribes an mRNA encoding CGRP whilst in *Styela* a calcitonin mRNA is produced. Thus the potential for tissue-specific RNA processing is quite clearly present in the protochordate ancestors of vertebrates and may represent a unique opportunity for the study of the switching mechanism.

In cephalochordates, studies concentrating on *Branchiostoma* have confirmed the presence of a brain-gut axis. As in tunicates there is no pancreas and the pre-pancreatic zymogen cells line the gut epithelium. Scattered in this epithelium are found endocrine cells which are immunoreactive for insulin, somatostatin, PP, VIP, calcitonin, gastrin/CCK, glucagon and neurotensin (Reinecke, 1981; Van Noorden, 1984). The neuronal location of peptides is also well established with gastrin/CCK-(Fig. 4), calcitonin- and PP-like immunoreactivity being evident in brain and nerve cord (Thorndyke and Bevis, 1981; Van Noorden, 1984).

The phylogeny of islet hormones

Protochordates

With regard to putative pancreatic islet hormones, there are no discrete islet clusters in tunicates. Insulin, somatostatin and pancreatic polypeptide immuno-reactivities have been localised in typical gut endocrine cells, the latter two also being found in the neural ganglion (Bevis and Thorndyke, 1978; Fritsch *et al.*, 1982). At present there is no evidence for the presence (or absence) of glucagon in urochordates. The insulin-like cells are of particular interest since they are found dispersed in the gut epithelium, although there is a tendency for them to be concentrated in the foregut (Bevis and Thorndyke, 1978). Furthermore, while many of these cells are of the 'open' type usually considered most primitive

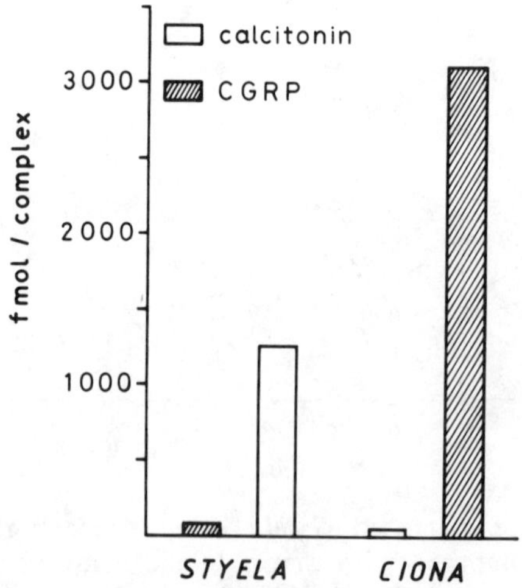

Fig. 3. CGRP- and calcitonin-like immunoreactivity in extracts from the neural complex of the ascidians *Styela clava* and *Ciona intestinalis*.

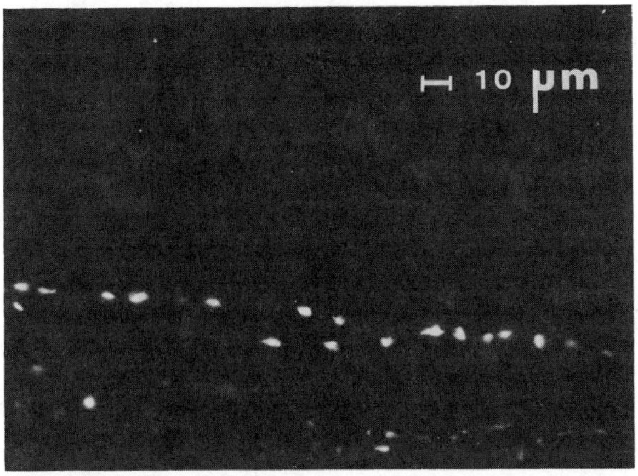

Fig. 4. Gastrin/CCK-like immunoreactive fibres in the nerve cord of *Branchiostoma lanceolatum*.

(Falkmer *et. al.*, 1984) there are some which are undoubtedly closed (Fig. 5) and could, perhaps be taken to have begun the transition towards the isolated islet cell. In cephalochordates, as in urochordates, presumptive islet cells are scattered in the gut epithelium and there is evidence here, the first in protochordates, for the presence of glucagon-like immunoreactivity (Van Noorden, 1984). Interestingly, there is also the suggestion that glucagon may co-exist with gastrin-like material (Van Noorden and Pearse, 1976).

Cyclostomes, cartilaginous fish

It is at the level of the earliest and most primitive vertebrates, the Agnatha, that the pattern of islet evolution first takes shape. A detailed appraisal of islet cell evolution may be found in recent reviews and will be dealt with only briefly here (Falkmer and Van Noorden, 1983; Falkmer *et al.*, 1984). In the Agnatha, even in the absence of discrete exocrine pancreatic tissue, islet organs appear as outgrowths from the bile duct. Essentially this is a two hormone parenchyma comprising insulin (99%) and somatostatin (1%)cells. The majority of somatostatin cells are to be found in the mucosa of the bile duct as a mixture of both closed and open cells, where they are accompanied by a few, closed, insulin cells. Glucagon and PP cells remain as open endocrine cells scattered in the gut epithelium along with a few somatostatin cells (Falkmer *et al.*, 1984; Falkmer, 1985). It is of great interest that *Myxine* represents one of the few primitive vertebrate species where complete identification, receptor binding characteristics and biological potency tests have been carried out on one of the islet hormones, insulin. This topic is covered in detail elsewhere in this volume (Chapter by Emdin). With the emergence of the first jawed vertebrates, the islets became associated with the first discrete exocrine acinar pancreas. Thus in holocephalans, a group usually considered the closest living relatives to the earliest of gnathostomes, one may find well developed islet organs (Falkmer *et al.*, 1981). In two of the three species studied this is a three-

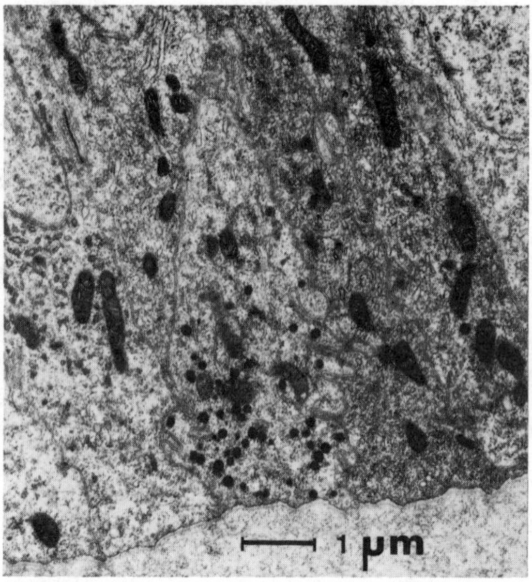

Fig. 5. Electron micrograph showing an endocrine cell of the closed type in the oesophagus of the ascidian *Styela clava*.

hormone parenchyma, with glucagon cells accompanying insulin and somatostatin cells in *Chimaera monstrosa* and *Hydrolagus colliei*. PP cells are restricted to the gut mucosa and the long pancreatic duct, along with additional glucagon and somatostatin cells (Falkmer and Van Noorden, 1983). In the other holocephalan studied, *Callorhynchus millii*, PP cells also appear as an islet component (Falkmer *et al.*, 1984). The condition in *Callorhynchus* foreshadows that seen in the largest surviving group of cartilaginous fishes, the elasmobranchs. Here, in sharks and rays, the pancreas comprises a well-developed exocrine gland although, unlike the holocephalan pancreas, it remains closely associated with the gastrointestinal tract (Falkmer *et al.*, 1981). The islet clusters which are closely duct-associated are clearly four hormone organs, in that insulin, somatostatin, glucagon as well as PP cells are present. As before, with the exception of insulin, all other islet hormones have representative cells in the gut mucosa.

Bony fish, other vertebrate phyla

This characteristic distribution appears to be maintained with only minor qualitative variations but with more extensive quantitative variations throughout the remaining vertebrate line. The wide variations in pancreatic organisation which exist in bony fishes make the continuing assessment of islet evolution through to Amphibia the most difficult aspect of these investigations. Much of the variation is likely due to the extensive adaptive radiation seen in this group, but nevertheless, in some species concentrations of islet parenchyma known as principal islets or Brockmann bodies may be found. One species, *Cottus scorpius*, has been studied in some detail (Falkmer *et al.*, 1981,1984) and here the pyloric or principal islet typically comprises all four hormones, with PP cells characteristically located in the peripheral region. Interestingly, the remaining splenic islet is almost completely devoid of PP cells (Falkmer *et al.*, 1981,1984). The outstanding significance of this lies in the fact that it reflects a similar, regionally qualitative, variation in islet components seen in higher vertebrates, including mammals. Thus, the splenic lobe of the pancreas in birds contains relatively few PP cells and a larger number of glucagon cells. In other areas, PP cells are infrequent, and the islets take on a more typical composition, although in birds, there is a tendency for glucagon cells to predominate.

The trend in vertebrate islet evolution is the gradual concentration of first insulin then somatostatin, glucagon and finally PP producing cells in discrete islet structures. Of these peptides, the latter three may be found also in typical gut endocrine cells. Insulin cells remain restricted to the islet parenchyma, although under certain pathological conditions they are found in the gut mucosa (Falkmer *et al.*, 1984). It could be that this represents a reversion to the primitive and immature condition (Alumets *et al.*, 1981).

Gastrointestinal peptides

This represents a vast area and several aspects of gut peptide evolution in vertebrates are discussed in accompanying chapters. Here an attempt will be made to give an overall assessment of the problem, together with concluding sections, each covering one of the major and topical areas of gut peptide research.

In lower vertebrates, especially fishes, the list of peptides both in gut endocrine cells and the gastrointestinal innervation is now extensive and includes most of those thought to comprise the full mammalian system. Moreover, the evidence currently available incorporates bioassay as well as RIA and ICC data. Thus in teleosts, material immunoreactive to substance P, glucagon/glicentin, gastrin/CCK, somatostatin, neurotensin, VIP, bombesin, enkephalin and PP have been located in the gut (Langer *et al.*, 1979; Holmgren *et al.*, 1982; Rombout and Taverne-Thiele, 1982). Some of these, such as VIP, appear to be characteristic of the gut innervation only, while others, such as substance P, have a dual location in nerves as well as endocrine cells. In elasmobranchs the list is shorter, with only bombesin-, gastrin/CCK-, somatostatin- and VIP-like immunoreactivities being noted and here VIP occurs in both nerves and endocrine cells (Falkmer *et al.*, 1980; Fouchereau-Peron *et al.*, 1980; Holmgren and Nilsson, 1983a). In holosteans (*Lepidosteus*) only bombesin-like, neurotensin-like and VIP-like activities have been described (Holmgren and Nilsson, 1983b). Investigations using other assay methods are rather few. Heterologous bioassays (in rats, guinea pigs or cats) have found both secretin- and gastrin/CCK-like activity in gut extracts from the agnathan *Myxine glutinosa* and the holocephalan, *Chimaera monstrosa* (Nilsson, 1970; 1973), and gastrin/CCK-like activity in *Eptatretus stouti* (Vigna, 1979). Secretin/VIP-like activity was shown in a similar fashion in extracts from the teleost *Esox lucius* (Dockray, 1974). In the majority of cases, these studies have been taken no further than the confirmation of presence of the peptide-like material. In a few instances, however, some effort has gone into a careful characterisation of the peptide moeity and in this way some trends in neurohormonal evolution can be evidenced.

The evolution of gastrin/CCK-like peptides has attracted particular interest in the last few years, due in no small part to the biological significance of the common C-terminal pentapeptide sequence shared by these molecules and in which resides the C-terminal tetrapeptide sequence necessary for any appreciable biological activity. This fact has proved to be a potent tool for biologists, since it has led to the development of a range of region-specific antisera which allow the identification of this biologically important region, as well as having the ability to discriminate between gastrin-like and CCK-like products. As pointed out earlier, gastrin/CCK-like molecules are already part of the brain-gut axis in protochordates. In the first vertebrates, the Agnatha, gastrin/CCK-like activity has been demonstrated in the gut by all three of the important criteria of bioassay, RIA and immunocytochemistry (Nilsson, 1973; Van Noorden *et al.*, 1971; Van Noorden and Pearse, 1974; Ostberg *et al.*, 1975; Vigna, 1979). Moreover, RIA studies on the brain (Holmquist *et al.*, 1979) indicate its presence there too. Perhaps the most outstanding problem yet to be resolved in this area is that of the origin of gastrin and CCK as separate products. Gastrin/CCK-like immunoreactivity has been detected in the gastrointestinal tract of many fish species including both teleosts and elasmobranchs (*op. cit.*). Its presence is also confirmed in the brain (Notenboom *et al.*, 1981). However, in most instances, the antisera used were directed towards the C-terminus and therefore unable to discriminate between gastrin and CCK. The situation is further complicated by the presence in amphibians of a skin-derived peptide, caerulein, which shares its C-terminal sequence with gastrin and CCK. In a study of the cod and two species of the frog, Larsson and Rehfeld (1977) used a selection of region-specific antisera to determine the character and distribution of gastrin-like and CCK-like peptides. Their conclusion was that, in bony fishes as well as in amphibians, cells produce a molecule which is both gastrin- and CCK-like and it is only with the emergence of the reptiles that gastrin and CCK occur as products of separate cells. This hypothesis includes the idea that gastrin and CCK evolved from a common caerulein-like molecule. Notwithstanding the possiblity of species variability in fishes, this idea can be challenged with the observation that Langer and colleagues (1979) successfully stained cells in the upper midgut of several teleost species using an antibody specific for the N-terminus of gastrin, while tests with antisera directed against the C-terminus of gastrin and the middle region of CCK proved negative.

More recent studies on amphibians have, in part, clarified the situation. Using a combination of immunocytochemistry, RIA and chromatographic techniques, Dimaline and Dockray (Dimaline, 1982; Dockray and Dimaline, 1984) demonstrate that caerulein is a unique product of the skin in certain amphibian species, with the brain and gut elaborating a peptide with CCK_8-like properties. Further studies by this group on reptilian and avian gastrin/CCK-like peptides indicate that part of the problem could be that "gastrins" in lower vertebrates are quite different chemically from mammalian gastrins, and it follows that antisera raised against mammalian peptides may well be incapable of detecting them. One of the most suitable ways to tackle this problem would be to assess the bioactivity of endogenous factors on their own putative target tissues. It is also imperative that an open-minded approach be used in such investigations, since endogenous factors in fishes need not necessarily subserve the same functions as indentified in mammals. The danger here is of the preconceived notion of function, and the finding of C-terminal gastrin-like activity in the stomachless fish (Rombout and Taverne-Thiele, 1982) should serve as an adequate warning. The value of the homologous bioassay has already been pointed out in an earlier section concerning CCK-like factor in the ascidian *Styela clava.* A variation on the bioassay approach is to use mammalian peptides and homologous tissue extracts as probes for receptors in lower vertebrates. A detailed assessment of this subject is outside the scope of this chapter and is, in any case, covered elsewhere in this volume (chapter by S.R. Vigna). Suffice it to say here that the significance of this approach is highlighted by the work of Holstein (Holstein and Humphrey, 1980; Holstein, 1982) on the control of gastric acid secretion in the cod. Here it seems mammalian gastrin/CCK-like peptides inhibit rather than stimulate gastric acid secretion, while bombesin is the only effective agonist amongst many tested. Clearly the isolation of the endogenous factors responsible for the stimulation of gastric acid secretion in fishes is an urgent requirement.

Vasoactive intestinal polypeptide, "rectin" and endogenous peptides in fishes

As mentioned above, VIP-like immunoreactivity has been found to be widespread in lower vertebrates, being localized in particular to neurones innervating the gastrointestinal tract (*op. cit.*). In mammals this peptide has been identified as having a number of peripheral roles including (a) control of local blood flow increases, by way of its vasodilatory effect, (b) relaxation of gut smooth muscle, (c) control of water, electrolyte and possibly protein secretion in the gut and associated glands (Said, 1980). Using such potential roles as a guide, there have been a number of attempts to identify the origins of these functions in lower vertebrates. In a continuing study of gastric acid secretion in the cod, Holstein (1983) showed that intramuscular exogenous VIP notably reduced gastric acid secretion. This effect was deemed, as it is in mammals, not to be due to a primary effect on mucosal blood supply, although its precise mechanism of action is yet to be identified. An apparently authentic role for VIP has, however, been ascertained in the cod swim bladder. VIP-like immunoreactivity has been localized to nerves innervating the swim bladder wall and oval edge as well as the coeliac and swim bladder arteries (Lundin and Holmgren, 1984). Gas resorption is controlled by muscular tension in the secretory mucosa and oval edge of the swim bladder, with a decrease in tension exposing more of the thin resorbing mucosa. Experiments utilizing exogenous VIP applied to isolated strips from this region suggest VIP is an effective agonist for this relaxation event (Lundin and Holmgren, 1984). Gas secretion is influenced by blood flow through the gas gland and, since VIP has been shown to increase this flow and have a hypotensive effect on isolated blood vessel strips, it seems highly likely that VIP innervation plays a significant part in the control of gas secretion (Lundin and Holmgren, 1984).

Although these investigations point to a genuine role for VIP in the cod which foreshadows its circulatory and gastrointestinal role in higher vertebrates, studies with VIP in its other potential spheres of influence have produced equivocal results and again brought into sharp focus the hazards associated with the use of heterologous peptides in phylogenetic studies. The role of VIP as an agonist for salt and water secretion in mammals prompted an investigation of its potential as a regulator of secretory activity in the elasmobranch rectal gland. An early examination of secretion in the isolated perfused rectal gland of *Squalus acanthias* showed that VIP was effective in stimulating secretion (Stoff *et al.*, 1979). However, it has since emerged that VIP may not in fact be the normal native

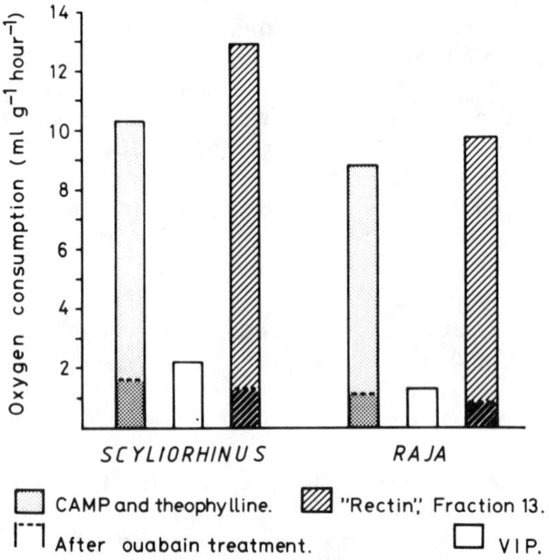

Fig. 6. Oxygen consumption of rectal gland slices following treatment with cAMP and theophylline (0.05 and 0.25 mmol l^{-1} respectively), VIP (0.1 mol l^{-1}) Fraction 13, "Rectin" (50 g ml^{-1}). Broken horizontal line indicates reduced level of oxygen consumption following ouabain (0.1 mmol l^{-1}) treatment. Ouabain-sensitive oxygen consumption is a recognized indicator of rectal gland secretory activity. Adapted from data in Shuttleworth and Thorndyke, 1984.

neurohormonal mediator of rectal gland secretion. Thus more recent work, taking advantage of the preferred, alternative approach of isolation of native peptides, has indicated that the natural secretagogue for elasmobranch rectal glands is a peptide other than VIP (Shuttleworth and Thorndyke, 1984; Thorndyke and Shuttleworth, 1985). These investigations have shown at the outset that VIP is effective only in *Squalus* and does not stimulate activity in *Scyliorhinus* or *Raja*. In sharp contrast, extracts prepared from the intestine of the spotted dogfish, *Scyliorhinus canicula* have proved to contain a peptide fraction which is a potent stimulant of rectal gland activity in *Squalus*, *Scyliorhinus*, and *Raja* (Shuttleworth and Thorndyke, 1984) (Fig. 6). This peptide is likely to have a major part to play in the regulation of rectal gland secretion *in vivo*, and the name 'Rectin' has been proposed for the putative hormone.

The confirmation that this material is quite distinct from elasmobranch VIP comes from studies carried out in parallel to those described above (Dimaline and Thorndyke, 1985). Analysis of the various fractions produced during the isolation of rectin have shown that VIP is present in only negligible quantities in the rectin fraction. Moreover this is not due to lack of cross reactivity of VIP antisera with dogfish VIP since large quantities of VIP-like immunoreactivity have been detected in other fractions of the extract (Dimaline and Thorndyke, 1985; unpublished observations). Furthermore, preliminary characterisation of this dogfish VIP indicates a peptide quite distinct from its mammalian counterpart. In this way, use of region-specific antisera and partial sequencing has established that while the N-terminal region of elasmobranch VIP resembles porcine VIP, the C-terminal sequence is likely to differ significantly. Quite clearly this has important implications for the origins and evolution of VIP, while also highlighting the dangers of relying upon the use of a "non-homologous" approach to peptide function in lower vertebrates.

The isolation of native fish neurohormonal peptides has in fact been taking place for a number of years and some aspects of this work may be found in the accompanying chapters of this volume. Perhaps the most significantly unique investigations in this area have been those concerned with the isolation and characterisation of peptides not from the gut, but from the caudal neurosecretory system. A complete appraisal of this topic is not possible within the confines of this chapter and details may be found in some recent reviews (Loretz *et al.*, 1981; Bern *et al.*, 1985). These factors do, however, warrant some attention because of their potential relationship to GEP peptides. To date, the teleost urophysis has yielded two distinct and novel peptide regulators and a third which is indistinguishable from arginine vasotocin (Lacanilao and Bern, 1972).

The first urotensin to be isolated and fully characterised was urotensin II (UII) (Pearson *et al.*, 1980) and its amino acid sequence indicated certain regional similarities with somatostatin-14. When urotensin I (UI) was finally isolated (Ichikawa *et al.*, 1982; Lederis *et al.*, 1982), it was shown to be homologous and analogous to mammalian corticotrophin releasing factor (CRF) and the amphibian skin peptide, sauvagine. Both UI and UII are considered to play an important part in epithelial transport phenomena and osmoregulation in teleosts, sometimes each exerting a similar effect such as in the inhibition of active sodium chloride efflux in *Tilapia* opercular membranes or stimulation of active sodium absorption in the goby urinary bladder. On other occasions they may be antagonistic as in the inhibition of active chloride efflux in goby skin by UII and its stimulation by UI (Bern *et al.*, 1985). As might be expected from their homologies to mammalian peptides, both UI and UII have notable effects in mammals. Indeed bioactivity based upon hypotensive effect on a rat hind limb preparation has been used extensively in the purification of UI (Ichikawa *et al.*, 1982).

In spite of the similarities, the importance of their relationship to mammalian peptides and its possible evolutionary significance have yet to be fully clarified. In this regard there would seem to be two crucial and interrelated areas in need of attention. First, as with brain-gut peptides, are urotensins to be found in locations peripheral to the urophysis? Moreover, and in view of the similarities to somatostatin and other peptides noted above, to what extent does the localization of, say, somatostatin-like immunoreactivity in the gut of many fishes in reality represent a gastrointestinal form of UII, rather than "mammalian" somatostatin?

Control of gastrointestinal motility and the evolution of transmitter interactions

In addition to secretory activity, the other major area where GEP neurohormonal peptides exert a controlling influence is in the regulation of gastrointestinal motility. The regulation of gastrointestinal motility in mammals has attracted increasing attention in recent years with the realisation that, in addition to the more traditional adrenergic and cholinergic factors, there is an important peptide (both neuronal and paracrine/endocrine) component which may well interact with the former regulatory agents (Furness and Costa, 1980; Ruppin and Domschke, 1980). In particular bombesin has attracted notice as an important regulator of gut function (Broccardo *et al.*, 1975; Hirschowitz and Gibson, 1979; Mayer *et al.*, 1982). Bombesin was first isolated from amphibian skin (Melchiorri, 1978) and this was followed rapidly by the identification of bombesin-like factors in mammals, and culminated in the characterisation of a closely related peptide from porcine gut, gastrin-releasing peptide (GRP) (McDonald *et al.*, 1979). Intensive investigation of the bioactivity of bombesin in mammals has established effects on the stimulation of gastric and pancreatic secretion which may be direct or indirect (McDonald *et al.*, 1979), together with an important role in the regulation of gut motility involving a direct myogenic component, as well as a more complex component where interaction with acetylcholine may be prevalent (Mayer *et al.*, 1982).

The situation in lower vertebrates is not yet clear, although there is evidence emerging which suggests that some of the complexities in the mammalian system may well have had their origins in fishes. Control of gut motility in fishes by classic cholinergic, aminergic and adrenergic mechanisms has been established for some time (Fänge and Grove, 1979). Exploration of the role of peptides in trout stomach has confirmed their potential as regulatory agents (Holmgren, 1983). These experiments and similar ones in *Cottus scorpius* (Fig. 7) have shown that a number of peptides, including bombesin, substance P and enkephalin stimulate gastric smooth muscle contraction, with some variation in response between circular and longitudinal preparations. In addition, it has been pointed out already that bombesin is one of the few effective stimulants of gastric acid secretion in the cod, although details of its mechanism of action are obscure (Holstein and Humphrey, 1980). These investigations, therefore, strongly suggest that bombesin is likely to be one of the more important peptide regulators in the primitive fish gut.

Against this background, and with the implication from mammalian studies that there is an interplay between bombesin and acetycholine, more recent investigations have concentrated on a possible interrelationship between bombesin and acetylcholine in the control of fish gut motility. Studies on this synergy in isolated gastric muscle strips from the sculpin, *Cottus scorpius* (Thorndyke and Falkmer, 1982; Thorndyke, 1983 unpublished observations) have shown that while bombesin treatment alone produces only a small increase in tension, when applied with a standard dose of acetylcholine (10^{-6} M) the response compared with either alone is considerably enhanced. Moreover this potentiation by bombesin is dose-dependent and substantially greater than the sum of the two separate effects (Fig. 7).

Interestingly, trials with the mammalian form of bombesin, GRP, show a similar effect, although dose for dose the potentiation with GRP is rather less than that seen with bombesin (Fig. 8). This work has been extended recently to include studies on the stomach of cod and trout (Thorndyke and Holmgren, 1985). These investigations confirmed the potentiation of the acetylcholine response by bombesin, with the effect being most marked in circular muscle from the pyloric

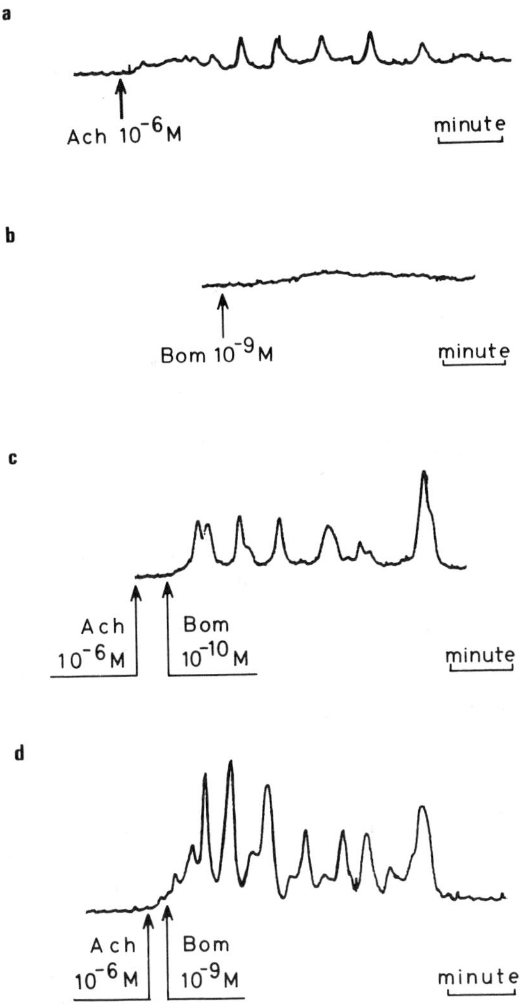

Fig. 7. Response of circular pyloric muscle strips from *Cottus scorpius* to: a) acetylcholine alone; b) bombesin alone; c) and d) ACh with two different doses of bombesin. Grass strain gauge, Washington oscillograph, 1 gm/cm sensitivity, 0.25 mm/sec chart speed. Method according to Thorndyke and Falkmer, 1982; Holmgren, 1983; Thorndyke *et al.*, 1984.

stomach. The specificity of the response was indicated in experiments where substance P was used in place of bombesin. Here, no enhancement of the cholinergic contraction was seen. Further tests where tetrodotoxin failed to block the potentiation would seem to suggest a mechanism which does not involve a presynaptic neuronal effect and, while the precise nature of the interaction remains

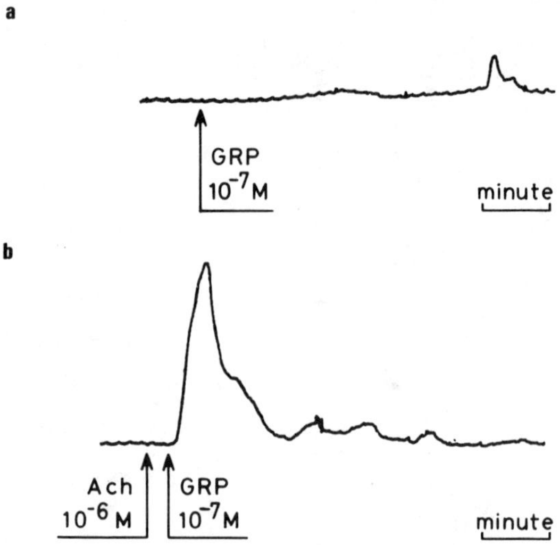

Fig. 8. Response of circular pyloric muscle strips from *Cottus scorpius* to a) gastrin-releasing peptide alone; b) acetylcholine plus GRP. Details as in Fig. 7.

to be determined, since atropine (10^{-5} M) effectively blocks the phenomenon, it would appear that a mechanism involving the muscarinic receptor might be one possibility.

Whatever the exact answer is, it is clear that the condition presently described for control of the fish stomach motility represents a suitably qualified pattern upon which the complex and sophisticated mammalian system may be based.

Conclusions

There can be no doubt that neurohormonal peptides are firmly established as important co-ordinators of gastrointestinal activity in primitive vertebrates. Perhaps one of the most substantial developments is the early emergence of the brain-gut axis and the concept that many chordate gut peptides had their origins in neurones of the invertebrate CNS (Van Noorden, 1984; Thorndyke, 1985). A fundamental issue to emerge from current studies is that any investigation of neurohormonal peptide evolution should be complemented by an equivalent assessment of target organ and receptor evolution. Moreover it is clear that gastrointestinal neurohormonal regulators each have the potential to fulfil a number of quite separate and varied roles, according to their location and/or target. The most urgent of present needs is for a synthesis of all current ideas, bringing together those investigations which approach the problem from the standpoint of peptide distribution with those using the alternative path of native peptide characterization with a functional examination of the gastrointestinal tract. Each of these are of value in their own right but only when they are brought together will the complete picture of neurohormonal evolution in the vertebrate gut be fully understood.

Acknowledgements

This chapter is based upon original work supported by grants from the Royal Society (UK), the Science and Engineering Research Council (Grant nos. B/RG 82919, GR/A 58852, GR/B 58787, GR/C 98296) and the Swedish Medical Research Council (Project no. 12X-718). The authors wish to acknowledge the following who have been involved in collaborative work: Peter Bevis, Rod Dimaline, Graham Dockray, Samia Girgis, Susanne Holmgren, Greg O'Neil, and Trevor Shuttleworth, as well as the Director and staff, Kristineberg Marine Biological Station, Sweden. We should also like to express gratitude to Ann Edwards for manuscript preparation, Zyg Podhorodecki for help with the figures, Tom McDonald for the gift of GRP and Steven Vigna for proofreading the manuscript.

Note added in proof

Recent work in the laboratory of one of the authors (O'Neil and Thorndyke, in prep.) has indicated the presence of insulin-like immunoreactivity in neuronal elements of the neural ganglion in the ascidian protochordate *Ciona intestinalis*. Thus, the brain-gut axis for insulin now appears to have continuity between invertebrates and the chordates, although 'brain' insulin is apparently absent from all chordates above the protochordates.

Literature cited

ALUMETS, J., P. ALM, S. FALKMER, R. HÅKANSON, O. LJUNGBERG, H. MÅRTENSSON, F. SUNDLER, and S. TIBBLIN. 1981. Immunohistochemical evidence of peptide hormones in endocrine tumors of the rectum. Cancer **48**: 2409-2425.

BAYLISS, W.M. and E.H. STARLING. 1903. The mechanism of pancreatic secretion. J. Physiol. (Lond.) **28**: 174-180.

BERN, H.A., D. PEARSON, B.A. LARSON, and R.S. NISHIOKA. 1985. Neurohormones from Fish Tails - the caudal neurosecretory system. I. "Urophysiology" and the caudal neurosecretory system of fishes. Rec. Prog. Horm. Res. **41**: (in press).

BEVIS, P.J.R., and M.C. THORNDYKE. 1978. Endocrine cells in the oesophagus of the ascidian *Styela clava*, a cytochemical and immunofluorescence study. Cell Tissue Res. **187**: 153-158.

BEVIS, P.J.R., and M.C. THORNDYKE. 1979. A cytochemical and immunofluorescence study of endocrine cells in the gut of the ascidian *Styela clava*. Cell Tissue Res. **199**: 139-144.

BEVIS, P.J.R., and M.C. THORNDYKE. 1981. Stimulation of gastric enzyme secretion by porcine cholecystokinin in the ascidian *Styela clava*. Gen. comp. Endocrinol. **145**: 458-464.

BROCCARDO, M. G. FALCONIERI ERSPAMER, P. MELCHIORRI, and L. NEGRI. 1975. Relative potency of bombesin-like peptides. Br. J. Pharmacol. **55**: 221-227.

DIMALINE, R. 1982. Different distributions of CCK- and caerulein-like peptides in the brain and gut of two amphibians. Regulatory Peptides **4**: 360.

DOCKRAY, G.J. 1974. Extraction of a secretin-like factor from the intestines of pike (*Esox lucius*). Gen. comp. Endocrinol. **23**: 340-347.

DOCKRAY, G.J., and R. DIMALINE. 1984. Evolution of the Gastrin/CCK family. pp. 313-333 *In* Falkmer, S., R. Håkanson, and F. Sundler [eds.] Evolution and tumor pathology of the neuroendocrine system. Elsevier, Amsterdam.

FALKMER, S. 1985. Phylogenetic aspects of the brain gut axis, with special reference to islet hormones in invertebrates and lower vertebrates. pp. 317-325 *In* Kobayashi, H., H.A. Bern and A. Urano [eds.] Neurosecretion and the biology of neuropeptides. Jap. Sci. Soc. Press, Tokyo.

FALKMER, S., and S. VAN NOORDEN. 1983. Ontogeny and phylogeny of the glucagon cell. Handb. exp. Pharmacol. **66**:81-119.

FALKMER, S., J. FAHRENKRUG, J. ALUMETS, R. HÅKANSON, and F. SUNDLER. 1980. Vasoactive intestinal polypeptide (VIP) in epithelial cells of the gut mucosa of an elasmobranchian cartilaginous fish, the ray. Endocrinol. Japon (Suppl.)**27**: 31-35.

FALKMER, S., R.E. CARRAWAY, M. EL-SALHY, S.O. EMDIN, L. GRIMELIUS, J.F. REHFELD, M. REINECKE, and T.F.W. SCHWARTZ. 1981. Phylogeny of the gastro-entero-pancreatic neuroendocrine system. A review with special reference to the occurrence of CCK-like and neurotensin-like polypeptides in lower vertebrates and invertebrates. UCLA Forum Med. Sci. **23**: 21-42.

FALKMER, S., M. EL-SALHY, and M. TITLBACH. 1984. Evolution of the neuroendocrine systems in vertebrates: A review with particular reference to the phylogeny and postnatal maturation of the islet parenchyma. pp. 59-87 *In* Falkmer, S., R. Håkanson, and F. Sundler [eds.] Evolution and tumor pathology of the neuroendocrine system. Elsevier, Amsterdam.

FÄNGE, R. and D.J. GROVE. 1979. Digestion. pp. 161-260 *In* Hoar, W.S., and D.J. Randall [eds.] Fish physiology, vol. VIII. Academic Press, New York.

FOUCHEREAU-PERON, M., M. LABURTHE, J. BESSON, G. ROSSELIN, and Y. LE GAL. 1980. Characterization of the the vasoactive intestinal polypeptide (VIP) in the gut of fishes. Comp. Biochem. Physiol. **64A**: 489-492.

FRITSCH, H.A.R., S. VAN NOORDEN, and A.G.E. PEARSE. 1982. Gastro-intestinal and neurohormonal peptides in the alimentary tract and cerebral complex of *Ciona intestinalis* (Ascidiaceae). Cell Tissue Res. **223**: 369-402.

FURNESS, J.B., and M. COSTA. 1980. Types of nerves in the enteric nervous system. Neuroscience **5**: 1-20.

GROSSMANN, M.I. 1979. Chemical messengers; a view from the gut. Fed. Proc. **38**: 2341-2343.

HIRSCHOWITZ, B.I., and R.G. GIBSON. 1979. Stimulation of gastrin release and gastric secretion: effect of bombesin and a nonapeptide in fistula dogs with and without fundic vagotomy. Digestion **18**: 227-239.

HOLMGREN, S. 1983. The effects of putative non-adrenergic, non-cholinergic autonomic transmitters on isolated strips from the stomach of the rainbow trout, *Salmo gairdneri*. Comp. Biochem. Physiol. **74C**: 229-238.

HOLMGREN, S., and S. NILSSON. 1981. On the non-adrenergic, non-cholinergic innervation of the rainbow trout stomach. Comp. Biochem. Physiol. **70C**: 65-69.

HOLMGREN, S., and S. NILSSON. 1983a. Bombesin-, gastrin/CCK-, 5-hydroxytryptamine-, neurotensin-, somatostatin-, and VIP-like immunoreactivity and catecholamine fluorescence in the gut of the elasmobranch, *Squalus acanthias*. Cell Tissue Res. **234**: 595-618.

HOLMGREN, S., and S. NILSSON. 1983b. Bombesin- and neurotensin-like immunoreactivity in neurons of the holostean fish, *Lepisosteus platyrhincus*. Acta Zool. (Stockh.) **64**: 25-32.

HOLMGREN, S., C. VAILLANT, and R. DIMALINE. 1982. VIP-, substance P-, gastrin/CCK-, bombesin-, somatostatin- and glucagon-like immunoreactivities in the gut of the rainbow trout, *Salmo gairdneri*. Cell Tissue Res. **223**: 141-153.

HOLMQUIST, A.L., G.J. DOCKRAY, G.L. ROSENQUIST, and J.H. WALSH. 1979. Immunochemical characterization of cholecystokinin-like peptides in lamprey gut and brain. Gen. comp. Endocrinol. **37**: 474-481.

HOLSTEIN, B. 1982. Inhibition of gastric acid secretion in the Atlantic cod, *Gadus morhua*, by sulphated and desulphated gastrin, caerulein and CCK-octapeptide. Acta Physiol. Scand. **114**: 453-459.

HOLSTEIN, B. 1983. Effect of vasoactive intestinal polypeptide on gastric acid secretion and mucosal blood flow in the Atlantic cod, *Gadus morhua*. Gen. comp. Endocrinol. **52**: 471-473.

HOLSTEIN, B., and C.S. HUMPHREY. 1980. Stimulation of gastric acid secretion and suppression of VIP-like immunoreactivity by bombesin in the Atlantic codfish, *Gadus morhua*. Acta Physiol. Scand. **109**: 217-223.

ICHIKAWA, T., D. McMASTER, and K. LEDERIS. 1982. Isolation and amino acid sequence of urotensin I, a vasoactive and ACTH-releasing neuropeptide, from the carp (*Cyprinus carpio*) urophysis. Peptides **3**: 859-867.

JORNVALL, H. 1984. Evolutionary principles in peptides and proteins. pp. 165-180 *In* Falkmer, S., R. Hakanson, and F. Sundler [eds.] Evolution and tumor pathology of the neuroendocrine system. Elsevier, Amsterdam.

LACANILAO, F., and H.A. BERN. 1972. The urophysial hydrosmotic factor in fishes. III. Survey of fish caudal spinal cord regions for hydrosmotic activity. Proc. Soc. exp. Biol. Med. **140**: 1252-1253.

LANGER, M., S. VAN NOORDEN, J.M. POLAK, and A.G.E. PEARSE. 1979. Peptide hormone-like immunoreactivity in the gastrointestinal tract and endocrine pancreas of eleven teleost species. Cell Tissue Res. **199**: 493-508.

LARSON, L.-I., and J.F. REHFELD. 1977. Evidence for a common evolutionary origin of gastrin and cholecystokinin. Nature **269**: 335-338.

LARSON, B.A., and S. VIGNA. 1983. Species and tissue distribution of cholecystokinin/gastrin-like substances in some invertebrates. Gen. comp. Endocrinol. **50**: 469-475.

LEDERIS, K., A. LETTER, D. McMASTER, G. MOORE, and D. SCHLESINGER. 1982. Complete amino acid sequence of urotensin I, a hypotensive and corticotrophin-releasing neuropeptide from *Catostomus*. Science **218**: 162-164.

LORETZ, C.A., H.A. BERN, J.K. FOSKETT, and J.R. MAINOYA. 1981. The caudal neurosecretory system and osmoregulation in fish. pp. 319-328 *In* Farner, D.S., and K. Lederis [eds.] Neurosecretion, molecules, cells, systems. Plenum Press, New York.

LUNDIN, K., and S. HOLMGREN. 1984. Vasoactive intestinal polypeptide-like immunoreactivity and effects of VIP in the swim bladder of the cod, *Gadus morhua*. J. comp. Physiol. **154**: 627-633.

MAYER, E.A., J. ELASHOFF, and J.H. WALSH. 1982. Characterization of bombesin effects on canine gastric muscle. Amer. J. Physiol. **243**: G141G-G147.

McDONALD, T.J., H. JORNVALL, G. NILSSON, M. VAGNE, M. GHATEI, S.R. BLOOM, and V. MUTT. 1979. Characterization of a gastrin-releasing peptide from porcine non-antral gastric tissue. Biochem. Biophys. Res. Commun. **90**: 227-233.

MELCHIORRI, P. 1978. Bombesin and bombesin-like peptides of amphibian skin. pp. 534-540 *In* Bloom, S.R., and J.M. Polak [eds.] Gut hormones. Churchill-Livingstone, Edinburgh.

NEGRI, L., and V. ERSPAMER. 1973. Action of caerulein and caerulein-like peptides on "short circuit current" and acid secretion in the isolated gastric mucosa of amphibians. Naunyn-Schmiedebergs Arch. Pharmakol. **277**: 401-412.

NILSSON, A. 1970. Gastrointestinal hormones in the holocephalan fish, *Chimaera monstrosa* (L.). Comp. Biochem. Physiol. **32**: 387-390.

NILSSON, A. 1973. Secretin-like and cholecystokinin-like activity in *Myxine glutinosa* L. Acta Reg. Sci. Gothenburg Zool. **8**: 30-32.

NOTENBOOM, C.D., J.C. GARAUD, J. DOERR-SCHOTT, and M. TERLOU. 1981. Localization by immunofluorescence of a gastrin-like substance in the brain of the Rainbow trout, *Salmo gairdneri*. Cell Tissue Res. **214**: 247-255.

OSTBERG, Y., S. VAN NOORDEN, and A.G.E. PEARSE. 1975. Cytochemical, immunofluorescence and ultrastructural investigations on polypeptide hormone localisation in the islet parenchyma and bile duct mucosa of a cyclostome, *Myxine glutinosa*. Gen. comp. Endocrinol. **25**: 274-291.

PEARSON, D., J.E. SHIVELY, B.R. CLARK, I.I. GESCHWIND, M. BARKLEY, R.S. NISHIOKA, and H.A. BERN. 1980. Urotensin II: a somatostatin-like peptide in the caudal neurosecretory system of fishes. Proc. Natl. Acad. Sci. U.S.A. **77**: 5021-5024.

POLAK, J.M., and S. VAN NOORDEN. 1985. Immunocytochemistry, practical applications in pathology and biology, 2nd ed. John Wright and Sons Ltd., Bristol (in press).

REHFELD, J.F. 1984. Some biochemical and semantic issues in the study of hormone families. pp. 225-230 *In* Falkmer, S., R. Hakanson, and F. Sundler [eds.] Evolution and tumor pathology of the neuroendocrine system. Elsevier, Amsterdam.

REINECKE, M. 1981. Immunohistochemical localization of polypeptide hormones in endocrine cells of the digestive tract of *Branchiostoma lanceolatum*. Cell Tissue Res. **219**: 445-456.

ROMBOUT, J.H.W.M., and J.J. TAVERNE-THIELE. 1982. An immunocytochemical and electron microscopical study of endocrine cells in the gut and pancreas of a stomachless teleost fish, *Barbus conchonius* (Cyprinidae). Cell Tissue Res. **227**: 557-593.

ROSENFELD, M.G., J.J. MERMOD, S.G. AMARA, L.W. SWANSON, P.E. SAWCHENKO, J. RIVIER, W.W. VALE, and R.M. EVANS. 1983. Production of a novel neuropeptide encoded by the calcitonin gene via tissue-specific RNA processing. Nature **304**: 129-135.

RUPPIN, H., and W. DOMSCHKE. 1980. Gastrointestinal hormones and motor function of the gastrointestinal tract. pp. 587-612 *In* Glass, G.B.J. [ed.] Gastrointestinal hormones. Raven Press, New York.

SAID, S.I. 1980. Vasoactive intestinal polypeptide (VIP): Isolation, distribution, biological actions, structure-function relationships and possible functions. pp.

245-273 *In* Glass, G.B.J. [ed.] Gastrointestinal hormones. Raven Press, New York.

SHUTTLEWORTH, T.J., and M.C. THORNDYKE. 1984. An endogenous peptide stimulates secretory activity in the elasmobranch rectal gland. Science **225**: 319-321.

STOFF, J.S., R. ROSA, R. HALLAC, P. SILVA, and F.H. EPSTEIN. 1979. Hormonal regulation of active chloride transport in the dogfish rectal gland. Amer. J. Physiol. **237**: F138-F144.

TATEMOTO, K., and V. MUTT. 1980. Isolation of two new candidate hormones using a chemical method for finding naturally occurring polypeptides. Nature **285**: 417-418.

TATEMOTO, K., and V. MUTT. 1981. Isolation and characterisation of the intestinal peptide porcine PHI (PHI-27), a new member of the glucagon-secretin family. Proc. Natl. Acad. Sci. U.S.A. **78**: 6603-6607.

THORNDYKE, M.C. 1982. Cholecystokinin (CCK) gastrin-like immunoreactive neurones in the cerebral ganglion of the protochordate ascidians *Styela clava* and *Ascidiella aspersa.* Regulatory Peptides **3**: 281-289.

THORNDYKE, M.C. 1985. Immunocytochemistry and evolutionary studies. *In* Polak, J. M. and S. Van Noorden [eds.] Immunocytochemistry, practical applications in pathology and biology, 2nd ed. John Wright and Sons Ltd., Bristol (in press).

THORNDYKE, M.C., and P.J.R. BEVIS. 1985. Peptide systems in protochordates. *In* Lofts, B. [ed.] Proceedings of the ninth international symposium on comparative endocrinology. Hong Kong University Press, Hong Kong (in press).

THORNDYKE, M.C., and S. FALKMER. 1982. Preliminary studies on the effect of bombesin on gastric muscle in the daddy sculpin, *Cottus scorpius.* Regulatory Peptides **4**: 382.

THORNDYKE, M.C., and P.J.R. BEVIS. 1984. Comparative studies on the effects of cholecystokinins, caerulein, bombesin 6-14 nonapeptide, and physalaemin on gastric secretion in the ascidian *Styela clava.* Gen. comp. Endocrinol. **55**: 251-259.

THORNDYKE, M.C., S. HOLMGREN, S. NILSSON, and S. FALKMER. 1984. Bombesin potentiation of the acetylcholine response in isolated strips of fish stomach. Regulatory Peptides **9**: 350.

THORNDYKE, M.C., and S. HOLMGREN. 1985. Bombesin potentiates the effect of acetylcholine on isolated strips of fish stomach. (in preparation).

THORNDYKE, M.C., and T.J. SHUTTLEWORTH. 1985. Biochemistry and physiology of peptides from the elasmobranch gut. Peptides (in press).

VAN NOORDEN, S. 1984. The neuroendocrine system in prostomian and deuterostomian invertebrates and lower vertebrates. pp. 7-38 *In* Falkmer, S., R. Håkanson, and F. Sundler [eds.] Evolution and tumor pathology of the neuroendocrine system. Elsevier, Amsterdam.

VAN NOORDEN, S., and A.G.E. PEARSE. 1974. Immunoreactive polypeptide hormones in the pancreas and gut of the lamprey. Gen. comp. Endocrinol. **23**: 311-324.

VAN NOORDEN, S., and A.G.E. PEARSE. 1976. The localisation of immunoreactivity to insulin, glucagon and gastrin in the gut of *Amphioxus (Branchiostoma) lanceolatus.* pp. 163-178 *In* Grillo, T.A.I., L. Liebson, and A. Epple [eds.] The evolution of pancreatic islets. Pergamon Press, Oxford.

VAN NOORDEN, S., and S. FALKMER. 1980. Gut-islet endocrinology - some evolutionary aspects. Invest. Cell Pathol. **3**: 21-35.
VAN NOORDEN, S. J. GREENBERG, and A.G.E. PEARSE. 1971. Cytochemical and immunofluorescence investigations on polypeptide hormone. Gen. comp. Endocrinol. **19**: 192-199.
VIGNA, S.R. 1979. Distinction between cholecystokinin-like and gastrin-like biological activities extracted from gastro-intestinal tissue of some lower vertebrates. Gen. comp. Endocrinol. **29**: 512-520.

FUNCTIONAL EVOLUTION OF GASTROINTESTINAL HORMONES

Steven R. Vigna

UCLA School of Medicine
Center for Ulcer Research and Education
Veterans Administration Medical Center, Los Angeles, CA

Introduction

The gastrointestinal tracts of vertebrates are useful systems in which to study the functional evolution of chemical regulatory systems because they provide a rich substrate of anatomical and physiological variability upon which selection pressures may act. The physiological problem of acquiring food and rendering it usable by incorporating it into the body of the organism is fundamental to all forms of life. Food is not available for nutrition until it has been absorbed across the wall of the intestine and enters the circulatory system. Topographically, food in the intestinal lumen is outside of the body. Vertebrates, including primitive fishes, have evolved systems for ensuring that ingested foods are processed efficiently in the various regions of the gut so that they are available at the appropriate times, in the appropriate gut segments, and in the appropriate chemical and physical forms to be absorbed and serve as the nutrients required for supporting the metabolic and behavioral activities of the organism.

Gastrointestinal hormones play important roles in regulating this chemical traffic in the vertebrate digestive tract. The aim of this communication is to describe the evidence suggesting roles for gastrointestinal hormones in the evolution of digestive mechanisms in vertebrates with primary focus on how the functions of these hormones changed during phylogeny.

New target organs -- old hormones

One phenomenon that seems to have occurred in the functional evolution of the gastrointestinal endocrine system is the "recruitment" of new target organs for pre-existing or old hormones. For example, the intestinal hormone cholecystokinin (CCK) appears to have been involved with stimulation of digestive enzyme secretion for a very long time in animals, at least from the level of protochordates through vertebrates, but only later in phylogeny to have become a stimulant of gallbladder contraction (Vigna, 1983; see also chapter by Thorndyke and Falkmer). In this case, the "old" hormone, CCK, somehow cultivated a new target organ, the gallbladder, and this seems to have occurred sometime after the first appearance of the gallbladder as a distinct abdominal organ because the gallbladder of an agnathan, the hagfish *Eptatretus stouti*, is insensitive to mammalian CCK (Vigna and Gorbman, 1979). Other interpretations of the apparent lack of CCK stimulation of the hagfish gallbladder are also possible. For example, it may be that the hagfish gallbladder has secondarily lost its responsiveness to CCK. Also, it remains possible that the endogenous hagfish CCK (Vigna, 1979) can stimulate the hagfish gallbladder whereas mammalian CCK cannot; that is, that there is marked species specificity in the actions of various CCKs. This possibility seems remote for two reasons. First, the biological activity of CCK resides in a C-terminal pentapeptide fragment of the molecule which is highly conserved in evolution (Crim and Vigna, 1983) and therefore probably is present in the hagfish CCK molecule in much the same form as it is in mammalian CCK. Second, mammalian CCK is capable of stimulating digestive enzyme secretion from the hagfish intestine (Vigna and Gorbman, 1979) and thus that lack of effect of CCK on the gallbladder is unlikely to be due to marked differences in the properties of hagfish *versus* mammalian CCK receptors.

Another example of the apparent recruitment of new gut target organs by gastrointestinal hormones in evolution is the control of the stomach by CCK. We have seen that CCK is associated with control of intestinal and pancreatic digestive enzyme secretion in all vertebrates and the few protochordates examined (Vigna, 1983). However, the stomach evolved in vertebrates apparently in the lineage leading to gnathostomes after their divergence from the Agnatha (Barrington, 1942). Thus, the postulated recruitment of the stomach as a target organ for CCK in vertebrate evolution (Vigna, 1983) represents another example of the opportunism exhibited by "old" hormones when new organs evolve. Whether or not this phenomenon will prove to be of general importance in the evolution of physiological control systems will require extensive documentation in a variety of different systems. However, it is an attractive working hypothesis because it is parsimonious -- it is easier to imagine that pre-existing hormones develop new target organs than to postulate that newly evolving physiological systems require the appearance *de novo* of new regulatory mechanisms to govern their activities.

New cellular sources -- old hormones

Another potential mechanism for generating new functions in regulatory systems is the development of new cellular sources of old hormones. This phenomenon could occur in any of several different forms. For example, a pre-existing hormone could begin to be expressed by an endocrine cell in a new tissue or organ, resulting in regulation of new physiological functions. This mechanism would be difficult to distinguish from migration of "old" endocrine cells to new tissue locations during ontogenesis. A good example illustrating these possibilities is the evolution of the vertebrate endocrine pancreas (see chapter by Thorndyke and Falkmer). All four hormones of the vertebrate endocrine pancreas originate from intestinal endocrine cells in protochordates. In the higher vertebrates, three of these hormones can be found in intestinal as well as pancreatic endocrine cells; only insulin is strictly of pancreatic origin. Did this pattern arise by differential migration during embryogenesis of insulin *versus* other pancreatic endocrine cell types, or did entirely new cell types evolve with the ability to express these peptide hormones? Current evidence is not sufficient to distinguish between these two possible mechanisms.

Another example of new cellular origins for old hormones is the apparent evolution of the sources of vasoactive intestinal peptide (VIP) and bombesin from endocrine cells in lower vertebrates to strictly neurons in mammals (Reinecke *et al.*, 1981; Dockray *et al.*, 1979). Unfortunately, the physiological roles of these substances in lower vertebrates, and even in mammals, are not well-defined and so it is not possible yet to ascertain if this evolution from an endocrine to an apparent neurotransmitter mode of action is related to changes in function for these two regulatory peptides.

Recent studies of the cellular origins and biological actions of CCK, gastrin, and bombesin in lower vertebrates have revealed another possible example of the role that evolution of new cellular origins for old hormones has played in changing physiological function. In mammals, the primary control over gastric acid secretion is exerted by the stomach hormone, gastrin, but many other regulatory substances also are involved; these factors act *via* endocrine, neurocrine, and paracrine routes (Soll and Grossman, 1978). In particular, bombesin-like peptides (the mammalian analogues of bombesin are called gastrin-releasing peptides or GRP) can also stimulate gastric acid secretion in mammals, probably through a neurocrine mechanism or mechanisms. However, recent elegant studies by Holstein have demonstrated that gastrin and its close chemical and biological homologue, CCK, inhibit (Holstein, 1982), whereas bombesin stimulates (Holstein and Humphrey, 1980) acid secretion from the bony fish stomach. Can we trace the pattern of evolution of control of gastric acid secretion from bony fishes to mammals?

Figure 1 illustrates the known relationships among the cellular origins of CCK, bombesin, and the acid-secreting oxyntic cell in the bony fish stomach, as well as the effects of the two peptides on acid secretion. Bony fish represent a stage in vertebrate phylogeny before the first appearance of a separate gastrin-like peptide from an ancestral CCK (see below). Also, CCK cells are found only in the intestinal epithelium (Holmgren *et al.*, 1982; Vigna *et al.*, in press) and not the gastric antrum of bony fish, although this conclusion is somewhat controversial (Larsson and Rehfeld, 1977). The weight of the currently available evidence, then, suggests that the primary stimulatory control over gastric acid secretion in bony fish is exerted by blood-born bombesin secreted by endocrine cells in the antrum of the stomach and that when food passes from the stomach to the intestine, CCK is secreted from intestinal endocrine cells and acts to inhibit further gastric acid secretion.

A somewhat different scenario can be constructed for the situation in Amphibia (Fig. 2). First of all, the bombesin cells in the frog stomach are not typical endocrine cells because they do not span the epithelium from basal lamina to lumen and do not extend microvilli into the gut lumen (characteristics of so-called open endocrine cells) as did the bombesin cells in the bony fish gastric antrum. Instead, bombesin cells in the frog gastric epithelium are found in both the antrum and the

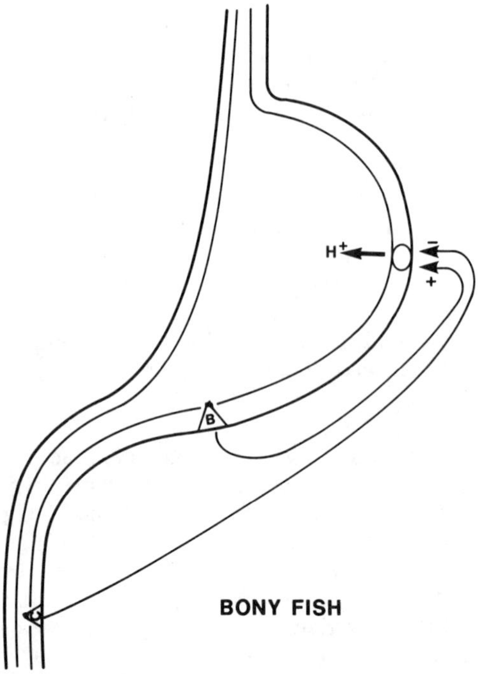

Fig. 1. Diagrammatic representation of the relationships among CCK- (*C*), bombesin- (*B*), and acid-secreting oxyntic cells in the gut of bony fishes. The oxyntic cells are in the oxyntic gland region of the stomach, the bombesin cells are in the antral region of the stomach, and the CCK cells are in the small intestine. Both CCK and bombesin are secreted by open endocrine cells, depicted as extending the full width of the epithelium and projecting microvilli into the gut lumen. Both CCK and bombesin are transported in the blood to the oxyntic cells; however, bombesin stimulates and CCK inhibits acid secretion.

oxyntic epithelium and seem to consist of so-called closed cells; that is, cells which rest on the basal lamina of the epithelium but do not extend to the lumen (Lechago *et al.*, 1978; Lechago *et al.*, 1981). Also, CCK-like peptides and cells are present in the gastric antrum as well as in the intestine (Larsson and Rehfeld, 1977). Finally, unlike the situation in bony fishes, CCK-like peptides stimulate acid secretion in frogs (Negri and Erspamer, 1973). Recent studies have suggested both a direct and a possible indirect role for bombesin in control of amphibian gastric acid secretion. Ayalon *et al.* (1981) have demonstrated that bombesin can directly stimulate the acid-secreting oxyntic cell in the frog stomach, suggesting that the bombesin-containing closed endocrine cells in the oxyntic epithelium release bombesin which diffuses to the oxyntic cells *via* a paracrine mechanism. Similarly, we have shown (Vigna, unpublished studies) that bombesin can stimulate the release of CCK-like peptides from the frog gastric antrum, presumably by a paracrine mechanism.

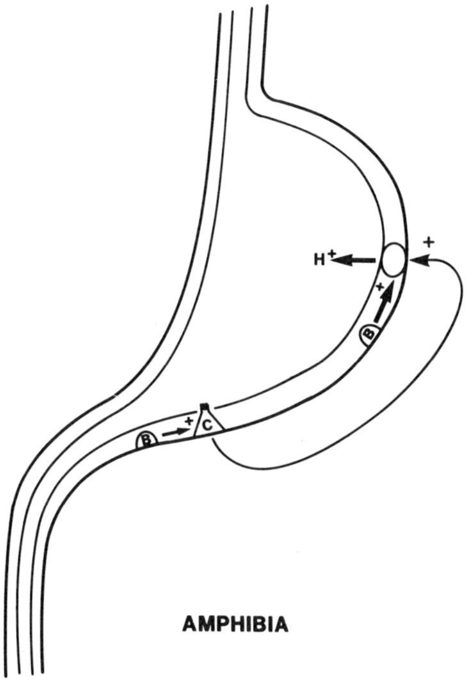

Fig 2. Diagrammatic representation of the relationships among CCK-, bombesin-, and acid-secreting oxyntic cells in the gut of amphibia. In amphibia, CCK cells are found in the antral region of the stomach as well as in the small intestine (not shown) and CCK stimulates acid secretion. Bombesin originates in closed endocrine cell types (depicted as cells lying on the basal lamina of the gastric epithelium but not extending to the gastric lumen) in the oxyntic as well as antral region of the stomach. CCK stimulates acid secretion via an endocrine mechanism, whereas bombesin stimulates acid secretion by two different paracrine mechanisms: an indirect effect via stimulation of CCK secretion and a direct effect on oxyntic cells. Symbols and conventions are described in the Fig. 1 legend.

Thus, bombesin is involved in the stimulation of gastric acid secretion in bony fish and Amphibia, but the cellular source of the peptide and its route of delivery is quite different in the two groups. It has a direct effect in both fish and Amphibia, but its direct effect is *via* a blood-born endocrine mechanism in fish *versus* an interstitial fluid-born paracrine mechanism in frogs. Superimposed on this, bombesin also has an indirect paracrine effect in frogs which appears to be lacking in fish.

Much the same pattern is seen in birds (and probably reptiles, although there is little experimental data available for reptiles) as was found in Amphibia (Fig. 3). The major difference is that CCK cells have been replaced in the antrum by gastrin

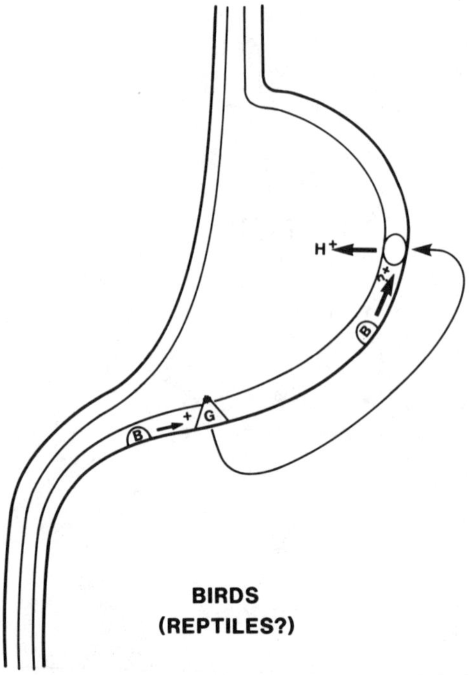

Fig. 3. Diagrammatic representation of the relationships among gastrin- (*G*), bombesin-, and acid-secreting bombesin cells in the gut of birds and possibly reptiles. In birds and reptiles, gastrin cells have replaced CCK cells in the gastric antrum. As in amphibia, bombesin originates in closed endocrine cell types in the oxyntic and antral regions of the gastric epithelium. Gastrin stimulates acid secretion via an endocrine mechanism. Bombesin stimulates acid secretion indirectly via a paracrine stimulation of gastrin secretion; whether the bombesin cells in the oxyntic mucosa also directly stimulate oxyntic cells is unknown. Symbols and conventions are as described in the Fig. 1 legend.

endocrine cells of the open type. This is accompanied by the replacement of CCK by gastrin as the major stimulatory endocrine substance regulating gastric acid secretion (see below). As was the case in Amphibia, the bombesin-containing cells in the avian oxyntic stomach (the proventriculus) are of the closed type (Vaillant *et al.*, 1979; Erspamer *et al.*, 1979) and thus presumably act *via* a paracrine mechanism. Linari *et al.* (1975) have shown that bombesin stimulates gastric acid secretion in chickens, but it is not yet known if endogenous bombesin-like peptides act *via* direct or indirect routes, or possibly both pathways in birds.

Figure 4 summarizes the relationships among bombesin, gastrin, and oxyntic cells in the mammalian stomach. The major difference between the mammalian and avian arrangement is that there appears to be no bombesin-containing endocrine

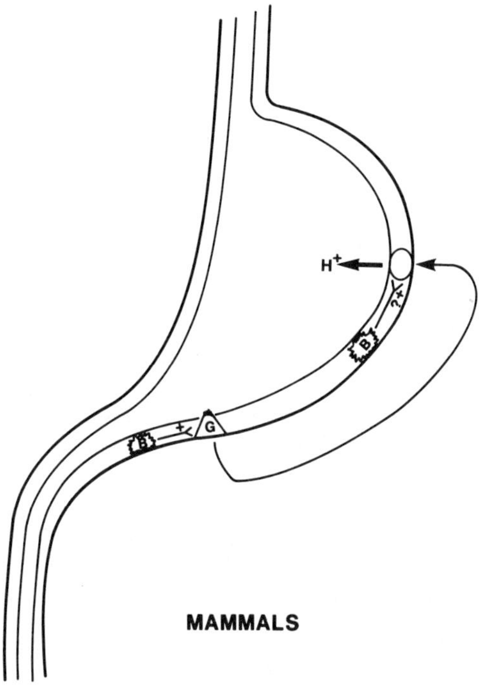

Fig. 4. Diagrammatic representation of the relationships among gastrin-, bombesin-, and acid-secreting oxyntic cells in the gut of mammals. In mammals, bombesin is present only in neurons in the wall of the stomach (depicted as stellate cells with a projecting nerve fiber). Gastrin stimulates acid secretion via an endocrine mechanism as it does in birds. Bombesin stimulates acid secretion indirectly via a neurocrine stimulation of gastrin secretion; whether the bombesin-containing neurons in the oxyntic mucosa also directly stimulate oxyntic cells in unknown. The bombesin neuronal cell bodies are depicted in the gastric epithelium for diagrammatic purposes only; their actual location is unknown. Symbols and conventions are as described in the Fig. 1 legend.

or paracrine cells of the open or closed type in the mammalian gastric mucosa. Instead, only bombesinergic nerve fibers are found (Dockray *et al.*, 1979). Bombesin retains the ability to stimulate acid secretion in mammals indirectly *via* a direct stimulatory action on antral gastrin (Varner *et al.*, 1981; Schubert *et al.*, 1985); this effect, however, is a neurocrine action in mammals in contrast to the paracrine action seen in Amphibia and birds. Whether or not the bombesinergic nerve fibers seen in the mammalian oxyntic mucosa directly stimulate acid secretion similarly to the direct paracrine stimulation of amphibian oxyntic cells remains to be determined.

What we have seen, then, in this proposed scenario for the evolution of the control of gastric acid secretion in vertebrates, is one constant: a stimulatory role for bombesin. Cholecystokinin appears to be inhibitory in bony fish and originates from the intestine, not the antrum; gastrin replaces antral CCK in amniotes as a primary effector. Even bombesin, however, displays changing cell types of origin while apparently retaining a role in stimulating acid secretion. If bombesin is an important regulator of gastric acid secretion as a blood-born hormone in bony fishes, what is gained by exerting the same control as a locally diffusible paracrine agent in Amphibia and birds and as a neurotransmitter in mammals? The overall pattern discernable here for bombesinergic control is evolution toward ever more precise delivery of the peptide to the target cell -- both in anatomical and temporal terms. It is clear that bombesin has a very large repertory of biological activities in vertebrates, including effects on thermoregulation, pituitary hormone secretion, food and water intake, and gastrointestinal (endocrine and exocrine) secretion and motility (Walsh, 1983). It is possible that as the regulatory repertoire of bombesin increased in evolution, selection pressure also increased for localized delivery in space and time of the peptide to its target cells in order not to interfere with other effects of the peptide that may have been nonadaptive if they occurred simultaneously or in close proximity. Viewed in this way, the changing cellular sources of an old hormone, bombesin, may be seen as contributing to the functional evolution of gastrointestinal hormones by resulting in an increase in the diversity of regulatory effects of the peptide. Whether similar arguments can be made for other systems, such as VIP for example, await the accumulation of more experimental data.

Old target organs -- new hormones

The stomach hormone, gastrin, appears to have evolved from a CCK-like ancestral peptide at the level of the divergence of the reptilian from the amphibian lineages during vertebrate phylogeny (Larsson and Rehfeld, 1977). We have just seen that CCK and gastrin are involved in control of gastric acid secretion in vertebrates from bony fishes through mammals. From the level of Amphibia through mammals, either CCK or gastrin is used as the primary endocrine stimulant of gastric acid secretion. Why then should gastrin have replaced CCK as the antral hormone of physiological importance in controlling gastric acid secretion? A case can be made that this phenomenon is highly adaptive in increasing the efficiency of digestion by precisely separating the gastric from the intestinal phases of digestion. It seems clear that gut CCK arose first as an intestinal peptide involved in the regulation of important components of the intestinal portion of digesting a normal meal. Subsequently, CCK endocrine cells appeared in the gastric antral epithelium but did not give up their place in the intestinal epithelium. Thus, CCK endocrine cells were now exposed to ingested food in both the stomach and the intestine. Clearly, if CCK is secreted when food is present in the stomach as well as the intestine, it would be impossible for CCK to separately regulate the gastric and intestinal phases of digestion. Therefore, it seems likely that the replacement of antral CCK cells by gastrin cells in the amniotes was highly adaptive and probably resulted in some increase in the efficiency of digestion. It certainly seems reasonable to argue that increased efficiency of digestion results in the availability of increased energy sources to the individual; increased ability to assimilate energy in turn must have been required to support the higher metabolic demands associated with the evolution of endothermy (Karasov and Diamond, 1985).

Whether or not the evolution of new hormones has played a wider role in the functional evolution of the gut is not known. It certainly seems likely because the gastrointestinal endocrine system consists of several extended molecular families of peptide hormones. This also applies to the enteric nervous system. Examples of such molecular families are the separate CCK, secretin, and tachykinin families. There have been few studies of the parent-offspring relationships among these or other molecular families that would contribute to such an analysis.

Old target organs -- new hormone receptors

Another example of a mechanism for evolution of function in the gastrointestinal endocrine system is the appearance of new hormone receptors on old target cells. In the example above, of the evolution of gastrin from CCK, we may ask what kind of receptors this new hormone, gastrin, was able to interact with on, say, the acid-secreting oxyntic cells of primitive reptiles? If gastrin acted on the same receptor that CCK did previously, then no increase in digestive efficiency would be gained because CCK could obviously continue to act on this receptor as well. New receptors must evolve for interaction with new hormones. The temporal relationship of appearance of new hormones and their receptors has been discussed elsewhere (Vigna, Amer. Zool., in press).

In recent studies, we have shown that there are differences in the properties of brain and pancreas CCK receptors among vertebrates (Vigna, Thorndyke and Williams, unpubl. manuscript). In birds and mammals, the pancreatic CCK receptor exhibits great specificity, in terms of high affinity interaction, for sulfated forms of CCK. The brain CCK receptor in birds and mammals, on the other hand, interacts nearly equally well with all forms of CCK and gastrin, whether sulfated or unsulfated. Quite a different pattern emerged when we examined the brain and pancreas CCK receptors in the ectothermic vertebrates. In particular, we found evidence for only one pattern of binding specificity for CCKs and gastrins in both the brain and pancreas CCK receptors. This binding site bound gastrins and CCKs nearly equally well if they were sulfated. Unsulfated forms of CCK and gastrin were only weak ligands.

From these data we constructed a proposed model for the evolution of the brain and pancreas CCK receptor in vertebrates (Fig. 5). It seems likely that the ectothermic receptor is primitive and gave rise to the bird and mammal type of pancreatic receptor by developing specificity for a sulfate group found in the position invariant in all known CCK molecules - 7 amino acid positions from the C-terminus. The bird and mammal type of brain CCK receptor could also be derived from the hypothetical ancestral receptor by losing completely any requirement for sulfation at all, rendering all forms of CCK and gastrin nearly equipotent at this binding site.

What would these changes gain for the organism in terms of physiological adaptiveness? It seems likely that this mechanism could account for the appearance

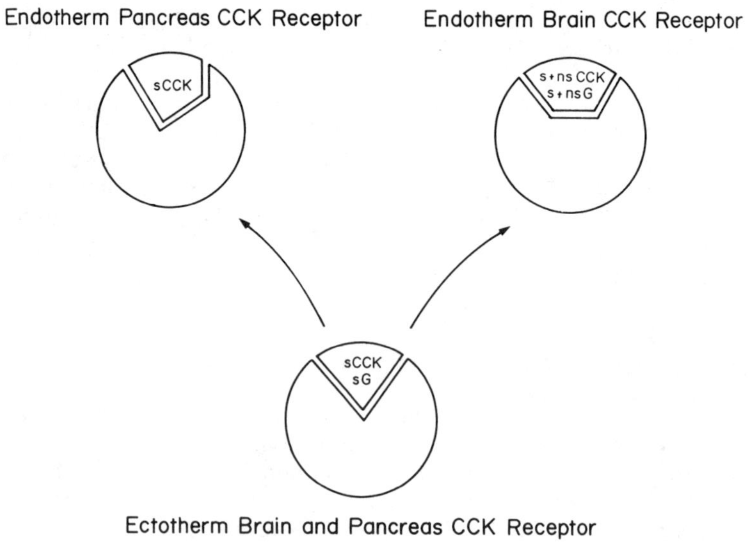

Fig. 5. Proposed model for the evolution of the endotherm brain and pancreas CCK receptors from a common ancestral receptor type found in ectotherms. The receptor in the ectotherm brain and pancreas interacts with high affinity only with sulfated forms of CCK (*sCCK*) and gastrin (*sG*). The endotherm pancreas receptor retains specificity for sulfated ligands, but only interacts with high affinity with sulfated CCKs. In contrast, the endotherm brain CCK receptor has apparently lost its specificity for sulfated ligands because it interacts nearly equally well with sulfated and nonsulfated CCKs (*s + nsCCK*) and sulfated and nonsulfated gastrins (*s + nsG*).

of new hormone receptors and thus allow newly evolved hormones, like gastrin, to act independently from their ancestral, but nevertheless still present, peptides. For example, the ectothermic CCK receptor cannot distinguish sulfated CCKs from sulfated gastrins and thus cells containing this binding site could not be regulated by one but not the other type of peptide. In the endotherms, conversely, the pancreas is highly efficient in interacting with CCK and not gastrin by virtue of the specificity of its receptor, whereas the brain receptor in endotherms should be able to interact with both CCKs and gastrins. Thus, the endotherm brain cells but not pancreatic acinar cells should be susceptible to the action of gastrin, whereas the pancreatic acinar cells can only be regulated by CCK *via* this receptor.

Conclusions

Gastrointestinal hormones and their actions provide a rich substrate of experimental material for studies of the functional evolution of physiological systems. Our understanding of the functional evolution of the gastrointestinal endocrine system is at a rudimentary level. However, several distinct phenomena giving rise to functional evolution in the endocrine system of the gut can be identified, such as recruitment of new target organs, changes in the cellular sources of the hormones, and appearance of new hormones and their receptors. It seems likely that these phenomena and others yet to be described have played an important role in the success of vertebrates. The technical tools and the theoretical framework necessary to pose meaningful and answerable questions in this field are at hand. Further progress requires studies of the properties of endogenous peptides, their receptors, their cells of origin, and their target cells in a wide variety of phylogenetically important species.

Acknowledgements

Unpublished studies described in this paper were supported by National Science Foundation grant number DCB-8542227

Literature cited

AYALON, A., R. YAZIGI, P.G. DEVITT, and P.L. RAYFORD. 1981. Direct effect of bombesin on isolated gastric mucosa. Biochem. Biophys. Res. Comm. **4**: 1390-1397.

BARRINGTON, E.J.W. 1942. Gastric digestion in the lower vertebrates. Biol. Rev. **14**: 1-27.

CRIM, J.W., and S.R. VIGNA. 1983. Brain, gut and skin peptide hormones in lower vertebrates. Amer. Zool. **23**: 621-638.

DOCKRAY, G.J., C. VAILLANT, and J.H. WALSH. 1979. The neuronal origin of bombesin-like immunoreactivity in the rat gastrointestinal tract. Neuroscience **4**: 1561-1568.

ERSPAMER, V., G. FALCONIERI ERSPAMER, P. MELCHIORRI, and L. NEGRI. 1979. Occurrence and polymorphism of bombesin-like peptides in the gastrointestinal tract of birds and mammals. Gut **20**: 1047-1056.

HOLMGREN, S., C. VAILLANT, and R. DIMALINE. 1982. VIP-, substance P-, gastrin/CCK-, bombesin-, somatostatin- and glucagon-like immunoreactivities in the gut of the rainbow trout, *Salmo gairdneri*. Cell Tissue Res. **223**: 141-153.

HOLSTEIN, B. 1982. Inhibition of gastric acid secretion in the Atlantic cod, *Gadus morhua*, by sulphated and desulphated gastrin, caerulein, and CCK-octapeptide. Acta physiol. scand. **114**: 455-461.

HOLSTEIN, B., and C.S. HUMPHREY. 1980. Stimulation of gastric acid secretion and suppression of VIP-like immunoreactivity by bombesin in the Atlantic codfish, *Gadus morhua*. Acta physiol. scand. **109**: 217-223.

KARASOV, W.H., and J.M. DIAMOND. 1985. Digestive adaptations for fueling the cost of endothermy. Science **228**: 202-204.

LARSSON, L.-I., and J.F. REHFELD. 1977. Evidence for a common evolutionary origin of gastrin and cholecystokinin. Nature **269**: 335-338.

LECHAGO, J., B.G. CRAWFORD, and J.H. WALSH. 1981. Bombesin(like)-containing cells in bullfrog gastric mucosa: immunoelectronmicroscopic characterization. Gen. comp. Endocrinol. **45**: 1-6.

LECHAGO, J., A.L. HOLMQUIST, G.L. ROSENQUIST, and J.H. WALSH. 1978. Localization of bombesin-like peptides in frog gastric mucosa. Gen. comp. Endocrinol. **36**: 553-558.

LINARI, G., M. BALDIERI, and L. ANGELUCCI. 1975. The action of bombesin on gastric secretion of the chicken. Eur. J. Pharmacol. **34**: 143-150.

NEGRI, L. and V. ERSPAMER. 1973. Action of caerulein and caerulein-like peptides on "short circuit current" and acid secretion in the isolated gastric mucosa of amphibians. Naunyn-Schmiedebergs Arch. Pharmakol. **227**: 401-412.

REINECKE, M., P. SCHULTER, N. YANAIHARA, and W.G. FORSSMANN. 1981. VIP immunoreactivity in enteric nerves and endocrine cells of the vertebrate gut. Peptides **2**(suppl. 2): 149-156.

SCHUBERT, M., B. SAFFOURI, J.H. WALSH, and G. MAKHLOUF. 1985. Inhibition of neurally-mediated gastrin secretion by bombesin antiserum. Amer. J. Physiol. **248**: G456-G462.

SOLL, A.H., and M.I. GROSSMAN. 1978. Cellular mechanisms in acid secretion. Ann. Rev. Med. **29**: 495-507.

VAILLANT, C., G.J. DOCKRAY, and J.H. WALSH. 1979. The avian proventriculus is an abundant source of endocrine cells with bombesin-like immunoreactivity. Histochemistry **64**: 307-314.

VARNER, A., I. MODLIN, and J.H. WALSH. 1981. High potency of bombesin for stimulation of human gastrin release and gastric acid secretion. Regul. Peptides **1**: 289-296.

VIGNA, S.R. 1979. Distinction between cholecystokinin-like and gastrin-like biological activities extracted from gastrointestinal tissues of some lower vertebrates. Gen. comp. Endocrinol. **39**: 512-520.

VIGNA, S.R. 1983. Evolution of endocrine regulation of gastrointestinal function in lower vertebrates. Amer. Zool. **23**: 729-738.

VIGNA, S.R., and A. GORBMAN. 1979. Stimulation of intestinal lipase secretion by porcine cholecystokinin in the hagfish, *Eptatretus stouti*. Gen. comp. Endocrinol. **38**: 356-359.

WALSH, J.H. 1983. Bombesin-like peptides. pp. 941-960 *In* Krieger, D., M. Brownstein, and J. Martin [eds.] Brain peptides. John Wiley & Sons, New York.

HORMONAL PEPTIDE EVOLUTION*

Yves-Alain Fontaine

Laboratoire de Physiologie générale et comparée du Muséum national d'Histoire naturelle; Laboratoire d'Endocrinologie comparée associé au C.N.R.S., Paris, France

Hormonal function is made possible for a naturally-circulating peptide by the existence in given cells (target cells) of receptors for this molecule. Receptors for peptides are generally located on the cell membrane; they are probably peptidic structures which specifically bind the hormone. The receptors then undergo changes which, in turn, induce modifications of cell activity. In the course of evolution, such situations may have arisen when a "fit" occurred between adequate secretory proteins and cell regulatory membrane proteins. Then this primitive hormonal function evolved further, by changes at the level of both the hormone and the receptor, reflecting changes in the structure and expression of the genome. Precise description and understanding of these events are quite difficult for several reasons. The main obstacle to the rebuilding of this past history is that only the study of endocrinology of presently living animals is within reach. In order to surmount this difficulty, one tries to infer the properties and the succession of ancestors by considering today's animals in order of their evolutionary appearance (*e.g.* lampreys, then teleosts, amphibians and finally mammals). This is indeed a very suspect approach because modern animals are generally quite different from their corresponding primitive ancestors. "Old" taxa, like lampreys, have undergone a long evolution, and they may exhibit recent or young characters which should not be mistaken for ancestral characters. Another difficulty lies in the scatter of the experimental data in view of the number of species and hormones to be considered. Finally, the definitive responses to the basic questions will probably depend on concepts and data from comparative molecular genetics, which are just emerging.

---

* The expression "hormonal peptide" will be used in a broad sense. We will consider here polypeptides, proteins, glycoproteins as well as small peptides. Also, it will be seen that comparative studies make very indistinct the boundary between hormones and paracrine substances acting locally, such as neurotransmitters.

In view of these difficulties it is not surprising that this paper is highly hypothetical and incomplete. Rather than review all available data on fish peptide hormones, I shall try to illustrate some possible patterns and mechanisms of the evolution of hormonal peptides. Three topics will be developed, namely molecular evolution, the strategies of functional evolution and some aspects of these phenomena in fish. I shall limit myself to certain groups of peptides, especially pituitary hormones (but not opiomelanocortins), some central nervous system peptides which may be involved in pituitary control, and calcium-regulating hormones. The large group of gastro-entero-pancreatic peptides is dealt with in other chapters of this book. Finally, there will be no reference to the ontogeny of hormonal function, though this would certainly be of interest.

Hormonal peptide families: the search for phylogenetic trees and ancestral molecules

General aspects of peptide molecular evolution

Amino acid sequences of a number of hormonal (mainly mammalian) peptides have been determined in the last 15 years. It has been shown that analogous hormones (*i.e.* endowed with a similar biological activity) from various species are different, but generally homologous (*i.e.* their sequences exhibited important similarities). Surprisingly, an important homology sometimes also was demonstrated between hormones which are not analogous. Such data led to the concept of families of homologous peptides, each of these families containing molecules derived from a presumptive ancestral molecule (*i.e.* coded by genes deriving from a same ancestral gene.) Moreover, when several of these homologous peptides are found in the same animal (*e.g.* LH, FSH and TSH*) one is led to assume that their past history included gene duplication(s).

Homologous peptides may be orthologous or paralogous (Wilson *et al.*, 1977). They are orthologous if they diverged at the same time that the species did (for instance, bovine and porcine GH's). They are paralogous when this condition is not fulfilled (for instance, bovine TSH and porcine LH diverged long before the separation of the two species, as we shall see later).

In order to illustrate more precisely the historical relationship between homologous peptides, a number of authors have constructed phylogenetic trees, based on mathematical comparisons of sequences. Let us consider the simplest example of two homologous peptides. The first step is to calculate the phylogenetic distance between them, *i.e.* the number of accepted mutations (in percent of the total number of amino acids). Even at this stage, choices have to be made: are all the substitutions equivalent? How does one treat deletions? Also, is it clear that calculated values are minimal estimations of the distances? Most importantly, this method implies that point mutations are the dominant mechanisms of evolution, although it appears more and more probable that other mechanisms such as unequal crossover, DNA transposition and reverse transcription may play important roles (Miller and Eberhardt, 1983).

---

* Key to abbreviations is located at the end of the text.

The second step is to determine the time of the node at which the two lineages leading to the present peptides diverged. Authors arbitrarily use a point equally distant between the two known sequences, at least "in the absence of any evidence to the contrary" (Dayhoff *et al.*, 1972). The same is done for duplications when such events have to be inserted. The final, more or less explicit, goal is to introduce a time scale in these trees. This is first done by calculating an absolute evolutionary rate between two relatively recent groups (generally mammalian orders) for which the fossil record precisely indicates the separation time (as pointed out by Wilson *et al.* 1977, such calculations of absolute evolutionary rates must be made by comparing orthologous sequences only; this represents a new limitation because orthology is often assumed rather than proven). Then, the authors extrapolate the evolutionary rate onto the entire tree and calculate the *minimal* durations of the branchings, as well as the *earliest* time of divergences and/or duplications. This extrapolation is based on the concept of the evolutionary clock, according to which the evolutionary rate appears to be constant for a given type of protein. The reality of the evolutionary clock was demonstrated for several proteins such as albumin in frogs and mammals (see Wilson *et al.*, 1977). However, one can wonder how absolute it is, and especially to what degree it applies to peptides, such as hormones, which are under strong functional constraints.

Given all the assumptions which have been listed, it should be clear that a calculated phylogenetic tree is only one of very many possible configurations, and that it must undergo important changes as new data and concepts become available. Indeed, one role of these trees is to raise questions, particularly when they are confronted with other kinds of evidence.

Trees for three hormonal peptide families

The glycoprotein pituitary hormones, GTHs and TSHs are composed of two subunits; α and ß; the α subunits are identical and the different ß subunits are homologous (references in Fontaine, 1980). A phylogenetic tree of these ß subunits was constructed by Hunt and Dayhoff (1976) on the basis of a few mammalian sequences (Fig. 1A). From the common ancestral molecular lineage, first the TSH structure and then (50-100 million years later) the FSH structure would have diverged. This general pattern is in agreement with our hypothesis that TSH and only one GTH exist in fishes (Fig. 1B, Fontaine, 1980a). However, there are striking problems as far as time is concerned. Hunt and Dayhoff (1976) had to assume that LH is experiencing mutations at almost four times the rate of TSH, in obvious contradiction to the evolutionary clock; this made the position of the first duplication even more empirical than usual. As far as lower vertebrates are concerned, only a partial sequence of carp GTH ß is available (Jolles *et al.*, 1977). For this portion of the molecule, the distance relative to bLH is only roughly two times greater than the distance between bLH and hLH, which does not appear consistent with an evolutionary clock.

Such discrepancies were observed and discussed in greater detail in the case of two other homologous pituitary hormones, GH and PRL. A first tree was elaborated by Hunt and Dayhoff (1976) which indicated a divergence of the two

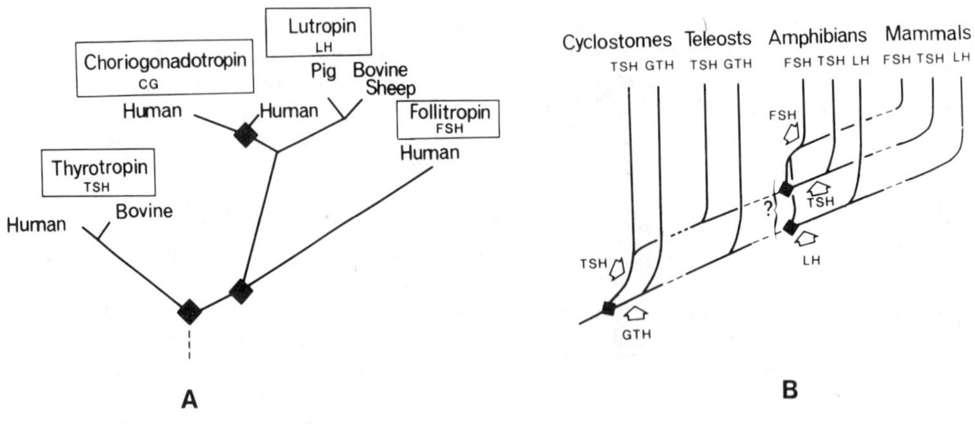

Fig. 1. Two different expressions of the phylogenetic relationship within the gonadotropin-thyrotropin family. A. "Molecular" phylogenetic tree of the ß subunits established by Hunt and Dayoff (1976) on the basis of sequence comparison; black squares indicate duplications. "The point of earliest time for the TSH-GTH divergence has been placed on the assumption that the rate of change has continuously increased on the line from TSH to LH. If this assumption is true, the TSH structure would have diverged first, approximately 320 MY ago". B. "Biological" tree (modified from Fontaine and Burzawa-Gérard (1977), based on the existence and various properties of the hormones in diverse vertebrate classes. It is assumed that TSH exists in cyclostomes and that FSH arose in primitive amphibians, either from the GTH-LH or from the TSH lineage.

lineages 350 million years ago; this *earliest* time, also reported by Miller and Mellon (1983), is obviously too recent because GH and PRL are present in teleosts and possibly in cyclostomes as well (see below). Wallis (1981) published a more detailed tree and insisted on the apparent changes of evolutionary rates which occurred in several instances, *i.e.* an acceleration in the lineage leading to hGH. Such a result may mean that paralogous rather than orthologous molecules are compared (*i.e.* primate GH diverged before the recorded divergence of primates and, therefore, its actual evolutionary rate is lower than the calculated value), or the evolutionary clock does not apply. Miller and Mellon (1983) and Miller and Eberhardt (1983) also indicated various inconsistencies; moreover, they reviewed recent work on mammalian GH/PRL genes and cDNA structures; these data suggest differences between the GH and PRH lineages with regard to the number of genes (one for PRL, several for GH) and to the number of intervening sequences. Therefore, according to Miller and Eberhardt (1983), "it is possible that the prolactin and growth hormone genes are evolving by several mechanisms, and that the dominant mechanism may differ between the two hormones and among various species". It seems interesting to observe (see below) that functional evolution also appears to differ in GH and PRL lineages.

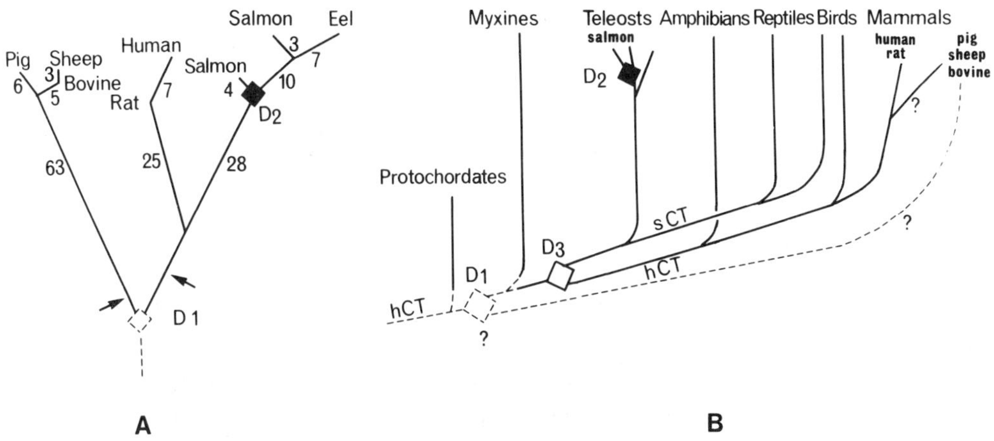

Fig. 2. Two different expressions of the phylogenetic relationship within the calcitonins. A. "Molecular" tree established by Hunt *et al.* (1978) on the basis of sequence comparison. The arrows indicate an approximate age of 500 MY. The empty square (D_1) indicates a possible ancient gene duplication. The black square indicates a recent duplication in teleosts. B. Tree based on the existence and various properties of calcitonins in diverse vertebrate classes, according to Perez-Cano *et al.*, 1982. A main duplication (D_3) would have occurred in fish ancestors, giving rise to two lineages (hCT and sCT). The artiodactyl CT may have arise from a very ancient duplication (D_1, ---) according to Hunt *et al.* (1978) or by a recent divergence from the human-rat lineage (——). The black square indicates a recent duplication in teleosts (see text).

All of the above-mentioned considerations are based on data from mammals. It is of great interest that Kawauchi *et al.* (1983) recently established the sequence of a salmon PRL. Its distance relative to hPRL is not less than to hGH, which also raises questions.

An evolutionary tree for calcitonins was constructed by Hunt *et al.* (1978). As shown in Figure 2, the authors were led to the hypothesis of a very ancient duplication, with one lineage persisting in fish, humans and rats, and the other in artiodacytls. Hunt and Dayhoff (1976) explained the very large distance between the CT's of these two mammalian groups by postulating that these molecules are paralogous. It seems interesting to compare such a tree with data on the existence of various CT forms in various vertebrates, as discussed by Perez-Cano *et al.* (1982). In particular, these authors showed that there are two calcitonin-like molecules in birds, which implies a primitive duplication that gave rise to the so-called hCT and sCT (Fig. 2). The artiodactyl CT has not been observed so far in other vertebrates, so that the hypothesis of Hunt *et al.* (1978) may be questioned. Alternatively, a very rapid evolution might have occurred in this lineage (Fig. 2). Gene studies are also in progress for this peptide family; a partial sequence of a chicken (apparently sCT type) calcitonin mRNA was established by Lasmoles *et al.* (1985).

From these examples, it seems difficult to believe that the evolutionary clock principle always applies strictly to the evolution of peptide hormones. It will be of interest to look for the genetic mechanisms of the probable exceptions, and also for a possible correlation with functional evolution.

Prehistory of vertebrate hormonal peptides

There has been a tendency to imagine that ancestors of the vertebrate hormones appeared in primitive fishes at the same time as the great lines of the vertebrate organization. This is no longer tenable, at least as a general rule, because data have accumulated which show the presence in invertebrates of representatives of the so-called "vertebrate hormone families", most of the evidence being gained by immunological approaches.

A number of hormonal peptide familes are represented in protochordates *e.g.* PRL (Pestarino, 1984), CT (Fritsch *et al.*, 1979, 1980; Girgis *et al.*, 1980; Pestarino, 1984), LHRH (Georges and DuBois, 1980) and SRIF (Fritsch *et al.*, 1979; Pestarino, 1983). Indeed, substances related to mammalian hypothalamic hormones were detected in various other invertebrate phyla, *e.g.* SRIF-like substances in insects (Doerr-Schott *et al.*, 1978), planaria (Bautz *et al.*, 1980) and gastropods (Grimm-Jorgensen, 1983), and CRH-like substances in insects (Verhaert *et al.*, 1984). AVT-like immunoreactivity was demonstrated in insects and molluscs (Remy *et al.*, 1979; Muhlethaler *et al.*, 1984) and even in hydra (Grimmelikhuizen *et al.*, 1982). Further biochemical characterization has been carried out for this peptide family. Although the AVT-like factor present in *Aplysia* behaves like AVT with HPLC (Moore *et al.*, 1981), it is not identical to this hormone (Sawyer *et al.*, 1984). The tri-peptide TRH may constitute a special case because its mode of synthesis (from a genetically coded prohormone or by a non-ribosomal mechanism) is still under discussion (Morley, 1981); TRH-like material was found in protochordates (Jackson and Reichlin, 1974) and gastropods (Grimm-Jorgensen *et al.*, 1975). Biochemical characterization of the invertebrate factors needs much further work. Even though certain previous immunological data may then be questioned, it is likely that profound changes will have to be introduced in the phylogenetic trees for "vertebrate" hormones.

Another problem may be raised by observations carried out in micro-organisms. Some of them were shown to contain factors similar to adrenocorticotropin, insulin (see Roth *et al.*, 1982) or hCG (Maruo *et al.*, 1979). The similarity concerns not only immunological properties, but also several biochemical characteristics, and even their biological activities. Also yeast mating pheromone is homologous to LHRH (see Loumaye *et al.*, 1982).

These data may suggest that genes for these types of peptides were present very early in evolution and have been highly conserved (Roth *et al.*, 1982). However, another possibility is that microorganisms secondarily gained these genes from higher animals later on in evolution by a natural process of DNA recombination, a kind of event which may have been much more frequent than imagined a few years ago (Syvanen, 1985). This second hypothesis seems to be a more likely way to explain the actual data, especially the extent of the similarity between the peptides from microorganisms and higher vertebrates. This is especially striking in the case of hCG. We have seen (Fig. 1) that this hormone was thought to have diverged recently in mammals, from the LH lineage. Whereas the α subunits are probably identical, hCGß mainly differs from hLHß by the presence of some 25 supplementary residues at the C-terminal end, the presence of which allows for the specific radioimmunoassay of hCG. In such an assay, bacterial culture extract reacted exactly like hCG whereas hLH was not recognized. Also the molecular weights and the electric behaviours of bacterial and human CG appeared identical. Both materials displayed a similar biological activity (Maruo *et al.*, 1979). Thus, to hold a hypothesis of a common, very ancient, primitive ancestor for two orthologous lineages, one should conclude from this extraordinary likeness that hCG did not evolve appreciably for more than 10^9 years. Also hCG should likely be present in various intermediary phyla, which so far has not been observed. Let us recall that the C-terminal end of teleost GTH resembles that of hLH and not that of hCG (Jolles *et al.*, 1977).

Hormonal function: the game between peptide hormones and receptors

Homologous peptides from a single family often exhibit quite different biological activities, either from structural changes in a given lineage or from an increase in the number of lineages with differentiated activities. In this latter event, hormone gene duplication plays a major role: "While the original hormone continues to carry out its functional role, the duplicate gene is free to mutate and to acquire the structural properties necessary to interact with a different set of receptors. Thus the organism gains a new hormone" (Niall, 1982). In all cases two main mechanisms seem to be involved and will be considered now.

Changes in the hormone-receptor interaction

Let us consider the simple case where a peptide hormone with the same function is present throughout representatives of a large number of vertebrate classes (*e.g.* TSH). Then, one could imagine that hormonal molecular evolution is not concerned with the sites involved in the biological activity. Studies on zoological specificity of biological action give some indications in this regard. The point is to compare the biological activities of zoologically different hormones on different vertebrate receivers. The results permit speculations on the presence or absence of differences in the structures involved in the biological action, at the level of both hormone and receptors (Table I). In the case of TSHs, the zoological specificity of action seems low within mammals (example A in Table I). In constrast, a teleost TSH, compared to bovine TSH, is about 300 times less active in mice than in trout (see Fontaine, 1980b), a case similar to example C in Table I.

Therefore, both the "active sites" of the TSH molecule and the specificity of recognition of the receptors are different in teleosts and in mammals. What is the meaning, if any, of such differences? I have postulated (see Fontaine, 1980a, c) that they reflect evolutionary changes leading to a more restricted physiological specificity, *i.e.* to the elimination of possible "background" stimulations of thyroid

Table I. Interpretation of data on the zoological specificity of hormonal action, in terms of hormone and receptor differences: a schematic example.

	Activity* ratios of two species-different analogous hormones on two species - different receivers (I,II)		Probable implication with regard to the "active sites" of hormones and and receptors
	I	II	
Example A	1	1	Hormones are identical
Example B	5	5	Hormones, but not receptors are different
Example C	0.1	10	Both hormones and receptors are different

* It is assumed that the biological response does not depend on other phenomena than the HR reaction.

by peptides other than TSH. In primitive vertebrates, the specificity of thyroidal receptors would have been relatively low, and then would have increased for TSH during evolution. This hypothesis may appear to contradict the fact that in the modern groups of vertebrates (even in teleosts) the thyroid physiologically responds quite specifically to TSH (*i.e.* it is not significantly stimulated by endogenous GTH). However, another pattern emerges if one considers not only the *physiological* specificity but also the *general* specificity (towards various exogenous homologous peptides). In some groups, and especially in teleosts, this general specificity is still low (indeed, mammalian GTHs exert a strong heterothyrotropic action in these animals) (Fontaine, 1958). A low general specificity of thyroid receptors was also shown in certain reptiles and birds (MacKenzie and Licht, 1984). I suggest that a low *general* specificity may, at least in some cases, reveal a primitive, low *physiological* specificity. Then, as evolution proceeds, changes at the levels of both TSH and TSH receptors would increase this physiological specificity in the various lineages, for instance by increasing affinity or by the development of negative specificities (Combarnous and Hengé, 1981) towards peptides other than TSH. It is likely that such results can be attained by very different evolutionary routes. Yet, it is not so astonishing if some vertebrates but not others have, by chance, retained the possibility to respond to certain foreign TSHs or TSH-like peptides. Even the general specificity of TSH receptors appears high in mammals, suggesting an especially efficient evolution towards specificity in this class.

Somewhat similar ideas could be developed in the case of several other hormonal lineages where a considerable zoological specificity of action also has been demonstrated: GH, PRL and the LH and FSH type GTHs; some of these examples will be considered later.

To the contary, it is interesting to note that in some cases the situation is quite different. Insulin underwent molecular evolution, but its receptors in various animals have different specificities (corresponding to the example B in Table I); this might reflect the probable antiquity of the insulin receptor (Muggeo *et al.*, 1979).

Changes in the location of hormone production and of receptors

It has been commonly thought that each hormone originated from one well-defined endocrine gland. Comparative data and the progress of immunohistochemistry reveal that this concept is no longer tenable. Several hormonal peptide families known as the gastro-entero-pancreatic group are represented in the central nervous system, and several of these are also in amphibian skin (see Erspamer, 1984). Parathyroid glands *sensu stricto* exist only in tetrapods. Yet a hormone homologous to PTH was discovered in teleosts, where it is secreted by organs located on, or close to, the kidneys, the Stannius corpuscles (Milet *et al.*, 1980); moreover, these organs and the tetrapod parathyroids show similarities (Lopez *et al.*, 1984) even though their embryological origins must be different. The ultimobranchial hormone, CT, was demonstrated in the central nervous system of many vertebrates from myxines to mammals (Girgis *et al.*, 1980; Galan-Galan *et al.*, 1981). It may act as a neuro-endocrine transmitter (MacInnes *et al.*, 1982) and hypophysiotropic functions have been suggested for CT in mammals (*e.g.* Mitsuma *et al.*, 1984). Indeed, the site of production of a hormone is likely to influence its function in several ways. Paracrine-like effects obviously depend on location. Also, there may be modifications in the control, the rate and the mode of secretion of the hormone according to the cells where it is produced. Even in mammals, the synthesis of certain hormones, especially insulin, appear more and more to be ubiquitous; the placenta secretes almost every peptide hormone for which it has been examined (Niall, 1982). All of this suggests that genes of peptide hormones can be expressed, more or less efficiently, in a number of cell types. As suggested by Niall (1982), gene repression may not be an all-or-none phenomenon.

Evolutionary changes in the locations of receptors are obvious in many cases where a striking functional evolution is observed within a hormone lineage, such as PRL (Clarke and Bern, 1980). In teleosts, for instance, PRL acts on gills and prevents, in fresh water, the loss of sodium; PRL specific binding sites have been found in various tissues, such as liver, gonad, intestine, and gill (Edery *et al.*, 1984). In birds it stimulates the activity of the crop-sac (perhaps in part by the mediation of a liver "synlactin" as suggested by Nicoll *et al.*, 1984). The mammotropic, and sometimes luteotropic, effects of PRL in mammals are well documented. Thus, depending on the evolutionary stage, the PRL receptor gene has been expressed in a variety of cell types. Other similar examples are those of PTH and TRH. Parathyrin possesses, in mammals, several targets including bone; in teleosts, it acts on gills (Milet *et al.*, 1979), but probably not on bone (Lopez, 1973). The neuropeptide TRH stimulates TSH and PRL release in mammals. It does not stimulate TSH release in fish (Eales, 1979; Jackson, 1979), whereas it was shown to activate PRL cells in teleosts (Batten and Wigham, 1984). Thus, TRH receptors of TSH cells probably appeared later in evolution, probably in amphibians (Darras and

Kühn, 1982) where, on the other hand, a clear effect on MSH-release was demonstrated (Tonon *et al.*, 1980). A primitive neurotransmitter function was suggested for TRH (Hardisty and Baker, 1982), and TRH receptors are detectable in teleost brain and pituitary (Burt and Ajah, 1984).

General case and possible strategies of the game

The evolution of two additional hormonal families (the GTH-LH-FSH family and the neuropituitary hormones), illustrate well the game between hormones and receptors. Studies carried out with teleost GTH hormone have showed the existence of specific binding sites in gonads (ref. in Van Der Kraak, 1983; Salmon *et al.*, 1984, 1985a). The properties of GTH receptors were indirectly characterized by studying the *in vitro* gonadotropic stimulation of cAMP production in immature fish ovary (Salmon *et al.*, 1985a,b). By comparing the effects of a fish GTH and of mammalian LH (or hCG) we were led to the hypothesis that the pool of receptors for the fish GTH was not homogenous, but consisted of two different classes of "isoreceptors", only one of which also recognized mammalian hormones. This hypothesis was supported by the results of cross-desensitization experiments with hCG and carp GTH (Salmon *et al.*, 1985a). We do not know if the pool of GTH receptors which recognizes hCG/LH has a special cellular localization, but it is endowed with unique properties with regard to cAMP release in the medium as well as the associated phosphodiesterase activity and/or the metabolism of the H-R complexes (Salmon *et al.*, 1985b). The differentiation of two types of receptors, the physiological significance of which is not known, may be a recently acquired character, or it may reflect a primitive situation in fishes which would have preceded the appearance of a second GTH in primitive amphibians. In amphibians, FSH is present in addition to LH, and the possible physiological interest of this novelty has been discussed elsewhere (Fontaine, 1980b, 1984). It is of interest to note that in these animals, receptors for the (new) FSH often appear to have a low physiological specificity: they also recognize LH, whereas some LH receptors do not recognize FSH (Fontaine, 1980b). Results from binding studies (Takada and Ishii, 1985) are in agreement with this pattern which may be interpreted in terms of a recent "duplication" of LH receptors: some of them would begin to differentiate and would no longer recognize the new hormone, FSH. In mammals, the physiological specificity of FSH and LH is generally high; however it has been suggested that FSH receptors have a less strict general specificity than LH receptors (Salmon *et al.*, 1982) and this could reflect the relative youth of the FSH specific receptors.

The comparative biochemistry of neuropituitary hormones is relatively well known (Acher *et al.*, 1981), but we still lack precise data on their physiology in lower vertebrates (Sawyer and Pang, 1979; Fontaine, 1980a). The situation appears to be as follows: in cyclostomes only one neuropituitary hormone (AVT) is present; it persists in almost all other groups where it is accompanied by other, homologous, peptides. Results in cyclostomes suggest that vascular smooth muscles were the first target tissues for AVT. In teleosts isotocin exists in addition to AVT, and some smooth muscles may be privileged targets, but there is no clear functional difference between the two hormones. In amphibians, AVT and mesotocin are present and act on smooth muscles (in blood vessels and also oviduct and ovary); moreover, receptors are present in epithelia (skin, kidney tubules); mesotocin may be more active than AVT on smooth muscles, but no clear functional difference between them has so far been demonstrated. Indeed, such a difference exists in mammals between vasopressin and oxytocin. Another point relevant to this topic is that specific binding sites for vasopressin were found in various mammalian tissues (*e.g.* kidney, brain, liver, testis) and that a gonadal production of "neuropituitary" hormones was suggested (Meidan and Hsueh, 1985).

An important trend in endocrine evolution is the progressive increase in the number of functions regulated independently, due to a progressive distribution of specific tasks between several hormones. Along with hormonal evolution, receptors progressively differentiate, both in their specificity and in their location. In our present state of knowledge (which is changing very quickly) no precise description of receptor evolution can be achieved. However, it is tempting to speculate further on the basis of some obvious phenomenological similarites between hormonal evolution and receptor evolution. As proposed by Niall (1982), it seems likely that receptors for hormones of a given family (and possibly others) are homologous, *i.e.* they are derived from a common ancestor, possibly by gene duplication; the copies independently evolved and eventually acquired different properties. We can make supplementary assumptions: genes for slightly different receptors of the same hormone can be present in one organism and can be differentially expressed in various cell types. If this were true, the two events previously described (specificity and location changes) could, indeed, be connected. For instance, let us suppose that a hormone (H) acts on a target (T) where receptors (R) are expressed with a relatively low specificity. If a more specific homologous receptor (R') happens to be expressed in another cell type, one can conceive that this tissue (T') will tend to become the principal functional target of H (by increase in the expression of R' and decrease in the expression of R); or, if a hormonal duplication occurs, H and H' may be capable of regulating T and T' respectively (by changes in the specificity of the HR interactions).

Evolution within fish

In view of the title of this Symposium, the situation within the fish group should be considered in more detail. Unfortunately, the available data on fish endocrinology, even though expanding rapidly, are still scattered among the diverse zoological forms. It seems beyond the scope of this paper to review these data exhaustively. I will illustrate only some general approaches and some of the questions raised, *i.e.* functional evolution, endocrine systematics and endocrine aspects of evolutionary trends.

Thyrotropic and gonadotropic functions

This topic has been dealt with in several reviews (*e.g.* Eales, 1979; Jackson, 1979; Ball *et al.*, 1980; Fontaine, 1980b; Dodd, 1983; Gorbman, 1983; Peter, 1983) and I shall limit myself to a few points. A thyroid gland was probably present in primitive pre-vertebrates. When did control by pituitary TSH begin? Physiological evidence for such early control has so far not been obtained in cyclostomes (see also Hardisty and Baker, 1982). However, Gorbman and his group, working with myxines, showed the possible existence of a bioactive pituitary

TSH, as well as a stimulation of the thyroid by mammalian TSH (see Dickhoff and Gorbman, 1977). On the other hand, mammalian TSH immunoreactivity was detected in some cells of the lamprey pituitary (Wright, 1984). With regard to GTH, convergent, although still limited data, indicate it is present in lampreys (Larsen and Rothwell, 1972; Wright, 1983; Sower *et al.*, 1983) but probably not in hagfish (Gorbman, 1983). These results suggest two hypotheses: either TSH appeared first in ancestors of the cyclostomes, whereas GTH appeared later (after the myxine stage), in common ancestors of lampreys and other vertebrates, or GTH was secondarily lost in hagfish because of their special, rather constant, environment and the absence of a seasonally-defined reproductive cycle (Gorbman, 1980, 1983).

In selachians, as well as in teleosts, the existence of bioactive TSH and GTH seems beyond doubt. With regard to the central nervous control of GTH function, it seems to exist, and to be exerted by, a LH-RH-like substance in all the groups where GTH itself is present, *e.g.* in lampreys but not in myxines (Crim *et al.*, 1979).

The situation is more complex for TSH control. All available data indicate that TRH, although probably present in all fishes (Jackson, 1979), does not stimulate pituitary TSH cells in these animals (see above). Physiological data suggest that, in teleosts, TSH function is under a negative central control (which might be exerted through SRIF; Peter and McKeown, 1975). This is somewhat puzzling, as it is also under the negative feedback control of thyroid hormones (Eales, 1979).

Endocrine systematics

Homologous hormones are different within fishes (*e.g.* GTH, Fontaine, 1980b). Their molecular evolution will become clearer when more sequence data become available. Here, I shall summarize only a few facts which differentiate fish classes.

Selachians are quite original, characteristic or even unique (even relative to holocephalans) in several respects. They possess special neuropituitary hormones (glumitocin, aspartocin, valitocin; Acher *et al.*, 1981) which are not found elsewhere, as well as corticosteroid, 1 α -hydroxy corticosterone (Idler and Truscott, 1972) found in no other group. Dipnoi attract attention in a similar fashion. They possess a particular tetrapod neuropituitary hormone (mesotocin; Acher *et al.*, 1981) and corticosteroid (aldosterone; Idler and Truscott, 1972). Moreover, dipnoan TSH (Fontaine, 1958) and GH (Geschwind, 1967) exhibit a zoological specificity of action very different from that of their teleost counterparts; indeed they are much more efficient in mammals.

Some unique endocrine organs exist in some groups of fish, *e.g.* Stannius corpuscles in actinopterygians and a caudal neurosecretory system (urophysis) in Chondrichthyes and actinopterygians. The urophysis secretes two main peptides, urotensins I and II (Bern, 1982). Their histories are somewhat parallel and we shall consider the example of urotensin II. This hormone is homologous to SRIF and it is involved in osmoregulation (Pearson *et al.*, 1980; Bern, 1982, Ichikawa *et al.*, 1984). It is interesting to note that other, more classical SRIF-like substances have been detected in teleost brain and digestive tract (Olivereau *et al.*, 1984; Cook and Peter, 1984). Sequence studies have indicated that these substances are more homologous to mammalian SRIF than is urotensin II (Hobart *et al.*, 1980; Ogawa *et al.*, 1980); they probably exert the usual inhibitory effect on the secretion of certain hormones such as PRL (Grau *et al.*, 1982, Batten and Wigham, 1984), GH (Cook and Peter, 1984) or insulin. Moreover, such an effect was documented in hagfish (Stewart *et al.*, 1978), where (as well as in lampreys) SRIF-like substances were detected (Homma, 1983). Thus, one may consider that within the SRIF family, a main, ancient and long-lasting tendency is to inhibit pancreas and/or pituitary hormone secretions. In some fish, in addition, this family would be put to a different use, with the appearance of a new lineage with characteristic sequences, activities, and production sites of the molecules.

Endocrines and evolutionary trends

Some of the main vertebrate novelties are concerned with the establishment of an efficient homeostasy, and of an internal calcified skeleton. It should be emphasized that this began in the ancient, sea-dwelling fish and persisted when representatives of the various classes conquered fresh water.

With regard to osmoregulation, it is known that corticosteroids play a main role in seawater teleosts, but I shall not consider these hormones or those involved in their regulation (adrenocorticotropin and CRH). On the other hand, several data (Leloup and de Luze, 1985) point to the importance of thyroid hormones, the secretion of which is stimulated by TSH. This raises again the question of the control of TSH function in fish, namely the apparent lack of a stimulating mechanism (see above). In view of the role of the thyroid-TSH axis in osmoregulation one may wonder if a direct control of fish TSH cells by variations in blood ions could exist. A similar proposition was made by Bern (1980) for various endocrine cells.

The osmoregulatory role of PRL is especially important in fresh water fishes (Clarke and Bern, 1980), and this leads us to ask what was the first function of this hormone in a primitive seawater fish. In any case, it is likely that PRL played a role in the conquest of estuarine, then freshwater environments by marine fish.

The evolution of calcium regulating hormones (CT and possibly PTH) and of the calcified skeleton were probably correlated. In cyclostomes, however, an endocrine control of calcium metabolism by these hormones has not been demonstrated. Ultimobranchial CT has been detected in selachians and in teleosts (Lopez, 1984). In teleosts, CT is able to exert its classical hypocalcemic effect (Lopez *et al.*, 1976) by acting at several levels, *e.g.* gills (Peignoux-Deville *et al.*, 1978; Fouchereau-Peron *et al.*, 1981) and bone (Lopez *et al.*, 1976). The hypercalcemic effect described in selachians (Glowacki *et al.*, 1985) could reflect not so much a fundamental class difference, but rather the physiological state of the animals. Indeed, opposite actions of CT on calcium fluxes through the teleost intestine, depending on the initial values of the fluxes, were described (Chartier *et al.*, 1983). In fish, PTH has so far been characterized only in teleost Stannius corpuscles. What, if any, are its sites of production in animals which do not possess these organs? This is one of the many questions which have arisen in this paper.

Abreviations and definitions of the hormonal peptides considered in the text

Anterior pituitary hormones: TSH: thyroid-stimulating hormone (glycoprotein, MW#30,000, made of two subunits α and ß); GTH: gonadotropic hormone (glycoprotein, MW#30,000, made of two subunits α and ß); LH: lutropin, one of the tetrapod GTHs; FSH: follitropin, one of the tetrapod GTHs; GH: growth hormone (MW#20-25,000); PRL: prolactin (MW#20-25,000).

Posterior pituitary hormones: AVT: arginine vasotocin (nanopeptide).

Central nervous system: TRH: TSH-stimulating hormone (tripeptide); LHRH: lutropin and follitropin-releasing hormone (decapeptide); GnRH: gonadotropin-releasing hormone (defined as LHRH in mammals); SRIF: somatostatin, GH-release inhibitor (14, or more, residues); CRH: Adrenocorticotropin-releasing hormone (41 residues).

Calcium regulating hormones: CT: calcitonin, produced by ultimobranchial cells (32 residues); PTH: parathyrin, produced by parathyroid gland (MW#9-10,000).

Others: CG: chorionic gonadotropin (h = human).

Acknowledgement

The author is very much indebted to Professor A. Gorbman for critical reading and English correction of this manuscript.

Literature Cited

ACHER, R., J. CHAUVET, and M.T. CHAUVET. 1981. Neurohypophysial hormones and Neurophysins: structures, precursors and evolution. *In* De Las Hera, F.G., and S. Vega [eds.] Medicinal Chemistry Advances. Pergamon Press, Oxford. pp. 473-485.

ANDREWS, P.C., M.H. PUBOLS, M.A. HERMODSON, B.T. SHEARES, and J.E. DIXON. 1984. Structure of the 22-residue somatostatin from catfish. J. biol. Chem. **259**: 13267-13272.

BALL, J.N., T.F.C. BATTEN, and G. YOUNG. 1980. Evolution of hypothalamo-adenohypophysial system in lower Vertebrates. pp. 45-46 *In* Ishii, S. *et al.* [eds.] Hormones, adaptation and evolution. Japan Sci. Soc. Press. Tokyo/Springer-Verlag, Berlin.

BATTEN, T.F.C., and T. WIGHAM. 1984. Effects of TRH and somatostatin on releases of prolactin and growth hormone *in vitro* by the pituitary of *Poecilia latipinna.* Cell Tissue Res. **237**: 595-603.

BAUTZ, A., J. SCHILT, J.P. RICHOUX, AND M.P. DUBOIS. 1980. Détection immunocytologique, dénombrement et localisation des cellules à somatostatine (SRIF) chez deux espèces de Planaires, *Dugesia lugubris* et *Dendrocoelum lacteum* (Turbellaries, Triclades). C.r. hebd. Séanc. Acad. Sci. (Paris) Ser. D **291**: 833-836.

BERN, H.A. 1980. Primitive control of endocrine systems. pp. 25-33 *In* Ishii, S. *et al.* [eds.] Hormones, adaptation and evolution. Japan Sci. Soc. Press. Tokyo/Springer-Verlag, Berlin.

BERN, H.A. 1982. The caudal neurosecretory system of fishes: the beginnings of "urophysiology". Gen. comp. Endocrinol. **46**: 349-350.

BURT, D.R., and M.A. AJAH. 1984. TRH receptors in fish. Gen. comp. Endocrinol. **53**: 135-142.

CHARTIER, M.M., E. MARTELLY, E. LOPEZ, and C. MILET. 1983. Effet de la calcitonine de saumon sur l'absorption intestinale du calcium chez l'anguille (*Anguilla anguilla* L.). C.r. hebd. Séanc. Acad. Sc. (Paris) sér. III. **296**: 1117-1120.

CLARKE, C.W., and H.A. BERN. 1980. Comparative endocrinology of prolactin. pp. 105-197 *In* Li, C.H. [ed.] Hormonal proteins and peptides, vol. 8, pt. 4. Academic Press, New York.

COMBARNOUS, Y., and M.H. HENGÉ. 1981. Equine follicle-stimulating hormone. Purification, acid dissociation and binding to equine testicular tissue. J. biol. Chem. **256**: 9567-9572.

COOK, F.A., and R.E. PETER. 1984. The effects of somatostatin on serum growth hormone levels in the Goldfish, *Carassius auratus*. Gen. comp. Endocrinol. **54**: 109-113.

CRIM, J.W., A. URANO, and A. GORBMAN. 1979. Immunocytochemical studies of luteinizing hormone-releasing hormone in brains of Agnathan fishes. I - Comparisons of adult Pacific Lamprey (*Entosphenus tridentata*) and the Pacific hagfish (*Eptatretus stoutii*). Gen comp. Endocrinol. **37**: 294-305.

DARRAS, V.M., and E.R. KÜHN. 1982. Increased plasma levels of thyroid hormones in a frog, *Rana ridibunda* following intravenous administration of TRH. Gen. comp. Endocrinol. **48**: 469-475.

DAYHOFF, M.O., C.M. PARK, and P.J. McLAUGHLIN. 1972. Building a phylogenetic tree: cytochrome C. pp. 7-16 *In* Dayhoff, M.O. [ed.] Atlas of protein sequence and structure, vol. 5, suppl. 3. NBRF, Georgetown University Medical Center, Washington.

DICKHOFF, W.W., and A. GORBMAN. 1977. *In vitro* thyrotropic effect of the pituitary of the Pacific hagfish, *Eptatretus stoutii*. Gen. comp. Endocrinol. **31**: 75-79.

DODD, J.M. 1983. Reproduction in cartilaginous fishes (Chondrichthyes). pp. 31-95. *In* Hoar, W.S., D.J. Randall, and E.M. Donaldson. [eds.] Fish physiology, vol. IX. Academic Press, New York.

DOERR-SCHOTT, J., L. JOLY, and M.P. DUBOIS. 1978. Sur l'existence dans la pars intercerebralis d'un insecte (*Locusta migratoria* R. et F.) de cellules neurosécrétrices fixant un antisérum antisomatostatine. C.r. hebd. Séanc. Acad. Sci. (Paris) **286D**: 93-95.

EALES, J.G.. 1979. Thyroid function in Cyclostomes and fishes. pp. 340-436 *In* Barrington, E.J.W. [ed.] Hormones and evolution, vol. 1. Acad. Press, New York.

EDERY, M., G. YOUNG, H.A. BERN., and S. STEINY. 1984. Prolactin receptors in Tilapia (*Sarotherodon mossambicus*) tissues: binding studies using ^{125}I-labelled ovine prolactin. Gen. comp. Endocrinol. **56**: 19-23.

ERSPAMER, V. 1984. Half a century of comparative research on biogenic amines and active peptides in Amphibian skin and molluscan tissues. Comp. Biochem. Physiol. **79C**: 1-17.

FONTAINE, Y.A. 1958. Quelques caractéristiques de l'activité thyréotrope hypophysaire d'un Dipneuste (*Protopterus annectens* Owen) comparée à celle d'un Téléostéen et de Tétrapodes. J. Physiol (Paris) **50**: 281-284.

FONTAINE, Y.A. 1980a. Hormones et évolution. Ann. Biol. **19**: 337-366.

FONTAINE, Y.A. 1980b. Les hormones gonadotropes de l'hyophyse: biochimie et biologie comparées: spécificité et évolution. Reprod. Nutr. Develop. **20**: 381-418.

FONTAINE, Y.A. 1980c. Evolution of pituitary gonadotropins and thyrotropins. pp. 261-270 *In* Ishii, S. *et al.*, [eds.] Hormones, adaptation and evolution. Japan Sci. Soc. Press. Tokyo/Springer-Verlag, Berlin.

FONTAINE, Y.A. 1984. Les hormones et l'évolution. La Recherche. **153**: 310-320.

FONTAINE, Y.A., and E. BURZAWA-GÉRARD. 1977. Esquisse de l'évolution des hormones gonadotropes des Vertébrés. Gen. comp. Endocrinol. **32**: 341-347.

FOUCHEREAU-PERON, M., M.S. MOUKHTAR, Y. LEGAL, and G. MILHAUD. 1981. Demonstration of specific receptors for calcitonin in isolated trout gill cells. Comp. Biochem. Physiol. **68A**: 417-421.

FRITSCH, H.A.R., S. VAN NOORDEN, and A.G.E. PEARSE. 1979. Localization of somatostatin-, substance P- and calcitonin- like immunoreactivity in the neural ganglion of *Ciona intestinalis* L. (Ascidiaceae). Cell Tissue Res. **202**: 263-274.

FRITSCH, H.A.R., S. VAN NOORDEN, and A.G.E. PEARSE. 1980. Calcitonin-like immunological staining in the alimentary tract of *Ciona intestinalis* L. Cell Tissue Res. **205**: 439-444.

GALAN-GALAN, F., R.M. ROGERS, S.I. GIRGIS, and I. MacINTYRE. 1981. Immunoreactive calcitonin in the central nervous system of the pigeon. Brain Res. **212**: 59-66.

GEORGES, D., and P.M. DUBOIS. 1980. Mise en évidence par les techniques d'immunofluorescence d'un antigène de type LH-RH dans le système nerveux de *Ciona intestinalis* (Tunicier asidiacé). C.r. hebd. Séanc. Acad. Sci. (Paris) **290D**: 29-31.

GESCHWIND, I.I. 1967. Growth hormone activity in the lungfish pituitary. Gen. comp. Endocrinol. **8**: 82-83.

GIRGIS, S.I., F. GALAN-GALAN, T.R. ARNETT, R.M. ROGERS, Q. BONE, M. RAVAZZOLA, and I. MacINTYRE. 1980. Immunoreactive human calcitonin-like molecule in the nervous systems of protochordates and a cyclostome, *Myxine*. J. Endocrinol. **87**: 375-382.

GLOWACKI, J., J. D'SULLIVAN, M. MILLER, D.W. WILKIE, and L.J. DEFTOS. 1985. Calcitonin produces hypercalcemia in leopard sharks. Endocrinology. **116**: 827-829.

GORBMAN, A. 1980. Endocrine regulation in Agnatha: primitive or degenerate? pp. 81-92 *In* Ishii, S. *et al.* [eds.] Hormones, adaptation and Evolution. Japan Sci. Soc. Press. Tokyo/Springer-Verlag Berlin.

GORBMAN, A. 1983. Reproduction in cyclostome fishes and its regulation. pp. 1-29 *In* Hoar, W.S., D.J. Randall, and E.M. Donaldson. [eds.] Fish physiology, vol. IX. Academic Press, New York.

GRAU, G.E., R.S. NISHIOKA, and H.A. BERN. 1982. Effects of somatostatin and urotensin II on Tilapia pituitary prolactin release and interactions between somatostatin, osmotic pressure, Ca^{2+}, and adenosine 3',5'- monophosphate in prolactin release *in vitro*. Endocrinology. **110**: 910-915.

GRIMMELIKHUIZEN, C.J.P., K. DIERICKX, and G. Y. BOER. 1982. Oxytocin/vasopressin-like immunoreactivity is present in *Hydra*. Neuroscience **7**: 3191-3199.

GRIMM-JØRGENSEN, Y. 1983. Immunoreactive somatostatin in two pulmonate gastropods. Gen. comp. Endocrinol. **49**: 108-114.

GRIMM-JØRGENSEN, Y., J.F. McKELVY, and I.M.D. JACKSON. 1975. Immunoreactive thyrotropin-releasing factor in gastropod circum oesophageal glandia. Nature **254**: 620.

HARDISTRY, M.W., and B.I. BAKER. 1982. Endocrinology of lampreys. pp. 1-115 *In* Hardisty, M.W., and I.C. Potter [eds.] The biology of lampreys, vol. 4b. Acad. Press, New York.

HOBART, P., R. CRAWFORD, L.P. SHEN, R. PICTET, and W.J. RUTTER. 1980. Cloning and sequence analysis of cDNAs encoding two distinct somatostatin precursors found in the endocrine pancreas of anglerfish. Nature **288**: 137-141.

HOMMA, S. 1983. Physiology and pharmacology of putative transmitters in lamprey central nervous sytem. Prog. Neurobiol. **20**: 287-311.

HUNT, L.T., and M.O. DAYHOFF. 1976. Hormones and active peptides. pp. 113-146 *In*: Dayhoff, M.O. [ed.] Atlas of Protein Sequence and Structure, vol. 5 suppl. 3. NBRF, Georgetown University medical center, Washington.

HUNT, L.T., F.D. LEDLEY, and M.O. DAYHOFF. 1978. Hormones and active peptides. pp. 145-164. *In* Dayhoff, M.O. [ed.] Atlas of Protein Sequence and Structure, vol., 5 suppl. 3. NBRF, Georgetown University medical center, Washington.

ICHIKAWA, T., K. LEDERIS, and H. KOBAYASHI. 1984. Primary structures of multiple forms of urotensin II in the urophysis of the carp, *Cyprinus carpio*. Gen. comp. Endocrinol. **55**: 133-141.

IDLER, D.R., and B. TRUSCOTT. 1972. Corticosteroids in fish. pp. 127-252 *In* Idler, D.R. [ed.] Steroids in non mammalian vertebrates. Academic Press, New York

JACKSON, I.M.D. 1979. The releasing factors of the hypothalamus. pp. 723-790 *In* Barrington, E.J.W. [ed.] Hormones and evolution, vol. 2. Academic Press, New York.

JACKSON, I.M.D., and S. REICHLIN. 1974. Thyrotropin-releasing hormone (TRH) distribution in hypothalamic and extrahypothalamic brain tissues of mammalian and submammalian chordates. Endocrinology. **95**: 854-862.

JOLLES, J. E. BURZAWA-GERARD, Y.A. FONTAINE, and P. JOLLES. 1977. The evolution of gonadotropins: some molecular data concerning a non-mammalian pituitary gonadotropin, the hormone from a teleost fish. Biochimie. **59**: 893-898.

KAWAUCHI, H, K.I. ABE, A. TAKAHASHI, T. HIRANO, S. HASEGAWA, N. NAITO, and Y. NAKAI. 1983. Isolation and properties of Chum Salmon prolactin. Gen. comp. Endocrinol. **49**: 446-458.

LARSEN, L.O., and B. ROTHWELL. 1972. Adenohypophysis. pp. 1-67 *In* Hardisty, M.W., and I.C Potter [eds.] The biology of lampreys. Academic Press, New York.

LASMOLES, F., A. JULIENNE, C. DESPLAN, G. MILHAUD, and M.S. MOUKHTAR. 1985. Structure of chicken calcitonin predicted by partial nucleotide sequence of its precursor. FEBS Lett. **180**: 113-116.

LELOUP, J., and A. DE-LUZE. 1985. Environmental effects of temperature and salinity on thyroid function in teleost fishes pp. 23-32 *In* Follet, B.K., S. Ishii,

A. Chandola [eds.] The endocrine system and the environment. Japan Sci. Soc. Press, Tokyo
LICHT, P. 1980. Relationship between receptor binding and biological activities of gonadotropins. pp. 167-174 *In* Ishii, S. *et al.* [eds.] Hormones, Adaptation and Evolution. Japan Sci. Soc. Press. Tokyo/Springer-Verlag, Berlin.
LOPEZ, E. 1973. Etude morphologique et physiologique de l'os cellulaire des poissons téléostéen. Mem. Mus. Nat. Hist. Nat. ser. A. 80. 90 p.
LOPEZ, E. 1984. Evolution of Ca regulating hormones in Vertebrates. Calcif. Tiss. Int. (suppl. 2) 36. S11.
LOPEZ, E., J. PEIGNOUX-DEVILLE, F. LALLIER, E. MARTELLY-BAGOT, and C. MILET. 1976. Effects of calcitonin and ultimobranchialectomy (UBX) on calcium and bone metabolism in the eel, *Anguilla anguilla* L. Calcif. Tiss. Res. **20**: 173-186.
LOPEZ, E., E. TISSERAND-JOCHEM, B. VIDAL, C. MILET, F. LALLIER, and I. MacINTYRE. 1984. Les corpuscules de Stannius sont-ils les glandes parathyroides des poissons Téléostéens? Arguments ultrastructuraux, cytologiques et immunocytochimiques. C. r. hebd. Séanc. Acad. Sci. (Paris) sér. III. **298**: 359-364.
LOUMAYE, E., J. THORNER, and K.J. CATT. 1982. Yeast mating pheromone activates mammalian gonadotrophs: evolutionary conservation of a reproductive hormone? Science. **218**: 1323-1325.
MacINNES, D.G., I. LASZLO, I. MacINTYRE, and G. FINK. 1982. Salmon calcitonin in lizard brain: a possible neuroendocrine transmitter. Brain Res. **251**: 371-373.
MacKENZIE, D.S., and P. LICHT. 1984. Studies on the specificity of thyroid responses to pituitary glycoprotein hormones. Gen. comp. Endocrinol. **56**: 156-166.
McLAUGHLIN, P.J., and M.O. DAYHOFF. 1972. Evolution of species and proteins: a time scale. pp. 47-52 *In* Dayhoff, M.O. [ed.] Atlas of protein sequence and structure, vol. 5 suppl. 3. NBRG, Georgetown University medical center, Washington.
MARUO, T., H. COHEN, S.J. SEGAL, and S.S. KOIDE. 1979. Production of choriogonadotropin-like factor by a microorganism. Proc. Natl. Acad. Sci. U.S.A. **76**: 6622-6626.
MEIDAN, R., and A.J.W. HSUEH. 1985. Identification and characterization of arginine vasopressin receptors in the rat testis. Endocrinology. **116**: 416-423.
MILET, C., J. PEIGNOUX-DEVILLE, and E. MARTELLY. 1979. Gill calcium fluxes in the eel, *Anguilla anguilla* (L.). Effects of Stannius corpuscles and ultimobranchial body. Comp. Biochem. Physiol. **63A**: 63-70.
MILET, C., C.J. HILLYARD, E. MARTELLY, S. GIRGIS, I. MacINTYRE, and E. LOPEZ. 1980. Similitudes structurales entre l'hormone hypocalcémiante des corpuscules de Stannius (PCS) de l'anguille, *Anguilla anguilla* L. et l'hormone parathyroidienne mammalienne. C.r. hebd. Séanc. Acad. Sci., (Paris) sér. D, **291**: 977-980.
MILLER, W.L., and N.L. EBERHARDT. 1983. Structure and evolution of the growth hormone gene family. Endocrinol. Rev. **4**: 97-130.
MILLER, W.L., and S.H. MELLON. 1983. Evolution and regulation of genes for growth hormone and prolactin pp. 177-202 *In* McKerns, K.W. [ed.] Biochemical Endocrinology. Plenum Press, N.Y.
MITSUMA, T., T. NOGIMORI, and M. CHAYA. 1984. Peripheral administration

of eel calcitonin inhibits thyrotropin secretion in rats. Eur. J. Pharmacol. **102**: 123-128.

MORLEY, J.E. 1981. Neuroendocrine control of thyrotropin secretion. Endocrinol. Rev. **2**: 396-436.

MUGGEO, M., B.H. GINSBERG, J. ROTH, D.M. NEVILLE, JR., P. DE MEYTS., and R.C. KAHN. 1979. The insulin receptor in vertebrates is functionally more conserved during evolution than insulin itself. Endocrinology. **104**: 1393-1402.

NIALL, H.D. 1982. The evolution of peptide hormones. Ann. Rev. Physiol. **44**: 615-624.

NICOLL, C.S., T.R. ANDERSON, N. HEBERI, and E.M. SPENCER. 1984. Comparative aspects of prolactin's growth promoting actions: evidence for synergism with an insulin-like growth factor (IGF)/somatomadin (SM). Proc. of the International Congress on "Prolactin". Charlottes-Ville. abstract 85.

NINIO, J. 1979. Approches moléculaires de l'evolution. Masson, Paris. 131 p.

OGAWA, H., R.A. BRADSHAW, O.J. BATES, and A. PERMUTT. 1980. Amino acid sequence of catfish pancreatic somatostatin I. J. biol. Chem. **255**: 2251-2254.

OLIVEREAU, M. F. OLLEVIER, F. VANDESANDE, and W. VERDONCK. 1984. Immunocytochemical identification of CRF-like and SRIF-like peptides in the brain and the pituitary of cyprinid fish. Cell Tissue Res. **237**: 379-382.

PEARSON, D., J.E. SHIVELY, B.R. CLARK, I.I. GESCHWINDM, M. BARKELY, R.S. NISHIOKA, and H.A. BERN. 1980. Urotensin II: a somatostatin-like peptide in the caudal neurosecretory system of fishes. Proc. Natl. Acad. Sci. U.S.A. **77**: 5012-5024.

PEIGNOUX-DEVILLE, J., C. MILET, and E. MARTELLY. 1978. Effects de l'ablation du corps ultimobranchial et de la perfusion de calcitonine sur les flux de calcium au niveau des branchies de l'anguille (*Anguilla anguilla* L.). Ann. Biol. Anim. Biochem. Biophys. **18**: 119-126.

PEREZ-CANO, R., S.I. GIRGIS, F. GALAN-GALAN, and I. MacINTYRE. 1982. Identification of both human and salmon calcitonin-like molecules in birds suggesting the existence of two calcitonin genes. J. Endocrinol. **92**: 351-355.

PESTARINO, M. 1983. Somatostatin-like immunoreactive neurone in a protochordate. Experientia **39**: 1156-1157.

PESTARINO, M. 1984. Immunocytochemical demonstration of prolactin-like activity in the neural gland of the ascidian *Styela plicata.* Gen comp. Endocrinol. **54**: 444-449.

PETER, R.E. 1983. The brain and neurohormones in teleost reproduction. pp. 97-135 *In* Hoar, W.S., D.J. Randall, and E.M. Donaldson [eds.] Fish physiology, vol. IX. Academic Press, New York.

PETER, R.A. 1983. Evolution of neurohormonal regulation of reproduction in lower vertebrates. Amer. Zool. **23**: 685-695.

PETER, R.E., and B.A. McKEOWN. 1975. Hypothalamic control of prolactin and thyrotropin secretion in teleosts with special reference to recent studies on the goldfish. Gen. comp. Endocrinol. **25**: 153-165.

ROTH, J., D. LEROITH, J. SHILOACH, J.L. ROSENZWEIG, M.A. LESNIAK, and J. HAVRABKOVA. 1982. The evolutionary origins of hormones, neurotransmitters, and other extracellular chemical messengers. New Engl. J. Med. **306**: 523-527.

SALMON, C., N. DELERUE-LE BELLE, and Y.A. FONTAINE. 1982. Effects d'une hormone gonadotrope de poisson téléostéen sur l'adénylate cyclase d'ovaire de ratte et sur sa stimulation par les gonadotropines ovines. C.r. Soc. Biol. **176**: 787-794.

SALMON, C., H. KAGAWA, S. ADACHI, Y. NAGAHAMA, and Y.A. FONTAINE. 1984. Mise en évidence de sites de liason spécifique de la gonadotropine de saumon chum (*Oncorhynchus keta*) dans des préparations membranaires de granulosa d'ovaire de saumon Amago (*Oncorhynchus rhodurus*). C.r. hebd. Séanc. Acad. Sci. (Paris) sér. III **298**: 337-340.

SALMON, C., J. MARCHELIDON, E. FONTAINE-BERTRAND, and Y.A. FONTAINE. 1985a. Human chorionic gonadotropin and immature fish ovary: characterization and mechanism of the *in vitro* stimulation of cyclic adenosine monophosphate accumulation. Gen. comp. Endocrinol. 58: (in press).

SALMON, C, J. MARCHELIDON, E. FONTAINE-BERTRAND, and Y.A. FONTAINE. 1985b. Accumulation du monophosphate cyclique d'adénosine dans l'ovaire d'anguille (*Anguilla anguilla* L.), *in vitro* sous l'effet de la gonadotropine de carpe ou de la lutropine ovine: cinétique et thermodépendance. Biochimie (in press).

SAWYER, W.H., and P.K.T. PANG. 1979. Responses of vertebrates to neurohypophysial principles. pp. 493-523 *In* Barrington, E.J.W. [ed.] Hormones and evolution, vol. 2. Academic Press, New York.

SOWER, S.A., W.W. DICKHOFF, A. GORBMAN, J.E. RIVIER, and W.W. VALE. 1983. Ovulatory and steroidal responses in the lamprey following administration of salmon gonadtropin and agonistic and antagonistic analogues of gonadotropin-releasing hormone. Can. J. Zool. **61**: 2653-2659.

STEWART, J.K., C.J. GOODNER, D.J. KOERKER, A. GORBMAN, J. ENSINK, and M. KAUFMAN. 1978. Evidence of a biological role of somatostatin in the Pacific hagfish, *Eptatretus stoutii*. Gen. comp. Endocrinol. **36**: 408-414.

SYVANEN, M. 1985. Cross species gene transfer: implications for a new theory of evolution. J. theor. Biology. **112**: 333-344.

TAKADA, K., and S. ISHII. 1985. Specific gonadotropin binding sites in the bullfrog testis. Gen. comp. Endocrinol. in press.

TONON, M.C., P. LEROUX, F. LEBOULENGER, C. DELARUE, S. JEGOU, and H. VAUDRY. 1980. Thryrotropin-releasing hormone stimulates the release of melanotropin from frog neurointermediate lobes *in vitro*. Life Sci. **26**: 869-875.

VAN DER KRAAK, G. 1983. An introduction to gonadotropin receptor studies in fish. pp. 405-441 *In* Hoar, W.S., D.J. Randall, and E.M. Donaldson. [eds.] Fish physiology, vol. IX. Academic Press, New York.

VERHAERT, P. S. MARIVOET, F. VANDESANDE, and A. DE LOOF. 1984. Localization of CRF immunoreactivity in the central nervous system of three vertebrate and one insect species. Cell Tissue Res. **238**: 49-53.

WALLIS, M. 1981. The molecular evolution of pituitary growth hormone, prolactin and placental lactogen: a protein family showing variable rates of evolution. J. mol. Evol. **17**: 10-18.

WILSON, A.C., S.S. CARLSON, and T.J. WHITE. 1977. Biochemical evolution. Ann Rev. Biochem. **46**: 573-639.

WRIGHT, G.M. 1983. Immunocytochemical study of luteinizing hormone in the pituitary of the sea lamprey, *Petromyzon marinus* L., during its upstream migration. Cell Tissue Res. **230**: 225-228.

WRIGHT, C.M. 1984. Immunocytochemical study of growth hormone, prolactin, and thyroid-stimulating hormone in the adenohypophysis of the sea lamprey, *Petromyzon marinus* L., during its upstream migration. Gen. comp. Endocrinol. **55**: 269-274.

TISSUE DISTRIBUTION OF HORMONAL PEPTIDES IN PRIMITIVE FISHES

Masumi Nozaki

Primate Research Institute
Kyoto University
Inuyama, Aichi 484 Japan

Introduction

Anatomically, the pituitary gland of the cyclostomes consists of the same two principal elements that are found in all other vertebrates: a neurohypophysis develops from the floor of the diencephalon as an infundibular extension, and an adenohypophysis develops from the epithelium that comes in contact with this infundibulum (see reviews by Hardisty, 1979; Gorbman, 1983b). Functionally, the role of the cyclostome pituitary has proven difficult to define. The enigma of the cyclostome pituitary is that evolution of a composite organ with such a complex double developmental origin must have been associated with some functionally adaptive value. Yet demonstration of this adaptive value in the cyclostomes themselves remains dubious. The most striking feature of the cyclostome pituitary is that the neurohypophysis and the pars distalis (or entire adenohypophysis in hagfish) are separated by a thick sheet of virtually avascular connective tissue (see review by Gorbman, 1980). Accordingly, one of several serious concerns about the cyclostome pituitary is how hypophysiotropic material (if it exists) could reach the adenohypophysis. Furthermore, gonadotropic activity is undetectable or may be limited to stimulation of steroidogenesis in cyclostomes (see review by Gorbman, 1983a). Weak ACTH activity in pituitary and brain tissues has been reported in both the lamprey (Eastman and Portanova, 1982; Baker and Buckingham, 1983) and the hagfish (Buckingham *et al.*, 1985). However, these apparently low levels of ACTH were determined by procedures that themselves require validation for use in measuring heterologous hormones (Nozaki and Gorbman, 1984). As to thyrotropin, prolactin, and growth hormone, there is no clear evidence to suggest the presence of such hormones (see reviews by Larsen and Rothwell, 1972; Hardisty, 1979; Hardisty and Baker, 1982). The only clear results have been obtained for the presence of MSH activity in the lamprey (Baker and Buckingham, 1983).

Immunocytochemistry has provided a new approach to the study of evolution of functional properties of the pituitary gland. This review, while focussing upon information from our own immunocytochemical studies with cyclostomes, will outline other current information available at this time. The information reported herein may provide insights into the perplexing brain and pituitary relationship in the cyclostomes, and may also provide a phylogenetic basis for better understanding the function of several neuropeptides in the brain and/or pituitary.

Pro-opiocortin-related peptides in lamprey pituitary and brain

Although it is inconclusive, there is some evidence that suggests the presence of ACTH and MSH in the lamprey (see review by Hardisty and Baker, 1982). Therefore, it could be expected that ACTH and its precursor pro-opiocortin-related peptides might be found in the pituitary and/or brain of the lamprey. We applied a series of antibodies to peptides that are related by virtue of the fact that they are subunits of the same precursor pro-opiocortin (Fig. 1), to anadromous adults of two species of lampreys, *Petromyzon marinus* and *Entosphenus tridentata*. Specificities and cross-reactivities of these antibodies have been described elsewhere (Nozaki and Gorbman, 1984).

Results obtained are summarized in Figure 2.

Pars distalis

In both species of lampreys, most cells of the rostral pars distalis (RPD) and some cells of the caudal pars distalis (CPD) showed an intense positive reaction toward anti-Met-enkephalin (Figs. 2 and 3a, d). Some of these cells also showed positive reaction toward anti-γ-endorphin (Fig. 2). However, results for pro-γ-MSH, ACTH, α-MSH or ß-endorphin were consistently negative in the lamprey pars distalis. The Met-enkephalin positive reaction in the lamprey pituitary was

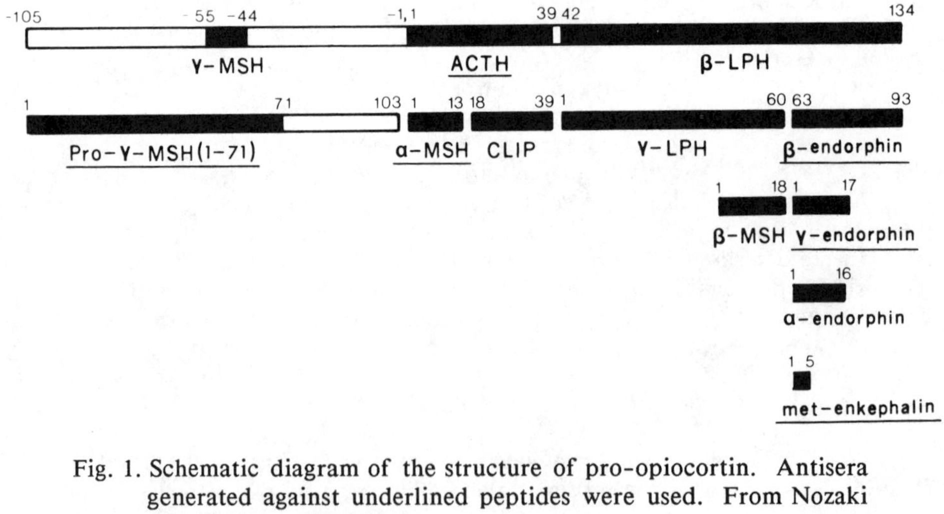

Fig. 1. Schematic diagram of the structure of pro-opiocortin. Antisera generated against underlined peptides were used. From Nozaki and Gorbman (1984).

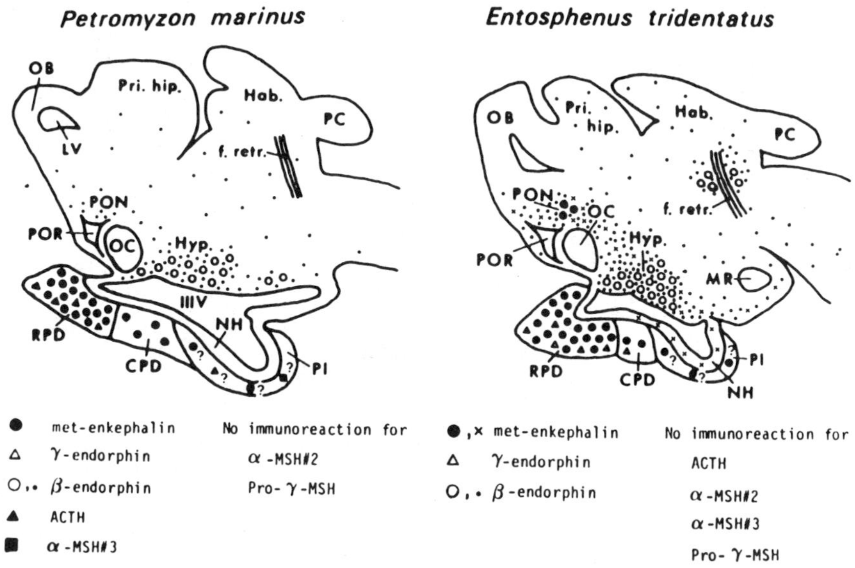

Fig. 2. Diagrammatic nearly-midsagittal sections of the brain of *Petromyzon marinus* and *Entosphenus tridentata*, showing the occurrence and localization of immunoreactive sites for several components of pro-opiocortin. Large symbols indicate adenohypophysial cells and nerve perikarya bearing immunoreactivities for corresponding peptides, and small symbols (x and .) show nerve fibers bearing immunoreactivities for Met-enkephalin and ß-endorphin, respectively. From Nozaki and Gorbman (1984).

eliminated by preabsorption with synthetic Met-enkephalin, but in order to eliminate the positive reaction in the lamprey (in contrast to the rat) a more than ten times greater amount of Met-enkephalin was needed. Furthermore, the Met-enkephalin-positive reaction was not eliminated by preabsorption with Leu-enkephalin, if the amount was very large. In the rat, preabsorption with Leu-enkephalin resulted in complete elimination of the Met-enkephalin immunoreactivity. In further disagreement with the results in rats, in the lamprey the γ-endorphin-positive reaction was eliminated by the preabsorption with Met-enkephalin as well as γ-endorphin. In the rat pars distalis, preabsorption with Met-enkephalin had no effect. Thus, it could be concluded that although the Met-enkephalin/γ-endorphin-positive material in the lamprey pituitary is immunologically related to Met-enkephalin, it evidently is not identical with Met-enkephalin nor γ-endorphin. Furthermore, this Met-enkephalin/γ-endorphin-positive material in the lamprey pars distalis is not sufficiently related to other pro-opiocortin constituents to permit immunological cross-reaction. Thus, the Met-enkephalin/γ-endorphin-positive cells do not correspond to corticotrophs of more advanced vertebrates.

Pars intermedia

In both species, the reaction for α-MSH or ACTH in the pars intermedia was questionable or absent (Fig. 2). In *Petromyzon*, apparently positive though weak α-MSH-like immunoreactivity was found in some cells of the pars intermedia, but was demonstrable by only one (anti-α-MSH#3) of two anti-α-MSH antibodies (Fig. 2). In *Petromyzon*, a similar slight and questionable type of ACTH-like immunoreactivity was found in some cells of the pars intermedia (Fig. 2). In *Entosphenus*, either α-MSH-like or ACTH-like immunoreactivity was absent altogether (Fig. 2). On the other hand, Met-enkephalin-positive reaction was consistently found in some cells of the pars intermedia of both lamprey species (Fig. 2). However, certain features of immunoreaction such as inconsistency of staining intensities among cells, diffusiveness of stained material within the cytoplasm and lack of cross-reaction to anti-γ-endorphin suggested that a cross-reaction to some other peptides, rather than the specific reaction, had occurred. Accordingly, the Met-enkephalin-positive material in the pars intermedia cells does not seem to be identical to that in the pars distalis. Results of the applications of other antisera were consistently negative in the pars intermedia of either species of lampreys (Fig. 2).

Hypothalamus and neurohypophysis

In contrast to the adenohypophysis, ß-endorphin-like immunoreactivity was a consistent feature in the brain (Fig. 2). In both species, ß-endorphin-positive perikarya were found in the ventral hypothalamus, and the positive fibers were distributed in many parts of the brain (Fig. 2). In the neurohypophysis, however, such positive fibers were not observed, while they were numerous in the adjacent hypothalamic region (Fig. 2). In *Entosphenus*, but not in *Petromyzon*, ß-endorphin-positive perikarya were also found in the dorsal thalamus (Fig. 2). Surprisingly, these ß-endorphin-positive neurons also exhibited positive reaction to anti-somatostatin, as mentioned later. In *Entosphenus* only, Met-enkephalin-positive material was observed in certain neurons of the preoptico-neurohypophysial system (Fig. 2), and ß-endorphin-positive and Met-enkephalin-positive materials were distributed in different neuronal elements (Fig. 2). However, results for other pro-opiocortin constituents were consistently negative in the brain of either species of lampreys (Fig. 2).

Met-enkephalin- and substance P-responses in adult and larval lampreys

The surprisingly low ACTH bioactivity (Baker and Buckingham, 1983) and immunoreactivity (Nozaki and Gorbman, 1984), in the presence of Met-enkephalin-like immunoreactivity in the pars distalis of the lamprey (Nozaki and Gorbman, 1984) prompted the further study of this question in *Petromyzon marinus* in specimens at two stages of the life cycle: anadromous adults and free-living ammocoete larvae. In addition, we have studied pituitary localization of material immunoreacting with anti-substance P (SP) antibody. We found such immunoreactivity in a preliminary test, and note that SP-like immunoreactivity has been reported in the guinea pig thyrotroph cells by DePalatis *et al.* (1982). Furthermore, the regional association between SP and Met-enkephalin has been shown by Hökfelt *et al.* (1977) in the mammalian brain, and these two peptides have mutually antagonistic physiological action in the brain (Jessel and Iversen, 1977).

Adults

As mentioned before, an immunoreaction to anti-Met-enkephalin was found in most cells of the RPD and a few cells of the CPD (Fig. 2 and 3a, d). In addition, an immunoreaction to one (anti-SP#1) of three anti-SP sera (for characterization of these anti-SP sera, see Nozaki and Gorbman, 1985) was found in certain pars distalis cells. However, the positive response to anti-SP#1 in *Petromyzon* pituitary was not eliminated by preabsorption with SP or SP-related peptides. Thus, the results obtained by preabsorption tests and lack of immunoreaction to other anti-SP sera, indicate that anti-SP#1-positive material in *Petromyzon* pituitary is not related to SP. The chemical nature of this material cannot be deduced at the present time. However, like a histological stain, the staining response in the pars distalis cells was selective and differential. By this means, the SP response was found in about half of the CPD cells (Fig. 3c, f). Most of the stained cells were limited to the dorsal portion, and the number of stained cells decreased gradually in the ventral direction (Fig. 3f). In the RPD, only a few scattered cells were stained with anti-SP#1 (Fig. 3c).

To better relate anti-Met-enkephalin- and anti-SP#1-positive cells to a more classical index of glycoprotein hormone distribution, Gomori's aldehyde fuchsin (AF) stain was applied, followed by the counterstains chromotrope 2R, orange G, and light green. In adult *Petromyzon*, a majority of cells in the RPD were AF-positive/light green positive (Fig. 3b, e). It was apparent that this predominant cell type is Met-enkephalin-like immunoreactive as well, to judge from the cell numbers and their position. However, there seemed to be a tendency in pituitaries of individuals exhibiting weak staining with anti-Met-enkephalin for a relatively stronger AF-positive reaction and *vice versa.* A majority of the CPD cells were chromophobic with the AF-stain: a few scattered cells contained AF-positive material (Fig. 3b). Cells stained by anti-SP#1 corresponded to one of the chromophobes, and cells containing Met-enkephalin-like immunoreactivity corresponded to the AF-positive cells or to a second type of chromophobe.

Ammocoetes

When anti-Met-enkephalin was applied to the larval *Petromyzon*, most cells of the RPD and a few solitary cells of the CPD showed intense positive reaction (Fig. 4a, b). The proportion of Met-enkephalin-positive cells and intensities of immunoreaction in the pars distalis cells of the ammocoetes were similar to or greater than in the adults (Fig. 4a, b). Accordingly, it appears that Met-enkephalin-positive cells in the pars distalis are as active in larvae as in adults.

On the other hand, the SP-response was limited to a few cells of the CPD, and no cells in the RPD were stained (Fig. 4d, e). The apparent intensities of such SP-positive cells were also less than in adults (Fig. 4d, e). Thus, the CPD cells reacting with anti-SP#1 appear at very low level in the larvae and grow in number and intensity of staining in a time pattern that parallels development of reproductive capacity.

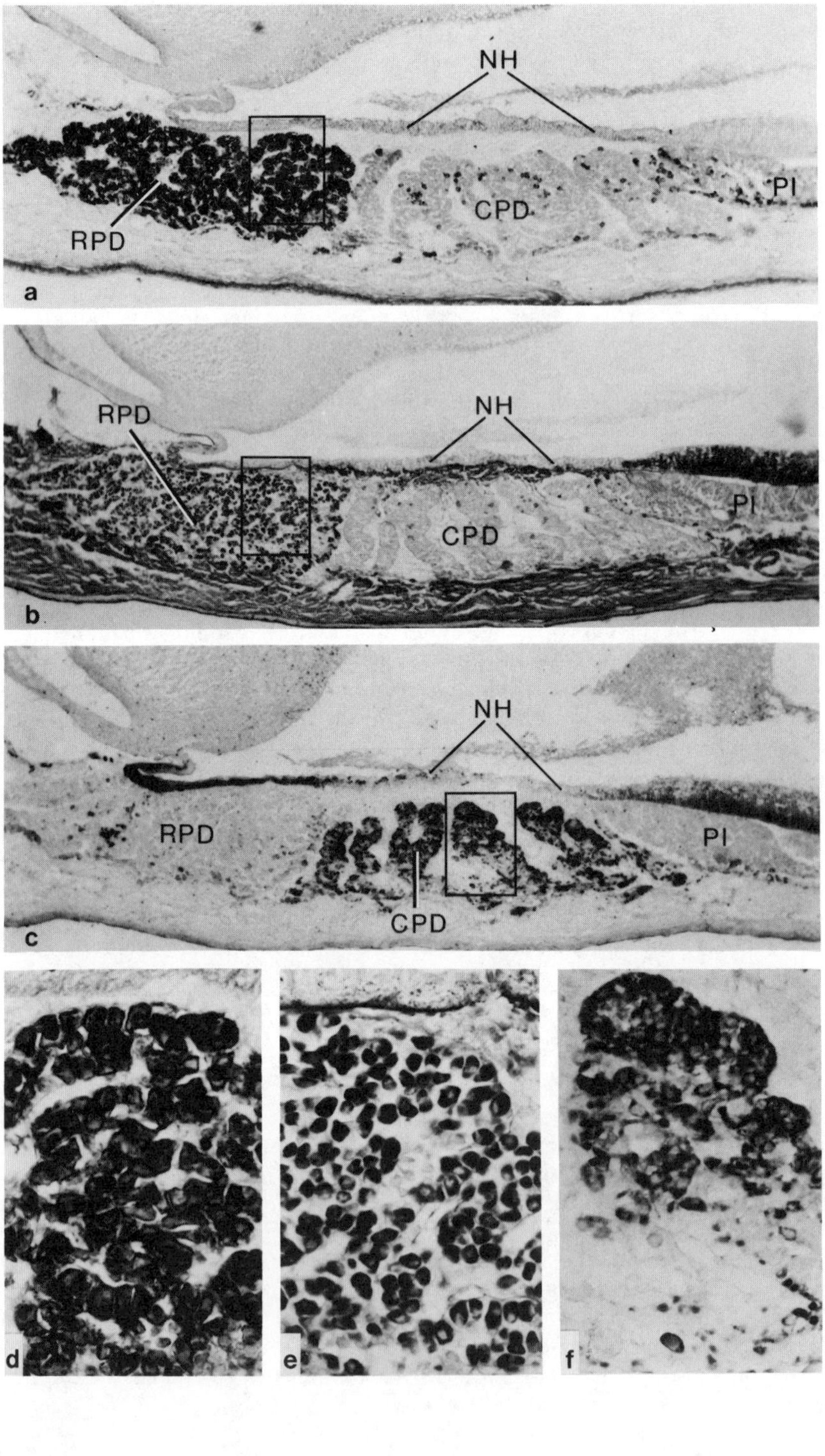
NH
RPD
CPD
PI
a
RPD
NH
CPD
PI
b
NH
RPD
CPD
PI
c
d
e
f

When adjacent sections were stained with Gomori's AF, no AF-positive cellular material was found in the adenohypophysis. In the RPD, the dominant cell type was light green-positive (fig. 4c), but a considerable proportion of chromophobes also was observed (Fig. 4c). Thus, in the ammocoetes both light green-positive and chromophobic cells correlated with Met-enkephalin-like immunoreactivity.

General discussion on the lamprey pituitary

Our study shows that in two species of lampreys the pars distalis lacks ACTH-like immunoreactivity, but it clearly reacts with antibodies for Met-enkephalin and γ-endorphin. In both species the reaction for α-MSH in the pars intermedia is questionable or absent, while Met-enkephalin-like immunoreactivity is a consistent feature there. A similar study has been done by Dores *et al.* (1984) in adult *Lampetra lamotteni.* They also found Met-enkephalin-like immunoreactivity in cells of the RPD and in the pars intermedia. Moreover, they observed that Met-enkephalin-positive cells of the RPD were also reactive to one of several anti-ACTH sera which was directed against the middle portion of the ACTH molecule, and further that Met-enkephalin-positive cells of the pars intermedia were reactive to another kind of anti-ACTH serum which was directed against the N-terminal portion of ACTH and α -MSH. Both our and their studies suggest that if a pro-opiocortin-related prohormone exists in the lamprey, it is appreciably different from those of more advanced vertebrates. The difference of MSH molecules between lamprey and other higher vertebrates has also been shown by the study of Baker and Buckingham (1983), who reported that extracts of neurointermediate lobe of *Lampetra fluviatilis* have MSH activity in an *Anolis* skin bioassay but they are not reactive in an immunoassay using an α-MSH antibody, and further that the electrophoretic Rf value of lamprey MSH activity was distinct from both α-MSH and des-Ac-α-MSH. In the same paper, Baker and Buckingham (1983) reported that ACTH activity of the pars distalis extracts of *Lampetra fluviatilis* was approximately 1000 times less than those found in mammals, and that brain extracts showed only low MSH activity, and again no immunoreactivity. Taking all findings mentioned above into consideration, pars distalis cells reactive to antibodies for Met-enkephalin and the middle portion of ACTH, and pars intermedia cells reactive to antibodies for Met-enkephalin and α-MSH seem to be the most likely sources of the ACTH activity and MSH activity, respectively.

Our study also shows that Met-enkephalin-positive cells of the RPD are as active in larvae as in adults. In agreement with this, Percy *et al.* (1975) have

Fig. 3. Three adjacent, but not exactly successive sagittal sections (*a-c*) passing through the hypothalamo-hypophysial region of an adult *Petromyzon marinus* showing Met-enkephalin-like immunoreactivity (*a*), Gomori's AF-positive material (*b*), and positive response to anti SP#1 (*c*) in the pars distalis cells. The rectangular areas in *a-c* are enlarged and shown in *d-f*, respectively. From Nozaki and Gorbman (1985).

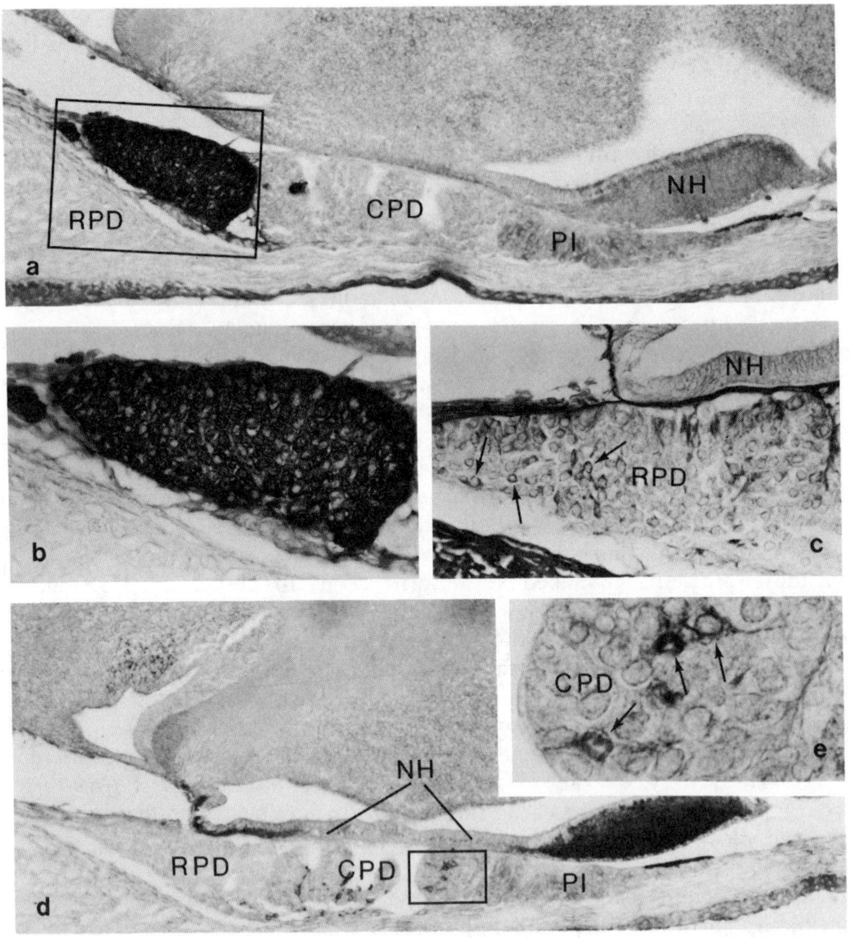

Fig. 4. Three sagittal sections *a, c,* and *d*) prepared from the same specimen passing through the hypothalamo-hypophysial region of the larval *Petromyzon marinus*. They were stained with anti-Met-enkephalin (*a*), Gomori's AF, followed by counterstains chromotrope 2R, orange G and light green (*c*), and anti-SP#1 (*d*). The rectangular areas in *a* and *d* are enlarged and shown in *b* and *e*, respectively. Note that in *a* and *b*, most cells of the RPD show intense Met-enkephalin-positive reaction, whereas in *c*, several cells of the RPD are stained with light green (arrows), but AF-positive material is absent. Also note that in *d* and *e*, a few cells of the CPD show positive response to anti-SP#1 (arrows). From Nozaki and Gorbman (1985).

reported that, in *Petromyzon marinus*, on the basis of electron microscopy, granulated cells can be detected in the RPD of the ammocoetes, even in the younger larvae within two years of hatching, while the CPD appears inactive and is almost completely devoid of granulated cells up to the onset of metamorphosis. It is most likely that our Met-enkephalin-positive cells correspond to the granulated cells of the rostral pars distalis of Percy *et al.* (1975). These findings strongly suggest that Met-enkephalin-positive cells may be involved in functions other than reproduction. Thus, this view may also support the possibility that the Met-enkephalin-positive cells may be the source of ACTH activity found in the lamprey pituitary by Baker and Buckingham (1983).

In contrast with our view, it has been proposed that basophils of the rostral pars distalis of the lamprey are possibly gonadotrophs, because they characteristically develop during the period of sexual maturation (see review by Larsen and Rothwell, 1972; Hardisty and Baker, 1982). As clearly shown in this study, Met-enkephalin-positive cells of the rostral pars distalis are basophilic with respect to the histological stain used. Thus, they may correspond to the presumptive gonadotrophs of earlier studies. This discrepancy seems to derive in part from the correlation, or negative correlation of AF-positive material and Met-enkephalin-like immunoreactivity: AF-positive material is completely absent from the RPD in the ammocoetes, while Met-enkephalin-like immunoreactivity is very intense there in the same specimens. Furthermore, mammalian TSH-like immunoreactivity has been shown in basophils of the RPD (Wright, 1984), which may correspond to our Met- enkephalin-positive cells. However, there is indeed little or no direct evidence that the lamprey pituitary controls thryroid function (Holmes and Ball, 1974; Pickering, 1976). Clearly, further studies and additional information are required to evaluate the possible function of so- called "basophils" of the lamprey RPD, which show Met-enkephalin-like, ACTH-like and TSH-like immunoreactivities (Nozaki and Gorbman, 1984, 1985; Dores *et al.*, 1984; Wright, 1984).

The cells of the CPD of the lamprey are more difficult to interpret than those of the RPD and this is especially true of the several kinds of active chromophobes (see review by Hardisty, 1979). Our immunocytochemical data show that in adult *Petromyzon* the CPD cells stained with anti-SP#1 are mainly limited to the dorsal half of the region and such cells stained with anti-Met-enkephalin are relatively few in number. Accordingly, most cells of the ventral half of the CPD remain uncharacterized as to immunostaining affinity. Therefore, one or more additional types of cells seem to be present in the CPD. Ultrastructural observations which have been made on the pituitary of the adult lamprey concur with our observations: electron microscopy has revealed three to four types of cells in the CPD (see reviews by Hardisty, 1979; Hardisty and Baker, 1982). The following immunoreactive materials toward anti-mammalian pituitary hormones have been demonstrated there: LH-like (Wright, 1983), growth hormone-like (Wright, 1984), prolactin-like (Wright, 1984), γ-LPH-like (Dores *et al.*, 1984) and Met-enkephalin-like immunoreactivities (Nozaki and Gorbman, 1984). Among these, only Met-enkephalin-positive cells and growth hormone-positive cells appear to correspond to the basophils and lead-hematoxylin-positive cells of standard light microscope stain, respectively. Cells containing other immunoreactivities may correspond to the chromophobes of that region. As is obvious from all of the literature that has appeared during the last two years, this field is now being pursued actively, and still other immunoreactivities may be found in the lamprey CPD. Accordingly, it is possible that some of these immunoreactivities may coexist in the same cells.

Our study has revealed that the CPD cells reacting with anti-SP#1 are few in larvae, and grow in number and intensity of staining in a time pattern that parallels development of reproductive capacity. Thus, this type of cell is at least a candidate for involvement in reproductive function. Larsen's hypophysectomy experiments seem to support this possibility: extirpation of the rostral pars distalis alone did not prevent the attainment of sexual maturity, but complete inhibition of sexual maturity occurred when both the caudal and rostral pars distalis were removed (Larsen, 1965, 1969; Larsen and Rothwell, 1972). However, the same possibility could hold true for other type(s) of cells in the CPD beyond those we have immunostained so far. Thus, the mere correlation of such immunoreactivity with passive adenohypophysial hormonal function clearly remains to be evaluated.

Pro-opiocortin-related peptides in hagfish pituitary

We have applied the following antibodies toward pro-opiocortin constituents to the pituitary of the hagfish (*Eptatretus burgeri* and *Eptatretus stouti*): antisera generated against pro-γ-MSH, ACTH, α-MSH, endorphin, ß-endorphin, α-endorphin and Met-enkephalin (for characterizations of these antibodies, see Nozaki and Gorbman, 1984; Nozaki *et al.*, 1984b). It was found that none of the antibodies showed a positive reaction in the hagfish adenohypophysis.

In contrast to our negative results, Buckingham *et al.* (1985) have recently reported low levels of ACTH activity in the extracts of the pituitary and brain of the hagfish. As Buckingham *et al.* (1985) have suggested, corticotrophic factor in the hagfish may differ structurally and immunochemically from its mammalian counterpart. In this connection, the observations of Jirikowski *et al.* (1984) are of interest. They have demonstrated enkephalin-related FMRF-amide-like immunoreactivity in both the brain and adenohypophysis of the hagfish. This material may have an ACTH activity.

Neurohypophysial hormone

We used antibodies for arginine vasopressin (AVP) and oxytocin. In both lamprey (*Petromyzon marinus*) and hagfish (*Eptatretus stouti*), anti-AVP yielded positive reaction in the brain, while anti-oxytocin failed to do so. Since arginine vasotocin (AVT) is the only neurohypophysial hormone in the cyclostomes (Acher, 1974), and our anti-AVP reacts with both AVP and AVT, but not with lysine vasopressin or oxytocin, it is highly probable that AVP-positive reaction in the cyclostome brain is due to AVT.

By this means, two discrete regions were found in the lamprey presumptive AVT-containing perikarya: one was located in the arc-shaped (in a sagittal plane) preoptic nucleus and the other in the posterior hypothalamic nucleus (Fig. 5).

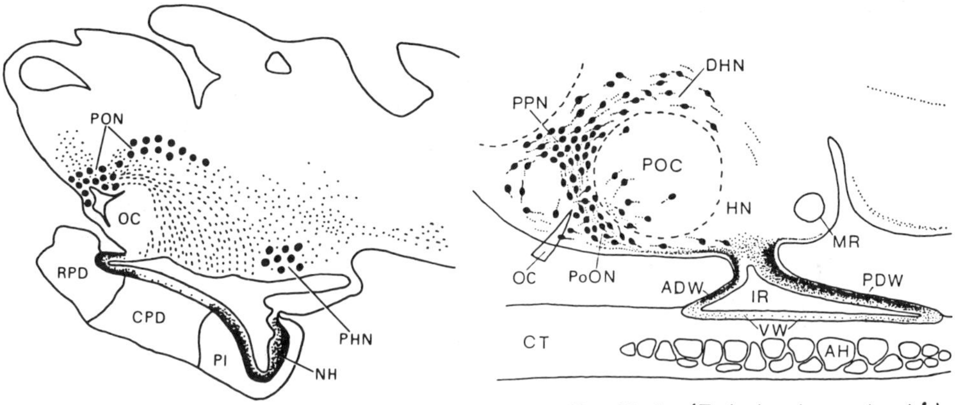

Lamprey *(Petromyzon marinus)* Hagfish *(Eptatretus stouti)*

Fig. 5. Topographic distributions of presumed AVT-containing perikarya (circles) and fibers (broken lines) in the brain of the sea lamprey (left) and Pacific hagfish (right), projected on nearly mid-sagittal planes. Lamprey, from Nozaki *et al.* (1984b), and hagfish from Nozaki and Gorbman (1983).

Positive fibers from the preoptic nucleus proceeded primarily to the neurohypophysis, with some fibers reaching the lower brainstem (Fig. 5). In the neurohypophysis, they were grouped together in the rostral part of the anterior neurohypophysis and posterior neurohypophysis (Fig. 5). Accordingly, only a few fibers could be found in the caudal part of the anterior neurohypophysis (Fig. 5). The ultimate destination of the fibers from the posterior hypothalamic nucleus could not be determined. The above-mentioned results are quite consistent with data from earlier studies using the traditional methods of staining for neurosecretory materials (Oztan and Gorbman, 1960; Sterba, 1972), and also agree well with those reported in *Lampetra fluviatilis* by Goossens *et al.* (1977) who used a specific antibody for AVT.

In the hagfish, presumptive AVT-positive perikarya were distributed in an extended area from the posterior part of the preoptic nucleus more caudally to the anterior part of the hypothalamic nucleus (Fig. 5). Most of the positive perikarya were located close to the paired prehypophysial arterial network near the anterior end of the postoptic nucleus (Fig. 5). In the neurohypophysis, positive fibers were concentrated along the dorsal walls with a few along the ventral wall (Fig. 5). Thus, in the hagfish, AVT may be released (1) directly from the perikarya into the capillaries of the prehypophysial plexus, from which portal vessels drain toward the neurohypophysis (Gorbman *et al.*, 1963), and (2) from the nerve terminals of the neurohypophysis into the hypophysial vein. The prehypophysial plexus, a puzzlingly placed portal system in the hagfish, thus may represent an evolutionary anatomical precursor to the neurohypophysis, and a more primitive neurosecretory arrangement.

LHRH

We used two different anti-mammalian LHRH antibodies (anti-LHRH#1 and #2). Anti-LHRH#1 can recognize both N-terminal and C-terminal regions of the LHRH molecule, but can bind more strongly to the C-terminal region, whereas anti-LHRH#2 can bind only to the N-terminal region of the LHRH molecule (Nozaki *et al.*, 1984a). For better understanding of the localization of LHRH-like immunoreactivity in the brain of lower vertebrates in general, results obtained in the Japanese eel (*Anguilla japonica*), leopard shark (*Triakis scyllia*), lamprey (*Entosphenus japonicus*, *Petromyzon marinus*), and hagfish (*Eptatretus burgeri*, *E. stouti*) are described.

In the Japanese eel, anti-LHRH#1 and #2 gave similar results. In the eel, LHRH-positive perikarya were found in the distal and proximal ganglia of the nervus terminalis (terminal nerve), and ventro-lateral portions of the ventral telencephalon and preoptic area (Fig. 6). The LHRH-positive fibers projected primarily to the neurohypophysis, where most of such fibers terminated in the caudal part of the anterior neurohypophysis just dorsal to the proximal pars distalis (Fig. 6). Some positive fibers proceeding toward the olfactory epithelium, rostral telencephalon, retina, optic tectum, and lower brainstem were also observed (Fig. 6). These results obtained in the eel brain generally agree with those obtained in other teleostean species and also with those reported in higher vertebrates (see reviews by Barry, 1979; Nozaki *et al.*, 1984a).

In the shark, anti-LHRH#1 and #2 also gave similar results. However, in the shark, positive reaction was almost limited to the nervus terminalis system (Fig. 6): a pair of thick LHRH-positive fiber bundles, composing the nervus terminalis, enter the brain at the level of the pars septi of the telencephalon and diverge into several pathways at the rostral part of the forebrain stalk (Fig. 6). Accordingly, numerous immuno-positive fibers can be found in the telencephalon (Fig. 6). Some of these fibers terminate near the blood vessels which are distributed on the ventral surface of the forebrain stalk (Fig. 6). Although a few positive perikarya were found in the preoptic nucleus, positive fibers were scarce in the hypothalamus, and no such fibers were found in the median eminence (Fig. 6). Thus, the results obtained in the shark are somewhat unusual, since other gnathostome vertebrates so far studied have always showed the heaviest accumulation of positive fibers in the median eminence or the median eminence area of the neurohypophysis (see review by Nozaki, 1984a). This difference may be important when we consider that in the selachians gonadotropin-producing cells are located mainly in the ventral lobe, which is far distant from the median eminence, and has a blood supply completely separate from the median eminence system (see review by Ball, 1981). Further detailed studies are needed to elucidate the following problem in the selachians: from where is LHRH released into the systematic circulation or how could LHRH reach the ventral lobe?

In contrast to the eel and shark, in the lamprey a different distribution of substances reactive with anti-LHRH#1 and #2 was obtained. When anti-LHRH#1 was applied, positive perikarya were found in the preoptic nucleus and their fibers were projected to the neurohypophysis (Fig. 6). In the neurohypophysis, immuno-positive fibers were distributed throughout the external layer (Fig. 6). On the other

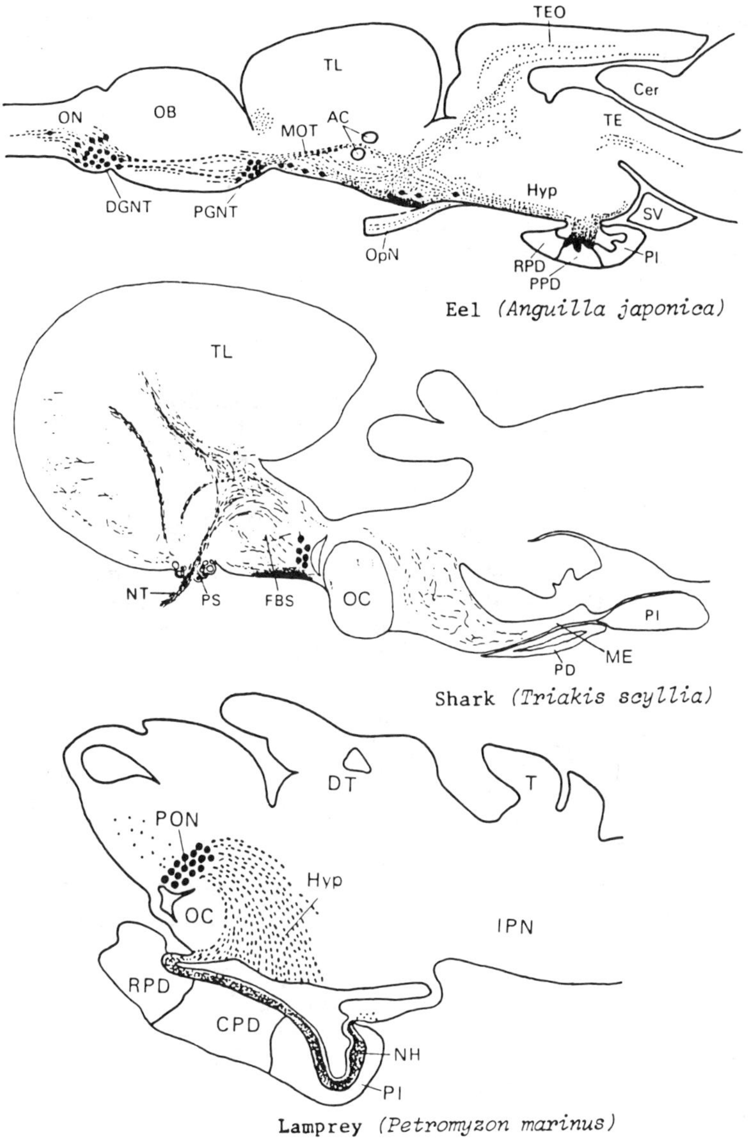

Fig. 6. Topographic distributions of LHRH-positive perikarya (circles) and fibers (broken lines or dots) in the brain of the Japanese eel (top), leopard shark (middle), and sea lamprey (bottom), projected on nearly mid-sagittal planes. Eel, from Nozaki *et al.* (1985), and shark and lamprey, from Nozaki *et al.* (1984b).

hand, anti-LHRH#2 revealed no positive perikarya or fibers in the brain, except for a few fibers in the neurohypophysis (Nozaki and Kobayashi, 1979). This finding suggests that the nature of immunoreactive LHRH of the lamprey is somewhat different from that of more advanced vertebrates, in which anti-LHRH#1 and #2 gave similar results (Nozaki *et al.*, 1984a). This view is supported by recent findings by Sherwood and Sower (1985), who reported that lamprey LHRH has a distinct HPLC elution pattern compared with dogfish shark, salmon and trout.

In the lamprey as well as the hagfish, anatomical structures for the transfer of hypothalamic influences to the pars distalis are lacking (see reviews by Hardisty, 1979; Ball, 1981). The finding that in the lamprey immunoreactive LHRH is present throughout the external layer may provide insights into the function of this perplexing anatomical relationship: LHRH may reach the pars distalis (1) by diffusion across the connective tissue sheet interposed between the anterior neurohypophysis and the pars distalis, or (2) via systemic circulation.

In the hagfish, no immunoreaction with either anti-LHRH#1 or #2 was found in the brain, including the neurohypophysis (Nozaki and Kobayashi, 1979). Similar negative results have been obtained in *Eptatretus stouti* by Crim *et al.* (1979: immunocytochemistry) and by Sherwood and Sower (1985: radioimmunoassay system). To explain the lack of LHRH-like immunoreactivity in the hagfish, two mutually exclusive possibilities could be considered. The hagfish may possess an LHRH-like substance that is undetectable by current immunochemical techniques because of lack of cross-reactivity with anti-mammalian LHRH, or an insufficient amount for visualization. Alternatively, the hagfish may actually lack LHRH-like substance. The latter possibility may be supported by the finding that total hypophysectomy in *Eptatretus stouti* provided no clear change in gonadal function (*i.e.*, histology of gonad, plasma testosterone and estradiol values: Matty *et al.*, 1976). This possibility is confounded, however, by the observations that partial hypophysectomy in *Eptatretus burgeri* resulted in slight retardation of spermatogenesis (Patzner and Ichikawa, 1977). Further studies are required to clarify these alternatives.

The nervus terminalis is now known to be present in some members of each class of gnathostome vertebrates, excepting the birds (Bullock and Northcutt, 1984). This cranial nerve, largely forgotten for over half a century, has suddenly regained prominence in neuroendocrinology, olfaction and sexual behavior and several other fields in the life sciences (Demski and Northcutt, 1983; Stell *et al.*, 1984). Particularly significant are reports that the nervus terminalis may mediate the reproductive responses toward sex pheromones (Demski and Northcutt, 1983). Our finding that the nervus terminalis system of the eel and shark contains LHRH-like immunoreactivity supports this hypothesis.

Somatostatin

We used two kinds of anti-somatostatin sera: one was generated against mammalian somatostatin, and the other against salmon somatostatin. To permit generalization, comparison is made here among several lower vertebrates: the Japanese eel (*Anguilla japonica*), leopard shark (*Triakis scyllia*), lamprey

(*Petromyzon marinus* and *Entosphenus tridentata*), and hagfish (*Eptatretus stouti*). In all species examined, anti-mammalian somatostatin and anti-salmon somatostatin gave essentially the same results.

In the Japanese eel, somatostatin-positive perikarya were found in several regions of the brain (Fig. 7): (1) telencephalon, where they were scattered throughout various regions of the hemisphere, (2) nucleus preopticus periventricularis, where they were concentrated, (3) nucleus lateralis tuberis, where they were scattered along the walls of the third venticle, (4 and 5) dorsomedial hypothalamus and dorsal thalamus, containing a few positive perikarya, and (6 and 7) two locations of the rhombencephalon. The heaviest accumulation of somatostatin-positive fibers was found in the neurohypophysis close to the proximal pars distalis (Fig. 7), with a few fibers in the neurohypophysis close to the rostral pars distalis or the pars intermedia (Fig. 7). A very dense network of positive fibers was observed also in the ventral hypothalamus and preoptic area (Fig. 7). Such fibers were also numerous in the telencephalon, dorsal thalamus and lower brainstem; in fact, some could be seen in virtually any part of the brain, though rarely in the olfactory bulb or cerebellum (Fig. 7). The precise origin of these somatostatin-fibers is still unclear. Above-mentioned results in the eel brain agree well with those noted in other teleostean species (Dubois *et al.*, 1979; Olivereau *et al.*, 1984), and are also very similar to those in the frog (Vandesande and Dierickx, 1980).

In the shark, somatostatin-positive perikarya were also observed in several brain regions (Fig. 7): (1) forebrain stalk, where several positive perikarya were scattered, (2) preoptic nucleus, where numerous such perikarya were concentrated, (3) infundibular region, containing a relatively large number of perikarya along the walls of the third ventricle, and (4) interpeduncular nucleus with numerous positive perikarya. The rhombencephalon caudal to the interpeduncular nucleus was not examined. There was an accumulation of somatostatin-positive terminals in the external layer of the posterior median eminence (Fig. 7), but such terminals were rare in the anterior median eminence. In the anterior median eminence many positive fibers were found, but they proceeded caudally to the posterior median eminence. Many positive fibers were also found in the forebrain stalk, preoptic area, infundibular region, mammillary body, and interpeduncular nucleus (Fig. 7). Thus, the topographic distribution of somatostatin-like immunoreactivity in the shark brain is virtually the same as that observed in the eel, although minor differences between the two species were observed in the dorsal thalamus and the dorsomedial hypothalamus.

In the lamprey, somatostatin-positive perikarya were found in the ventral hypothalamus, dorsal thalamus, and two locations of the rhombencephalon, but not in the preoptic nucleus (Fig. 7). In the ventral hypothalamus, numerous positive perikarya were found in the nuclear zone extending from a point just caudal to the optic chiasma to the level of the mammillary recess (Fig. 7). Somatostatin-positive perikarya of the dorsal thalamic group were concentrated about the fasciculus retroflexus (Fig. 7), while those of the rhombencephalic groups were scattered about. Somatostatin-positive fibers were abundant in the preoptic nucleus, ventral hypothalamus, tectum and interpeduncular nucleus (Fig. 7). In the neurohypophysis, however, no positive fibers were observed, although they were numerous in

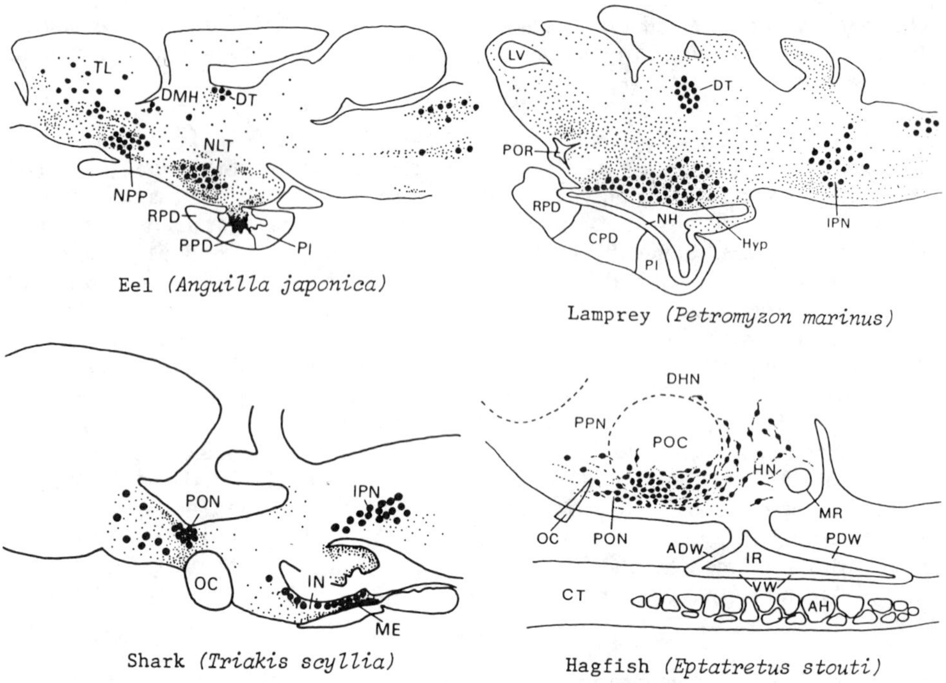

Fig. 7. Topographic distributions of somatostatin-positive perikarya (circles) and fibers (dots) in the brain of the Japanese eel (upper left), leopard shark (lower left), sea lamprey (upper right) and Pacific hagfish (lower right), projected on nearly mid-sagittal planes. Eel, shark and lamprey, from Nozaki *et al.* (1984b), and hagfish, from Nozaki and Gorbman (1983).

the adjacent hypothalamic region (Fig. 7). A possible explanation for the lack of somatostatin-positive fibers in the neurohypophysis of the lamprey will be presented below together with the description of the hagfish. In addition, in the lamprey, but not in other species, somatostatin-like immunoreactivity and ß-endorphin-like immunoreactivity coexist in the same neurons of both the hypothalamus and the dorsal thalamus.

In the hagfish, somatostatin-positive perikarya were found only in the ventral hypothalamus (Fig. 7). Although several short, stained fibers were observed in the vicinity of the perikarya, positive fibers were not found in the neurohypophysis, nor in any other part of the brain (Fig. 7).

Our data show that in both lamprey and hagfish, somatostatin-positive fibers are not found in the neurohypophysis, while they are present in the adjacent hypothalamic region. Since the topographic distribution of somatostatin-positive perikarya was somewhat similar among the fish species examined, our data may provide insight into the evolution of the function of somatostatin: that is, somatostatin may have evolved originally as a regulatory factor involved in brain and/or gut function, and later it may have developed a hypophysiotropic function. This may possibly explain the lack of somatostatin-fibers in the neurohypophysis of the lamprey and hagfish.

Coexistence of somatostatin-like and ß-endorphin-like immunoreactivities in the lamprey brain

During the course of the study, we noted that distributions of somatostatin-like and ß-endorphin-like immunoreactivities show a high degree of similarity in the brain of the lamprey, particularly in *Entosphenus tridentata* (cf., Fig. 2 *vs*. Fig. 7). In other species so far examined (*i.e.*, rat, chicken, snake, frog, eel, and shark), however, these immunoreactivities show quite distinct localizations. Therefore, localizations of somatostatin-like and ß-endorphin-like immunoreactivities were examined carefully in the brain of *Entosphenus tridentata* using pairs of thin adjacent sections: one section of each pair was stained with anti-mammalian somatostatin, while the adjacent section was stained with anti-ß-endorphin.

By this means, both in the ventral hypothalamus and in the dorsal thalamus of *Entosphenus*, most neurons that stained with anti-somatostatin were also stained with anti-ß-endorphin, whereas in the rhombencephalon only weakly stained neurons with anti-somatostatin were observed. These latter stainings were eliminated only when antibodies were preabsorbed with corresponding antigens. Thus, our data apparently show the coexistence of somatostatin-like and ß-endorphin-like immunoreactivities in the brain of *Entosphenus*. However, similarity of overall distributions of both immunoreactivities in the brain of the lamprey suggests that both immunoreactivities may form different parts of a common larger brain peptide. If this possibility is correct, a peptide containing somatostatin-like immunoreactivity of the lamprey brain seems to be somewhat different from its mammalian counterpart (somatostatin itself or somatostatin precursor).

Substance P

Three kinds of anti-substance P sera (anti-SP#1, #2 and #3) with specificities for different regions of the SP molecule were used (for characterizations of these antibodies, see Nozaki and Gorbman, 1985).

When these anti-SP sera were applied to the lampreys (*Petromyzon marinus* and *Entosphenus tridentata*), the two (anti-SP#1 and #2) which were directed against the C-terminal portion of the SP molecule showed positive reaction, while the other antiserum (#3) which was directed against the middle portion of the SP molecule did not. Following the preabsorption of anti-SP#1 or anti-SP#2 with SP or its related peptides, it was found that eledoisin-related peptide (Lys-Phe-Ile-Gly-Leu-Met-NH_2) was the most active in elimination of the positive reaction in the lamprey brain, and authentic "SP" itself was questionable. These results, together with the lack of immunoreaction to anti-SP#3, strongly suggest that SP-positive material in the lamprey brain is more closely related in terms of immunological determinants to eledoisin than to SP.

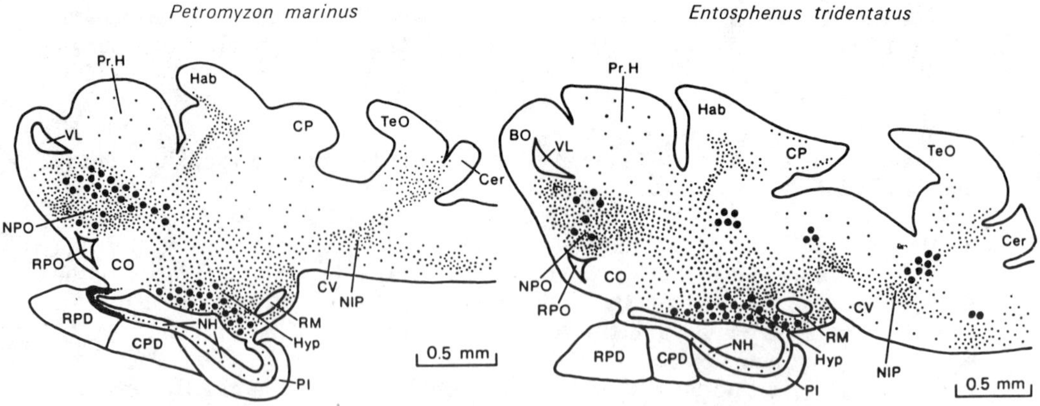

Fig. 8. Topographic distributions of substance P-positive perikarya (circles) and fibers (dots) in the brain of the lampreys, *Petromyzon marinus* (left) and *Entosphenus tridentata* (right), projected on nearly mid-sagittal planes. From Nozaki and Gorbman (unpublished).

By this means, as shown in Figure 8, in *Petromyzon* SP-positive perikarya were found in the ventrolateral telencephalon and ventral hypothalamus whereas in *Entosphenus* they were found in the ventral thalamus and three locations of the brainstem as well as the above-mentioned two regions. Nevertheless, the distributions of SP-positive fibers in brain regions other than the neurohypophysis were very similar between the two species (Fig. 8): SP-positive fibers were found in many brain locations, and were especially rich in the periventricular subependymal zone of the ventral telencephalon and of the diencephalon, preoptic area, hypothalamus and interpeduncular nucleus. In the neurohypophysis of *Petromyzon*, a heavy accumulation of positive fibers was observed in the rostral part of the anterior neurohypophysis (Fig. 8), but in *Entosphenus* no stained fibers were observed there (Fig. 8). These results suggest the presence of a definite neuronal system containing an SP-related peptide, of unknown function, in the brain of the lamprey.

In the hagfish (*Eptatretus stouti*), no immunoreaction was found in the brain after the applications of these anti-SP sera.

Conclusion

Our study has shown that various neuropeptide-like materials similar to those found in more advanced gnathostome vertebrates can be found in the lamprey brain and/or pituitary, but the chemical natures of most such materials are somewhat different from their mammalian counterparts (*i.e.*, pro-opiocortin-related peptides, LHRH, SP, and probably somatostatin as well). Thus, the lamprey may possess ancestral stem molecules of such neuropeptides. To further explore the evolution of the function of such neuropeptides and the unusual brain to pituitary relationships in the cyclostomes, the elucidation of the primary structures of lamprey neuropeptides is now required.

On the other hand, the hagfish has yielded largely negative results in tests for the presence of a variety of neuropeptides, most of which are found in the lamprey (*i.e.*, pro-opiocortin-related peptides, LHRH, SP, present study; TRH, neurotensin, Tsukahara *et al.*, 1983; Nozaki *et al.*, 1984b). Various neuropeptide-like materials reactive with antibodies to mammalian brain and/or gut peptides have been demonstrated even in certain species of several phyla of invertebrates (*i.e.*, tunicates, Fritsch *et al.*, 1979, 1982; molluscs, Schot *et al.*, 1981). For the hagfish, during its adaptive evolution to very stable living conditions, a progressive regression may have created what seems now to be a simple organization of the brain and other organs. It is possible that a number of peptides in the hagfish may have been eliminated during evolution, or more precisely, regression.

Abbreviations in Figures 1-8.

AC: anterior commissure; **ADW**: anterior dorsal wall of the neurohypophysis; **AH**: adenohypophysis; **BO**: olfactory bulb; **Cer**: cerebellum; **CO**: optic chiasma; **CP**: posterior commisure; **CPD**: caudal pars distalis; **CT**: connective tissue; **CV**: ventral commissure; **DGNT**: distal ganglion of the nervus terminalis; **DHN**: dorsal hypothalamic nucleus; **DMH**: dorsomedial hypothalamus; **DT**: dorsal thalamus; **FBS**: forebrain stalk; **f. retr.**: fasciculus retroflexus; **Hab**: *habenula;* **HN**: hypothalamic nucleus; **Hyp**: hypothalamus; **IN**: infundibular nucleus; **IPN**: interpeduncular nucleus; **IR**: infundibular recess; **LV**: lateral ventricle; **ME**: median eminence; **MOT**: medial olfactory tract; **MR**: mammillary recess; **NH**: neurohypophysis; **NIP**: nucleus interpeduncularis; **NLT**: nucleus lateralis tuberis; **NPO**: nucleus preopticus; **NPP**: nucleus preopticus periventricularis; **NT**: nervus terminalis; **OB**: olfactory bulb; **OC**: optic chiasma; **ON**: olfactory nerve; **OpN**: optic nerve; **PC**: posterior commissure; **PD**: pars distalis; **PDW**: posterior dorsal wall of the neurohypophysis; **PHN**: posterior hypothalamic nucleus; **PI**: pars intermedia; **Pit**: pituitary; **POC**: postoptic commissure; **PGNT**: proximal ganglion of the nervus terminalis; **PON**: preoptic nucleus; **PoOT**: postoptic nucleus; **POR**: preoptic recess; **PPD**: proximal pars distalis; **PPN**: posterior part of the preoptic nucleus; **Pr. H.**: primordium hippocampi; **Pri. Hip.**: primordium hippocampi; **PS**: pars septi of the telencephalon; **RM**: mammillary recess; **RPD**: rostral pars distalis; **RPO**: preoptic recess; **SV**: saccus vasculosus; **T**: optic tectum; **TE**: mesencephalic tegmentum; **TEO**: optic tectum; **TeO**: optic tectum; **TL**: telencephalon; **VL**: lateral ventricle; **VW**: ventral wall of the neurohypophysis; **IIIV**: third ventricle.

Literature Cited

ACHER, R. 1974. Chemistry of the neurohypophysial hormones: an example of molecular evolution. pp. 119-130 *In* Greep, R.O., Astwood, E.B., Knobil, E., Sawyer, W.H., and S.R. Geiger [eds.] Handbook of physiology. Section 7: Endocrinology, vol. 6: The pituitary gland and its neuroendocrine control. Part 1. American Physiological Society. Washington, D.C.

BAKER, B.I., and J.C. BUCKINGHAM. 1983. A study of corticotrophic and melanotrophic activities in the pituitary and brain of the lamprey *Lampetra fluviatilis*. Gen. comp. Endocrinol. **52**: 283-290.

BALL, J.N. 1981. Hypothalamic control of the pars distalis in fishes, amphibians, and reptiles. Gen. comp. Endocrinol. **44**: 135-170.

BARRY, J. 1979. Immunohistochemistry of luteinizing hormone-releasing hormone-producing neurons of the vertebrates. Int. Rev. Cytol. **60**: 179-221.

BUCKINGHAM, J.C., J.H. LEACH, E. PLISETSKAYA, S.A. SOWER, and A. GORBMAN. 1985. Corticotrophin-like bioactivity in the pituitary gland and brain of the Pacific hagfish, *Eptatretus stouti*. Gen. comp. Endocrinol. **57**: 434-437.

BULLOCK, T.H., and R.G. NORTHCUTT. 1984. Nervus terminalis in dogfish (*Squalus acanthias*, Elasmobranchii) carries tonic efferent impulses. Neurosci. Lett. **44**: 155-160.

CRIM, J.W., A. URANO, and A. GORBMAN. 1979. Immunocytochemical studies of luteinizing hormone-releasing hormone in brains of agnathan fishes. I. Comparisons of adult Pacific lamprey (*Entosphenus tridentata*) and the Pacific hagfish (*Eptatretus stouti*). Gen. comp. Endocrinol. **37**: 294-305.

DEMSKI, L.S., and R.G. NORTHCUTT. 1983. The terminal nerve: a new chemosensory system in vertebrates? Science. **220**: 435-437.

DePALATIS, L.R., R.P. FIORINDO, and R.H. HO. 1982. Substance P immunoreactivity in the anterior pituitary gland of the guinea pig. Endocrinology. **110**: 282-284.

DORES, R.M., T.E. FINGER, and M.R. GOLD. 1984. Immunohistochemical localization of enkephalin- and ACTH-related substances in the pituitary of the lamprey. Cell Tissue Res. **235**: 107-115.

DUBOIS, M.P., R. BILLARD, B. BRETON, and R.E. PETER. 1979. Comparative distribution of somatostatin, LH-RH, neurophysin, and -endorphin in the rainbow trout: an immunocytochemical study. Gen. comp. Endocrinol. **37**: 220-232.

EASTMAN, J.T., and R. PORTANOVA. 1982. ACTH activity in the pituitary and brain of the least brook lamprey, *Lampetra aepyptera*. Gen. comp. Endocrinol. **47**: 346-350.

FRITSCH, H.A.R., S. VAN NOORDEN, and A.G.E. PEARSE. 1979. Localization of somatostatin-, substance P- and calcitonin-like immunoreactivity in the neural ganglion of *Ciona intestinalis* L. (Ascidiaceae). Cell Tissue Res. **202**: 263-274.

FRITSCH, H.A.R., S. VAN NOORDEN, and A.G.E. PEARSE. 1982. Gastrointestinal and neurohormonal peptides in the alimentary tract and cerebral complex of *Ciona intestinalis* (Ascidiaceae). Cell Tissue Res. **223**: 360-402.

GORBMAN, A. 1980. Evolution of the brain-pituitary relationship: Evidence from the Agnatha. Can. J. Fish. Aquat. Sci. **37**: 1680-1686.

GORBMAN, A. 1983a. Reproduction in cyclostome fishes and its regulation. pp. 1-29 *In* Hoar, W.S., and D.J. Randall [eds.] Fish physiology, vol. 9A. Academic Press, New York.

GORBMAN, A. 1983b. Early development of the hagfish pituitary gland: evidence of the endodermal origin of the adenohypophysis. Amer. Zool. **23**: 639-654.

GORBMAN, A., H. KOBAYASHI, and H. UEMURA. 1963. The vascularization of the hypophysial structures of the hagfish. Gen. comp. Endocrinol. **5**: 505-514.

GOOSSENS, N. K. DIERICKX, and F. VANDESANDE. 1977. Immunocytochemical demonstration of the hypothalamo-hypophysial vasotocinergic system of *Lampetra fluviatilis*. Cell Tissue Res. **177**: 317-323.

HARDISTY, M.W. 1979. Biology of the cyclostomes. Chapman and Hall, London.

HARDISTY, M.W., and B.I. BAKER. 1982. Endocrinology of lampreys. pp. 1-115 *In* Hardisty, M.W., and I.C. Potter [eds.] The biology of lampreys, vol. 4b. Academic Press, New York.

HÖKFELT, T., Å. LJUNGDAHL, L. TERENIUS, R. ELDE, and G. NILSSON. 1977. Immunohistochemical analysis of peptide pathways possibly related to pain and analgesia: enkephalin and substance P. Proc. Natl. Acad. Sci. U.S.A. **74**: 3081-3085.

HOLMES, R.L., and J.N. BALL. 1974. The pituitary gland: a comparative account. Cambridge Univ. Press, London.

JESSEL, T.M., and L.L. IVERSEN. 1977. Opiate analgesics inhibit substance P release from rat trigeminal nucleus. Nature. **268**: 549-551.

JIRIKOWSKI, G., G. ERHART, C.J.P. GRIMMELIKHUIJZEN, J. TRIEPEL, and R.A. PATZNER. 1984. FMRF-amide-like immunoreactivity in brain and pituitary of the hagfish *Eptatretus burgeri* (Cyclostomata). Cell Tissue Res. **237**: 363-366.

LARSEN, L.O. 1965. Effects of hypophysectomy in the cyclostome, *Lampetra fluviatilis* (L.) Gray. Gen. comp. Endocrinol. **5**: 16-30.

LARSEN, L.O. 1969. Effects of hypophysectomy before and during sexual maturation in the cyclostome, *Lampetra fluviatilis* (L.) Gray. Gen. comp. Endocrinol. **12**: 200-208.

LARSEN, L.O., and B. ROTHWELL. 1972. Adenohypophysis. pp. 1-67 *In* Hardisty, M.W., and I.C. Potter [eds.] The biology of lampreys, vol. 2. Academic Press, New York.

MATTY, A.J., K. TSUNEKI, W.W. DICKHOFF, and A. GORBMAN. 1976. Thyroid and gonadal function in hypophysectomized hagfish, *Eptatretus stouti*. Gen. comp. Endocrinol. **30**: 500-516.

NOZAKI, M., I. FUJITA., N. SAITO, T. TSUKAHARA, H. KOBAYASHI, K. UEDA, and K. OSHIMA. 1985. Distribution of LHRH-like immunoreactivity in the brain of the Japanese eel (*Anguilla japonica*) with special reference to the nervus terminalis. Zool. Sci. **2(4)**: (in press).

NOZAKI, M., and A. GORBMAN. 1983. Immunocytochemical localization of somatostatin and vasotocin in the brain of the Pacific hagfish, *Eptatretus stouti*. Cell Tissue Res. **229**: 541-550.

NOZAKI, M., and A. GORBMAN. 1984. Distribution of immunoreactive sites for several components of pro-opiocortin in the pituitary and brain of adult lampreys, *Petromyzon marinus* and *Entosphenus tridentata*. Gen. comp. Endocrinol. **53**: 335-352.

NOZAKI, M., and A. GORBMAN. 1985. Immunoreactivity for Met-enkephalin and substance P in cells of the adenohypophysis of larval and adult sea lampreys, *Petromyzon marinus*. Gen. comp. Endocrinol. **57**: 172-183.

NOZAKI, M., and H. KOBAYASHI. 1979. Distribution of LHRH-like substance in the vertebrate brain as revealed by immunohistochemistry. Arch. Histol. Jap. **42**: 201-219.

NOZAKI, M., T. TSUKAHARA, and R. KOBAYASHI. 1984a. Neuronal systems producing LHRH in vertebrates. pp. 3-27 *In* Ochiai, K., Y. Arai, T. Shinoda, and M. Takahashi [eds.] Endocrine correlates of reproduction. Japan Sci. Soc. Press. Tokyo/Springer-Verlag, Berlin.

NOZAKI, M., T. TSUKAHARA, and H. KOBAYASHI. 1984b. An immunocytochemical study on the distribution of neuropeptides in the brain of certain species of fish. Biomed. Res. **4**(Suppl.): 135-145.

OLIVEREAU, M., F. OLLEVIER, F. VANDESANDE, and J. OLIVEREAU. 1984. Somatostatin in the brain and the pituitary of some teleosts. Cell Tissue Res. **238**: 289-296.

ÖZTAN, N., and A. GORBMAN. 1960. The hypophysis and hypothalamo-hypophysial neurosecretory system of larval lampreys and their response to light. J. Morphol. **106**: 243-261.

PATZNER, R.A., and T. ICHIKAWA. 1977. Effects of hypophysectomy on the testis of the hagfish, *Eptatretus burgeri* Girard (Cyclostomata). Zool. Anz. **5/6**: 371-380.

PERCY, R., J.F. LEATHERLAND, and F.W.H. BEAMISH. 1975. Structure and ultrastructure of the pituitary gland in the sea lamprey, *Petromyzon marinus* at different stages in its life cycle. Cell Tissue Res. **157**: 141-164.

PICKERING, A.D. 1976. Iodide uptake by the isolated thyroid gland of the river lamprey, *Lampetra fluviatilis* L. Gen. comp. Endocrinol. **28**: 358-364.

SCHOT, L.P.C., H.H. BORE, D.F. SWAAB, and S. VAN NOORDEN. 1981. Immunocytochemical demonstration of peptidergic neurons in the central nervous system of the pond snail *Lymnaea stagnalis* with antisera raised to biologically active peptides of vertebrates. Cell Tissue Res. **216**: 273-291.

SHERWOOD, N.M., and S.A. SOWER. 1985. A new family member for gonadotropin-releasing hormone. Neuropeptides. (in press).

STELL, W.K., S.E. WALKER, K.S. CHOHAN, and A.K. BALL. 1984. The goldfish nervus terminalis: a luteinizing hormone-releasing hormone and molluscan cardioexcitatory peptide immunoreactive olfactory pathway. Proc. Natl. Acad. Sci. U.S.A. **81**: 940-944.

TSUKAHARA, T., S. SHIODA, Y. NAKAI, and H. KOBAYASHI. 1983. Somatostatin and arginine vasotocin revealed by immunohistochemistry in the hypothalamo-hypophysial region of the hagfish, *Eptatretus burgeri*. Zool. Mag. (Doubutsugaku Zasshi) **92**: 386-392.

VANDESANDE, F. and K. DIERICKX. 1980. Immunocytochemical localization of somatostatin-containing neurons in the brain of *Rana temporaria*. Cell Tissue Res. **205**: 43-53.

WRIGHT, G.M. 1983. Immunocyctochemical study of luteinizing hormone in the pituitary of the sea lamprey *Petromyzon marinus* L., during its upstream migration. Cell Tissue Res. **230**: 225-228.

WRIGHT, G.M. 1984. Immunocytochemical study of growth hormone, prolactin, and thyroid-stimulating hormone in the adenohypophysis of the sea lamprey, *Petromyzon marinus* L., during its upstream migration. Gen. comp. Endocrinol. **55**: 269-274.

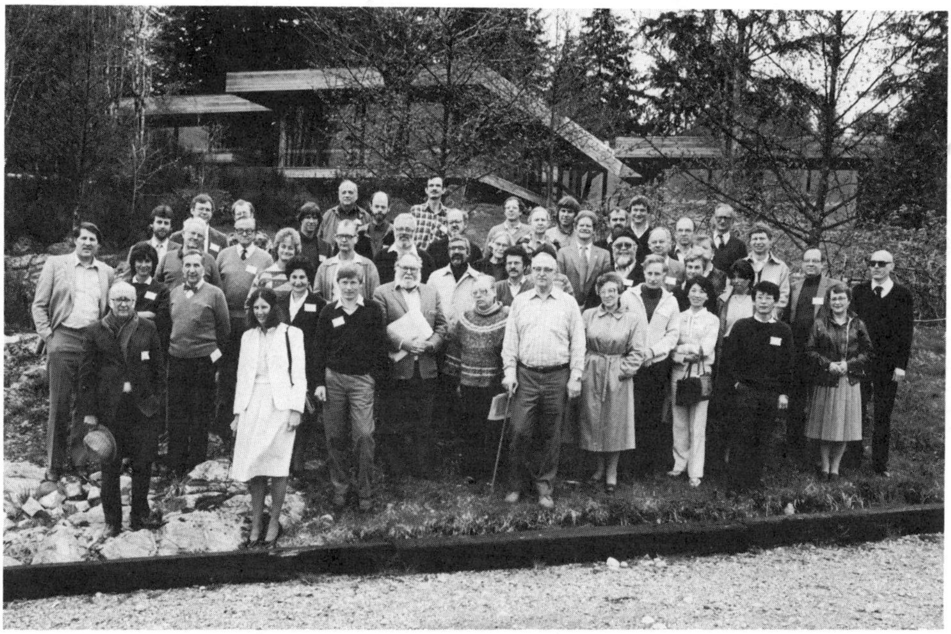

Group photograph of participants

left to right -- R. Foreman, M. Jollie, A. Buchan, M. Thorndyke, A. Gorbman, H. Copp, S. Vigna, J. Dodd, S. Emdin, S. Sower, S. Van Noorden, S. Geldiay, R. Griffith, J. Steffensen, R. Olsson, A. Tamarin, B. Fernholm, G. Brown, C. Gans, G. Rijkers, L. Saldanha, G. Northcutt, S. Brown, Mrs. Prosser, J. Youson, M. Bianchini, N. Wilimovsky, M. McEnroe, C. Prosser, J. Mallatt, E. Donaldson, E. Plisetskaya, J. Leatherland, D. Jensen, R. Beamish, G. Eales, Y. Fontaine, L. Smith, H. Nishimura, J. Joss, D. Randall, G. Bertmar, A. Ramos, J. Cech, M. Nozaki, B. McMahon, M. Dodd, H. Bjerring, Missing: W. Burggren.

CONTRIBUTORS AND PARTICIPANTS

R. J. Beamish, Pacific Biological Station, Nanaimo, B. C., CANADA, V9R 5K6

G. Bernardi, Institut Jaques Monod, Université Paris VII, Tour 43-2, Place Jussieu, 75221 Paris, Cedex 05, FRANCE

G. Bertmar, Department of Ecological Zoology, Umeå University, S-901, 87 Umeå, SWEDEN

M. Bianchini, c/o IPRA-CNR, Via Nizza, 128, 00198 Roma, ITALY

H. C. Bjerring, Section of Palaeozoology, Swedish Museum of Natural History, S-104 05, Stockholm, SWEDEN

G. W. Brown, School of Fisheries, University of Washington, WH-10, Seattle, Washington, USA

S. G. Brown, School of Fisheries, University of Washington, WH-10, Seattle, Washington, USA

A. Buchan, Department of Physiology, University of British Columbia, Vancouver, B. C., CANADA, V6T 1W5

W. Burggren, Zoology Department, University of Massachusetts, Amherst, Massachusetts, USA, 01003

J. J. Cech, Jr., Wildlife and Fisheries Biology, University of California Davis, Davis, California, USA, 95616

H. H. Copp, Department of Physiology, University of British Columbia, Vancouver, B. C., CANADA, V6T 1W5

J. M. Dodd, School of Animal Biology, University College of North Wales, Bangor, Gwynedd LL57 2UW, U.K.

M. H. I. Dodd, School of Animal Biology, University College of North Wales, Bangor, Gwynedd LL57 2UW, U.K.

E. M. Donaldson, West Vancouver Laboratory, Department of Fisheries and Oceans, 4160 Marine Drive, West Vancouver, B. C., CANADA V7V 1N6

J. G. Eales, Department of Zoology, University of Manitoba, Winnipeg, Manitoba, CANADA, R3T 2N2

S. O. Emdin, Department of Pathology, University of Umeå, S-901 87, Umeå, SWEDEN

S. Falkmer, Department of Pathology, Karolinska Institutet, Karolinska Sjukhuset, S-104 01, Stockholm, SWEDEN

R. Fänge, Department of Zoophysiology, University of Göteborg, S400-33, Göteborg, SWEDEN

B. Fernholm, Research Department, Swedish Museum of Natural History, S-104 05, Stockholm, SWEDEN

Y. A. Fontaine, Museum National d'Historie Naturalle, 7 rue Cuvier, 75005 Paris, FRANCE

R. E. Foreman, Bamfield Marine Station, Bamfield, B. C. CANADA, V0R 1B0

C. Gans, Zoology Department, University of Michigan, Ann Arbor, Michigan, USA 48109

S. Geldiay, Department of Zoology, EGE University, Bornova, Izmir, TURKEY

A. Gorbman, Zoology Department NJ-15, University of Washington, Seattle, Washington, USA 98195

R. W. Griffith, Biology Department, Southeastern Massachusetts University, North Darmouth, Massachusetts, USA 02747

W. S. Hoar, Department of Zoology, University of British Columbia, Vancouver, B. C., CANADA, V6T 1W5

D. D. Jensen, Department of Psychology, University of Nebraska, Lincoln, Nebraska, USA 68588

K. Johansen, Department of Zoophysiology, University of Aarhus, DK-8000, Aarhus C, DENMARK

M. Jollie, Department of Biological Sciences, Northern Illinois University, DeKalk, Illinois, USA 60115

J. Joss, Biological Sciences, Macquarie University, North Ryde NSW 2113, AUSTRALIA

J. F. Leatherland, Department of Zoology, University of Guelph, Guelph, Ontario, CANADA, N1G 2W1

J. Mallatt, Department of Zoology, Washington State University, Pullman, Washington, USA 99164

M. McEnroe, Department of Wildlife and Fisheries, University of California Davis, Davis, California, USA 95616

B. McMahon, Department of Biology, University of Calgary, Calgary, Alberta, CANADA, T2N 1N4

H. Nishimura, Center for the Health Sciences, University of Tennessee, 894 Union Ave., Memphis, Tennessee, USA 03816

G. R. Northcutt, Division of Biological Sciences, University of Michigan, Ann Arbor, Michigan, USA 48109

M. Nozaki, Primate Research Institute, University cf Kyoto, Inuyama, Aichi 484, JAPAN

R. Olsson, Department of Zoology, University of Stockholm, S-106 91, Stockholm, SWEDEN

E. Plisetskaya, Zoology Department NJ-15, University of Washington, Seattle, Washington, USA 98195

C. L. Prosser, Department of Physiology, University of Illinois, 407 S. Goodwin Ave., Urbana, Illinois, USA 68101

M. A. Ramos, Institute Nationale de Investigacao das Pescas, Avenue de Brazilia, 1400 Lisbon, PORTUGAL

D. J. Randall, Department of Zoology, University of British Columbia, Vancouver, B. C., CANADA, V6T 1W5

G. T. Rijkers, Wilhelmina Childrens Hospital, P.O. Box 18009, 3501 CA Utrecht, The NETHERLANDS

L. Saldanha, Department de Zoology E Antropologie , Faculdade de Ciencias, Rua de Escola, Politecnica, 1200 Lisboa, PORTUGAL

L. S. Smith, School of Fisheries, University of Washington, Seattle, Washington, USA 98195

S. A. Sower, Department of Zoology, University of New Hampshire, Durham, New Hampshire, USA 03824

J. F. Steffensen, Department of Zoology, University of British Columbia, Vancouver, B. C., CANADA, V6T 1W5

A. Tamarin, Department of Oral Biology SB22, University of Washington, Seattle, Washington, USA 98195

M. Thorndyke, Department of Zoology, Royal Holloway College, Egham Hill, Egham, Surrey, TW20 0EX, ENGLAND

S. Van Noorden, Royal Postgraduate Medical School, Hammersmith Hospital, Ducane Rd., London W12 0HS, ENGLAND

S. R. Vigna, C.U.R.E., Bldg. 115, V.A. Wadsworth Hospital Center, Los Angeles, California, USA 90073

N. J. Wilimovsky, Institute of Animal Resource Ecology, University of British Columbia, Vancouver, B. C., CANADA, V6T 1W5

M. Wolowyk, Department of Pharmacology, University of Alberta, Edmonton, Alberta, CANADA, T6G 2E9

J. H. Youson, Department of Zoology, University of Toronto, West Hill, Ontario, CANADA, M1C 1A4

INDEX